Essentials in Ophthalmology

Series Editor

Arun D. Singh, Cleveland Clinic Foundation, Cole Eye Institute,
Cleveland, OH, USA

Essentials in Ophthalmology aims to promote the rapid and efficient transfer of medical research into clinical practice. It is published in four volumes per year. Covering new developments and innovations in all fields of clinical ophthalmology, it provides the clinician with a review and summary of recent research and its implications for clinical practice. Each volume is focused on a clinically relevant topic and explains how research results impact diagnostics, treatment options and procedures as well as patient management.
The reader-friendly volumes are highly structured with core messages, summaries, tables, diagrams and illustrations and are written by internationally well-known experts in the field. A volume editor supervises the authors in his/her field of expertise in order to ensure that each volume provides cutting-edge information most relevant and useful for clinical ophthalmologists. Contributions to the series are peer reviewed by an editorial board.

More information about this series at https://link.springer.com/bookseries/5332

Jorge L. Alió • H. Burkhard Dick
Robert H. Osher
Editors

Cataract Surgery

Advanced Techniques for Complex and Complicated Cases

Springer

Editors
Jorge L. Alió
Division of Ophthalmology
School of Medicine
Miguel Hernandez University
Alicante, Spain

Cornea, Refractive and Cataract
Surgery Unit
Vissum Miranza Alicante, Spain

Robert H. Osher
Cincinnati Eye Institute
University of Cincinnati
Video Journal of Cataract, Refractive &
Glaucoma Surgery
Cincinnati, OH, USA

H. Burkhard Dick
Ruhr University Eye Clinic
Bochum, Germany

ISSN 1612-3212 ISSN 2196-890X (electronic)
Essentials in Ophthalmology
ISBN 978-3-030-94529-9 ISBN 978-3-030-94530-5 (eBook)
https://doi.org/10.1007/978-3-030-94530-5

This Springer imprint is published by the registered company Springer Nature Switzerland AG
The registered company address is: Gewerbestrasse 11, 6330 Cham, Switzerland

Foreword

Cataract surgery remains the most common ophthalmic procedure performed worldwide. Intravitreal injections are a close second, but they are often performed by a retinal sub-specialist. Cataract surgery remains the bread and butter of the comprehensive ophthalmologist, the cornea sub-specialist, and the glaucoma sub-specialist, and is also frequently performed by our retina-vitreous and pediatric sub-specialist colleagues. In 2020, as many as 4,000,000 cataract surgeries were performed in the USA and nearly 28,000,000 globally. In spite of those large numbers, every year there are more patients suffering from reduced vision that could be corrected with cataract surgery. If the 8 per 1000 population cataract surgeries performed each year in Europe is the appropriate number, we would need to increase cataract surgery procedures performed per year in the world to twice that done today, or 56,000,000 per year, to fully meet the demand.

At ophthalmology meetings worldwide, attendance at educational programs that relate to cataract surgery are dominant. While many patients with cataract present without significant co-morbidities, over 50% have one or another additional diagnosis that make the surgery more complex. Ocular surface disease(OSD), especially dry eye disease and blepharitis/meibomian gland dysfunction, impacts over 50% of the senior population presenting with cataract. While not a significant factor intraoperative, it is critical to manage OSD in the preoperative period to achieve good biometry and rapid and high-quality recovery of vision. Glaucoma or ocular hypertension is present in 15–20% of patients with cataract. Some evidence of macular disease, often only uncovered with ocular coherence tomography, is observable in at least another 25%. Corneal topographic abnormalities are common. One or another systemic disorder including diabetes mellitus, hypertension, and arteriosclerotic vascular disease are more often present than absent in the patient over age 65. A multitude of other co-morbidities, from keratoconus to axial myopia, all impact the cataract surgeon's plan and their patient's intraoperative and postoperative course. When I see a patient with a visually significant cataract, I expect to place one or more other diagnosis in my clinical record in nearly every case. This makes management of the complex and complicated cataract patient more the rule than the exception.

It takes years of training and experience to become expert at managing the broad array of complexities that challenge us cataract surgeons every week. To help us better prepare, Professor Jorge Alio, MD, of Spain, Professor Burkhard Dick, MD, of Germany, and Robert Osher, MD, of the United

States, have joined together with a rare group of surgeons who are superb teachers and highly experienced in the management of complex and complicated cataracts. The end result is the book *Cataract Surgery in Complicated and Complex Cases*. This book is recommended reading for every cataract surgeon, from trainee to master surgeon. It is a book that belongs on every cataract surgeon's desk, and it will be opened frequently in the course of everyday practice.

Richard L. Lindstrom, MD
Founder and Attending Surgeon: Minnesota Eye Consultants
Minneapolis, MN, USA

Adjunct Professor Emeritus: University of Minnesota
Department of Ophthalmology, Minneapolis, MN, USA

Visiting Professor: University of California Irvine
Gavin Herbert Eye Institute, Irvine, CA, USA

Preface

When I look back at my career, it's hard for me to believe that I performed my first cataract surgery as a second-year resident at the Bascom Palmer Eye Institute in Miami, Florida, in 1978. It seems like yesterday! Although phacoemulsification had been introduced by Charles Kelman, MD, almost a decade before, it was still very unpopular and "off limits" to the residents. It seemed so obvious to me that a smaller incision would reduce the risk of complications, and I would sneak up to the operating room in the evening and practice emulsifying the lens in Eye Bank eyes. I waited until Dr. Ed Norton, our famous chairman, was supposed to be out of town and then scheduled a patient to be the first phacoemulsification performed by a resident at Bascom Palmer. I am still haunted by the fact that in a middle of a case, I heard Dr. Norton's voice over my shoulder say "Bobby, this better go well!" Had it not, I would probably be engaged in the practice of neuro-ophthalmology today.

It has been amazing to witness the evolution of small incision cataract surgery over the last four decades. Incisions have shrunk, sutures are gone, and patients can return to their normal activities almost immediately. Innovations are the hallmark of this subspecialty, and every year, we see the debut of sophisticated diagnostics, better IOL formulae, improved machines, new intraocular lens options, novel devices and instrumentation, and safer surgical techniques. I cannot imagine a subspecialty that has had more exciting changes, and I am so grateful that I went into ophthalmology rather than proctology!

Cataract surgeons have hit the jackpot for other reasons. What could possibly be more satisfying than taking a patient who is legally blind and giving them the opportunity to enjoy crystal clear vision the day following surgery. Our patients are extremely happy and appreciate the recovery of the gift of sight. Our work is delicate and rarely marred by complications. How lucky we are to have chosen this subspecialty!

Yet even with unprecedented surgical success, every cataract surgeon will eventually encounter anxiety-provoking challenging cases. Cataract surgeons are familiar with challenges. We have learned to tackle the mature lens, the white lens, and the loose lens. We have tamed the once-dreaded posterior polar cataract. We are comfortable managing very large eyes and very small eyes as well as coexisting corneal, retinal, and glaucoma comorbidities. Small pupils can be managed by pharmacologic or mechanical solutions, and damaged irises can be reconstructed almost as good as new. While complications are less frequent today than ever before, they still happen. However, the cataract surgeon can achieve excellent outcomes in both challenging and complicated cases by sound knowledge, meticulous preparation, and skillful dexterity.

I am honored to serve as a co-author of this book with Drs. Jorge Alio and Burkhard Dick. Each of these extraordinary surgeons has spent his career making cutting-edge contributions and has devoted an enormous amount of time to teaching colleagues how to perform better and safer cataract surgery. I am confident that this book will expand the expertise of the reader and enhance the joy that every cataract surgeon should experience throughout his or her career.

Robert H. Osher, MD
Professor of Ophthalmology
University of Cincinnati
Cincinnati, OH, USA

Medical Director Emeritus
Cincinnati Eye Institute
Cincinnati, OH, USA

Editor, Video Journal of Cataract,
Refractive & Glaucoma Surgery
Cincinnati, OH, USA

Contents

Contributors

Ahmed A. Abdelghany Ophthalmology Department, Faculty of Medicine, Minia University, Minia, Egypt

Iqbal Ike Ahmed Department of Ophthalmology and Vision Sciences, Faculty of Medicine, University of Toronto, Toronto, ON, Canada

Jorge Alió del Barrio Cornea, Refractive and Cataract Surgery Unit, Vissum Miranza Alicante, Spain

Division of Ophthalmology, School of Medicine, Miguel Hernandez University, Alicante, Spain

Jorge L. Alió Division of Ophthalmology, School of Medicine, Miguel Hernandez University, Alicante, Spain

Cornea, Refractive and Cataract Surgery Unit, Vissum Miranza Alicante, Spain

Olena Al-Shymali Cornea, Refractive and Cataract Surgery Unit, Vissum Miranza Alicante, Spain

Division of Ophthalmology, School of Medicine, Miguel Hernandez University, Alicante, Spain

Ehud I. Assia Center for Applied Eye Research, Department of Ophthalmology, Meir Medical Center, Kfar Saba, Israel, affiliated with the Sackler School of Medicine, Tel Aviv University, Tel Aviv, Israel

Ein-Tal Eye Center, Tel Aviv, Israel

Gerd U. Auffarth Department of Ophthalmology, University of Heidelberg, Heidelberg, Germany

The David J. Apple International Laboratory for Ocular Pathology, Heidelberg, Germany

A. J. Augustin Department of Ophthalmology, Staedtisches Klinikum Karlsruhe, Karlsruhe, Germany

Graham D. Barrett University of Western Australia, Centre for Ophthalmology and visual Science, Lions Eye Institute, Sir Charles Gairdner Hospital, Perth, WA, Australia

George H. H. Beiko Division of Ophthalmology, Department of Surgery, Faculty of Health Sciences, McMaster University, Hamilton, ON, Canada

Department of Ophthalmology and Vision Sciences, University of Toronto, Toronto, ON, Canada

Bahram Bodaghi Department of Ophthalmology, IHU FOReSIGHT, Sorbonne-APHP, Paris, France

Karl Thomas Boden Eye Clinic Sulzbach, Knappschaft Hospital Saar, Sulzbach/Saar, Germany

Lucio Buratto CAMO Centro Ambrosiano Oftalmico – Milano, Milan, Italy

Thierry Burtin Department of Ophthalmology, IHU FOReSIGHT, Sorbonne-APHP, Paris, France

David F. Chang University of California, San Francisco, San Francisco, CA, USA

Andrew Cho Advanced Vision Care, Los Angeles, CA, USA

C. Cursiefen Department of Ophthalmology, University of Cologne, Faculty of Medicine and University Hospital Cologne, Cologne, Germany

Division for Dry-Eye and Ocular GVHD, Department of Ophthalmology, University of Cologne, Faculty of Medicine and University Hospital Cologne, Cologne, Germany

Center for Molecular Medicine Cologne (CMMC), University of Cologne, Cologne, Germany

Francesco D'Oria Vissum Miranza Alicante, Alicante, Spain

Division of Ophthalmology, Universidad Miguel Hernández, Alicante, Spain

Section of Ophthalmology, Department of Basic Medical Science, Neuroscience and Sense Organs, University of Bari, Bari, Italy

Michael J. daSilva Stein Eye Institute, University of California Los Angeles (UCLA) School of Medicine, Los Angeles, CA, USA

Uday Devgan Stein Eye Institute, University of California Los Angeles (UCLA) School of Medicine, Los Angeles, CA, USA

E. Di Carlo Department of Ophthalmology, Staedtisches Klinikum Karlsruhe, Karlsruhe, Germany

H. Burkhard Dick Ruhr University Eye Clinic, Bochum, Germany

Kendall E. Donaldson Cornea/External Disease/Cataract/Refractive Surgery, Bascom Palmer Eye Institute in Plantation, Plantation, FL, USA

Carlos G. Figueiredo D'Olhos Day Hospital, S. J. Rio Preto, Brazil

Gabriel B. Figueiredo D'Olhos Day Hospital, S. J. Rio Preto, Brazil

Marta S. Figueroa Ophthalmology Department, Ramon y Cajal University Hospital, Alcala de Henares University, Madrid, Spain

Nicole R. Fram Advanced Vision Care, Los Angeles, CA, USA

Gerd Geerling Department of Ophthalmology, University Hospital Duesseldorf, Duesseldorf, Germany

Ronald D. Gerste University Eye Clinic, Bochum, Germany

Andrea Govetto Oftalmico Hospital, ASST-Fatebenefratelli-Sacco, Milan, Italy

Maximilian Hammer The David J. Apple International Laboratory for Ocular Pathology, Heidelberg, Germany

Ken Hayashi Hayashi Eye Hospital, Fukuoka, Japan

Christoph Holtmann Department of Ophthalmology, University Hospital Duesseldorf, Duesseldorf, Germany

Arjan Hura Cleveland Eye Clinic, Brecksville, OH, USA

Wen Fan Hu The University of Utah John A. Moran Eye Center, Salt Lake City, UT, USA

Ananya Jalsingh Advanced Vision Care, Los Angeles, CA, USA

Ahmed M. Khalafallah Ophthalmology Department, Faculty of Medicine, Minia University, Minia, Egypt

Douglas D. Koch Cullen Eye Institute, Baylor College of Medicine, Houston, TX, USA

Friedrich E. Kruse Department of Ophthalmology, Friedrich-Alexander-University of Erlangen-Nürnberg, Erlangen, Germany

Marissa Larochelle The University of Utah John A. Moran Eye Center, Salt Lake City, UT, USA

Phuc LeHoang Department of Ophthalmology, IHU FOReSIGHT, Sorbonne-APHP, Paris, France

Adi Levy Ein-Tal Eye Center, Tel Aviv, Israel

John Liu Department of Ophthalmology and Vision Sciences, Faculty of Medicine, University of Toronto, Toronto, ON, Canada

Victoria Liu University of Ottawa Eye Institute, Ottawa Hospital Research Institute, University of Ottawa, Ottawa, ON, Canada

Division of Ophthalmology, Department of Surgery, Faculty of Health Sciences, McMaster University, Hamilton, ON, Canada

Zala Lužnik Eye Hospital, University Medical Centre, Ljubljana, Slovenia

Jingyi Ma Department of Ophthalmology and Vision Sciences, Faculty of Medicine, University of Toronto, Toronto, ON, Canada

Boris Malyugin S. Fyodorov Eye Microsurgery Federal State Institution, Moscow, Russian Federation

Miha Marzidovšek Eye Hospital, University Medical Centre, Ljubljana, Slovenia

Samuel Masket Stein Eye Institute, Geffen School of Medicine UCLA, Los Angeles, CA, USA

Advanced Vision Care, Los Angeles, CA, USA

Jessie McLachlan Advanced Vision Care, Los Angeles, CA, USA

Anirudh Mukhopadhyay Baylor College of Medicine, Houston, TX, USA

Siddharth Nath Department of Ophthalmology and Visual Sciences, McGill University, Montréal, Québec, Canada

Tadas Naujokaitis Department of Ophthalmology, University of Heidelberg, Heidelberg, Germany

The David J. Apple International Laboratory for Ocular Pathology, Heidelberg, Germany

Ali Nowrouzi Cornea, Cataract and Refractive Surgery Unit, Department of Ophthalmology, Hospital Quironsalud Marbella, Alicante, Spain

Thomas A. Oetting University of lowa, Department of Ophthalmology, Iowa City, IA, USA

Gregory S. H. Ogawa University of New Mexico, Department of Ophthalmology, Albuquerque, NM, USA

Randall Olson The University of Utah John A. Moran Eye Center, Salt Lake City, UT, USA

Jeb Alden Ong Department of Ophthalmology and Vision Sciences, Faculty of Medicine, University of Toronto, Toronto, ON, Canada

James M. Osher Cincinnati Eye Institute, University of Cincinnati, Cincinnati, OH, USA

Robert H. Osher Cincinnati Eye Institute, University of Cincinnati, Cincinnati, OH, USA

Mark Packer Packer Research Associates, Inc., Boulder, CO, USA

Jeff Pettey The University of Utah John A. Moran Eye Center, Salt Lake City, UT, USA

Vladimir Pfeifer Eye Hospital, University Medical Centre, Ljubljana, Slovenia

Christopher D. Riemann Cincinnati Eye Institute, University of Cincinnati, Cincinnati, OH, USA

Zsofia Rupnik Advanced Vision Care, Los Angeles, CA, USA

Samantha L. Schockman Cincinnati Eye Institute, Cincinnati, OH, USA

Tal Sharon Center for Applied Eye Research, Department of Ophthalmology, Meir Medical Center, Kfar Saba, Israel, affiliated with the Sackler School of Medicine, Tel Aviv University, Tel Aviv, Israel

Ein-Tal Eye Center, Tel Aviv, Israel

M. Victoria De Rojas Silva Department at Complexo Hospitalario Universitario A Coruña, A Coruña, Spain

Victoria de Rojas Instituto Oftalmológico, Policlínica Assistens, A Coruña, Spain

Michael E. Snyder Cincinnati Eye Institute, University of Cincinnati, Cincinnati, OH, USA

P. Steven Department of Ophthalmology, University of Cologne, Faculty of Medicine and University Hospital Cologne, Cologne, Germany

Division for Dry-Eye and Ocular GVHD, Department of Ophthalmology, University of Cologne, Faculty of Medicine and University Hospital Cologne, Cologne, Germany

Peter Szurman Eye Clinic Sulzbach, Knappschaft Hospital Saar, Sulzbach/Saar, Germany

Volkan Tahmaz Department of Ophthalmology, University of Cologne, Faculty of Medicine and University Hospital Cologne, Cologne, Germany

Division for Dry-Eye and Ocular GVHD, Department of Ophthalmology, University of Cologne, Faculty of Medicine and University Hospital Cologne, Cologne, Germany

Theofilos Tourtas Department of Ophthalmology, Friedrich-Alexander-University of Erlangen-Nürnberg, Erlangen, Germany

Argyrios Tzamalis 2nd Department of Ophthalmology, Aristotle University of Thessaloniki, Papageorgiou General Hospital, Thessaloniki, Greece

Veronica Vargas Cornea, Cataract and Refractive Surgery Department, VISSUM Alicante, Alicante, Spain

Research & Development Department, VISSUM Alicante, Alicante, Spain

Abhay R. Vasavada Iladevi Cataract & IOL Research Centre, Raghudeep Eye Hospital, Ahmedabad, India

Vaishali Vasavada Iladevi Cataract & IOL Research Centre, Raghudeep Eye Hospital, Ahmedabad, India

Angela Verkade Department of Ophthalmology, Baylor College of Medicine, Houston, TX, USA

Ophthalmology, Winston Salem, NC, USA

Li Wang Cullen Eye Institute, Baylor College of Medicine, Houston, TX, USA

Mitchell Weikert Baylor College of Medicine, Houston, TX, USA

Julia M. Weller Department of Ophthalmology, Friedrich-Alexander-University of Erlangen-Nürnberg, Erlangen, Germany

Kate Xie Cullen Eye Institute, Baylor College of Medicine, Houston, TX, USA

Motoaki Yoshida Hayashi Eye Hospital, Fukuoka, Japan

Koichi Yoshimura Hayashi Eye Hospital, Fukuoka, Japan

Key Elements in the Risk Evaluation

1

Wen Fan Hu, Marissa Larochelle, Randall Olson, and Jeff Pettey

Bullet Point

- Preoperative risk assessment is fundamental to safe and efficient ocular surgery.
- A systematic approach to surgical evaluation is the primary safeguard against errors and missed diagnoses to guide surgical care.
- A thorough history with focus on past ocular history can identify obstacles to routine and uncomplicated surgery.
- Each step of the slit lamp and ophthalmic exam can identify unique risk factors for each surgical patient.
- Identifying improvements in your systematic approach to surgical evaluation will lead to improved surgical results and patient outcomes.

Introduction of Key Elements in the Risk Evaluation

Preoperative risk assessment is fundamental for surgical planning, for intraoperative decision making, and for the patient's informed consent and pre-procedure counseling. Eliciting critical elements of a patient history and performing the appropriate physical examination are fundamental to our roles as physicians and surgeons. While diagnosing cataract is elemental, clearly elucidating and evaluating risk requires a well-developed skillful approach.

Edward Deming, a renowned engineer and statistician, famously quipped: "Every system is perfectly designed to give the result that it does." When surgeons fail to identify key risk factors in cataract evaluation, it is more likely to due to systemic flaws, rather than a lack of knowledge or skill in examination. A flawed systemic evaluation may be due to overreliance on physician extenders or a hurried or lackadaisical approach. In short, a high level of knowledge about risk factors for complicated cataract surgery is only as good as your system of evaluation.

While the chapter will focus on areas of medical knowledge and technical skill, one would be well served to thoughtfully evaluative your system's ability to identify or miss key risk factors in complex cataract surgery.

Supplementary Information The online version contains supplementary material available at [https://doi.org/10.1007/978-3-030-94530-5_1].

W. F. Hu · M. Larochelle · R. Olson (✉) · J. Pettey
The University of Utah John A. Moran Eye Center, Salt Lake City, UT, USA
e-mail: Wen_hu@urmc.rochester.edu; Marissa.Larochelle@hsc.utah.edu; Randall.Olson@hsc.utah.edu; Jeff.Pettey@hsc.utah.edu

J. L. Alió et al. (eds.), *Cataract Surgery*, Essentials in Ophthalmology,
https://doi.org/10.1007/978-3-030-94530-5_1

Risk Assessment

Risk assessment is the process of identifying and evaluating elements of risk and determining whether these risks outweigh the potential benefit of an intervention. The benefit of cataract surgery to a 20/15 emmetrope with a faint congenital cataract clearly does not outweigh the risks, while a "count fingers" cataract, even in the setting of pseudoexfoliation and intumescent cataract, is an entirely different calculation. However, inherent to both of these examples, every other patient who presents for surgery is the imperative to identify risk.

Once identified, the level of risk will vary for each surgeon, depending on their skillset and experience. Surgical educators frequently reference the Dreyfus model of skill acquisition to describe the learning curve of cataract surgeons. Novice surgeons painstakingly dissect and evaluate each step of surgery as if they were distinctly unique procedures. While expert surgeons seamlessly flow through surgery with nary a conscious thought given to hand position, approach angle, or instrument nomenclature. Similarly, experienced surgeons effortlessly evaluate the risk-benefit ratio as they glean the relevant elements of the history and physical examination.

However, as risk assessment becomes more intuitive and surgical cases routine, surgeons themselves risk becoming numb to important elements in risk assessment. As a surgeon's experience and skill grow, the relative importance of a detailed risk evaluation may take on less importance. We caution surgeons to remain vigilant in identifying risk and thoughtfully contemplating risk, as even the most experienced and skilled can best mitigate risk when armed with all available risk factors before they declare themselves during the surgery.

Our discussion is not a full review of all potential history and examination findings, rather a focused discussion on key and relevant findings for the preoperative cataract risk assessment.

History

History of Present Illness

Vision loss from age-related cataract development is classically characterized by slowly progressive, painless vision decline. Subjectively, patients report decreased visual acuity, increased glare, and an increased need for light over the course of years. There are, however, exceptions to this classic presentation, many of which highlight elements of potential increased perioperative and intraoperative risk for the cataract surgeon.

Cataract development is associated with aging, smoking, and ultraviolet exposure, and most patients present after the age of 50 [2]. Furthermore, cataract development is usually bilateral, though there may be mild-to-moderate asymmetry in the degree of cataract formation. In patients where there is rapid onset of vision loss, significant asymmetry in the degree of cataract-related vision change, or cataract formation in a young patient, the surgeon must search for alternative etiologies, such as trauma (Fig. 1.1), prior intraocular surgery, uveitic disease (Fig. 1.2) and its first-line therapy, and corticosteroids (whether topical, periocular injection, or oral). All of these entities can induce or accelerate cataract forma-

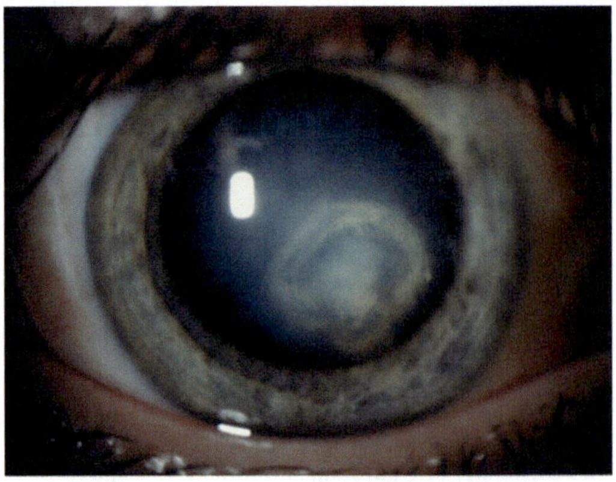

Fig. 1.1 Traumatic cataract following blunt trauma

tion. Of note, some patients may report a "pseudo-sudden" onset of vision loss where they abruptly notice vision loss despite the low vision being present for months or years. Often, this is more common if there is asymmetric disease and the better-seeing eye is suddenly occluded. Attributing this type of vision loss to cataract is a diagnosis of exclusion only after a full ophthalmic evaluation.

Cataract formation itself is a painless process. However, cataracts may cause secondary pain due to mechanical intraocular pressure elevation as seen with phacomorphic glaucoma or lens subluxation from trauma or zonular laxity (Fig. 1.3), or due to inflammation or inflammation-induced IOP elevation in phacolytic or phacoantigenic glaucoma. A prior history of redness and eye pain in an eye with cataract should also increase suspicion for an underlying uveitic process.

Past Ocular History

Ocular Trauma A history of trauma demands special attention, particularly in the setting of acute cataract. Any history of facial trauma, periorbital hematoma, or direct eye injury can greatly increase the risk of intraoperative complications. Zonulopathy (Figs. 1.4 and 1.5) is most frequently encountered complication from closed globe injuries, although its severity varies widely. Given that zonulopathy may not be detectable in even the most detailed exam, eliciting even

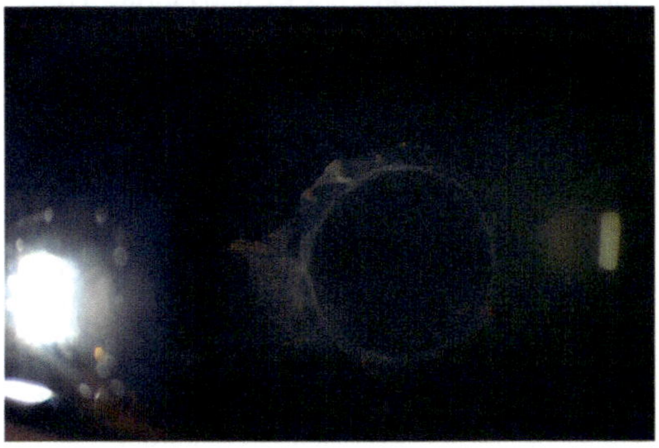

Fig. 1.2 Fibrin ring on anterior capsule in an eye with a history of uveitis

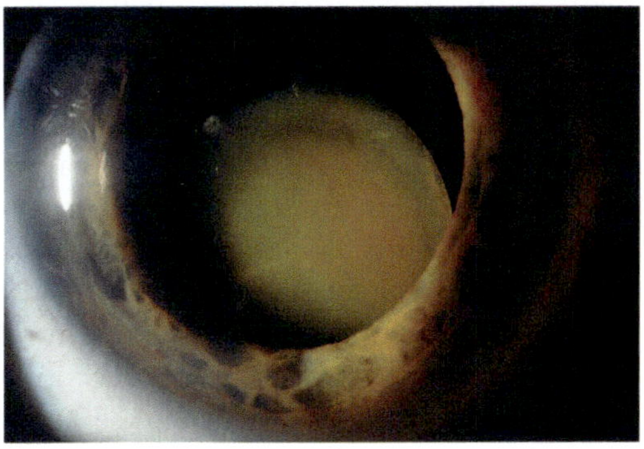

Fig. 1.4 Inferior subluxation of lens in setting of mature cataract and zonulopathy

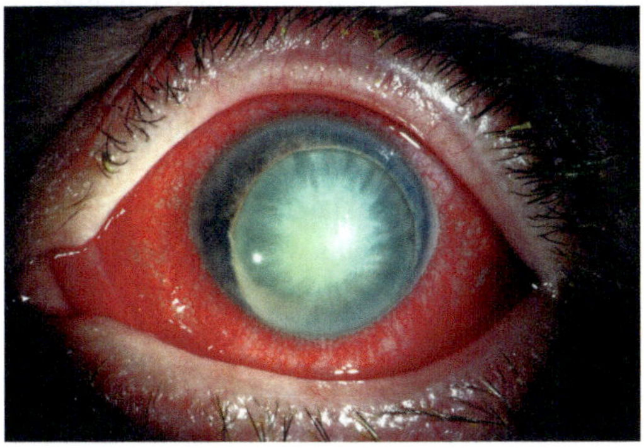

Fig. 1.3 Acute traumatic dislocation of crystalline lens into anterior chamber

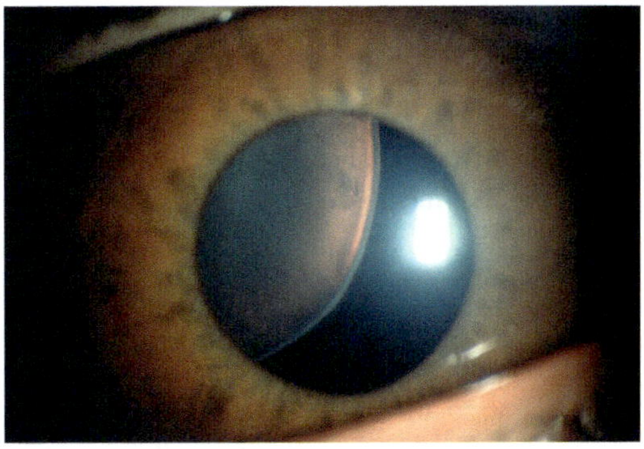

Fig. 1.5 Lateral subluxation of lens in setting of blunt trauma

remote histories of trauma alert the surgeon to potential intraoperative zonulopathy. Traumatic cataracts can also be intumescent and increase risk of complications during anterior capsulorhexis creation.

Uveitis A history of uveitis can affect preoperative, intraoperative, and postoperative management significantly. Preoperatively, patient may have a history of fluctuating macular edema, which can affect biometry measurements of axial length. Additionally, there are many sequelae of uveitic disease that may present intraoperative surgical challenges, including but not limited to band keratopathy, posterior synechiae, pupillary membrane, and fibrotic lens capsule. Finally, postoperatively, these patients are at increased risk for flares of their uveitic disease and postoperative CME. Different types of uveitis confer different levels of risk. Eyes with juvenile idiopathic arthritis (JIA)- associated uveitis have a high risk of forming posterior synechiae to the implanted intraocular lens, which can lead to pupillary membranes, IOL displacement, cocooning of the IOL, and ultimately pupillary block glaucoma [3]. To minimize the risks associated with cataract surgery in uveitis patients, general consensus within the uveitic community is to attain minimum of 3 months of disease quiescence whenever possible prior to proceeding with surgery [8, 9]. Furthermore, surgeons may consider preoperative topical corticosteroids and NSAIDs, a perioperative oral corticosteroid burst or periocular steroid injection, and/or intraoperative IV steroids. Herpetic ocular disease is a specific uveitic entity in which the surgeon should consider starting, or increasing, the dose of systemic antiviral medication perioperatively.

Glaucoma In patients with glaucoma, it is critical to assess the severity of their glaucoma and susceptibility of the optic nerve to further elevations in intraocular pressure. In mild-moderate cases of glaucoma, combined MIGS surgery should be considered. In more severe cases, particular care should be taken to avoid prolonged elevated intraocular pressure intraoperatively during phacoemulsification, as well as during femtosecond laser-assisted suction application, if applicable. Cataract surgery in patients with pseudoexfoliation glaucoma also requires specific attention to zonulopathy. Postoperatively, all glaucoma patients should be monitored more closely for elevations in intraocular pressure.

Diabetic retinopathy – Fluctuating macular edema can affect axial length biometry measurements prior to surgery. Furthermore, cataract surgery can induce or exacerbate cystoid macular edema, particularly in patients with existing diabetic retinopathy. Surgeons should consider use of topical NSAIDs perioperatively if it is not used routinely for their cataract surgery patients.

Corneal Disease Multiple corneal disease entities can cause corneal opacities leading to difficulty with intraoperative visualization. Trypan blue can be used to improve visualization during surgery. Additionally, the severity of Fuchs' endothelial dystrophy should be assessed as to the need for a combined endothelial transplant procedure. Care must be taken intraoperatively to decrease phacoemulsification energy and frequent application of dispersive viscoelastic to protect the endothelium.

High Myopia For patients with high myopia, it is critical to ascertain any history of prior ocular procedures, such as refractive surgery or prior retinal surgery (see below). Refractive targets may be unpredictable in axial myopes and IOL choices may be limited. Furthermore, myopia-associated macular disorders, such as choroidal neovascular membranes and their associated retinal edema, macular schisis, or staphyloma, may impact axial length measurements. Intraoperatively, patients with high myopia often exhibit deep anterior chambers and large, floppy lens capsules. Furthermore, they are prone to anterior chamber instability and lens-iris diaphragm retropulsion syndrome during surgery. Toric intraocular lenses are more prone to rotation in patients with high myopia, and may benefit from a capsular tension ring to help stabilize the IOL. Both at baseline and postoperatively, patients with high myopia are at increased risk for retina tears and detachment compared to the emmetropic patient, with postoperative rates of retinal detachment reported at between 0.4 and 5.0% [4]. Careful postoperative dilated fundus examinations should always be performed.

Past Ocular Surgical History

A history of ocular surgery can result in compromised ocular structures, corneal opacity, or any number of complicating factors for surgery. Identification of risk factors and preparation with capsule stains, iris or capsule stabilization measures, or specialized instrumentation can greatly improve the likelihood of successful surgery.

Prior Retinal Surgery Retinal surgery (whether scleral buckle or vitrectomy) and prior intravitreal injections all affect cataract surgery. In patients with a history of vitrectomy, intraoperative fluid dynamics change, leading to a floppy posterior capsule that tends to come forward. Special caution should be taken if the patient develops an acute cataract soon after PPV given concern for posterior capsule violation. Similarly, surgeons should be vigilant in patients with repeated intravitreal injections to be aware of possible posterior capsule weakness. There may also be fibrosis of the posterior capsule which may be better treated with YAG capsulotomy after surgery than polishing during surgery. In instances where silicone oil is or has been present in the eye, attention should be paid to the biometry and IOL calculations. Specifically, one must note whether the axial length was acquired on the silicone oil setting, and whether the IOL calculations are intended for permanent silicone oil placement or eventual removal of silicone oil. With silicone oil, intraoperatively, there can be intraoperative posterior pressure. Furthermore, presence of silicone oil can obscure the red reflex and use of trypan blue should be considered. In patients with prior scleral buckle surgery, refractive outcome can be difficult to predict, and consideration should be given to the status of the fellow eye to avoid anisometropia.

Prior Corneal Surgery Prior refractive surgery, such as LASIK or PRK, is an important consideration for IOL counseling, particularly regarding refractive outcomes and higher-order aberrations. IOL selection should be considered in the context of offsetting spherical aberrations. In patients with prior RK or PKP, the cornea is weakened at the prior incisions or graft-host junction. Decreasing intraocular pressure and fluid flow during surgery and being prepared for possible wound dehiscence are critical. Special attention to corneal opacities and the endothelial examination also directs surgical planning from capsule stains to unique surgical approach to allow visualization through small corneal windows of view. In patients with RK, PKP, or prior endothelial transplants, a scleral tunnel can be considered to place the wound further from the graft-host junction and/or to avoid prior incisions (Video 1.1).

Prior Glaucoma Surgery In patients with prior glaucoma tube shunt or trabeculoplasty, the location of the prior surgery must be taken into account, and wound location may need to be adjusted accordingly to avoid intersecting the conjunctival bleb or intraocular hardware. Gonioscopy should be performed to assess patency of bleb ostium or positioning of tube structures and the depth of the anterior chamber. These cases warrant close evaluation of the irido-lens-bag complex stability, corneal clarity, and pupillary dilation. Pachymetry and specular microscopy should also be performed where there is concern for endothelial dysfunction.

Past Medical History

Cataract surgery is considered an elective surgery, and as such, the surgeon must be cognizant of the patient's overall systemic health in order to fully assess the risks and benefits of undergoing anesthesia and surgery. There are many systemic diseases and medications that the surgeon must consider regarding anesthesia, preoperative planning, intraoperative complication, and postoperative concerns.

Anesthesia While cataract surgery is done under minimal anesthesia, there are nevertheless risks associated with even light sedation. Patients with cardiac or pulmonary disease such as CHF or COPD are at increased risk for hypoxia. Additionally, patients with a history of substance abuse may require more sedation than usual or react to anesthesia in an unexpected manner. If a surgeon elects for local anesthesia with a retrobulbar or peribulbar block, he/she should be aware of a patient's anticoagulation status. If anticoagulation cannot be stopped, sub-Tenon's block can be considered if topical anesthesia is insufficient. Finally, while uncommon, there may be reasons to elect general anesthesia for cataract surgery, such as in pediatric patients, patients with severe anxiety, or patients with intellectual disability.

Positioning – Because cataract surgery is so delicate and precise, patients need to be able to remain still for the duration of surgery. Supine positioning during surgery can be challenging for patients with back pain, neck pain, other spinal issues (particularly kyphosis), or large body habitus. Holding still may also be an issue for a patient with tremor (such as in Parkinson's disease), restless legs syndrome, or chronic cough. Finally, patients with claustrophobia may require creative arrangement of the sterile drape during surgery.

Intraoperative Challenges Patients with current or prior use of alpha-blockers (such as for prostate disease or nephrolithiasis) are at risk for intraoperative floppy iris syndrome. Additionally, young patients have a very elastic capsule that tends to run out during capsulorhexis creation and may have very soft nuclei, and pediatric patients may require a posterior capsulotomy at the time of surgery.

Postoperative Concerns Patients with diabetes are at increased risk of postoperative CME. Furthermore, patients with allergic conjunctivitis, intellectual disability, or self-injurious behavior may rub at their eyes and potentially reopen wounds; thus, it may be prudent to suture wounds in these situations.

Past Surgical History

While past non-ocular surgery generally does not affect cataract surgery, it is valuable to know if a patient has had prior issues with anesthesia.

Family History

General ocular family history and any family history of complications during eye surgery can help the surgeon understand the patient's expectations and/or fears regarding surgery. Family history regarding prior adverse reactions to anesthesia should also be elicited.

Social History

Understanding a patient's occupation and hobbies helps to guide appropriate lens choice and target refraction for cataract surgery. Alcohol or recreational drug use may affect a patient's response to intraoperative sedation, and smoking may cause chronic cough that can be difficult to control intraoperatively.

Review of Systems

A patient's health is dynamic. Thus, it is critical to reassess for any changes to a patient's general health on the day of surgery. Acute respiratory illness, abnormal vital signs, and unanticipated severe anxiety are just some of the reasons that may warrant postponing surgery or significantly changing the surgical or anesthetic plan.

Physical Examination

Unique among surgical specialists, ophthalmologists are able to directly visualize the affected tissue prior to an initial incision. The vast majority of essential information for surgery can be identified on slit lamp examination, with supplemental information gleaned from imaging modalities. A consistent and meticulous system of evaluation is paramount, and time spent improving your system of evaluation will likely yield more than reading every existing book chapter on the ophthalmic examination. The most common approach for slit lamp evaluation is an anatomic approach moving from the external examination progressing through each ocular tissue from anterior to posterior.

General Appearance

Much can be learned about a patient through simple observation of the patient during history-taking, in the exam chair, and how they position in the slit lamp. Body habitus, resting tremor, kyphosis, and neck mobility are just some of the factors that are important to consider preoperatively.

Visual Acuity

With experience, clinicians are able to correlate cataract severity with expected visual acuity. When visual acuity is significantly worse than a cataract would indicate, care should be taken to identify additional pathology or amblyopia responsible for vision loss.

Intraocular Pressure

Elevated intraocular pressure, especially if asymmetric, needs evaluation prior to cataract surgery. This includes gonioscopic evaluation of the angle specifically looking for signs of trauma (angle recession or cyclodialysis) or prior uveitis (peripheral anterior synechiae) which may affect cataract surgery planning and risk assessment. Typically, it is recommended to have intraocular pressure controlled, in the normal range prior to elective cataract surgery. Certain circumstances require proceeding with surgery despite high or low pressures such as refractory phacomorphic glaucoma or chronic hypotony. Intraocular pressure far outside of the normal range may affect how the eye behaves during the initial incision.

Pupil Examination

Iris corectopia or coloboma may indicate congenital or acquired pathology. Corectopia in particular may indicate iridocorneal endothelial syndrome, epithelial downgrowth, trauma, or prior herpetic uveitis.

Any asymmetry in pupil size and reactivity should be thoroughly evaluated. Presence of an afferent pupillary defect indicates additional ocular pathology that warrants assessment.

Pupil asymmetry due to a history of intraocular inflammation, trauma, and ocular ischemia is particularly relevant to cataract risk assessment. Pupil asymmetry, greater in bright light, indicates the larger pupil has a relative inability to constrict. A common cause of impaired constriction is traumatic mydriasis. Conversely, a smaller pupil that fails to dilate appropriately can be a clinician's first clue to the presence of posterior synechiae or a pupillary membrane. Poor pupillary dilation may also be associated with pseudoexfoliation and zonular weakness. Sub-optimal pupillary dilation may require intraoperative epinephrine and ketorolac, or a mechanical pupil expansion device.

Extraocular Motility

Any deficit in extraocular motility should be properly assessed before cataract surgery. A slight asymmetry in ductions could have resulted from prior muscle restriction related to orbital trauma and may raise the surgeon's suspicion for other trauma-related surgical challenges.

Misalignment of the eyes can also be a sign of prior trauma, childhood strabismus, or amblyopia that may limit visual outcomes after surgery.

Confrontation Visual Fields

Abnormalities in confrontation visual field testing may signify retina or optic nerve pathology that needs to be addressed prior to surgical intervention.

Red Reflex

The etiology of any asymmetry of the red reflex should be elucidated prior to surgery with a full-dilated exam. If media opacity (whether due to corneal, lenticular, or vitreal opacities) precludes adequate view of the fundus, ultrasound evaluation is recommended to rule out retinal detachment, ocular mass, or other posterior pathology.

External Structures

Orbit and Eyelid

Preoperatively, significant blepharitis should be treated, as this increases the risk of endophthalmitis. Similarly, lid malpositions such as entropion or ectropion may cause significant ocular surface pathology, leading to inaccurate biometry.

The anatomy of the orbit and eyelids can pose specific challenges during surgery. For example, enophthalmia or a deep brow may not be compatible with superior incisions, such as for a scleral tunnel. Additionally, individuals with small palpebral fissures may have difficulty tolerating a full size lid speculum during surgery, and a smaller size, such as a Miyoshi lid speculum, should be used.

The surgeon must also be aware of the tendency for pooling of fluids within the orbit causing visual distortions. Finally, proptosis, orbital adipose tissue prolapse, or very tight lids may predispose to positive pressure and anterior chamber shallowing during surgery.

Conjunctiva Sclera

Patients with prior conjunctival surgery, such as trabeculectomy or glaucoma tube implant, may necessitate altering the placement of corneal wounds. Furthermore, areas of scleral thinning may indicate prior episodes of scleritis.

Cornea

Careful evaluation of the cornea is essential to cataract surgery planning and risk assessment. Something as seemingly benign as superficial punctate keratitis or dry eye may alter corneal topography and decrease the reliability of intraocular lens calculations. A corneal scar can present intraoperative challenges by impeding visualization at the microscope or may hint at prior ocular trauma or herpetic disease that can alter surgical risk.

The presence of a pterygium can affect IOL choice, wound position, and timing of surgery. Pterygia causing significant astigmatism may require excision prior to surgery, and if planned, pterygium surgery should be done prior to cataract extraction with sufficient time for the corneal topography to stabilize. Similarly, anterior membrane dystrophy may cause significant astigmatism, which can be reduced or eliminated by a superficial keratectomy prior to proceeding to cataract surgery.

Band keratopathy, calcium deposits in the sub-epithelium, Bowman's layer, and the anterior stroma, is important for risk assessment during cataract surgery for several reasons. While sometime idiopathic, its presence often denotes a concurrent disease whether systemic (renal disease, hyperparathyroidism) or ocular (chronic uveitis or keratitis) of which the surgeon should be aware. If the corneal opacity is visually significant, removal with chelation may be required before cataract surgery, and ample time for the corneal surface to stabilize is necessary.

A detailed examination of the corneal endothelium is essential. The presence of keratic precipitates can indicate prior uveitis, whereas fine pigment such as Krukenberg's spindle may indicate pigment dispersion glaucoma. Surgeons should look carefully for corneal guttae as special attentions are warranted when operating on a patient with Fuchs' endothelial corneal dystrophy (FECD). FECD confers a higher risk of corneal decompensation after cataract surgery, especially in the presence of microcystic corneal edema, stromal thickening (central corneal thickness greater than 640 microns), and low endothelial cell counts [6]. These patients may benefit from combined cataract surgery with endothelial keratoplasty. At minimum, patients should be counseled about the increased risk of corneal decompensation, and the surgeon should take extra care intraoperatively to protect the endothelium by repeatedly injecting dispersive viscoelastic and minimizing phacoemulsification energy above the iris plane.

Patients with keratoconus present an interesting challenge for cataract surgeons both preoperatively in terms of accurate astigmatism and IOL power estimation and intraoperatively if corneal thinning and scarring are present. Corneas with advanced keratoconus are thinner and floppier which can increase likelihood of wound leak. Surgical techniques to address this include a well-constructed clear corneal incision with placement of a corneal suture, or a sclerocorneal tunnel to reduce change in corneal shape. Some experts advise choosing the placement of the corneal incision based on the location of scarring and peripheral corneal thickness, as follows: the main incision should be placed 90 degrees apart from the scar location while avoiding the quadrant with the steepest and thinnest cornea. The surgeon's view during cataract surgery can be compromised in cases with moderate to advanced keratoconus due to image distortion from scarring or steep K's – utilization of capsular staining dye is recommended to aid in visualization [1].

In cases of prior cornea transplant, whether full-thickness penetrating keratoplasty, endothelial transplants, or any form of transplant, careful assessment of corneal clarity, with focus on the layer of opacity, can guide intraoperative management. Any corneal opacity may warrant capsule stain, while superficial opacities such as Salzmann's nodules or thickened epithelium may be removed to improve the surgeon's view. Special attention to the endothelium should be given as discussed above. The depth, size, and centration of the transplanted tissue give critical cues to operative planning to avoid intersecting the graft tissue or detaching endothelial grafts. Surgical incisions should be made at appropriate clock hour or depth to allow adequate clearance from grafted tissue. Consideration may be given to specific viscoelastics, phacodynamic settings and instrumentation to minimize trauma to the graft.

Anterior Chamber

Depth Very shallow or deep anterior chambers present unique challenges during cataract surgery. A shallow AC limits the physical space for instruments and manipulation within the eye. This can increase the risk of iatrogenic damage to ocular structures such as corneal endothelium or iris. It can also change the angle of approach for instruments, potentially complicating the capsulorrhexis or phacoemulsification steps of surgery. Furthermore, risk of iris prolapse is greater given the proximity to the wound. In patients with shallow anterior chamber depth, care should be taken to avoid a short wound that is too posterior, and one can consider a more cohesive viscoelastic to maintain anterior chamber depth. Unusually deep chambers also make aspects of cataract surgery more challenging and are more susceptible to reverse pupillary block when infusion is introduced to the eye. To avoid deterioration of the surgeon's view from instruments distorting corneal tissue, surgeons should avoid long corneal incisions and to allow easier access to subincisional manipulations.

Cell/Flare Careful examination of the anterior chamber for cell or flare indicative of active intraocular inflammation is crucial before signing a patient up for cataract surgery. A minimum of 3 months with no active inflammation is associated with better outcomes among uveitic patients undergoing cataract surgery. Rare circumstances require proceeding with surgery before this period of quiescence is achieved such as refractory uveitis in a child with a cataract in the amblyogenic stage, or cataract obstructing view to retina in a case of unknown inflammatory or infectious etiology. In these instances, aggressive topical steroids or systemic steroids if appropriate are often utilized to control inflammation in the perioperative period.

Iris

Various iris findings can increase intraoperative and postoperative risk. Iris tears may indicate prior trauma. Presence of posterior synechiae, iris nodules, or a pupillary membrane indicates prior uveitic disease. Iris atrophy specifically points to a herpetic etiology. Poor dilation limits visualization and increases risk of complications during surgery. Furthermore, poor dilation, along with peripupillary transillumination defects and fibrillar material, may signal pseudoexfoliation syndrome and zonular weakness.

There are several intraoperative techniques to aid in dilation, such as intracameral pharmacologic dilation, viscodilation, stretching of the iris tissue with various instruments, and placement of iris hooks or a pupil expansion device, which will be discussed separately in a later chapter. Pupillary membranes may require peeling or cutting with intraocular forceps (Video 1.2)

Lens

Capsule The ideal anterior capsulorhexis is continuous, curvilinear, round, and centered. However, certain situations may make creating the perfect capsulorhexis more challenging. In adolescents and young adults, the capsule is more elastic with a tendency to run out during surgery; thus, the force vector applied during capsulorhexis creation must be directed more centrally or even reverse to the direction of the rhexis. In patients with uveitis, the anterior capsule may be focally or diffusely fibrotic, and in patients with traumatic violation of the anterior capsule with leakage of lens protein, the capsule may have run out already. Trying to create a continuous curvilinear capsulorhexis may require an irregularly shaped capsulorhexis. If the extent of fibrosis is significant and the capsulorhexis cannot be torn, or if the capsule has run out from traumatic violation, cutting the capsulorhexis with microscissors may be necessary (Fig. 1.6), though this may predispose to areas of weakness and possible anterior capsular tears (Video 1.3). Finally, both presence of pseudoexfoliation material on the anterior capsule and older age increase the risk of encountering zonular weakness during surgery.

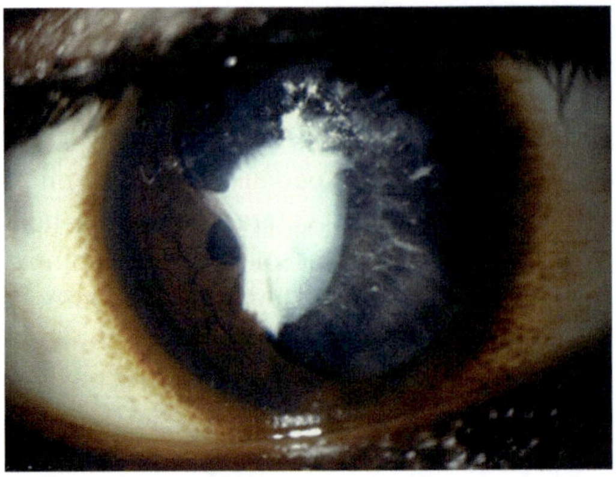

Fig. 1.6 Traumatic ocular injury with iridodialysis and with anterior capsule fibrosis and posterior synechiae

Cataract Type and Grade Careful evaluation of the type and severity of cataract will help a surgeon plan for potential intraoperative challenges. Dense nuclear sclerotic lenses will require additional phacoemulsification energy during surgery, and care should be taken to protect the corneal endothelium. In extremely dense brunescent cataracts, extracapsular extraction may be preferred. Significant cortical spoking may interfere with the red reflex and trypan blue staining will help highlight the anterior capsule. Finally, in posterior polar cataracts, there is a risk of a weak posterior capsule, and hydrodissection should be avoided and hydrodelineation performed instead.

Intumescent Bowing forward of the anterior capsule with a shallow chamber, particularly in the context of a white cataract, suggests intumescence and high intracapsular pressure. These cataracts are at high risk of anterior capsular run-out during capsulorhexis creation. Multiple techniques can help decrease this risk. First, trypan blue is an absolute must. Use of a more cohesive viscoelastic will also help maintain the anterior chamber pressure. Additionally, decompression of the lens can be taken with a 27 g needle through the paracentesis, prior to creating the main wound

(Video 1.4). This allows the anterior chamber pressure to be maintained. Alternatively, the main wound can be created and the capsule and lens directly decompressed with the phacoemulsification tip, or a double rhexis can be created, with the first smaller rhexis to decompress the lens and release the fluid trapped in the posterior intralenticular compartment, followed by a second, larger rhexis to achieve the final desired size [5].

Donesis Phacodonesis signifies zonular weakness, such as from pseudoexfoliation or trauma. Subtle signs on exam may suggest focal zonular weakness, including decentration of the fetal nucleus, focal iridodonesis, visualization of the lens equator in eccentric gaze, and presence of a gap between the iris border and the anterior surface of the crystalline lens [7]. For zonular weakness, capsular hooks, a capsular tension ring, Ahmed segment, or Cionni ring may be utilized to support the capsule during and after surgery.

Lens Subluxation Subluxation of the lens may indicate trauma, Marfan's syndrome, or homocystinuria (Fig. 1.7). Depending on the extent of subluxation, capsular hooks, a Cionni ring, or sutured Ahmed segment may be necessary. Additionally, combined surgery with retina may be necessary if there is significant vitreous prolapse, loss of zonule support, or need for primary fixated IOL.

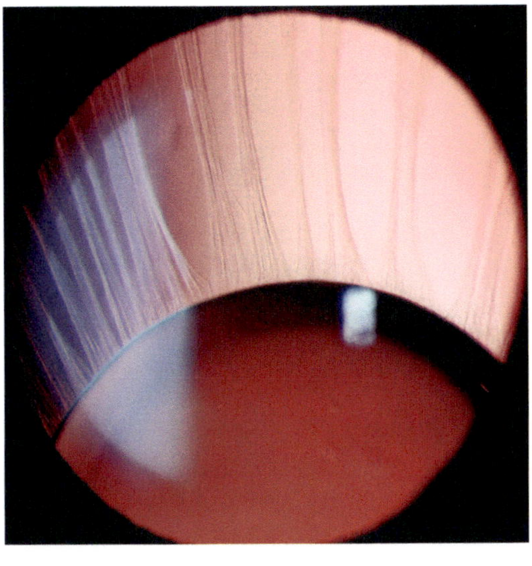

Fig. 1.7 Inferiorly subluxed lens with visible superior zonules

Vitreous

Presence of vitreous cells and haze may reveal underlying uveitis, whereas presence of vitreous hemorrhage may indicate prior trauma or proliferative diabetic retinopathy. Presence or absence of PVD may also impact appropriate counseling of patients regarding of expectations of postoperative floaters.

Optic Nerve

Evaluation of the optic nerve is critical to determine glaucoma risk. If workup indicates glaucoma, the patient may benefit from a combined MIGS procedure. In the presence of severe glaucoma, susceptibility to transient elevated IOP during surgery should be assessed.

Presence of optic nerve pallor, drusen, optic nerve pit, optociliary shunt vessels, or other pathology should be evaluated prior to surgery.

Fundus

A careful fundus examination is required in all patients prior to cataract surgery. It may alert a surgeon to any potential intraoperative challenges such as signs of prior trauma, or postoperative risk of cystoid macular edema, or retinal detachment. Furthermore, attention should be paid to the macular exam as it may alter appropriate counseling of postoperative outcome expectation and IOL choice.

Conclusion

There are several key factors that can be gleaned from a patient's history and careful examination. Perhaps the most important step to decrease patient risk is a systematic approach to identify unique risk factors. As your current system is perfectly designed to give the results you achieve, a periodic evaluation of your approach is time well spent. All surgeons would agree that intraoperative surprises are unwelcome. With a systematic and conscientious practice in place to evaluate a patient's risk factors, surgeons can plan accordingly and often reduce the likelihood of an adverse outcome.

Take-Home Notes

- Re-evaluating your systemic approach to the ophthalmic history and physical examination will improve your preoperative risk assessment.
- Ensure your process includes a surgery specific history and your referring providers and surgical staff are educated in relevant past medical and ocular history elements.
- Special focus on the anterior chamber anatomy including gonioscopy can alert surgeons to past trauma or potential ocular comorbidities.
- Ocular motility testing including cover and cross-cover testing should be performed to identify patients at risk for postoperative diplopia.
- Preoperative ancillary testing such as ocular coherence tomographic imaging of the macula can identify comorbidities affecting patient outcomes.

References

1. Aiello F, Nasser QJ, Nucci C, Angunawela RI, Gatzioufas Z, Maurino V. Cataract surgery in patients with keratoconus: pearls and pitfalls. Open Ophthalmol J. 2017;11:194–200.
2. Asbell PA, Dualan I, Mindel J, Brocks D, Ahmad M, Epstein S. Age-related cataract. Lancet. 2005;365:599–609.
3. Chan NS, Ti SE, Chee SP. Decision-making and management of uveitic cataract. Indian J Ophthalmol. 2017;65(12):1329–39.
4. Chong EW, Mehta JS. High myopia and cataract surgery. Curr Opin Ophthalmol. 2016;27:45–50.
5. Figueiredo CG, Figueiredo J, Figueiredo GB. Brazilian technique for prevention of the Argentinean flag sign in white cataract. J Cataract Refract Surg. 2012;38:1531–6.
6. Kaup S, Pandey SK. Cataract surgery in patients with Fuchs' endothelial corneal dystrophy. Community Eye Health. 2019;31(104):86–7.
7. Marques DMV, Marques FF, Osher RH. Subtle signs of zonular damage. J Cataract Refract Surg. 2004;30:1295–9.
8. Mehta S, Linton MM, Kempen JH. Outcomes of cataract surgery in patients with uveitis: a systematic review and meta-analysis. Am J Ophthalmol. 2014;158(4):676–92.e7.
9. Rojas B, Zafirakis P, Foster CS. Cataract surgery in patients with uveitis. Curr Opin Ophthalmol. 1997;8(1):6–12.

Technology and Devices Involved in Cataract Surgery in Special Cases

2

Mark Packer

Bullet Points
In this chapter, you will find advice on managing difficult and challenging cataract cases, including:

- Radial keratotomy.
- Small pupil.
- Eyes needing intraocular lens exchange.
- Patients with kyphosis.
- Eyes with corneal endothelial cell compromise.

Introduction

In this chapter you will learn my approach to addressing cataract in eyes with a history of radial keratotomy, small pupil, a need for intraocular lens exchange, corneal endothelial cell compromise, and patients with kyphosis. These approaches reflect my personal experience with techniques and technology that I have found to be useful in addressing difficult and challenging cases. Of course, other surgeons may prefer different approaches, and it is left to the reader to weigh and consider a variety of methods. Cataract surgery remains at least as much art as science, and the development of skill and judgment is a lifelong pursuit.

Status Post Radial Keratotomy

Patients with a history of corneal refractive surgery, including radial keratotomy (RK), photorefractive keratectomy (PRK), and laser in situ keratomileusis (LASIK), present unique challenges to the surgeon, not the least of which is their demonstrated desire for excellent vision without glasses or contact lenses. These patients' expectations for emmetropia as well as presbyopia correction after cataract surgery must be tempered by the limitations of our diagnostic measurements, power calculations, and intraocular lens designs.

The presence of radial, arcuate, and other types of incisions in the cornea poses particular challenges in surgical technique. The goal is to enter the anterior chamber without bisecting any of the preexisting corneal incisions, which have a propensity to split open if interrupted. If a radial incision does split, it will often require suture repair, most commonly using 10–0 nylon. When multiple radial incisions have been placed close

Supplementary Information The online version contains supplementary material available at [https://doi.org/10.1007/978-3-030-94530-5_2].

M. Packer (✉)
Packer Research Associates, Inc., Boulder, CO, USA
e-mail: mark@markpackerconsulting.com

J. L. Alió et al. (eds.), *Cataract Surgery*, Essentials in Ophthalmology,
https://doi.org/10.1007/978-3-030-94530-5_2

together, avoiding them can be a challenge. In these cases, the use of bimanual microincision (BMMI) surgical techniques can help avoid problems.

Using a 1.4 mm diameter diamond blade allows entry with 20-gauge instrumentation, including a phaco and irrigation tips (Duet, MST, Redmond, WA) such as those demonstrated in the attached video (2.1). The use of slit beam retroillumination (Carl Zeiss Meditec, Dublin, CA) is also highlighted to facilitate removal of posterior capsular cortical material. The IOL is then implanted through a fresh, 2.4 mm clear corneal incision placed between two radial incisions. Careful stromal hydration and Seidel testing are performed to ensure that all incisions are sealed. Sometimes, stromal hydration can lead to gaping of neighboring radial incisions. In order to avoid this problem, which can lead to temporary irritation and distorted vision, observe the nearby radial incisions while performing stromal hydration and discontinue hydration at the first sign of a gap appearing along the epithelial surface overlying the radial incisions.

Zonular Weakness

Ranging from mild pseudoexfoliation syndrome without significant compromise to lens stability to ectopia lentis with severe lens dislocation, zonular weakness poses challenges to the cataract surgeon. The capsular tension ring (CTR) and its various modifications have proven of inestimable value in conquering these difficulties. Insertion of a CTR may be accomplished most conveniently with an injector; alternatively, it may be placed using forceps. In either case, the leading tip of the CTR should be introduced into the capsule in the area of zonular weakness, such that it pushes against the weakened fibers and avoids further stretching or tearing of zonular fibers.

Although signs of zonulopathy are often discernible at the time of preoperative slit lamp examination, there are occasions when subtle signs may be missed, and an unexpected problem is encountered intraoperatively, as seen in the attached video (2.2). In this case, zonular weakness revealed itself during the initial instillation of OVD, as the lens moved laterally and posteriorly in response to the increasing pressure in the anterior chamber. Early placement of the CTR helped to stabilize the lens and achieve successful cataract extraction and IOL implantation without complications. In addition, the long-term presence of the CTR helped to stabilize the IOL postoperatively.

Occasionally, when zonulopathy is minimal, lens extraction may be accomplished without the CTR, and the ring can be implanted after completion of cortical cleanup. The advantage of this approach is that removal of the cortex is routine. If the CTR is placed prior to removal of cortex, a modification of technique is necessary because the ring may actually trap cortical material against the capsular equator. In this situation, engaging the cortex anteriorly with the aspiration port and then performing tangential stripping is effective. Attempting to strip cortex centripetally will meet with resistance in this situation. The modified Henderson CTR is designed with undulations to facilitate cortical removal.

Construction of the capsulorhexis is challenging in the presence of a weakened zonule because the forces that keep the capsule on stretch during the procedure are lacking. One approach to avoiding complications of capsulorhexis is to instead use a femtosecond laser to construct a capsulotomy [1].

Small Pupil

A small pupil must be enlarged enough to permit safe capsulorhexis or capsulotomy (in the case of femtosecond laser-assisted cataract surgery) and lens extraction. An important device in this regard is the pupil ring, such as the Malyugin ring (MST, Redmond, WA). The Malyugin ring, which is available in both 6.25 mm and 7.00 mm sizes, consists of a flexible plastic wire with four spiral corners that engage the pupil margin. The injector allows insertion and removal through a small incision. When injecting the ring, it is most convenient to engage the distal pupil margin first, and then capture the pupil margin to the left and right sequentially. The proximal pupil must often be captured by manipulating the ring with a hook.

When posterior synechiae prevent straightforward enlargement of the pupil, these synechiae must first be broken by viscodissection using a dispersive OVD agent. Another instance where the pupil ring cannot be directly applied is the fibrotic pupillary margin or membrane, which does not stretch. These stiff membranes must first be stripped from the pupil margin using appropriate forceps. Bleeding may occur during this procedure and can be tamponaded with additional OVD.

Other approaches to small pupil management such as stretching can result in tearing the pupillary sphincter and a mydriatic pupil. If an enlarged pupil causes unwanted optical side effects such as glare, or results in an untoward cosmetic appearance, a pupilloplasty can be performed [2].

IOL Exchange

There are multiple reasons why an intraocular lens must be exchanged for another. Many times, this procedure is performed for a refractive surprise, although implanting a piggyback lens or performing a corneal refractive procedure may provide a more predictable result. However, in the case of unwanted optical side effects from a multifocal or extended depth of focus IOL, exchange is the only viable course. Exchanging an IOL early in the postoperative course prior to capsular fibrosis is relatively straightforward and involves simply instilling a dispersive OVD agent beneath the edge of the capsulorhexis. As the OVD fills the capsular bag, the IOL will prolapse anteriorly where it can be safely bisected with microscissors (Packer Chang IOL Cutters, MST, Redmond, WA) and the halves can be pulled out of the eye through a clear corneal incision.

Later in the postoperative course, even years after the initial surgery, IOL exchange can still be accomplished, but greater care must be taken to preserve the now fibrotic capsule. Again, the procedure begins with instillation of a dispersive OVD beneath the margin of the capsulorhexis; however, the anterior capsule may be somewhat firmly adherent to the anterior surface of the IOL optic, so that a 25-gauge or smaller needle must be used first to insinuate itself between the capsule and the lens, gently elevate the capsule, and thus create a space for instillation of the OVD. The dispersive OVD should then be directed along the arms of the haptics, in the case of a C-loop design IOL. The critical step is freeing the haptic arms from the capsular equator. Using a micro forceps to grasp the IOL and attempt to pull it free from the bag, one must carefully observe the capsule itself to insure that one is not ripping the zonular fibers away from their attachments to the ciliary body or to the capsule rather than freeing the IOL.

Sometimes, releasing the haptics from the capsule is not possible. In this case, amputation of the haptics is necessary. One should attempt to cut the haptics as far peripherally as possible, to ensure that they do not reside within the visual axis, i.e., they are not centripetal to the margin of a physiologically mydriatic pupil. Particular IOLs are more prone to requiring haptic amputation because of their designs, including Crystalens and Trulign Toric IOLs (Bausch + Lomb, Rochester, NY) and AcrySof IOLs (Alcon, Ft. Worth, TX).

Following successful explantation, with an intact capsular bag, the new IOL is implanted in standard fashion. The fibrotic capsule, now expanded by viscodissection of the old IOL, will not again undergo contraction as it did after the primary surgery. Thus, the effective lens position of the new IOL is less predictable. One approach to achieving greater predictability is to select an IOL with a large overall diameter, such that it will come to rest at the capsule equator.

Kyphosis

Sometimes the challenges to successful surgery are not related to ocular anatomy, but rather to systemic conditions. For example, the inability of a patient to lie flat disrupts the routine approach to cataract surgery and requires adaptation on the part of the surgeon and the entire surgical team. Extreme kyphosis is one example of this situation. As shown in the attached video (2.3), the approach taken is to utilize an adjustable surgical bed and perform surgery with the patient practically sitting up. This approach makes the surgeon's viewing angle quite unfamiliar, particularly during capsulorhexis construction. One must proceed slowly and carefully in this novel environment; nevertheless, a successful outcome will be all the more appreciated. A similar approach has been described by Kooner and Barte [3].

Macular Degeneration

Although macular degeneration does not pose a particular challenge for lens extraction and IOL implantation, it does mean that the outcome with a standard IOL will not necessarily involve an improvement in visual acuity. Nevertheless, cataract surgery may be indicated, even in the setting of advanced macular degeneration, in order to improve peripheral vision. In these cases, it is critical to provide a detailed informed consent so that the patient does not have unreasonable expectations. Performing a potential acuity test may help inform the patient's decision in this setting.

Alternatively, special optical devices such as the implantable miniaturized telescope (IMT, VisionCare, Saratoga, CA) may be indicated in this population. As shown in the attached video (2.4), the IMT is a large intraocular device that requires not only an incision far beyond the dimensions of today's routine small incision cataract surgery but also a surgical iridectomy to prevent pupillary block. Given the requirement for a large incision, one might surmise that an older technique such as extracapsular cataract extraction might be appropriate. However, the risk of damage to the capsular bag with this older surgical technique precludes its use. Therefore, the optimal approach is to perform standard small incision, or, in this case, bimanual micro-incision and cataract surgery, and then enlarge the clear corneal incision for implantation. Of course, an incision of this size requires suture closure.

Corneal Endothelial Cell Compromise

Various situations can result in compromise to the corneal endothelium. Most commonly, loss of endothelial cells is associated with Fuchs dystrophy; however, prior intraocular surgery, including glaucoma and vitreoretinal procedures, may also be associated with endothelial cell loss. The corneal endothelium represents a "canary in the coal mine," i.e., an early warning of future decompensation. With today's endothelial transplantation techniques, the risk/benefit ratio has shifted toward intervention.

Visual inspection at the slit lamp and corneal pachymetry do not always provide a meaningful approximation of corneal endothelial cell density and function, because these findings do not show changes until the cell density is severely reduced. Even with a density of 500 cells/mm^2, the cornea will often maintain clarity and thickness within the normal range. In the setting of prior intraocular surgery or endothelial dystrophy, specular microscopy can be helpful in providing meaningful information to the surgeon and the patient regarding the expected outcomes of cataract surgery.

One of the times when corneal pachymetry can be helpful to understand outcomes is on postoperative day 1, when the change in pachymetry is highly correlated with the loss of endothelial cells [4]. Essentially, corneal edema and swelling in the immediate postoperative period indicate damage to corneal endothelial cells. The expected loss of endothelial cells due to cataract surgery is about 10 percent, although there is a wide range that depends on multiple factors, not the least of which is surgical technique. Risk factors for corneal endothelial cell loss include the following:

- Diabetes mellitus [5].
- Age >70 years [6].
- Shorter axial length (<23 mm) [7, 8].
- Shallow anterior chamber depth [9].
- Higher-grade nuclear sclerosis [10, 11].
- Higher ultrasound energy utilization as reported by cumulative dispersed energy (CDE) or effective phaco time (EPT) [12, 13].

The primary approach to protecting the corneal endothelium during lens extraction and IOL implantation is the use of appropriate dispersive OVD agents. In addition, surgical techniques which reduce the amount of ultrasound energy released in the eye will help to preserve the endothelium. In this regard, chopping techniques eliminate the need to make grooves in the lens material and reduce ultrasound use. Authors have also shown that the use of femtosecond laser-assisted cataract surgery may reduce endothelial cell loss [14]. Endocapsular phacoemulsification, rather than operating in the anterior chamber, is also useful in this setting.

Conclusion

The cataract surgeon benefits from many innovative technologies and techniques that have evolved over the years since Sir Harold Ridley implanted the first intraocular lens on February 8, 1950, and Charlie Kelman filed the first patent for phacoemulsification on July 25, 1967 [15]. It behooves surgeons to continually update their files and improve their approaches to difficult and challenging cases.

Take-Home Notes

- In eyes with a history of radial keratotomy, the goal is to enter the anterior chamber without bisecting any of the preexisting corneal incisions.
- Use of a pupil expander ring can convert a difficult case with a small pupil into a relatively routine procedure.
- Later in the postoperative course, even years after the initial surgery, IOL exchange can still be accomplished, but great care must be taken to preserve the now fibrotic capsule.
- Patients with challenging postural issues such as kyphosis can be managed through creative collaboration with surgery personnel to achieve adequate positioning for surgery.
- Use of appropriate OVD agents represents the key to protecting the corneal endothelium during lens extraction and IOL implantation.

References

1. Teshigawara T, Meguro A, Sanjo S, Hata S, Mizuki N. The advantages of femtosecond laser-assisted cataract surgery for zonulopathy. Int Med Case Rep J. 2019;11(12):109–16.
2. Narang P, Agarwal A. Single-pass four-throw technique for pupilloplasty. Eur J Ophthalmol. 2017;27(4):506–8.
3. Kooner KS, Barte FM. Intraocular surgery in kyphosis: an easier approach. Case Rep Ophthalmol. 2013;4(2):34–8.
4. Lundberg B, Jonsson M, Behndig A. Postoperative corneal swelling correlates strongly to corneal endothelial cell loss after phacoemulsification cataract surgery. Am J Ophthalmol. 2005;139(6):1035–41.
5. Hugod M, Storr-Paulsen A, Norregaard JC, Nicolini J, Larsen AB, Thulesen J. Corneal endothelial cell changes associated with cataract surgery in patients with type 2 diabetes mellitus. Cornea. 2011;30:749–53.
6. Orski M, Synder A, Pałenga-Pydyn D, Omulecki W, Wilczyński M. The effect of the selected factors on corneal endothelial cell loss following phacoemulsification. Klin Oczna. 2014;116(2):94–9.
7. Storr-Paulsen A, Norregaard JC, Ahmed S, Storr-Paulsen T, Pedersen TH. Endothelial cell damage after cataract surgery: divide-and-conquer versus phaco-chop technique. J Cataract Refract Surg. 2008;34(6):996–1000.
8. Yamazoe K, Yamaguchi T, Hotta K, Satake Y, Konomi K, Den S, Shimazaki J. Outcomes of cataract surgery in eyes with a low corneal endothelial cell density. J Cataract Refract Surg. 2011;37:2130–6.
9. Hasegawa Y, Nejima R, Mori Y, et al. Risk factors for corneal endothelial cell loss by cataract surgery in eyes with pseudoexfoliation syndrome. Clin Ophthalmol. 2016;10:1685–89. Published 2016 Aug 30.

10. Hayashi K, Hayashi H, Nakao F, Hayashi F. Risk factors for corneal endothelial injury during phacoemulsification. J Cataract Refract Surg. 1996;22(8):1079–84.
11. Bourne RR, Minassian DC, Dart JK, Rosen P, Kaushal S, Wingate N. Effect of cataract surgery on the corneal endothelium: modern phacoemulsification compared with extracapsular cataract surgery. Ophthalmology. 2004;111:679–85.
12. Pirazzoli G, D'Eliseo D, Ziosi M, Acciarri R. Effects of phacoemulsification time on the corneal endothelium using phacofracture and phaco chop techniques. J Cataract Refract Surg. 1996;22(7):967–9.
13. Berdahl JP, Jun B, DeStafeno JJ, Kim T. Comparison of a torsional handpiece through microincision versus standard clear corneal cataract wounds. J Cataract Refract Surg. 2008;34:2091–5.
14. Mayer WJ, Klaproth OK, Hengerer FH, Kohnen T. Impact of crystalline lens opacification on effective phacoemulsification time in femtosecond laser-assisted cataract surgery. Am J Ophthalmol. 2014;157(2):426–32.e1.
15. Packer M. Phaco has turned 40, gracefully. Expert Rev Ophthalmol. 2008;3(2):113–6. https://doi.org/10.1586/17469899.3.2.113.

The Hard Cataract

3

Angela Verkade and Kendall E. Donaldson

Objectives

- Discuss presurgical evaluation of the dense cataract.
- Review techniques for successful removal of the dense cataract.
- Outline how to optimize ultrasound settings for dense cataracts.
- Explore technologies available for complex cataract removal.
- Describe postoperative complications and ways to avoid them.

Supplementary Information The online version contains supplementary material available at [https://doi.org/10.1007/978-3-030-94530-5_3].

A. Verkade
Department of Ophthalmology, Baylor College of Medicine, Houston, TX, USA

Ophthalmology, Winston Salem, NC, USA

K. E. Donaldson (✉)
Cornea/External Disease/Cataract/Refractive Surgery, Bascom Palmer Eye Institute in Plantation, Plantation, FL, USA
e-mail: KDonaldson@med.miami.edu

The Preoperative Evaluation

The preoperative evaluation should always begin with the establishment of rapport and trust. It is a time of education for both the physician and the patient. The patient needs to be educated regarding what a cataract is and what is involved in cataract surgery, whereas the surgeon needs to be educated on the patient's history, expectations, and visual potential. This is particularly important in cases that may be complex or may involve a prolonged postoperative treatment course. Understanding the history of vision loss and any other prior confounding events (such as trauma, surgery, amblyopia, or other ocular disease) are key determinants of a patient's final visual outcome and may play a role in lens choice at the time of surgery. A patient with a rapid rate of vision loss or unilateral loss of vision should make the surgeon suspicious for other underlying conditions (such as chronic uveitis, retinal detachment, or an intraocular malignancy). Many patients present with a misconception that cataract surgery will fix other underlying conditions, such as the visual distortions from an epiretinal membrane or the foreign body sensation associated with their dry eye condition. Thus, providing a reasonable expectation for the outcome of the surgery is of utmost importance in the earliest portion of the consultation in order to eliminate postoperative dissatisfaction. It is not uncommon for patients with a purely brunescent nuclear cat-

J. L. Alió et al. (eds.), *Cataract Surgery*, Essentials in Ophthalmology,
https://doi.org/10.1007/978-3-030-94530-5_3

aract to have best corrected vision that is 20/40 or better. Ideally, in these patients, if a protracted course of recovery is anticipated, they should be counseled on the potential for delayed visual recovery, temporary worsening of vision, or extended need for drops postoperatively. Of course, we can't always anticipate the exact postoperative course, but we need to do our best to set reasonable expectations for our patients preoperatively.

The preoperative exam should include grading of the nuclear density. Developing a systematic approach to grading the lens prior to surgery allows for the surgeon to accurately predict surgical complexity. Using a standardized classification modality such as the Lens Opacities Classification System III eliminates subjective evaluation in order to facilitate consistent preoperative grading. Furthermore, standardized classification allows for consulting services and other surgeons to objectively communicate when referring a patient to higher levels of care in the setting of complex cataract removal [1]. Notation of color and opalescence of the nuclear cataract as well as identification of any associated posterior capsular or cortical component can help the surgeon determine if additional tools, such as trypan blue, may be required during surgery. While the LOCS III classification system is well accepted, some newer systems have attempted to utilize computer algorithms, quality of retinal imaging, as well as anterior segment optical coherence tomography, to determine the cataract grade [2].

Initial evaluation should also include a thorough eye exam, as dense or hypermature cataracts are often associated with a variety of comorbid conditions. These comorbid conditions are key determinants of visual outcome as well as the rate of recovery. Their detection preoperatively also allows time for creation of appropriate patient expectations, as well as time for the surgeon to prepare to have any anticipated tools available at the time of surgery. Corneal examination, in particular notation of guttae, corneal edema, and corneal scars, is of paramount importance. Corneal scarring may be suggestive of previous trauma or inflammation, and notation of this is key in order to determine potential for delayed healing or diminished best corrected visual acuity after surgery. A full dilated preoperative exam provides a wealth of information to prepare the surgeon for the case. Maximum degree of dilation should always be documented preoperatively in the chart. Any pupillary irregularities (such as transillumination defects or synechia) should also be well-documented. In addition, by having the patient look to the far periphery in each meridian can sometimes demonstrate zonular discontinuities or irregular movements of the lens that can be associated with a zonular weakness. Pigment on the anterior lens capsule or on the corneal endothelium can also be a sign of prior intraocular inflammation or pigment dispersion which may be associated with zonular fragility. It is important to note any signs of pseudoexfoliative material on the lens capsule, zonules, or pupillary margin so as to anticipate abnormal zonules in surgery. In addition, occasional vitreous prolapse may occur in an area of zonular discontinuity. Such patients may require a capsular tension ring, iris hooks, capsular hooks, or vitrectomy. Additionally, these patients may have a higher risk of pupillary block due to hydration of the vitreous during phacoemulsification through the open zonular apparatus.

In patients with a history of prior ocular surgery, the eye may behave in a less predictable manner. Many of our patients undergo serial intravitreal injections for macular degeneration, vascular occlusions, and diabetic retinopathy. On rare occasions, these patients have experienced needle penetration of the posterior capsule, which could lead to a dropped lens at the time of surgery (Fig. 3.1), In addition, many patients have undergone a vitrectomy in the past which may result in zonular compromise and/or weakening of the integrity of the posterior capsule. In these cases, the posterior capsule tends to be more friable and can prolapse anteriorly more easily toward the end of surgery. Similarly, our glaucoma patients who have undergone prior trabeculectomy or tube shunt surgery are at risk for lower endothe-

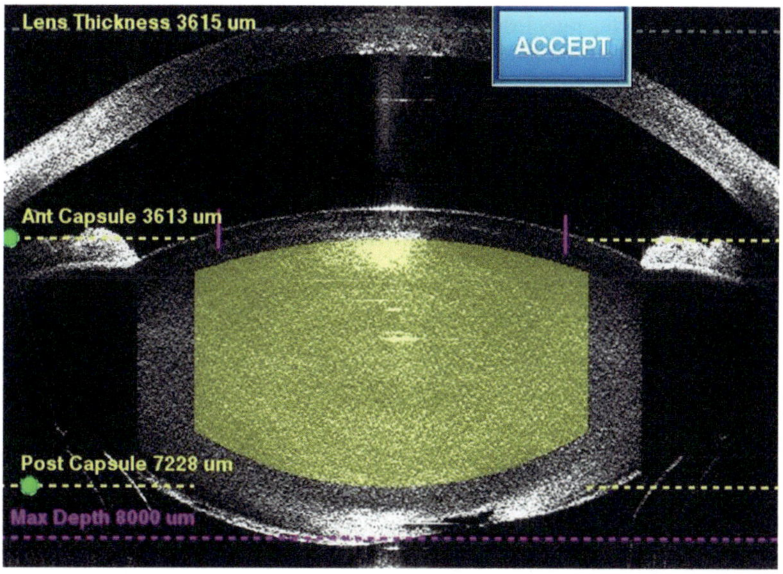

Fig. 3.1 Intraoperative optical coherence tomography scan revealing a violation of the posterior capsule. (LenSX, Alcon, Geneva, Switzerland)

lial cell counts and a higher incidence of postoperative corneal edema. It is best to recognize these issues preoperatively in order to be prepared to manage any potential surgical and postsurgical challenges.

Obtaining a thorough systemic history is also imperative because it can help elucidate any risk factors for "intraoperative floppy iris syndrome" (IFIS). Any history of hypertension or current treatment with alpha blockers, finasteride, benzodiazepines, or antipsychotics can affect degree of pupillary dilation [3]. These medications pose a potential risk for pupillary constriction and irregular iris behavior, characteristic of IFIS [4, 5]. Floppy iris syndrome may be associated with a higher risk of complications including vitreous loss, corneal edema, and damage to the iris during phacoemulsification. Other systemic disorders to consider include those with underlying inflammatory or autoimmune conditions. These conditions may place the patient at risk for prolonged inflammation after dense cataract removal. In these cases, one should consider preoperative pulse steroids or intraoperative subconjunctival injection versus intracameral injection of steroid, in addition to the typical prolonged topical therapy in the postoperative period.

Preoperative Testing

We are very fortunate to have an expansive array of technology that assists us in the preoperative evaluation of the cataract patient. Over the past decade, increasing importance has been placed on achieving emmetropia, by correction of both the spherical and astigmatic portion of the patient's refractive error. With premium lens technology, many surgeons are offering their patients an opportunity to upgrade to either monofocal or multifocal astigmatism correction. This has caused preoperative topography and/or tomography to become a standard component of the preoperative evaluation. In many patients, these tests can help facilitate the diagnosis and treatment of ocular surface disease in preparation for cataract surgery. Several studies have shown that the preoperative regularization of both the amount and the axis of astigmatism can be significantly altered by dry eye syndrome and other forms of ocular surface disease [6]. Corneal topography and placido disc technology also aid with the diagnosis and grading of anterior basement membrane syndrome, Salzmann's nodular degeneration, and any irregularities that may have been induced after prior refractive surgery.

In many cases, this may lead to pretreatment with a superficial keratectomy 6–8 weeks before cataract surgery in an attempt to make the corneal surface more regular and optimize it for intraocular lens measurements. In such cases, cataract surgery is delayed until the topography is deemed stable.

Preoperative specular microscopy is an essential tool for a variety of patients, but it is especially useful in patients with mature cataracts. In anticipating the increased need for high energy expenditure during surgery, a preoperative assessment of endothelial cell count and cell integrity is very helpful in setting expectations for rate of recovery and for the potential need for endothelial transplantation in rare cases [7–9].

Immersion A scan and intraocular lens (IOL) biometry are fundamental for lens power calculations needed in cataract surgery. Dense cataracts may not be amenable to IOL biometry due to the increased lens density; thus, it is common to revert to immersion A scan technology in these cases. In addition, if the preoperative view to the posterior segment is poor, a B scan ultrasound is an effective modality for elucidating integrity of the posterior segment, often ruling out retinal detachment, choroidal masses, and severe optic nerve cupping.

The ultimate goal of the preoperative assessment is to anticipate all of the intraoperative and postoperative potential needs and to communicate any limitations to the patient, so that both the surgeon and the patient can be best prepared throughout the cataract surgery and recovery experience. Any potential needs should also be shared with the operating room (OR) team in order to plan for the type of anesthesia, the length of case, any vitrectomy instrumentation, or other tools that may be required so as to avoid inconveniencing staff with unexpected needs throughout the case. More challenging cases, including dense cataract with their potentially complicated demands, should be placed toward the end of the surgical day, to avoid lengthening the wait time for other patients while also alleviating some degree of surgeon stress.

Intraoperative Tools and Techniques

Tools

As previously mentioned, successful surgery begins long before the patient enters the operating room, with proper preoperative testing and the gathering of any tools that may be needed during the case. Appropriate anesthesia for a complex case may deviate from the routine topical lidocaine gel. For any case in which a potential vitrectomy may be needed, the case duration may be prolonged, or if extensive iris manipulation and repair may be involved, a block consisting of either 2% or 4% lidocaine, with or without Marcaine, should be administered.

Trypan blue is one of the most commonly used tools to facilitate visualization, thus making the removal of a dense cataract safer and faster. Since dense cataracts may be associated with limited pupillary dilation, there are a variety of tools that can be used to expand the pupil. These include intracameral injection of preservative-free 1% lidocaine with phenylephrine, adding epinephrine to the irrigating solution, or placing intraoperative 1.0% phenylephrine/0.3% ketorolac in the irrigating solution (Omidria, Omeros, Inc.). On occasion, despite these interventions, it may be necessary to use other forms of mechanical pupil dilators, including mechanical expanders, rings, and hooks. Synechialysis may be indicated in some cases in which adhesions have formed between the anterior lens capsule and the iris, resulting in a small, fixed pupil. A small pupil can often make it difficult to stain the anterior capsule entirely with trypan blue. One technique the surgeon may use is staining with trypan blue prior to pupillary enlargement. The surgeon may then wash the trypan from the anterior chamber but reserve some for later re-staining. Subsequently, one may employ their chosen method of pupillary dilation solutions or devices. If the initial stain was insufficient and a cohesive ophthalmic viscosurgical device (OVD) was used, the surgeon can then either remove the OVD from the anterior chamber followed by reinjection of trypan blue, or they may use the trypan blue cannula to "paint" the stain between the OVD and the anterior capsule. If there is any concern for zonular weakness, a small amount of OVD can be injected in the area of weakness in order to create a barrier for trypan blue leakage into the posterior chamber. If the surgeon does not have access to trypan blue (or in addition to trypan blue), radiofrequency diathermy may be used to create a continuous curvilinear capsulorrhexis in the absence of a red reflex. Diathermy is particularly useful in the setting of elastic capsules as seen in pediatric cases or in fibrotic capsules which may have a tendency to tear irregularly. A technology called Zepto (Mynosys Cellular Devices, United States), when inserted through the main incision, uses a small amount of suction to adhere to the anterior capsule combined with electrical pulses delivered through a nitinol ring and offers a circular capsulorrhexis without the need for trypan blue or a red reflex [28]. Zepto technology can facilitate creation of a capsulotomy of a perfect size and shape while reducing the risk of radialization of a tear in an irregular capsule (which is commonly associated with mature cataracts).

In any case requiring prolonged operating time, especially in the setting of a dense cataract, or extra manipulation of the nuclear material, it is wise to stop and replenish dispersive OVD multiple times throughout the case to provide protection for the corneal endothelium. Replenishing OVD will also help to maintain the anterior chamber stability. It is important to use a "goldilocks" approach to refilling the anterior chamber with OVD, as over-pressurizing the anterior chamber may cause iris prolapse through the wounds or tension on fragile zonules. Additionally, overfilling with a dispersive OVD may cause clogging of the phacoemulsification tip, thereby increasing energy and heat release in the anterior chamber, which may cause endothelial damage. Our advice is to use just enough OVD to fill your working space or cover the corneal endothelium. This is particularly important in cases involving dense cataracts, due to the greater energy expenditure for nuclear disassembly without the added heat generated from OVD clogging the phacoemulsification tip. In addition, these lenses are often removed in the context of a compromised working space as a result of compression of anterior chamber depth associated with the progressively enlarging lens. The surgeon must pay particular attention when disassembling a dense lens and using the second instrument to prevent nuclear fragments from propelling against the corneal endothelium in order to prevent postoperative corneal edema and long-term endothelial damage.

Another useful tool is the miLOOP device (Carl Zeiss Meditec, Germany), which consists of a nitinol filament that can essentially "lasso" the nuclear material and cleave it into planes. Cleaving the cataract prior to phacoemulsification can significantly reduce ultrasound time and energy expenditure during the case [10]. Additionally, the miLOOP may be helpful in cleaving the leathery posterior plate often associated with dense lenses. In an extremely dense lens, it may be helpful to debulk the nuclear material first with phacoemulsification to create more working space before inserting the miLOOP device. A thorough hydrodissection and hydrodelineation facilitate movement and rotation of the nucleus which also create space for the miLOOP device [11]. Some surgeons prefer to use this device simply to create an initial cleavage plane and complete the rest of the nuclear cleavage manually. However, others will repeat the miLOOP maneuver multiple times to subdivide the nuclear material into multiple segments before attempting manual removal. Care should be taken to maintain central positioning of the device throughout use to avoid placing any additional stress on the zonules.

We are often unable to predict with 100% certainty if a patient will need a vitrectomy. However, at times we can anticipate this need based on our preoperative exam and, with this anticipation, may arrange for a retina specialist to be on standby if such a need were to occur. Many anterior segment surgeons are also skilled at both anterior vitrectomy and limited pars plana vitrectomy, which becomes useful for complex cases. A vitrectomy may be planned in special scenarios, including the need for posterior decompression with a pars plana approach in the setting of a dense cataract with short axial length (nanophthalmos). Additionally, vitrectomy may be planned if there is any concern for posterior capsular violation in any patient with a history of a posterior polar cataract, intravitreal injections, trauma, or posterior segment surgery. If a vitrectomy is performed, it is helpful to use dilute intravitreal or intracameral triamcinolone for visualization of any residual vitreous at the end of the case.

In mature cataracts with an unstable zonular complex, it is often still possible to place an intraocular lens (IOL) in the capsular bag with the use of a capsular tension ring or with sutured capsular segments [12]. If the surgeon does not feel comfortable placing a single-piece IOL in the bag, other alternatives include a three-piece IOL in the sulcus with or without optic capture. Optic capture is preferred for better lens stability within the sulcus when possible. If the entire bag complex is compromised, one may suture a three-piece lens to the iris or place an anterior chamber IOL. These fixation techniques are less desirable in younger patients, those with a history of endothelial compromise, or those with a history of uveitis. Lenses may also be secured to the sclera using the Yamane technique or a glued IOL technique or with sutures such as Gore-Tex or Prolene.

Surgical Techniques

Femtosecond Laser Pre-fragmentation of the Lens

The use of a femtosecond laser for pre-fragmentation of the lens in preparation for phacoemulsification is a technique which has been shown to significantly reduce the energy required for phacoemulsification [13, 16–18]. This conservation of energy has been shown relative to traditional phacoemulsification with all available laser platforms [9, 13]. Reducing the energy of phacoemulsification may preserve endothelial cells and may be associated with a more rapid visual recovery [8, 19]. There are multiple femtosecond platforms available, but when pre-fragmenting the rock-hard cataract, it is best to utilize a system that allows for multiple line fragmentation patterns (Fig. 3.2). Multiple line fragmentation may require more femtosecond energy due to the more intricate fragmentation pattern, but the increased femtosecond energy used to pre-fragment the lens will ultimately allow for less ultrasound energy when removing the dense cataract. Additionally, use of a femtosecond capsulotomy allows for consistent capsulotomy size when visualization is poor. Furthermore, the capsule can always be stained with trypan once surgery is started. An invariably round and precisely sized capsulotomy may save the surgeon in cases of posterior capsular rupture or complex nuclear removal allowing for optic capture and a more stable lens at the end of the case. The femtosecond laser capsulotomy also allows for visualization of centration as it allows for assessment of capsulotomy size and centration in reference to the pupil center and approximation based on the optical coherence tomography imaging of the lens itself [27]. The surgeon may elect to decenter the capsulotomy in reference to the pupil if there is irregular or poor dilation in order to allow for estimated centration over the lens center, ultimately providing adequate anterior capsule override over the IOL edge [27] (Fig. 3.2).

The Capsulorrhexis

If a femtosecond platform is not available, attention should be drawn to the accurate sizing of the capsulorrhexis in a dense lens. Sizing becomes important in the rock-hard cataract for a multitude of reasons. Too small of a capsulorrhexis, and the surgeon may have difficulty removing large dense fragments for phacoemulsification, or they may incidentally place undue tension on the anterior capsule when manipulating fragments with instruments, thus causing an anterior capsular tear. And while a large capsulorrhexis can make nuclear removal easier, the surgeon

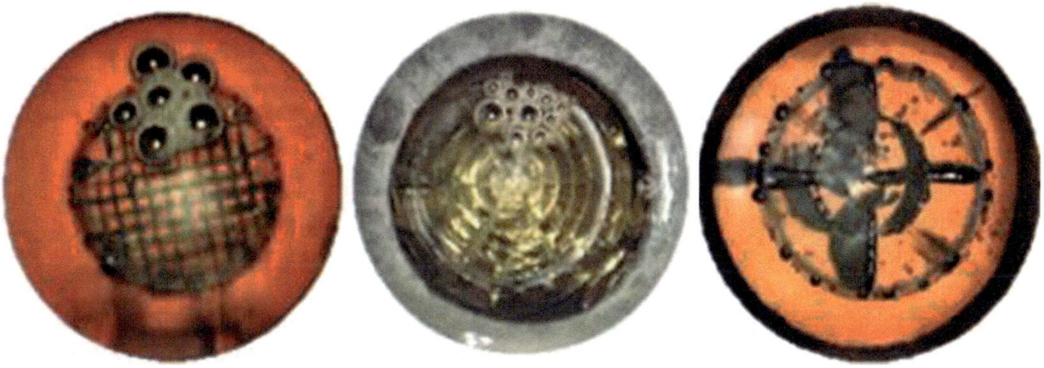

Fig. 3.2 Femtosecond laser lens fragmentation patterns. The first image demonstrates a grid or cube pattern. The second and third image demonstrate both cylindrical and pie/spoke patterns, with the third photo exhibiting fewer cuts

may have difficulty getting proper overlap of the anterior capsule over the lens optic, which may cause the optic to prolapse. Additionally, too large of a rhexis may prevent the surgeon from stabilizing a three-piece lens in the sulcus with optic capture. While a 5.0 to 5.5 mm rhexis diameter allows for sufficient lens-capsule overlap of most lenses, the surgeon can enlarge the rhexis to just under 6.0 if needed for a dense lens. A rhexis just under 6.0 mm in diameter allows the surgeon to utilize optic capture of the 6.0 mm lens optic in most cases. There are multiple tools available to aid in sizing of the capsulorrhexis including circular corneal markers, a ring light source projected through the operating microscope, and capsulorrhexis forceps with a marked edge for estimation [14]. Other tools that may become useful when creating the capsulorrhexis in the rock-hard cataract include intraocular forceps and scissors, as frequently, dense nuclear cataracts can be associated with anterior capsular fibrosis. These areas of fibrosis should be incorporated into the capsulorrhexis when able, but if there are areas of fibrosis along the path of the rhexis edge, intraocular scissors and forceps can be used to complete the tear through these fibrotic zones [15].

Hydrodissection

After creation of the "goldilocks"-sized capsulorrhexis, it is important to proceed with gentle but complete hydrodissection in the rock-hard cataract. Often dense nuclear cataracts may be associated with a thin layer of outer cortex or seemingly no remaining cortex at all, which leaves only a large dense nucleus filling the majority of the capsular bag. This creates little space for fluid waves and promotes the risk of posterior capsular blowout during hydrodissection. Gentle fluid waves with delicate decompressions in multiple quadrants prevent the risk of fluid buildup posterior to the lens and avoid the risk of sudden decompression through the posterior capsule [15]. Often it is impossible to hydrodelineate in ultra-dense cataracts, but if able, the surgeon may attempt limited hydrodelineation to create a shell of epinucleus to protect the posterior capsule during removal of the dense nuclear core.

Nuclear Removal

As with a standard cataract extraction, removal of the dense nuclear material can be performed in a number of ways. As stated previously, femtosecond nuclear fragmentation and the miLOOP device can allow for decreased phacoemulsification energy required during nuclear disassembly. There are instruments available to divide the lens into smaller pieces for removal without the use of sculpt mode. There are "prechoppers," which are designed to fragment the nucleus prior to insertion of the phacoemulsification probe, thereby reducing ultrasound energy used during removal of the dense cataract. Prechoppers like the Aguilar Prechopper (Katena Products, United States) and the Akahoshi Prechopper (Katena Products, United States) have thin blades at the tip that are combined with a "jaw-like motion," which when inserted into the nucleus will penetrate and crack the nucleus with minimal zonular stress and no ultrasound power. If the surgeon is more comfortable with using a chopper combined with the phacoemulsification probe, it is important to keep in mind the dense lens frequently has adherent nuclear fibers and often a leathery posterior plate. Choosing a chopper with a more tapered or thinner tip becomes useful for penetration of the hard cataract for chopping. Some examples include the Nagahara Chopper, Chang-Seibel, or the Hwang chopper (Katena Products, United States).

There are multiple customizations that can be made when choosing a phacoemulsification probe tip when approaching the rock-hard cataract. The surgeon may choose a curved or angled probe over a straight probe as it requires less torque of the wound and angulation within the surgeon's hand to allow for deeper grooves. The bevel may also be customized to have a 0 to 60 degree cut. The larger the degree allows for more surface area available for nuclear removal but a sharper edge to the probe. Additionally, the diameter of the probe may range from 19 to 23 gauge. The larger diameter probes allow for a higher flow rates and less vacuum when removing fragments but require a larger incision for use.

Some surgeons advocate first sculpting a wide but deep central groove to create space and allow for the first hemi-nuclear crack. This first groove must be deep enough in order to allow for splitting of the posterior plate, but always keeping in mind there is often very little lens cortex to protect the posterior capsule from ultrasound energy. The divide and conquer technique is certainly helpful to continue to create space within the capsular bag by making wide and deep grooves within each quadrant. This technique may allow for less zonular stress if the forces are placed tangentially. There is a tradeoff to the divide and conquer technique, as more ultrasound energy is required for sculpting each quadrant than that which is expended with chopping techniques. Both horizontal and vertical chop can be used to disassemble the dense lens. Chopping allows for mechanical splitting of the lens to be used in place of ultrasound energy, thereby decreasing total ultrasonic energy expenditure within the eye. Additionally, chopping allows for the surgeon to cleave the lens into smaller and smaller pieces for removal. In exceedingly dense lenses, vertical chopping maneuvers may be limited if the surgeon is unable to impale the nucleus and may place unwanted stress on the zonular fibers. Horizontal chopping in very dense lenses may place stress on, or cause tears in, the anterior capsule when trying to place the instrument peripheral to the lens [15]. No matter the choice of nuclear disassembly, it is important to be methodical when removing a dense nuclear lens.

Most dense cataracts require a longer surgical duration than the standard cataract removal. Maintaining a balanced and stable anterior chamber can mitigate risks such as wound burn and posterior capsular rupture in these complex surgeries. Equilibrium in these cases, requires fluid influx into the anterior chamber is equivalent to egress from the wounds. Multiple variations can be made during surgery in order to maintain anterior chamber stability. It is not only important to test the phacoemulsification hand piece outside the eye before wound entry but to also observe the phacoemulsification device on insertion into the anterior chamber. As OVD is removed, if the lens iris diaphragm "bounces" or there is shallowing with aspiration and phacoemulsification, the surgeon must make adjustments to their fluidics. Some systems allow the surgeon to raise the bottle height to allow for an increased inflow, while other systems require an increase in the maintained intraocular pressure target [15]. A leaky wound can be a source for rapid egress of fluid and loss of anterior chamber stability. Ensuring the appropriate wound size for your phacoemulsification hand piece and sleeve is of utmost importance to prevent leakage to create a stable anterior chamber environment for phacoemulsification. If the wound is too tight around the phacoemulsification sleeve, you are at risk for

Settings	Longitudinal Ultrasound (%)	Burst Mode (on time/off time ms)	Pulse Rate (Pulse per second)	Torsional Ultrasound (%)	Vacuum (mmHg)	Asp Flow (cc/min)	IOP (mmHg)
Sculpt	0	-	-	100	135	28	65 (88)
Chop	50	80/25	-	0	575	35	65 (88)
Quad	0	-	30	80	525	40	65 (88)
Epinucleus	0	-	10	25	425	35	65 (88)
Cortex	-	-	-	-	600	45	60 (82)
Polish	-	-	-	-	18	8	60 (82)
Visco	-	-	-	-	700	55	55 (75)

Fig. 3.3 Author's phacoemulsification settings for "dense cataract mode". (Centurion, Geneva, Switzerland)

poor egress of fluid and a potential resultant wound burn. The surgeon should be aware of the centration of their phacoemulsification probe within the wound. They should maintain a symmetric distance of the probe from the walls of the wound in order to prevent occlusion of irrigation through the sleeve when compressed against the walls of the wound. Occlusion of irrigation and proximity of the probe against the walls of the wound increase the risk of wound burn. If the chamber continues to shallow with increasing IOP or bottle height, the surgeon should stop and carefully inspect for any posterior capsular rupture or a "tense" eye suggestive of hemorrhagic choroidal or hydration of the vitreous space.

Other settings that may be manipulated during phacoemulsification of the dense cataract include vacuum, aspiration, and ultrasound power. Again, it is critical to keep in mind that any changes to ultrasound parameters require a balancing change to other settings. Increases in aspiration and vacuum settings for the dense cataract will also increase the amount of fluid required to irrigate throughout the case, but it is important to keep in mind that this will often cause quicker loss of OVD [15]. Judicious replenishing of OVD maintains endothelial health, but care must be taken not to overfill so as to not clog the phacoemulsification tip and risk thermal burn of the incision [15].

Phacoemulsification ultrasonic parameters can also be customized according to the density of nuclear material (Fig. 3.3). Surgeons that prefer sculpting the dense cataract often increase longitudinal ultrasound power and duty cycle during this stage [20]. This allows for more efficient debulking of the dense lens. As with normal sculpting, vacuum and bottle height/IOP remains low to normal. For segment removal, often vacuum levels are increased in order to maintain "holdability" of the lens fragments within in a small working space. In this stage, often aspiration is increased in order to allow pieces to easily flow to the phacoemulsification tip and subsequently bottle height/IOP rise in order to maintain a stable chamber [20]. The duty cycle, or the percentage "on" time of ultrasound energy, is frequently increased anywhere from 40% to 80% for a brunescent cataract [20].

Phacoemulsification machines depend on a pumping mechanism by which fluid is moved throughout the machine. Phacoemulsification machines are based on either a peristaltic or venturi pump system or a combination of the two. A thorough understanding of the phacoemulsification device allows the surgeon to adjust settings in order to maximize efficiency dependent on lens density. When using peristaltic devices in the setting of a rock-hard cataract, one may want to lower vacuum parameters in order to avoid a prolonged rise time in the phacoemulsification tubing, thereby reducing a sudden surge once the tip is no longer occluded. Fortunately, inflow and outflow tubing compliance has been progressively optimized in order to create a low-surge environment characterized by soft inflow tubing with high compliance and rigid outflow tubing with low compliance. This creates an environment in which the inflow is greater than the outflow which maintains anterior chamber volume and stability while reducing surge. Some phacoemulsification machines allow for combined peristaltic and venturi settings in order to better control vacuum levels without reliance on occlusion of the phacoemulsification tip.

Most surgeons prefer ultrasound burst mode or ultrasound pulse mode over continuous mode for these cases, so as to reduce total ultrasonic energy and allow for cooling between energy deliveries (Fig. 3.4) [15]. Pulse mode not only allows for cooling between pulses but also decreases cumulative ultrasound energy over time, allowing the surgeon to adjust the amount of energy delivered based on the lens density.

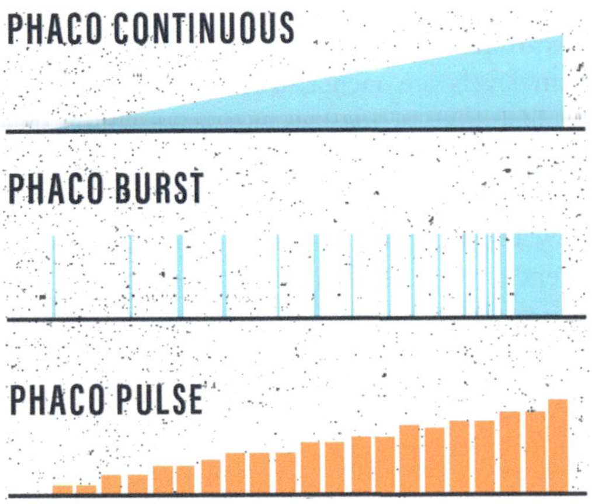

Fig. 3.4 Ultrasound power modes. Phacoemulsification continuous mode provides a continuous build of ultrasound energy as the pedal is depressed in foot position 3. Phacoemulsification burst mode allows for the same amount of ultrasound energy to be applied with each burst. The bursts become more frequent with further depression of the foot pedal into position 3. Similar to continuous mode, phacoemulsification pulse mode allows for the ultrasound energy to build with further depression into position 3, but the pulses allow for ultrasound "off time" between each pulse. https://millennialeye.com/articles/2017-sept-oct/phaco-power-fundamentals/. Figure reproduced with permission of Kate Xie, MD; Sumit "Sam" Garg, MD; and Bryn Mawr Communications. Xie K, Garg S. Phaco power fundamentals. *MillennialEYE.* September/October 2017 (accepted for use)

Burst mode allows the surgeon to control how frequently a particular quantity of ultrasound power is being delivered over a certain period of time. This allows for delivery of more frequent bursts in order to pulverize a large piece of nuclear material. Less frequent bursts are applied when burying into a large piece for improved mobility or for breaking apart smaller lens pieces. Both burst and pulse mode allow for customization of ultrasound energy depending on lens density and lens material remaining in the case, thus allowing for overall reduced energy utilization due to efficiency of energy delivery. Utilizing other modes of energy delivery such as torsional and elliptical patterns of the phacoemulsification tip may reduce chatter often seen with longitudinal phacoemulsification in the rock-hard lens [15]. Lastly, we advise every surgeon to learn about their own personal phacoemulsification machine and settings prior to approaching complex cataracts. Understanding how to alter these settings can help to avoid intraoperative complications.

While the evolution of phacoemulsification has allowed the cataract surgeon to tackle some extremely dense lenses, occasionally the surgeon may encounter a cataract that is not amenable to phacoemulsification. When the preoperative assessment of cataract density warrants excessive ultrasound energy, cataracts often deemed "black cataracts," employment of the manual small-incision cataract surgery (MSICS) technique may allow for better rehabilitation and quicker visual recovery. This technique utilizes a 5.5 to 7.5 mm superior scleral tunnel incision, often triplanar in nature, that when made properly acts as a self-sealing wound. The initial entry into the anterior chamber from the tunnel incision is made with a standard keratome single-entry incision. After the wound is made, routine steps are performed such as injection of OVD and creation of the capsulorrhexis, provided the rhexis is adequately sized to about 6.5 mm. Then after completion of the capsulorrhexis, the entry into the anterior chamber is enlarged to match the scleral tunnel, and hydrodissection is performed to prolapse the lens into the anterior chamber. The nucleus is then expressed through the scleral tunnel wound by a variety of mechanisms. The surgeon can express the lens material using an irrigating lens loop cannula, OVD, or manual expression with a hook or cannula [21]. Most surgeons will use extra OVD or an anterior chamber maintainer in this stage in order to protect the corneal endothelium and maintain anterior chamber stability. Then, the cortex is removed with irrigation and aspiration using the phacoemulsification machine or a Simcoe cannula [21]. The IOL can then be delivered into the capsular bag. Advantages of the MSICS technique include lesser or equal astigmatism rates when compared to traditional phacoemulsification, less operative time, and less energy expenditure inside the eye when compared to phacoemulsification [21, 22]. The disadvantages include a larger incision size, which may predispose to high risk of infection or wound leak, and iris damage if there is premature entry into the anterior chamber when creating the scleral tunnel [21]. It is important to weigh all risks and benefits in the preoperative period when a patient presents with a very dense cataract, as other techniques such as MSICS may benefit both the patient and surgeon when performed correctly.

Less commonly used techniques include both traditional extracapsular cataract extraction (ECCE) and supracapsular phacoemulsification. While these techniques are used infrequently, knowledge of these methods may come in handy when approaching a dense cataract with very poor zonular support. Surgeons may even consider consultation with a retina specialist for pars plana lensectomy in rare cases, but some may be limited by specialist availability. With extracapsular cataract extraction, a limbal entry wound is made and the standard steps such as OVD injection and capsulorrhexis are performed. The limbal wound is enlarged often to roughly 10 mm in length. Hydrodissection is performed, and the lens nucleus is delivered through the large limbal incision. Disadvantages of this technique include large incision size that often requires multiple sutures for closure and induction of astigmatism due to wound tension. This technique may become useful if there is evidence of scleromalacia preventing a scleral tunnel incision, as seen in MSICS, or if the lens appears remarkably unstable such that the surgeon anticipates need to remove some, or all, of the capsular complex with the lens. In supracapsular phacoemulsification, the standard steps of phacoemulsification are performed up to hydrodissection. The goal in this technique is to swiftly hydrodissect the lens nucleus, so as to prolapse the lens into the anterior chamber and remove the lens material in total, with phacoemulsification starting at the prolapsed lens margin. With this technique, one must create a large capsulorrhexis to aid in lens prolapse. Additionally, the surgeon must use copious OVD, as corneal edema is a common complication due to direct damage from lens-cornea touch and to the delivery of ultrasound energy in close proximity to the endothelium. These techniques may be used as a last resort when there is concern for significant capsule/zonular instability preventing the surgeon from using standard phacoemulsification. Luckily, with the advent of the MSICS technique and capsular stabilizing devices such as capsular hooks and segments, these techniques are rarely used.

Wound Integrity

After successful removal of the rock-hard cataract, ensuring wound closure is exceedingly important to prevent hypotony, endophthalmitis, or IOL instability. It has been demonstrated in the literature that complex cataract extraction with prolonged operative time, vitrectomy, or excessive wound manipulation, particularly in the dense cataract, is a setup for poor wound closure [23]. Apart from the standard stromal hydration, placement of a 10–0 nylon suture at the main wound or usage of corneal sealant may prevent these complications. Regardless of the method of wound closure used, assurance of wound integrity and avoidance of wound leak significantly reduce postop morbidity after dense cataract extraction. In addition, these cases are at higher risk of wound burn given the additional ultrasound energy required for phacoemulsification. If a wound burn occurs, wound closure may be very difficult to achieve, even with sutures. Fibrin glue with or without a bandage contact lens may be helpful to ensure adequate closure, thus reducing the risk of infection.

Postoperative Care

Frequently after dense cataract removal, there can be a protracted course of corneal edema following surgery [24]. Patients with preexisting corneal dystrophy or degenerations, particularly those with Fuchs' endothelial dystrophy, are at increased risk of corneal decompensation after dense cataract extraction. The surgeon can attempt to mitigate this risk by instituting an extended regimen for topical steroid after surgery. Not only is it often necessary to administer a longer course of topical steroid but also to administer more frequent steroid in the immediate postoperative period. Hourly topical steroid application in the first few days after surgery with a slow taper over a matter of 6 to 8 weeks is often required when there is evidence of significant corneal decompensation after surgery. It is important to monitor these patients every 2 to 3 weeks to avoid a steroid response with elevated intraocular pressure so that one can initiate treatment before damage to the optic nerve. Though every attempt may be made to support the endothelium both during surgery and after, pseudophakic bullous keratopathy is a common indication for partial thickness corneal endothelial grafting [24].

There is also a higher risk of postoperative cystoid macular edema (CME) after complex cataract removal [26]. This risk increases with addition of other predisposing conditions such as diabetes, vein occlusions, use of prostaglandin analogs, and uveitis [26]. Some studies have shown that perioperative use of topical nonsteroidal anti-inflammatory drugs (NSAIDs) in addition to postoperative use can lower the risk of cystoid macular edema (CME) after cataract removal [25]. Along with topical steroids, often the postsurgical use of NSAIDs may be required for several months in the setting of CME. While the incidence of postoperative CME after cataract extraction is low, suspicion should remain high in patients who are not correctable to 20/20 in an otherwise normal eye, as often the peak incidence of CME is around 4 to 6 weeks after surgery [26]. In these patients, we recommend screening with retinal optical coherence tomography (OCT), as commonly these cases can be subtle and difficult to appreciate on dilated fundus exam alone. The appropriate anticipation of these postoperative complications can avoid patient disappointment and dissatisfaction after complex cataract removal.

Conclusion

The modern ophthalmologist has a multitude of tools and techniques at their fingertips in order to tackle the removal of the rock-hard cataract. The proper surgical planning and anticipation of all possible complications allows the surgeon to feel more comfortable with the once dreaded dense cataract extraction. While not every case will require every tool or technique listed in this chapter, we hope that one or more of those mentioned may become helpful if standard techniques fail. Collaboration and communication between the surgeon and the clinical team, as well as between the surgeon and the patient, is essential for a successful surgical outcome with the rock-hard cataract.

Take-Home Notes

- The proper preoperative evaluation of the dense cataract can set up a surgeon for success once in the OR.
- The ophthalmologist has a multitude of tools available for successful avoidance of complications during dense cataract removal.
- Phacoemulsification of the dense cataract requires skilled and thoughtful technique during each and every step.
- Surgical complications can easily occur in even the most experienced hands, but it is important to anticipate these complications in order to be prepared to correct them.

References

1. Chylack LT Jr, Wolfe JK, Singer DM, et al. The lens opacities classification system III. The longitudinal study of cataract study group. Arch Ophthalmol. 1993;111(6):831–6.
2. Gali HE, Sella R, Afshari NA. Cataract grading systems: a review of past and present. Curr Opin Ophthalmol. 2019;30(1):13–8.
3. Chatziralli IP, Peponis V, Parikakis E, et al. Risk factors for intraoperative floppy iris syndrome: a prospective study. Eye (Lond). 2016;30(8):1039–44.
4. Enright JM, Karacal H, Tsai LM. Floppy iris syndrome and cataract surgery. Curr Opin Ophthalmol. 2017;28(1):29–34.
5. Lunacek A, Mohamad Al-Ali B, Radmayr C, et al. Ten years of intraoperative floppy iris syndrome in the era of α-blockers. Cent European J Urol. 2018;71(1):98–104.
6. Epitropoulos A, Matossian C, Berdy G, et al. Effect of tear osmolarity on repeatability of keratometry for cataract surgery planning. J Cataract Refract Surg. 2015;41:1672–7.
7. Takács AI, Kovacs I, Mihaltz K, et al. Central corneal volume and endothelial cell count following femtosecond laser-assisted refractive cataract surgery compared to conventional phacoemulsification. J Refract Surg. 2012;28:387–91.
8. Conrad-Hengerer I, Al Juburi M, Schultz T, et al. Corneal endothelial cell loss and corneal thickness in conventional compared with femtosecond laser-assisted cataract surgery: three-month follow-up. J Cataract Refract Surg. 2013;39:1307–13.
9. Al-Mohtaseb Z, He X, Yesilirmak N, et al. Comparison of corneal endothelial cell loss between two femtosecond laser platforms and standard phacoemulsification. J Refract Surg. 2017;33(10):708–12.
10. Diakonis VF, Cook BN, Desai NR, et al. Crystalline lens endocapsular fragmentation using an elastic loop filament. Eur J Ophthalmol. 2018;28(4):412–4.
11. Ianchulev T, Chang DF, Koo E, et al. Microinterventional endocapsular nucleus disassembly for phacoemulsification-free full-thickness fragmentation. J Cataract Refract Surg. 2018;44(8):932–4.
12. Ahmed IK, Teichman JC. Using the capsular tension segment: tips and pearls. AAO Curr. Insight. 2007;
13. Popovic M, Campos-Moller X, Schlenker MB, Ahmed II. Efficacy and safety of femtosecond laser-assisted cataract surgery compared with manual cataract surgery: a meta-analysis of 14 567 eyes. Ophthalmology. 2016;123:2113–26.
14. Dick HB, Pena-Aceves A, Manns M, et al. New technology for sizing the continuous curvilinear capsulorhexis: prospective trial. J Cataract Refract Surg. 2008;34(7):1136–44.
15. Foster GJL, Allen QB, Ayres BD, et al. Phacoemulsification of the rock-hard dense nuclear cataract: options and recommendations. J Cataract Refract Surg. 2018;44(7):905–16.
16. Abell RG, Darian-Smith E, Kan JB, et al. Femtosecond laser-assisted cataract surgery versus standard phacoemulsification cataract surgery: outcomes and safety in more than 4000 cases at a single center. J Cataract Refract Surg. 2015;41:47–52.
17. Abell RG, Kerr NM, Vote BJ. Toward zero effective phacoemulsification time using femtosecond laser pretreatment. Ophthalmology. 2013;120:942–8.
18. Abell RG, Kerr NM, Howie AR, et al. Effect of femtosecond laser-assisted cataract surgery on the corneal endothelium. J Cataract Refract Surg. 2014;40:1777–83.
19. Krarup T, Morten Holm L, la Cour M, Kjaerbo H. Endothelial cell loss and refractive predictability in femtosecond laser-assisted cataract surgery compared with conventional cataract surgery. Acta Ophthalmol. 2014;92:617–22.
20. Fishkind WJ, Wallace RB, Henderson BA, et al. Phaco machine settings. Cataract Refract Surg Today. 2008;1:1–7.
21. Singh K, Misbah A, Saluja P, et al. Review of manual small-incision cataract surgery. Indian J Ophthalmol. 2017;65(12):1281–8.
22. Venkatesh R, Tan CS, Sengupta S, et al. Phacoemulsification versus manual small-incision cataract surgery for white cataract. J Cataract Refract Surg. 2010;36(11):1849–54.
23. Matossian C, Makari S, Potvin R. Cataract surgery and methods of wound closure: a review. Clin Ophthalmol. 2015;9:921–8.
24. Chan E, Mahroo OA, Spalton DJ. Complications of cataract surgery. Clin Exp Optom. 2010;93(6):379–89.
25. Yavas GF, Ozturk F, Kusbeci T. Preoperative topical indomethacin to prevent pseudophakic cystoid macular edema. J Cataract Refract Surg. 2007;33(5):804–7.
26. Zur D, Loewenstein A. Postsurgical cystoid macular edema. Dev Ophthalmol. 2017;58:178–90.
27. Packer M, Teuma EV, Glasser A, Bott S. Defining the ideal femtosecond laser capsulotomy. Br J Ophthalmol. 2015;99(8):1136–42.
28. Chang DF. Zepto precision pulse capsulotomy: a new automated and disposable capsulotomy technology. Indian J Ophthalmol. 2017;65(12):1411–4.

4 Intumescent Cataract and Preventing the Argentinian Flag Sign

Gabriel B. Figueiredo and Carlos G. Figueiredo

Bullet Points
- Creation of a continuous curvilinear capsulorhexis in the white cataract is a challenge even for the experienced ophthalmic surgeon.
- Staining of the anterior capsule is mandatory.
- Different subtypes of the white cataract present different risks.
- The surgeon must always be attentive to the anterior segment pressure gradient – capsular bag vs anterior chamber.
- Glaucoma is often associated with the intumescent cataract.

Introduction

The white cataract can be a challenge even to the experienced surgeon. Particularly, the creation of a continuous curvilinear capsulorhexis is tricky due to the increased endolenticular pressure. Further challenges the surgeon may face include absence of the red reflex, shallow anterior chamber, and zonular fragility. Secondary glaucoma can develop through multiple mechanisms, and the adequate pre- and postoperative management is required.

Etiology

This chapter is aimed at the white cataract caused by aging. A white cataract can also rapidly develop following either ocular trauma (see Chap. 9) or iatrogenic puncture of the capsular bag.

Senile White Cataract

The senile white cataract is a type of mature cataract in which lens proteins denature and break down into smaller particles, increasing the number of osmotically active particles in the capsular bag. This osmotic gradient draws fluid into the bag (which is a semipermeable membrane) until the hydrostatic pressure within the bag balances the osmotic pressure. This process of lens hydration leads to a significant increase of the volume within the capsular bag.

Supplementary Information The online version contains supplementary material available at [https://doi.org/10.1007/978-3-030-94530-5_4].

G. B. Figueiredo (✉) · C. G. Figueiredo
D'Olhos Day Hospital, S. J. Rio Preto, Brazil
e-mail: gabrielfigueiredo@dolhos.com.br; carfig@dolhos.com.br

J. L. Alió et al. (eds.), *Cataract Surgery*, Essentials in Ophthalmology,
https://doi.org/10.1007/978-3-030-94530-5_4

Comorbidities

Glaucoma

Two pathophysiological mechanisms can lead to high intraocular pressure and secondary glaucoma in eyes with white cataract.

Phacomorphic Glaucoma

Phacomorphic glaucoma is a consequence of the excessive increase in lens thickness, causing obstruction of the trabecular meshwork by (1) the mass effect of the thickened lens physically crowding the posterior chamber and pushing the iris anteriorly and/or (2) totally or partially obstructing the physiological flow of the aqueous from the posterior chamber into the anterior chamber through the pupil due to the pupil border touching the anterior capsule, trapping aqueous in the posterior chamber, and consequently causing the peripheral iris to bow forward.

Phacolytic Glaucoma

Tiny proteins arising from the lens protein denature process can leak through the capsular bag into the aqueous. These proteins then precipitate a secondary glaucoma as phagocytizing macrophages and inflammatory debris, and the proteins themselves obstruct the trabecular meshwork.

Preoperative Management

Before proceeding to dilated exam, a thorough investigation for angle closure must be performed. Initially, the patient should be asked about previous symptoms compatible with episodes of angle closure – acute or intermittent ocular pain. Next, the surgeon should look for indirect signs of narrow angle on slit lamp exam including shallow anterior chamber and peripheral iris bowing, pupil atony/hypotony, iris atrophy, pigment deposition on the anterior capsule or endothelium, and anterior lens capsule opacities (glaukomflecken), findings suggestive of previous acute angle closure. Finally, one should always perform gonioscopy looking for an occludable angle – when the posterior trabecular meshwork is seen for less than 90° of the angle circumference; identifying the presence of peripheral anterior synechiae (PAS) is suggestive of previous angle closure. Once an occludable angle is diagnosed or there is suspicion of previous acute angle closure, a laser peripheral iridotomy should promptly be performed.

The mature, opaque lens makes fundus examination and axial length measurement through optical biometers impossible. Therefore, both A- and B-scan should be performed for axial length measurement and gross retinal changes, respectively. The mature cataract often slowly develops in an eye with previous impaired visual acuity, and the surgeon should attempt to figure out why the patient waited so long before seeking help. History of previous low vision, whether amblyopic or acquired, should be investigated for proper counseling. A potential acuity meter test can be performed, but the results are often misleading and the true visual acuity potential can only be assessed after surgery is performed.

Subtype Classification

The white cataract presents different features according to the stage [1] (Table 4.1) (Video 4.1). Correct subtype diagnosis is crucial for proper surgical management.

Pearly White Cataract

A big, hydrated nucleus is found in the pearly white cataract. Whitish fluid can be either absent or present in low to moderate amount. Several shades of white can be found on the anterior surface of the lens during slit lamp exam (Fig. 4.1). The anterior cortex may have a "frothy" appearance and a "flare" can occasionally be seen. Increased convexity of the anterior capsule is an indirect sign of the presence of fluid within the capsular bag and consequent increase in endolenticular pressure.

Table 4.1 Feature comparison of white cataract subtypes

	Pearly white		Morgagnian
	Without fluid	With fluid	
	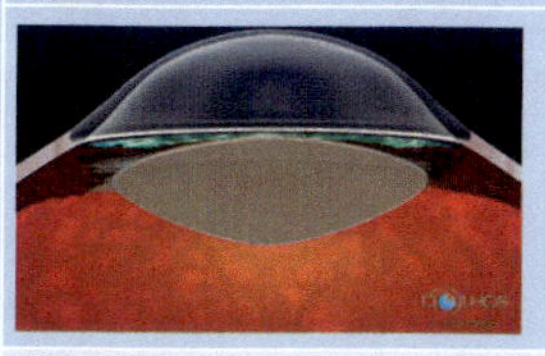	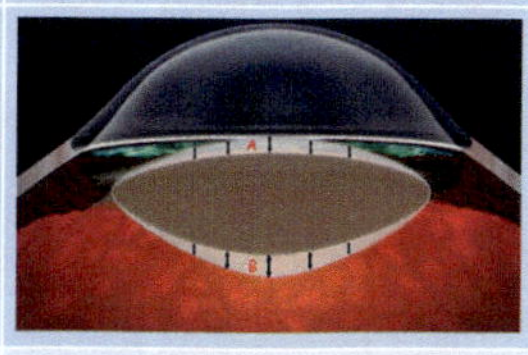	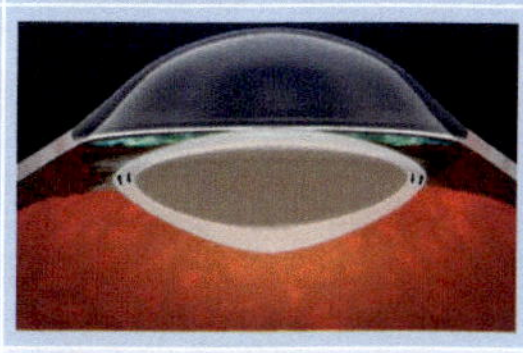
Nucleus	Big	Big	Small
Fluid	Absent	Low to moderate	Abundant
Endolenticular pressure	Normal to minimally elevated	High to extremely high	High
Equatorial block	Yes	Yes	No
Independent endocapsular spaces	No	Yes	No

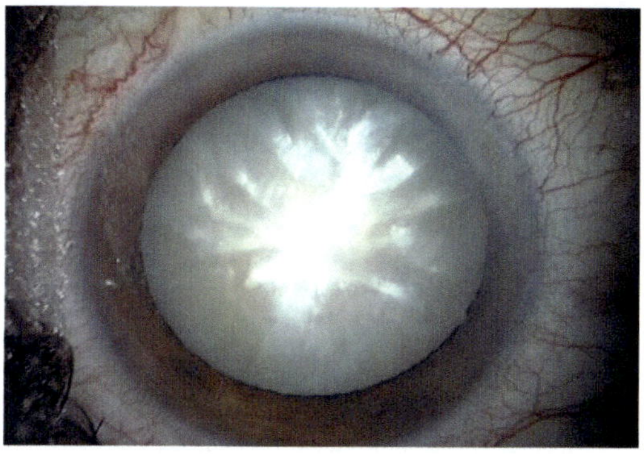

Fig. 4.1 Slit lamp picture of a pearly white cataract. Note the multiple shades of white throughout the anterior surface of the lens

Equatorial Block

Equatorial block occurs in the pearly white cataract with liquid. The fluid builds up within both the anterior and posterior subcapsular spaces, anteriorly and posteriorly to a large nucleus. This liquid accumulation leads the anterior and posterior capsules to bow anteriorly and posteriorly, respectively; consequently, the equatorial capsular bag is compressed against the nucleus, preventing the fluid from freely circulating between the two subcapsular spaces (Fig. 4.2). This process leads to the emergence of two independent hyperpressoric spaces within the capsular bag

Morgagnian Cataract

Morgagnian cataract is the most advanced stage of the white cataract, when most, or all, of the cortex is liquefied. The capsular bag is filled with a yellowish milky fluid and the small but very hard nucleus floats freely in the bag. On slit lamp exam, the anterior surface of the lens presents a homogeneous milky yellowish aspect, and the brown nucleus can occasionally be seen inferiorly (Fig. 4.3).

Surgical Procedure

Surgical Principles

The biggest challenge the anterior segment surgeon faces when approaching a white lens is the continuous curvilinear capsulorhexis. Several techniques have been described and we lack scientific consensus on the most appropriate one; different experienced surgeons have different techniques of choice to deal with the white cataract. Given the description of all of those techniques in a single chapter is not feasible, the author presents his preferred technique, based in his own personal surgical experience. Nevertheless, whichever technique one chooses, there are some fundamental surgical principles the surgeon should always keep in mind.

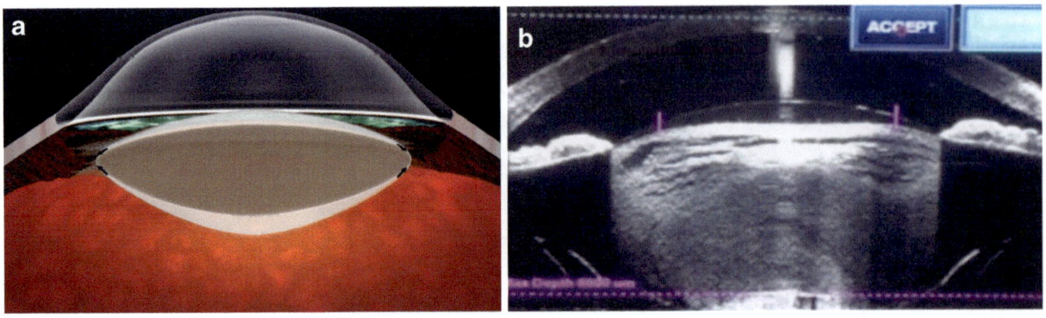

Fig. 4.2 (**a**) Illustration of a pearly white cataract demonstrating the equatorial block. Note the equatorial portion of the capsular bag compressed against the nucleus and the consequent accumulation of fluid in both the anterior and posterior subcapsular spaces. (**b**) Trapped fluid can clearly be identified in the anterior subcapsular space in an anterior segment OCT image of a pearly white cataract; although optical image capture of the posterior portion of the capsular bag is not possible, it is safe to assume a similar configuration is present

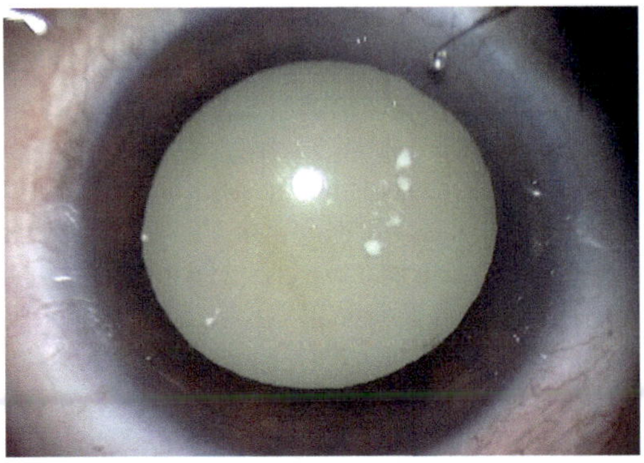

Fig. 4.3 Slit lamp picture of a morgagnian cataract. Note the homogeneously milky yellowish anterior surface of the lens

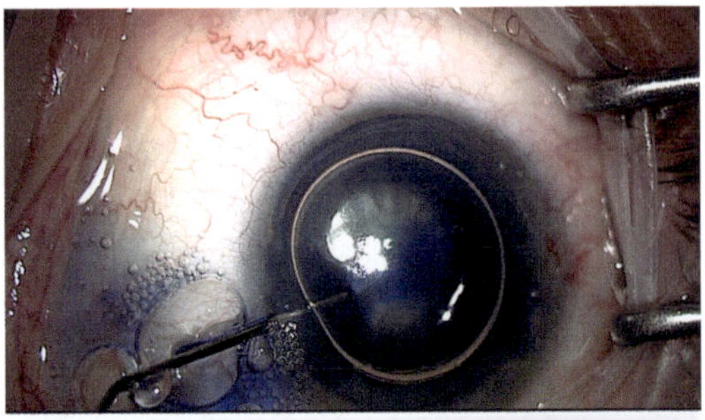

Fig. 4.4 Intraoperative picture demonstrating the injection of trypan blue under an air bubble in the anterior chamber of an eye with a white cataract to stain the anterior capsule. Trypan blue can also be injected directly into the anterior chamber without an air bubble

Capsule Staining

The white, opacified lens blocks the intraoperative red reflex. Therefore, the use of a capsular dye is mandatory to correctly identify the anterior capsule during creation of the capsulorhexis. The most utilized dye is trypan blue ophthalmic solution 0.06% [2]. The dye can be injected undiluted into the anterior chamber with or without an air bubble (Fig. 4.4). The anterior chamber is then washed after a few seconds with balanced salt solution, or directly with viscoelastic. Although staining of the anterior capsule is mandatory, trypan blue decreases elasticity of the capsule [3], which contributes to the increased risk of anterior capsule radial tear.

Pressure Gradient

The tendency for capsular tears to extend centrifugally toward the equator of the bag is due to a hydrostatic/hydrodynamic principle: the anterior segment pressure gradient – the difference between the anterior chamber and capsular bag pressures. The increased endolenticular volume leads to increased endolenticular pressure, causing the distension of the capsular bag and consequent increased convexity of the anterior capsule; the greater the convexity of the anterior capsule, the greater the tendency of the flap to run centrifugally. Simultaneously, as soon as the anterior capsule is pierced and a communication is created between the capsular bag and the anterior chamber, the content of both spaces will flow according to the pressure gradient, from the space of higher pressure to the space of lower pressure, until the pressure is equalized. Because the endolenticular pressure is greater than the intracameral pressure, the lenticular fluid will flow from the capsular bag into the anterior chamber, pushing the nucleus against the anterior capsule. Therefore, the surgeon should always be attentive to the fundamental principle of keeping the anterior chamber highly pressurized up until the capsulorhexis has been created and the endolenticular and intracameral pressures have been equalized.

Hydrodissection

Hydrodissection is contraindicated in a white lens. It is simply unnecessary in the morgagnian cataract, while it is a risk in the white pearly cataract. Due to the equatorial block present in the latter, the fluid injected under pressure reaches the posterior subcapsular space where it is trapped (Fig. 4.5). The additional increase in pressure in the posterior subcapsular space can lead either to a radial tear of the anterior capsule or even the explosion of the posterior capsule.

Capsular Fibrosis

In mature and hypermature cataracts, the anterior capsule may undergo degeneration, with deposition of calcium or the development of focal dense plaques. Ideally, when creating the capsulorhexis, the surgeon should direct the tear around these abnormalities. If not possible, then the surgeon can cut across the plaque with small gauge scissors. Multiple cuts can be performed across the plaque; however, one single and continuous cut should be made when clear capsule is being cut both when entering and exiting the plaque, to avoid the creation of zones of weakness.

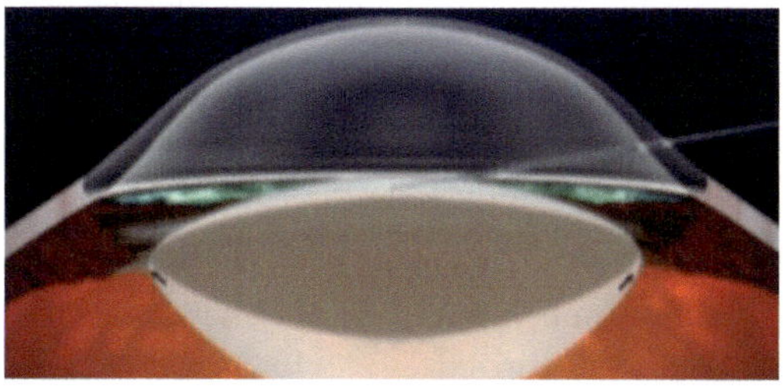

Fig. 4.5 Illustration of hydrodissection in a lens where equatorial block is present. Note that the BSS, injected under pressure, accumulates in the posterior subcapsular space. (*BSS* balanced salt solution)

Pearly White Cataract

The adequate surgical approach depends on the presence or absence of fluid within the capsular bag (Video 4.2). Even though one can look for signs of endolenticular liquid during slit lamp exam as discussed previously, this will be confirmed intraoperatively once the anterior capsule has been pierced. While there are multiple methods of initiating the procedure, we prefer the following steps:

- Make two corneal paracentesis at 12 and 6 o'clock.
- Inject trypan blue into the anterior chamber.
- Wash out the trypan blue and overfill the anterior chamber with viscoelastic to keep it highly pressurized.
- Puncture the anterior capsule with a cystotome (Fig. 4.6a).
- Attentively watch for white fluid leaking out of the bag and proceed accordingly (Fig. 4.6b).

Pearly White Cataract Without Fluid

Endolenticular pressure is normal or just slightly elevated in this stage. The surgeon should keep the anterior chamber pressurized with OVD and perform the capsulorhexis with his or her routine technique.

Pearly White Cataract with Fluid

This is the lens with the greatest risk for a radial capsular tear. Besides the elevated endolenticular pressure, there is also the presence of equatorial block and two independent and pressurized subcapsular spaces. Once the anterior capsule is open and the anterior subcapsular space pressure is equalized with the anterior chamber pressure,

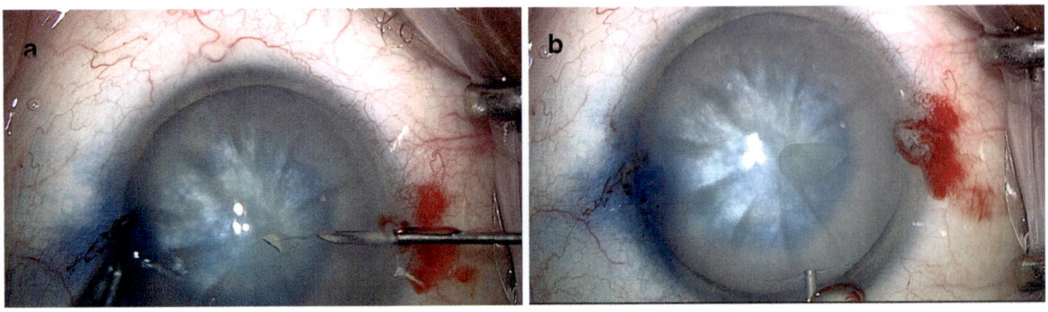

Fig. 4.6 Intraoperative pictures of the initial steps in a pearly white cataract. (**a**) The anterior capsule is pierced under a highly pressurized anterior chamber. (**b**) The surgeon must then attentively watch for any white fluid leakage from the capsular bag and proceed accordingly

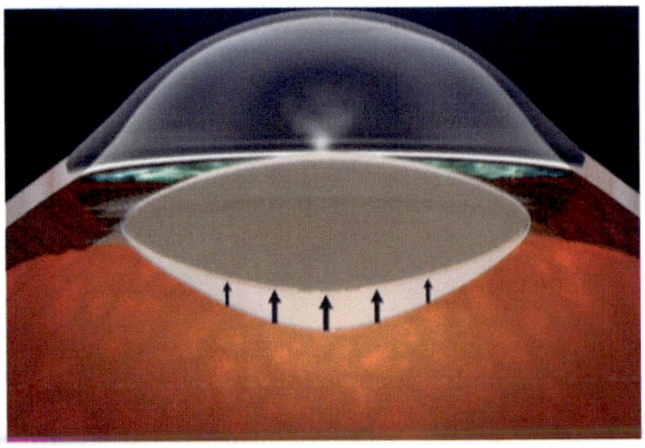

Fig. 4.7 Illustration of the anterior capsule piercing in a pearly white cataract with fluid. Note that the fluid in the anterior subcapsular space flows into the anterior chamber until the pressure in these two compartments is equalized; meanwhile, the fluid trapped in the posterior subcapsular space pushes the nucleus anteriorly against the anterior capsule

the fluid trapped in the posterior subcapsular space pushes the nucleus anteriorly against the anterior capsule (Fig. 4.7). The greater the gradient pressure between the posterior subcapsular space and the anterior chamber, the greater the force exerted by the nucleus onto the anterior capsule. The following steps have been proven safe and effective in our approach to this challenging cataract:

- Create a “mini-rhexis” (2.5–3.0 mm) with small gauge forceps through one of the paracenteses (Fig. 4.8a). If visualization of the flap gets clouded by the white fluid, clear the central area by injecting more viscoelastic.
- Use bimanual irrigation and aspiration to aspirate the fluid in the anterior subcapsular space. Next, use the aspiration handpiece to mobilize the nucleus posteriorly and peripherally, breaking the equatorial block and allowing the fluid in the posterior subcapsular space to flow anteriorly and be aspirated (Fig. 4.8b).
- Make the temporal main incision.
- Create a new flap using small gauge scissors (Fig. 4.8c).
- Enlarge the capsulorhexis to the desired diameter (Fig. 4.8d).
- Proceed with surgery according to surgeon’s routine (Video 4.3).

Morgagnian Cataract

Even though endolenticular pressure is usually elevated in these lenses, equatorial block is not present and pressure equalization can be achieved more easily.

- Create one paracentesis.
- Inject trypan blue into the anterior chamber.
- Wash out the trypan blue and overfill the anterior chamber with viscoelastic to keep it highly pressurized.
- Puncture the anterior capsule with a 27 g needle attached to a 3 cc syringe (Fig. 4.9a).
- Aspirate the endolenticular fluid (Fig. 4.9b).
- Refill the capsular bag with OVD separating the anterior and posterior capsules while

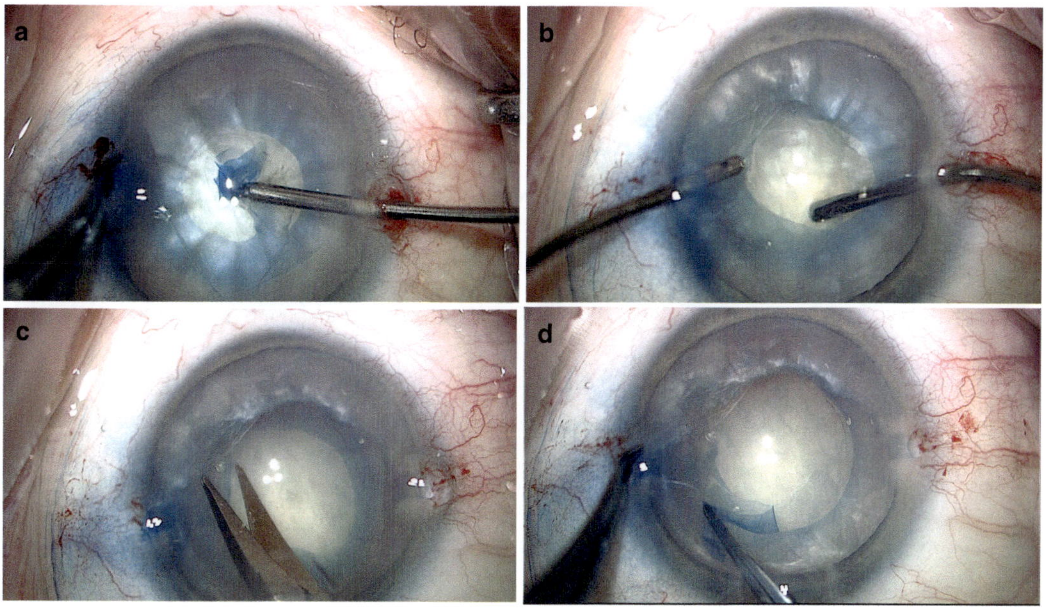

Fig. 4.8 Intraoperative pictures of key surgical steps in a pearly white cataract with fluid. (**a**) Creation of a "mini-rhexis" around 3 mm in diameter with a small gauge forceps through the paracentesis to avoid viscoelastic burping out. (**b**) Decompression of the capsular bag by aspiration of the fluid both in the anterior and posterior subcapsular spaces using bimanual irrigation and aspiration, the nucleus is balloted posteriorly and peripherally to break the nuclear block decompressing the posterior compartment. (**c**) Creation of a new anterior capsular flap. (**d**) Enlargement of the capsulorhexis to the desired diameter

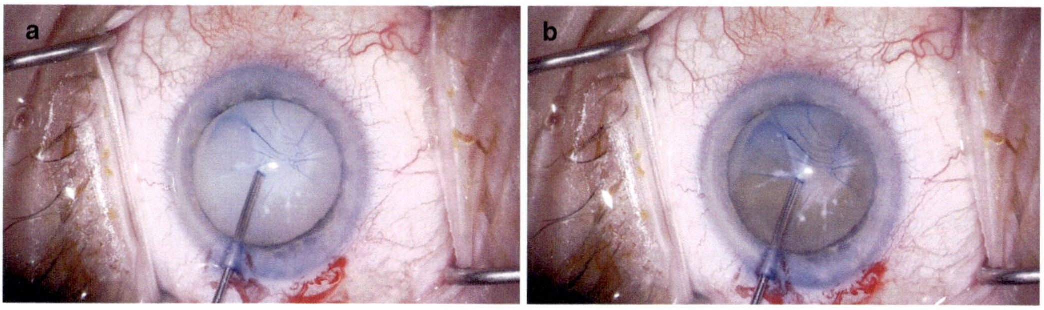

Fig. 4.9 Intraoperative picture (**a**) before and (**b**) after the aspiration of the fluid with a 27 g needle in a morgagnian cataract

creating some counterpressure to facilitate the capsulorhexis.

- Create the temporal main incision.
- Create the capsulorhexis to the desired diameter.
- Proceed with surgery according to surgeon's routine (Video 4.4).

Potential Complications

Argentinean Flag Sign

The most common complication in white cataracts is the radial tear of the anterior capsule, known as the Argentinean flag sign (Fig. 4.10).

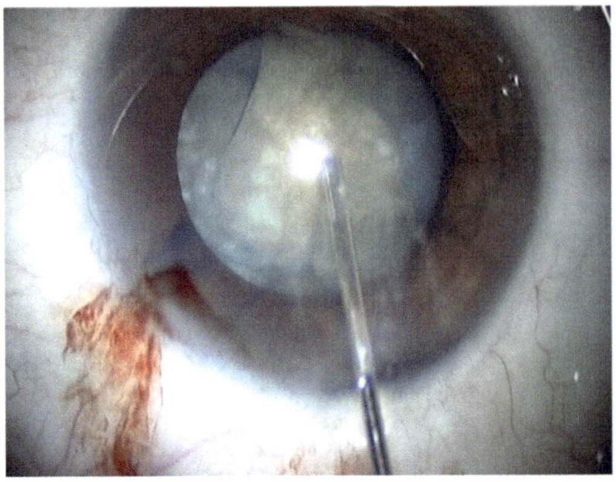

Fig. 4.10 Intraoperative picture of the Argentinean flag sign

To manage this complication, the surgeon can either (1) create a new flap with small gauge scissors in both "hemi-capsules" and create two "hemi-rhexis" or (2) resume opening the anterior capsule with the can opener technique with a cystotome. Next, one should proceed with phacoemulsification carefully, in a slow motion fashion with low parameters – "slow phaco" [4]. The radial tear might extend around the equator into the posterior capsule; therefore, the surgeon must remain vigilant for posterior capsule rupture signs (see Chap. 9).

Posterior Capsule Rupture

The posterior capsule, previously distended by the increased endolenticular volume, may be flaccid and with a tendency of "trampolining" anteriorly during phacoemulsification. Dispersive viscoelastic should be used to keep the posterior capsule posteriorly, and adequately sized incisions are mandatory to avoid BSS leakage during phacoemulsification.

Zonulopathy

Zonulopathy is frequently associated with these mature lenses. The surgeon should attentively look for signs of zonular fragility during preoperative evaluation. Further information on the management of weak zonules can be found in Chap. 9.

Take-Home Notes

- Creation of a continuous curvilinear capsulorhexis (CCC) is a challenge in the white cataract due to the elevated endolenticular pressure.
- Always stain the anterior capsule.
- During creation of the CCC, the surgeon should keep the anterior chamber highly pressurized to counterbalance the endolenticular pressure.
- The pearly white cataract with fluid is at the greatest risk for Argentinean flag sign due to presence of the equatorial block. The surgeon should keep in mind that the risk is only diminished once the posterior subcapsular space pressure has been alleviated.
- Angle closure and secondary glaucoma are often associated with the intumescent lens and should be managed accordingly.

References

1. Figueiredo CG, Figueiredo J, Figueiredo GB. Brazilian technique for prevention of the Argentinean flag sign in white cataract. J Cataract Refract Surg. 2012;38:1531–6. https://doi.org/10.1016/j.jcrs.2012.07.002.
2. Melles GRJ, de Waard PWT, Pameyer JH, Beekhuis HW. Trypan blue capsule staining to visualize the capsulorhexis in cataract surgery. J Cataract Refract Surg. 1999;25:7–9. https://doi.org/10.1016/S0886-3350(99)80004-2.
3. Dick BH, Aliyeva SE, Hengerer F. Effect of trypan blue on the elasticity of the human anterior lens capsule. J Cataract Refract Surg. 2008;34:1367–73. https://doi.org/10.1016/j.jcrs.2008.03.041.
4. Osher RH. Slow motion phacoemulsification approach. J Cataract Refract Surg. 1993;19:667. https://doi.org/10.1016/S0886-3350(13)80025-9.

Pediatric Cataract

5

H. Burkhard Dick

Bullet Points

- The global prevalence of congenital cataract is estimated to be about 4.24 per 10,000.
- In pediatric cataract surgery, the surgeon faces a morphology widely different from an adult patient: the capsule is extremely elastic, the cornea and sclera usually lack any noteworthy rigidity, and the nucleus is soft rather than hard.
- Primary posterior capsulotomy or capsulorhexis (PPC) is regarded as a necessary precaution to prevent posterior capsule opacification.
- The femtosecond laser is able to perform primary anterior and posterior with high accuracy and predictability.
- Glaucoma and inflammation are the most common postoperative complications.

Epidemiology and Pathology

Cataract presenting at birth or during early childhood is generally termed congenital and constitutes a major threat to a normal development of the visual system. Pediatric cataract is a global yet treatable cause of blindness and visual impairment. The global prevalence of congenital cataract is estimated to be about 4.24 per 10,000 with the highest prevalence in Asia and with an increasing tendency [1]. There is a large variety of etiological causes which in many cases will remain unknown. About half of congenital cataracts are believed to be caused by mutations of the protein-coding genes involved in building the structure of the lens [2]. Major causes are maternal infections such as toxoplasmosis, rubella, cytomegalovirus, herpes virus, and syphilis (TORCHS) as well as the exposition of the mother-to-be against certain toxic agents such as alcohol and probably aspirin [3]. Lens opacifications that appear in older children are usually caused by systemic and eye diseases, among the latter in particular uveitis, as well as by trauma and by exposure to drugs, most importantly to corticosteroids [4, 5].

There is a broad spectrum of morphology in pediatric cataracts, from minor punctate opacification to central opacities and complete, dense cataracts of the entire lens. Such total cataracts are not unusual in patients with Down syndrome and in cases when the mother was infected with

Supplementary Information The online version contains supplementary material available at [https://doi.org/10.1007/978-3-030-94530-5_5].

H. B. Dick (✉)
Ruhr University Eye Clinic, Bochum, Germany
e-mail: burkhard.dick@kk-bochum.de

J. L. Alió et al. (eds.), *Cataract Surgery*, Essentials in Ophthalmology,
https://doi.org/10.1007/978-3-030-94530-5_5

rubella. Anterior subcapsular cataracts are in general seen in patients with uveitis and atopic skin conditions as well as following trauma and irradiation. Partial opacities, generally described as wedge-shaped cataracts, are seen in diseases like neurofibromatosis type 2, Stickler syndrome, and Fabry's disease. Posterior subcapsular cataracts are typically steroid-induced or a consequence of radiotherapy for ocular and periocular tumors. Unilateral cataracts in particular are associated with persistent fetal vasculature (PFV) [6].

A unique form of pediatric cataract is the one caused by galactosemia which may present as posterior subcapsular cataract or with small nuclear opacifications. Unlike all other pediatric cataracts, this one is reversible by dietary modification [7].

Timing of Cataract Surgery

In cataract surgery, caring for pediatric patients confronts the surgeon with a unique situation. While adult cataract patients can expect a remaining lifespan measured in years or probably a decade or two and the emphasis in planning the operation is on best possible visual acuity, preferably without glasses and increasingly with the demand for good visual function in far, intermediate, and near distances at the same time (which has given rise to multifocal, EDOF, and other sophisticated IOL designs), the goal in young children is different and even more challenging. The surgeon has to initiate a long process that ensures the child's normal visual development and in doing so will determine the visual performance and thus the vision-related quality of life of the young patient for an extensive time period, given today's life expectancy of something close to a hundred years. The responsibility is high and so is the demand for meticulous planning – of surgery and of all the other steps that have to be taken by ophthalmologists and other specialists over the next couple of years.

Choosing the time to operate upon a newborn or a very young child always means weighing the risks and the benefits. After early surgery, massive axial elongation and a substantial myopic shift can be expected. Operating at a very young age, however, increases the likelihood of the major postoperative complication, glaucoma. Glaucoma and other postoperative complications occur at a much higher incidence when surgery takes places at an age younger than 4 weeks [8]. Waiting too long, on the other hand, can result in deprivation and consequently in amblyopia. A general recommendation might be – with all necessary caution – that unilateral congenital cataract is operated upon 4 to 6 weeks after birth and bilateral cataract between 6 and 10 weeks [9].

Whether bilateral cataracts should be operated simultaneously has been a matter of intense debate for quite a while. Arguments in favor of removing both cataracts in one session are a reduction of the anesthesia-related risk of complications (or even mortality), the reduction of hospital admissions, and the chance to achieve an improved visual acuity and binocular vision faster. Medicolegal reasons are points made against simultaneous surgery as are the risks of bilateral postoperative complications (like the worst-case scenario, endophthalmitis) and the inability of the physician to change his or her surgical plans for the second eye if complications should arise over time after surgery of the first eye [10]. When operated on different days, the time interval between both surgeries should be kept to a minimum.

To sum it up: the uncomfortable choice the cataract surgeon is facing is between the pitfalls of operating too early and operating too late. It is widely accepted knowledge that every additional week of waiting to a certain degree reduces the risk of glaucoma – and at the same time increases the risk of amblyopia [11].

Pre- and Intraoperative Considerations

As the saying goes, children are no downsized adults. This is particularly true for very young and their eye. Almost all of its anatomical structures are very different from the eye of a 70-something cataract patient: the capsule is extremely elastic, the cornea and sclera usually lack any noteworthy rigidity, the nucleus is soft rather than hard, and increased pressure from the vitreous can be expected.

In many respects, pediatric cataract surgery is different from adult cataract surgery on (in general) order patients. Removing the natural lens at a time when the eye and in particular the lens are still growing influences the development of the child's visual system profoundly. While elderly patients undergoing the procedure in most cases have been presbyopic for a long time (and often these days expect a cure from this condition by choosing an accommodative or any other kind of IOL that gives them at least a resemblance of accommodation), pediatric cataract surgery renders the child presbyopic for the rest of his or her life – or until the time in probably the intermediate future when true accommodation can be restored by some revolutionary, currently still unknown, technique. Wearing bifocal lenses will be part of the child's postoperative life, a fact the parents or caretakers should be thoroughly informed about.

In general, two small corneal or limbal incisions suffice; larger incisions are, of course, required if an IOL implantation is planned. The use of viscoelastic agents is helpful to prevent the collapse of the anterior chamber. Staining with trypan blue is essential in visualizing the anterior capsule in eyes without the red reflex; it might also diminish the elasticity of the capsule. Primary posterior capsulotomy or capsulorhexis (PPC) is regarded as a necessary precaution to prevent posterior capsule opacification (PCO) which in children develops rapidly and in almost 100% of our youngest patients. Manual PPC, however, is a challenging technique and not exactly well liked by many cataract surgeons. Performing it with the femtosecond laser is a viable and valuable alternative, where available. In a young child's eye, the likelihood of self-sealing is poor; therefore, sutures are more often than not required.

The lens can in most cases be removed by aspiration or vitrectomy cutter; the employment of phacoemulsification is only rarely necessary. After aspiration of the lens, posterior capsulotomy and anterior vitrectomy are performed. Removal of the central posterior capsule is warranted because of the almost violent development of opacification in younger children. Another technique frequently applied to lessen the chance of PCO is polishing the lens capsule in an attempt to restrict lens epithelial cell migration and proliferation [12].

There are a number of children in a peculiar situation with special needs and the necessity for some additional preoperative considerations. A group of young patients with a higher incidence of childhood cataract than the general population are those with Down syndrome. As Saifee et al. have stated based on their surgical experience, cataract extraction in pediatric patients with Down syndrome does not appear to have a higher rate of surgical complications than does cataract surgery in the general pediatric population [13]. There is no reason to assume that laser cataract surgery in these patients might be less effective or less safe than in children without this condition. Of particular concern for the anesthesiologist involved in the operation, however, is the fact that congenital heart comorbidities are common (92.3% in the cohort described by Saifee et al.) in children with Down syndrome.

Patients with Marfan syndrome are another special case: they may need surgery of the lens without actually suffering from cataract. Their vision is often compromised by a subluxation of the lens that may render the visual axis aphakic, by irregular astigmatism from the lens periphery, and also occasionally from lens opacity. Lens removal with capsule fixation and intraocular lens (IOL) implantation is a valuable strategy to address these problems. However, like in the younger infants with congenital cataract, challenges with manual capsulorhexis result from the high elasticity of the capsule which has a tendency toward posterior tears, damage to the zonules from stress during manipulation, and the fact that the desired position for capsulorhexis is off center, all too often resulting in increased intraoperative complications for these patients who undergo surgery at a relatively young age [14].

If PFV, also known as persistent hyperplastic primary vitreous, is present, the surgical technique has to be adapted to this pathology which, as Self et al. rightfully have pointed out, particularly in case of bilaterality may be associated with systemic disorders that should be further investigated. Depending on the morphology, capsule vitrectorhexis combined with lens aspiration may be required. If active blood vessels are to be found in this structure, intraocular diathermy may be required. IOL implantation may be possible in mild cases of PFV, but a number of complications such as vitreous hemorrhage, retinal detachment, and corneal decompensation might occur early during or following surgery; typical late complications are glaucoma, re-opacification, and even phthisis. Eyes with congenital cataract and persistent hyperplastic primary vitreous have a less favorable prognosis than those with cataract alone [11].

At the end of surgery, antibiotics are usually injected into the anterior chamber and steroids are also applied, either inside the anterior chamber or under the conjunctiva. In cases where the eye is left aphakic, some surgeons insert a contact lens at the conclusion of the operation, while in most cases, this is done a couple of days after surgery [15, 16].

Primary and Secondary IOL Implantation

One of the most controversial aspects of pediatric cataract surgery is to decide whether an intraocular lens should be implanted at the time of cataract surgery. Both IOLs and surgical techniques have immensely improved over the last two decades. The surgical procedure of implantation is hardly regarded a hurdle anymore. In general, IOL implantation in children older than 2 years has widely become the norm. In younger children, the propensity to inflammation has to be taken into account as has the small capsule size which in neonates has a diameter of just about 7 mm [11]. Some experts suggest that in children younger than 7 months, the eye should be left aphakic and a contact lens will be worn; the secondary implantation of an IOL is suggested to take place before or shortly after entering elementary school. The Infant Aphakia Treatment Study (IATS) in which 114 children younger than 7 months either received a primary IOL or were left aphakic and were then outfitted with contact lenses did not show a significant difference in visual acuity between both groups 5 years after surgery. Glaucoma as the most common complication was slightly more common in the contact lens group (35%) than in the IOL group (28%) [17]. In a secondary analysis of patients enrolled in this study, it turned out that delayed – i.e., secondary – IOL implantation which was performed at a mean age of 5.4 years resulted in a more predictable refractive outcome at 10 years of age though the range of refractive error was still considered to be relatively large [18]. The re-opacification of the visual axis in children younger than 2 years appears to be more common in pseudophakic than in aphakic eyes [19, 20].

In favor of primary implantation, it can be argued that every new intervention and thus any new anesthesia poses a risk for young children, particularly for those with comorbidities which are not uncommon among newborns with congenital cataract. Another factor is patient – and parents – compliance which is crucial in contact lens wear. Whether coping with contact lenses like fulfilling the hygienic requirements poses more stress for the parents than caring for child with an IOL has been cast into doubt by IATS which demonstrated higher stress levels in the latter group, most possibly due to additional interventions after primary IOL implantation [21]. A study from the USA contradicted the results of IATS and reported a relatively low rate of adverse events (21%) over a mean follow-up in patients that received primary IOL implantation at an age of 7 to 22 months. The group, however, was relatively small with 14 eyes if 10 patients [22].

It is difficult to give an overall recommendation when – and when not – to perform a primary IOL implantation; this will always be an individual decision which is to a large degree based on the support the child has at home, i.e., the competence and compliance of parents or caretakers. We are very reluctant to implant an IOL in children 6 months and younger. Even when performing primary implantation in older children (>2 years), one has to be aware that further surgical interventions are highly probable. Among the different materials, hydrophobic acrylate might probably offer the best solution given the long life expectancy of those young patients. Multifocal lenses are an option only in eyes that have fully grown, like at an age of 12 years and beyond. It should be kept in mind that currently there is no multifocal IOL for sulcus implantation.

The current IOL formulas have been developed for adults, not children. The Barrett formula has proven to be more reliable than other formulas [23, 24]. The ideal target refraction seems to be a slight myopia – very young infants are focusing on near objects like their toys, their rattle, or their mother's face. IOL implantation seems to be preferable when the cooperation necessary in dealing with contact lenses seems to be questionable. Bag-in-the-lens is an option in very young children – though challenging for the surgeon – which leave the anterior hyaloid membrane intact while otherwise an anterior vitrectomy is unavoidable. The latter, however, paves the way for the genesis of what is commonly called aphakic glaucoma, caused by an overpowering of the anterior segment, most of all the anterior chamber angle and the trabecular meshwork by the continuous liquefaction of vitreous. This pathogenesis is basically prevented when the vitreous is left intact. However, it is generally postulated that posterior capsulotomy and anterior vitrectomy are indispensible in pediatric cataract surgery to prevent PCO (as far as is possible). Regarding visual outcome, a recent meta-analysis by Chen et al. focusing on children younger than 2 years at the time of cataract surgery found a better visual acuity in those with primary IOL implantation but – as expected – also a higher prevalence of PCO [25].

Pediatric Cataract Surgery with the Femtosecond Laser

The introduction of the femtosecond laser into cataract surgery and the establishment of laser cataract surgery (LCS) have provided ophthalmologists with a new technology that has some advantages (at least from the view of those surgeons who use it) over manual procedures which seems to be particularly true for capsulotomy. Employing the femtosecond laser in pediatric cataract cases is, like so many interventions in the youngest patients, an off-label procedure. There are some requirements in pediatric cataract surgery that the surgeon has to be aware of before planning the intervention: the surgeon will encounter soft eye tissues and there will be a high degree of difficulty calculating the intraocular lens (IOL) power (Figs. 5.1 and 5.2). Chances of PCO (posterior capsule opacification) development in a relatively short timespan after surgery are not only high, but the occurrence of that complication is almost guaranteed. Finally, the surgeon must be able to perform vitrectomy.

The femtosecond laser has been used in a growing number of cases of pediatric cataract by specialized centers like the Bochum University

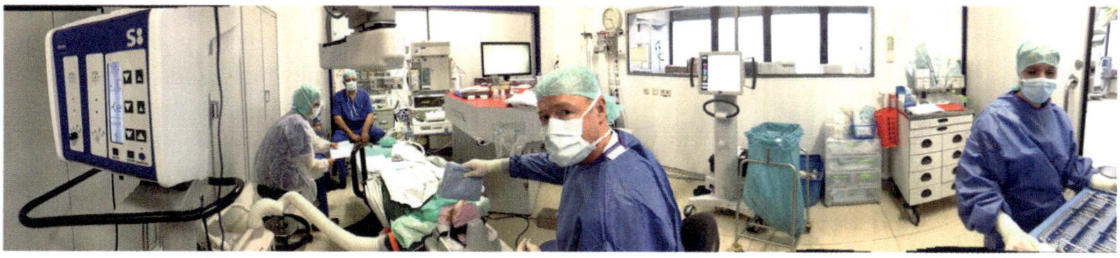

Fig. 5.1 Overview of the OR for LCS in pediatric cataract surgery: the femtosecond laser is placed in the same room. A specialized anesthesia team has patient warming tools available as well as an anesthesia machine for kids

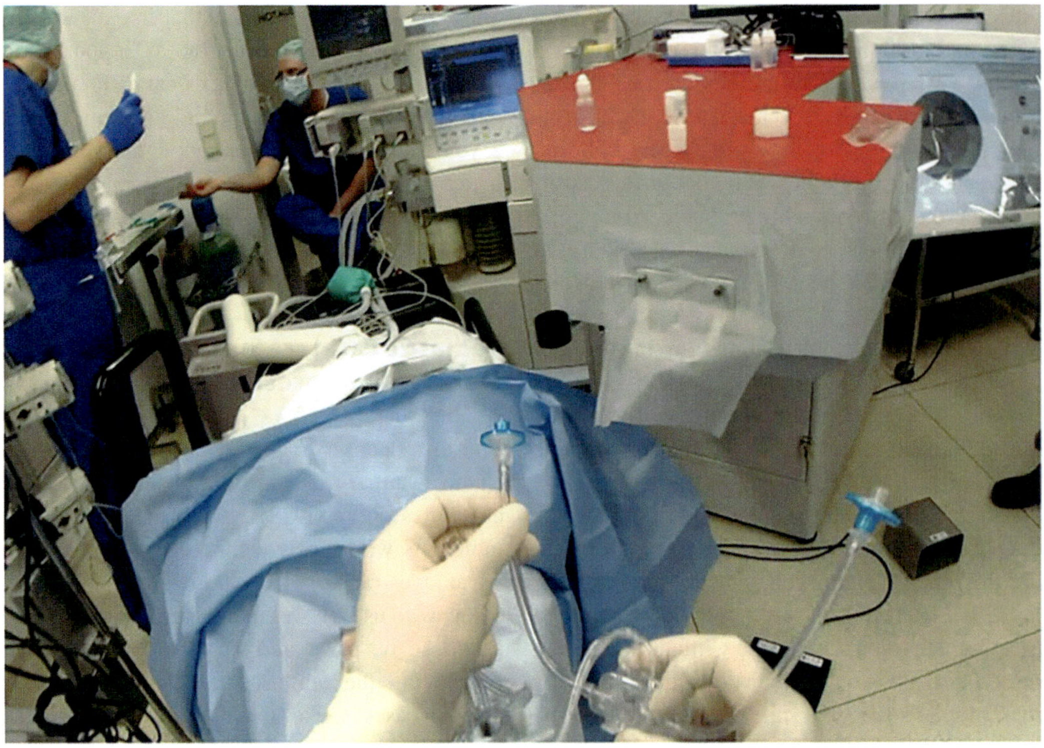

Fig. 5.2 The LCS system offers complete sterility in order to perform the complete procedure including redocking under sterile conditions

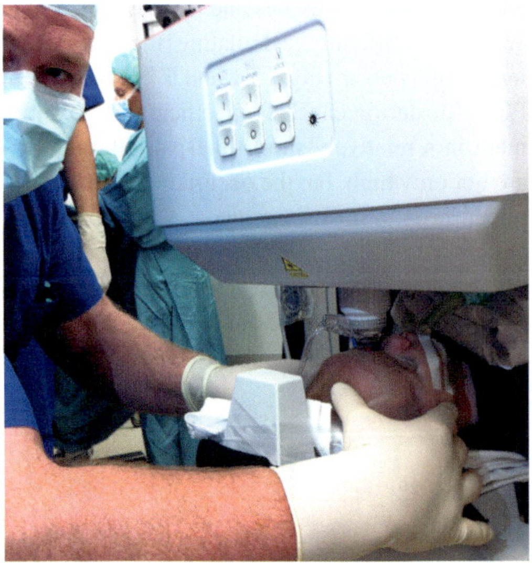

Fig. 5.3 Pediatric patient eye is docked under the femtosecond laser system

Eye Clinic, and the experience so far is a generally very positive one (Fig. 5.3). Unlike in cataract surgery of adults, the laser is not employed for lens fragmentation (this is done by phacoemulsification) but primarily to achieve a perfect capsulotomy which is so essential when primary IOL implantation is intended (Fig. 5.4).

Docking the femtosecond laser to the eye is the first step that is different from the same procedure in an adult – and a reminder that children indeed are no small grown-ups. Since none of the femtosecond laser systems were created for the treatment of small children, placing the interface between the laser and the globe can be difficult. Fortunately, at least one company so far has introduced a smaller interface especially for patients with tight palpebral fissure with a diameter of 12 versus the regular 14.1 mm (Fig. 5.5).

Performing the anterior capsulotomy with the laser in pediatric cases will probably be appreciated by every surgeon who ever tried manual continuous curvilinear capsulorhexis (CCC) in infants and small children. Their capsule tends to be extremely elastic and their intravitreal pres-

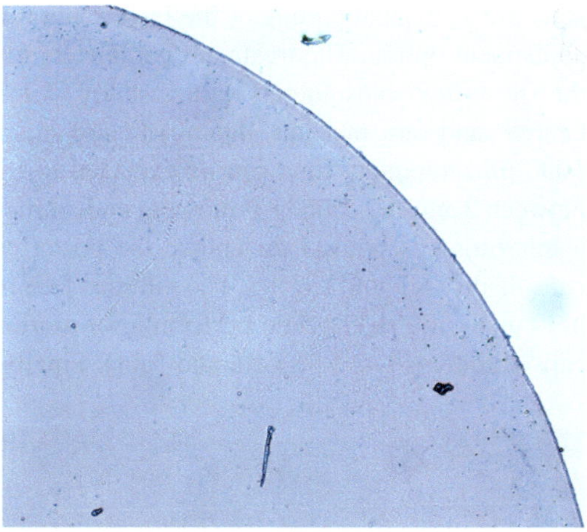

Fig. 5.4 Light microscopy of the pediatric anterior capsular edge after laser-assisted capsulotomy demonstrating a very smooth cut edge

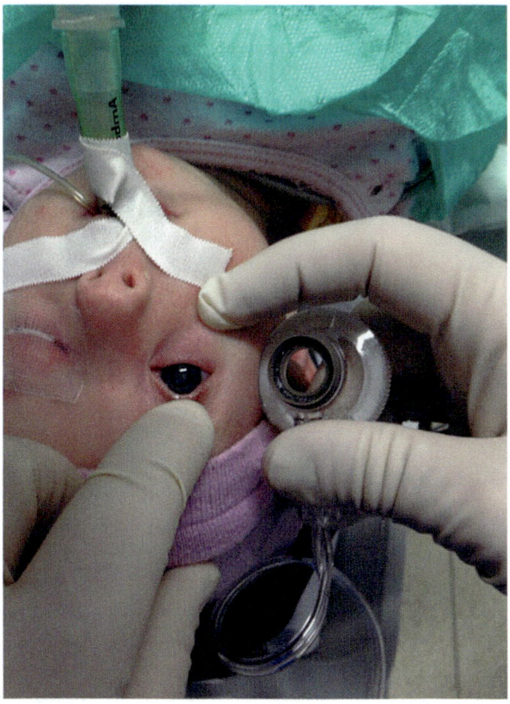

Fig. 5.5 Liquid optic interface diameter size matters in pediatric cataract surgery in order to allow sufficient docking even in the youngest patients

sure to be much larger than can be expected in an adult. Furthermore, children's pupils in general dilate rather poorly. Manual CCC thus is quite difficult in children. Besides the capsule's elasticity, the vitreous pressure which moves the entire lens anteriorly contributes to the problems that can lead to the "runaway rhexis," an inadvertent extension out to the lens equator. The failure rate to create an intact CCC has been reported by Vasavada et al. to be up to 80% [26].

Like in adult femto-cataract surgery, the interface is placed on the eye and vacuum is activated. The computer software creates a three-dimensional treatment plan based on the laser platform's imaging system. After the capsule and iris safety zones have been confirmed, the laser is activated. Usual settings would be, for instance, 4-μJ pulse energy and an incision depth of 600 mm. The whole anterior capsulotomy takes hardly more than one second. The laser then is undocked and removed. With anterior capsulotomy as a crucial step in the operation and for postoperative visual recovery, in the first pediatric laser cataract surgery (LCS) cases, an optimal circularity of femtosecond laser-created anterior and posterior capsulotomies was found. The size of the capsulotomy, however, did initially not turn out as planned because of the aforementioned elasticity. There was considerable widening of the capsule opening immediately after laser treatment (Fig. 5.6). Particularly in very young children, the capsulotomy diameter tends to turn out larger than planned. This led to the development of the Bochum formula which has proven its value in correcting for that aberration (Figs. 5.7 and 5.8).

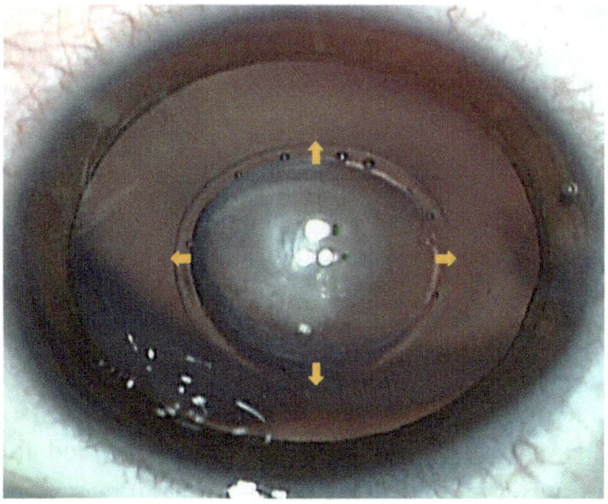

Fig. 5.6 The anterior capsulotomy diameter increases directly after performing LCS in a pediatric eye

$$\textit{capsulotomy enlargement factor} = 1.34 + (-0.09 * \textit{age})$$

A certain capsulotomy diameter can be achieved with the following formula:

$$\textit{programmed diameter} = \frac{\textit{aimed diameter}}{(1.34 + (-0.009 * \textit{age}))}$$

Fig. 5.7 Bochum ormula to calculate the capsulotomy diameter for the lasing depending on the actual patient's age

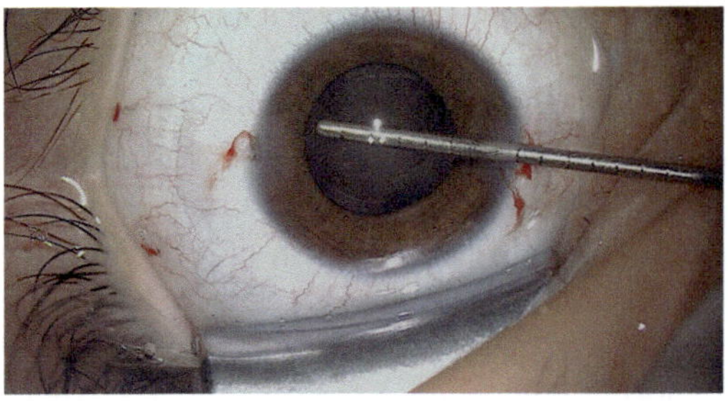

Fig. 5.8 View through the OR microscope: intraoperative measurement of the achieved capsulotomy diameter after LCS using the Engel device (Geuder, Germany)

Based on clinical experience with cases of pediatric cataract, the Bochum laser formula for pediatric cataract has the potential to become a valuable tool in achieving safe anterior and posterior capsulotomies of an exact precalculated diameter [27].

After performing laser capsulotomy and undocking, surgery of the lens is completed on the same bed, which is permanently mounted to the laser. Two 1.2-mm clear corneal side port incisions are made at 10 and 2 o'clock with a paracentesis knife. Trypan blue may be used to stain the anterior capsule for visibility. After ophthalmic viscosurgical device (OVD) injection, the free-floating capsulotomy disc is removed with forceps. The lens cortex and nucleus are removed with bimanual irrigation/aspiration (I/A). The anterior chamber is filled with OVD, and the side ports were hydrated and closed with 11–0 nylon suture where necessary in order to achieve absolutely watertight incisions. The same sterile patient interface is used to dock the eye again.

At present, there is no software adapted for posterior capsulotomy, which makes it necessary to position the treatment zones manually. Three-dimensional OCT scanning of the posterior capsule allows manual aiming of the laser using the adjustment option. The treatment parameters for the posterior capsulotomy are usually 4-mJ energy and an incision depth of maximum 1000 μm; treatment time can be expected to be between 2 and 10 seconds. Following undocking, a microforceps is used to remove the posterior capsule disc without tearing. The vitreous face is not cut by the laser while performing posterior capsulotomy (Figs. 5.9, 5.10, and 5.11). Finally,

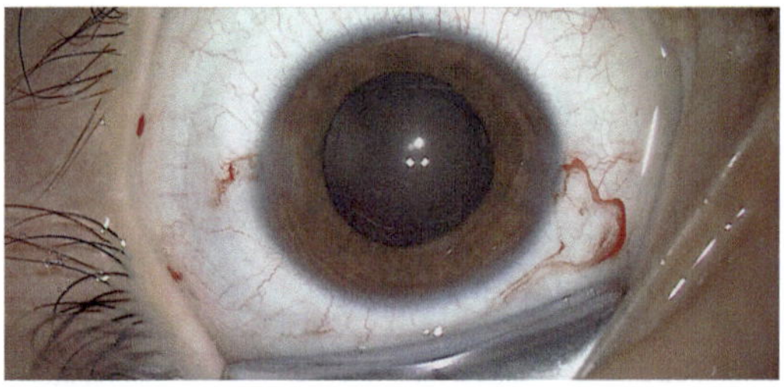

Fig. 5.9 Anterior and posterior capsulotomy perfectly centered and aligned to each other (before implantation of a bag-in-the-lens intraocular lens; the anterior vitreous surface is kept intact)

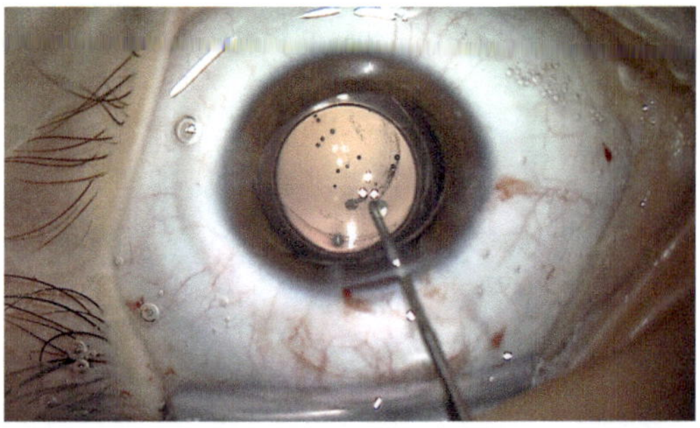

Fig. 5.10 Careful movement of the BIL haptics into the anterior and posterior capsule under OVD protection

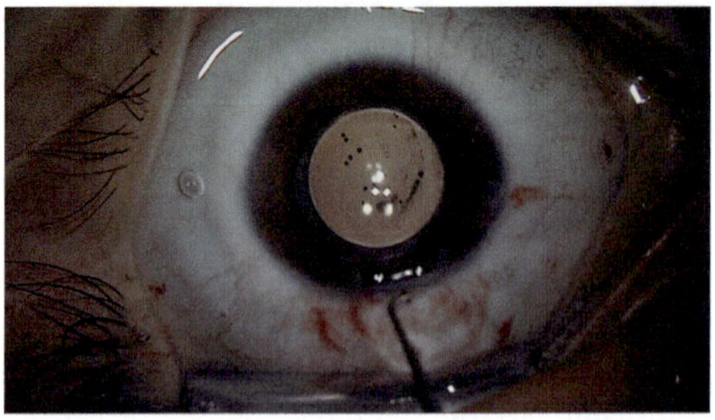

Fig. 5.11 BIL is positioned and fixed by the capsules after LCS in pediatric cataract

cautious 23-gauge central anterior vitrectomy can be performed bimanually through the side ports without removing the peripheral or posterior vitreous. In general, an experienced surgeon can expect a treatment time in pediatric laser cataract surgery of 15 to 30 minutes [28, 29].

Postoperative Management

Finishing surgery is just the first step in dealing with pediatric cataract. The children require a thorough follow-up, and among the complications that will in all likelihood manifest are at the foremost postoperative inflammation and posterior capsule opacification (PCO). To take a look from the bright side: cystoid macular edema (CME), so frequent in adult patients, is extremely rare in young children.

Following surgery, suppression of the inflammatory response that is so pronounced in young children and in those whose cataract is due to uveitis is a mainstay of medical treatment. Topical corticosteroids are usually employed for up to 6 weeks and in tapering dosage. The steroid regimen, however, can contribute to the rises in intraocular pressure which are so frequently seen in these children. In addition, an adrenal suppression can happen in young children even under topical steroid therapy which requires close cooperation with an endocrinologist. The insertion of punctum plugs may reduce systemic absorption and thus systemic adverse events in when applying steroid eye drops [30, 31].

Besides PCO, the occurrence of glaucoma is the foremost ocular pathology that requires a sometimes intense treatment and that threatens the visual results which successful pediatric cataract surgery hopes to achieve. It can be divided into early-onset secondary glaucoma which is usually caused by vitreous pupillary block or peripheral inflammation and can to a certain degree be prevented by modern surgery techniques and anti-inflammatory medications. Late-onset postoperative glaucoma is regarded as a secondary open-angle glaucoma of unknown pathogenesis in which probably trabeculitis and toxic agents released from the vitreous may play a role. In a major systemic review and meta-analysis based on a total of 892 eyes, primary IOL implantation was associated with a low long-term incidence of secondary glaucoma (9.5%) than in eyes with aphakia and secondary IOL implantation (15.1%). While there was no significant difference in eyes with unilateral cataract between those with primary and those with secondary implantation, there was a distinctively higher glaucoma incidence in patients with bilateral congenital cataract who had primary IOL implantation (6.7%) compared to those with secondary IOL implantation (16.7%).The fear of inducing secondary glaucoma should not influence the decision to perform pediatric cataract surgery in any way since such a delay may result in irreversible vision loss. Glaucoma, if it occurs, can and should be treated either with IOP-lowering medication or by surgical procedure. IOP measurement should be a major parameter in the long-term follow-up of children following cataract surgery [32].

The operation is the first step to visual recovery for a child with cataract, to be followed by long-term care provided by the ophthalmologist. The parents (or caretakers) must be educated about the need for continuous follow-up so that complications like inflammation, glaucoma, and posterior capsule opacification can be detected and treated as soon as they arise, and refractive errors can be corrected and amblyopia therapy pursued. Children with congenital cataract or acquired early childhood cataract must be cared for by a multidisciplinary approach in which specialists of all aspects of neurodevelopmental and visual function must be involved.

Conclusion

Pediatric cataract surgery is performed under the sword of Damocles: done too early, the risk of complications, most of all glaucoma, inflammation, and re-opacification, rises; done too late, amblyopia looms. Modern techniques and equipment, however, can overcome the problems the very young eye poses, and with appropriate surgical procedures and a meticulous and sometimes interdisciplinary postoperative management, good visual outcomes can be achieved. Our clinical experience convinces us that the femtosecond laser can play a valuable role in making this intervention precise, safe, and effective. We are probably just in the early stages of pediatric LCS and a number of issues have to be resolved. Pediatric cataract surgery might be the ultimate challenge for the surgeon: the results may last for almost a century.

Take-Home Notes

- Cataract surgery is only the first step in a long process to make the development of normal visual function possible; these patients require regular follow-up examinations and additional measures over many years.
- Manual continuous curvilinear capsulorhexis (CCC) in infants and small children is a challenge since the capsule tends to be extremely elastic and intravitreal pressure is usually much larger than can be expected in an adult.
- The time point of IOL implantation is recommended to take place between the age of 6 months and school enrollment. If the cataract occurs in the age over 6 years, the IOL can be implanted into the capsular bag usually without anterior vitrectomy. Time of implantation is based on an individual decision depending, e.g., on the cooperation of the parents.
- Laser cataract surgery (LCS) with the femtosecond laser has proven to be safe and effective in pediatric cataracts, even in special cases like in patients with Down syndrome and Marfan syndrome. It is generally an off-label procedure.
- Laser capsulotomies tend to be larger than planned, particularly in young children. The Bochum formula helps to overcome this aberration.
- IOL implantation in children older than 2 years has widely become the norm. In younger children, the propensity to inflammation has to be taken into account.

References

1. Wu X, Long E, Lin H, Liu Y. Prevalence and epidemiological characteristics of congenital cataract: a systematic review and meta-analysis. Sci Rep. 2016;6:28564.
2. Mohammadpour M, Shaabani A, Sahraian A, et al. Updates on managements of pediatric cataract. J Curr Ophthalmol. 2019;31:118–26.
3. Prakalapakorn SG, Rasmussen SA, Lambert SR, et al. Assessment of risk factors for infantile cataracts using a case-control study, National Birth Defects Prevention Study, 2000–2004. Ophthalmology. 2010;117:1500–5.
4. Ophthalmology AAO. Pediatric cataracts. Focal Points; 2018. https://www.aao.org/focalpointssnippetdetail.aspx?id¼46505fda7-f7e7-4d52-925b-bc5cad4feeae.
5. Rosenberg KD, Feuer WJ, Davis JL. Ocular complications of pediatric uveitis. Ophthalmology. 2004;111:2299–306.
6. Medsinge A, Nishal KK. Pediatric cataract: challenges and future directions. Clin Ophthalmol. 2015;9:77–90.
7. Beigi B, O'Keefe M, Bowell R, et al. Ophthalmic findings in classical galactosaemia – prospective study. Br J Ophthalmol. 1993;77:162–4.
8. Vishwanath M, Cheong-Leen R, Taylor D, et al. Is early surgery for congenital cataract a risk factor for glaucoma ? Br J Ophthalmol. 2004;88:905–10.
9. Vasavada V. Paradigms for pediatric cataract surgery. Asia-Pac J Ophthalmol. 2018;7:123–7.
10. Buchan JC, Donachie PHJ, Cassels-Brown A, et al. The Royal College of Ophthalmologists' National Ophthalmology Database study of cataract surgery: report 7, immediate sequential bilateral cataract surgery in the UK: current practice and patient selection. Eye. 2020;34:1866–74.
11. Self JE, Taylor R, Solebo AL, et al. Cataract management in children: a review of the literature and current practice across five large UK centres. Eye. Published online august 10. 2020. https://doi.org/10.1038/s41433-020-1115-6.
12. Luft N, Kreutzer TC, Dirisamer M, et al. Evaluation of laser capsule polishing for prevention of posterior capsule opacification in a human ex vivo model. J Cataract Refract Surg. 2015;41:2739–45.
13. Saifee M, Kong L, Jen KG. Outcomes of cataract surgery in children with down syndrome. J Ophthalmic Vis Res. 2017;12:243–4.
14. Schultz T, Ezeanosike E, Dick HB. Femtosecond laser-assisted cataract surgery in pediatric Marfan syndrome. J Refract Surg. 2013;29:650–2.
15. Trivedi RH, Wilson ME. Selection of an initial contact lens power for infantile cataract surgery without primary intraocular lens implantation. Ophthalmology. 2013;120:1973–6.
16. Koo EB, VanderVeen DK, Lambert SR. Global practice patterns in the management of infantile cataracts. Eye Contact Lens. 2018;44:S292–6.

17. Lambert SR, Lynn MJ, Hartmann EE, Infant Aphakia Treatment Study Group. Comparison of contact lens and intraocular lens correction of monocular aphakia during infancy: a randomized clinical trial of HOTV optotype acuity at age 4.5 years and clinical findings at age 5 years. JAMA Ophthalmol. 2014;132:676–82.
18. Van der Veen DK, Drews-Botsch CD, Nizam A et al. Outcomes of secondary intraocular lens implantation in the infant Aphakia treatment study. J Cataract Refract Surg. Published online September 7. 2020. https://doi.org/10.1097/j.jcrs.0000000000000412.
19. Solebo AL, Cumberland P, Rahi JS, British Isles Congenital Cataract Interest Group. 5-year outcomes after primary intraocular lens implantation in children aged 2 years or younger with congenital or infantile cataract: findings from the IoLunder2 prospective inception cohort study. Lancet Child Adolesc Health. 2018;2:863–71.
20. Plager DA, Lynn MJ, Buckley EG, Infant Aphakia Treatment Study Group. Complications in the first 5 years following cataract surgery in infants with and without intraocular lens implantation in the Infant Aphakia Treatment Study. Am J Ophthalmol. 2014;158:892–8.
21. Celano M, Hartmann EE, Drews-Botsch CD. Parenting stress in the infant aphakia treatment study. J Pediatr Psychol. 2013;38:484–93.
22. Struck MC. Long-term results of pediatric cataract surgery and primary intraocular lens implantation from 7 to 22 months of life. JAMA Ophthalmol. 2015;133:1180–3.
23. Chang P, Lin L, Li Z, et al. Accuracy of 8 intraocular lens power calculation formulas in pediatric cataract patients. Graefes Arch Clin Exp Ophthalmol. 2020;258:1123–31.
24. Xia T, Martinez CE, Tsai LM. Update on intraocular lens formulas and calculations. Asia Pac J Ophthalmol (Phila). 2020;9:186–93.
25. Chen J, Chen Y, Zhong Y, et al. Comparison of visual acuity and complications between primary IOL implantation and aphakia in patients with congenital cataract younger than 2 years: a meta-analysis. J Cataract Refract Surg. 2020;46:465–73.
26. Vasavada AR, Nihalani BR. Pediatric cataract surgery. Curr Opin Ophthalmol. 2006;17:54–61.
27. Dick HB, Schelenz D, Schultz T. Femtosecond laser-assisted pediatric cataract surgery: Bochum formula. J Cataract Refract Surg. 2015;41:821–6.
28. Dick HB, Schultz T. Femtosecond laser-assisted cataract surgery in infants. J Cataract Refract Surg. 2013;39:665–8.
29. Gerste RD, Schultz T, Dick HB. Pediatric cataract surgery with the femtosecond laser. In: Dick HB, Gerste RD, Schultz T, editors. Femtosecond laser surgery in ophthalmology. New York: Thieme; 2018. p. 162–6.
30. Lambert SR, Shah S. Adrenal suppression from topical and subconjunctival steroids after pediatric cataract surgery. Ophthalmology. 2018;125:1644–5.
31. Bangsgaard R, Main KM, Boberg-Ans G, et al. Adrenal suppression in infants treated with topical ocular glucocorticoids. Ophthalmology. 2018;125:1638–43.
32. Zhang S, Wang J, Li Y, et al. The role of primary intraocular lens implantation in the risk of secondary glaucoma following congenital cataract surgery: a systematic review and metaanalysis. PLOS one. Published April 1. 2019. https://doi.org/10.1371/journal.pone.0214684.

The Unstable Lens in the Adult Patient

6

M. Victoria De Rojas Silva

Introduction

Zonular compromise poses serious challenges at every step of cataract surgery. The continued refinement of phacoemulsification techniques and platforms and the development of novel devices for capsular bag stabilization, together with a thorough understanding of the challenges of subluxated lens, as well as their management strategies, allow to approach these cases with more safety and better outcomes through a 2 to 2.2 mm microincision, resulting in a rapid and safe visual recovery.

It is of paramount importance for the decision-making during surgery, to know the etiology of the condition, regarding mainly its stable or progressive nature, as surgical strategy will change. An exhaustive preoperative exploration and planification is mandatory, as well as a deep understanding of the mechanical challenges that this surgery poses to the surgeon together with the knowledge of each of the alternatives to stabilize the capsular bag, how each of them works, and how they can be combined.

Etiology

Subluxated lens is the term used to refer to any displacement of malposition of the crystalline lens of whatever cause or association.

The causes of lens subluxation are multiple and they have been classified based on different criteria. From the surgical point of view, the most important issue to consider is whether the condition is progressive or not [1]. For example, in trauma, which is the cause of more than 50% of cases [2] (Fig. 6.1), we know that the remaining zonules are healthy so that further increase

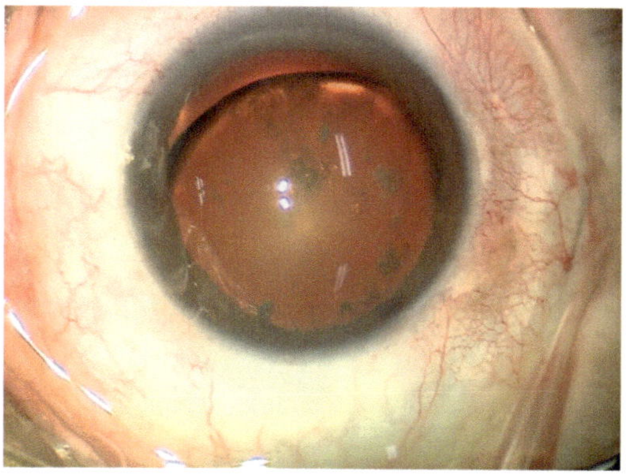

Fig. 6.1 Traumatic lens subluxation, with 180° of zonular dehiscence

Supplementary Information The online version contains supplementary material available at [https://doi.org/10.1007/978-3-030-94530-5_6].

M. V. D. R. Silva (✉)
Department at Complexo Hospitalario Universitario A Coruña, A Coruña, Spain

Victoria de Rojas Instituto Oftalmológico, Policlínica Assistens, A Coruña, Spain

J. L. Alió et al. (eds.), *Cataract Surgery*, Essentials in Ophthalmology,
https://doi.org/10.1007/978-3-030-94530-5_6

in zonular damage is not expected, neither during surgery nor afterward. The opposite occurs in pseudoexfoliation (Fig. 6.2), a progressive condition in which the surgery poses significant challenges, because of the generalized weakness of the zonules, together with the possibility of progression of the subluxation over the years (in-the-bag IOL dislocation) [3, 4]. The progressive nature of the disease in this and other cases (Marfan (Fig. 6.3), etc.) may change the surgeon's decisions during surgery, regarding scleral fixation to secure the capsular bag even in cases in which that fixation is not needed according to the degree of zonular dehiscence during surgery, due to the uncertain evolution in the future.

Another important point to consider regarding the etiology is the association of some conditions with systemic alterations that can be potentially severe (Marfan and cardiac involvement, cardiovascular abnormalities) [1, 2, 5].

The causes of lens subluxation are summarized in Table 6.1 [1].

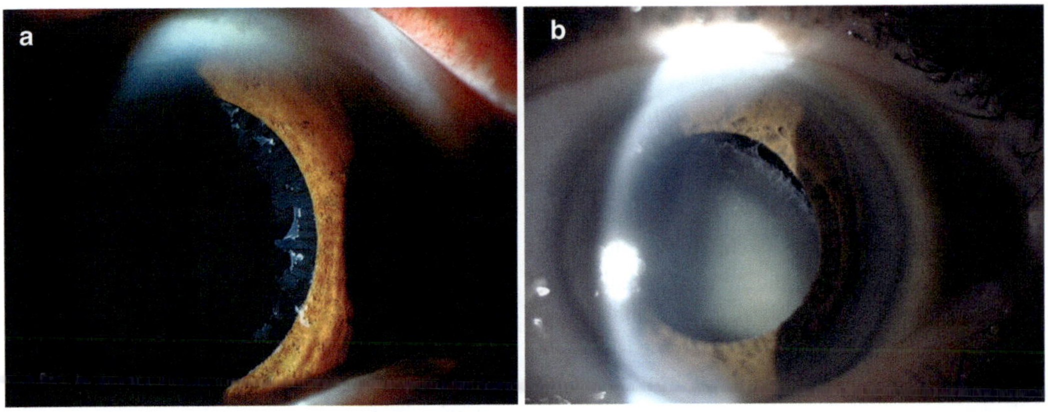

Fig. 6.2 (**a**) Pseudoexfoliation is characterized by generalized zonular weakness. Usually, significant subluxation is not observed, but frequently, pseudophacodonesis is observed before pupil dilation or anterior chamber asymmetry is detected. (**b**) Rarely, lens subluxation is observed, as in this case in which, in addition to present pseudoexfoliation, a blunt trauma triggered the subluxation

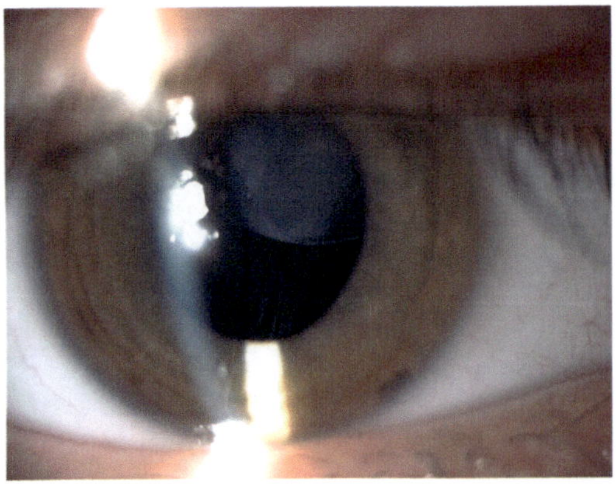

Fig. 6.3 Superior subluxation and elongated zonular fibers in Marfan syndrome

Table 6.1 Causes of lens subluxation

Traumatic	
Endogenous	
Hereditary	Marfan syndrome Homocystinuria Weill-Marchesani syndrome Deficit of sulfite oxidase Essential idiopathic familial ectopia Retinitis pigmentosa
Acquired conditions	Uveitis, myopia, glaucoma
Pseudoexfoliation	
Iatrogenic	Iridectomy, trabeculectomy, vitrectomy

Preoperative Evaluation

A detailed preoperative evaluation is mandatory, beginning with the anamnesis, including family history, any relevant trauma, and onset and types of visual symptoms. Since several hereditable syndromes have associated systemic anomalies, patients should be referred to their primary physician for systemic examination and metabolic workup (Marfan syndrome, homocystinuria, etc.) [1, 2, 5]. Also, in these hereditable conditions, family should be informed. The main symptom is the decrease of visual acuity.

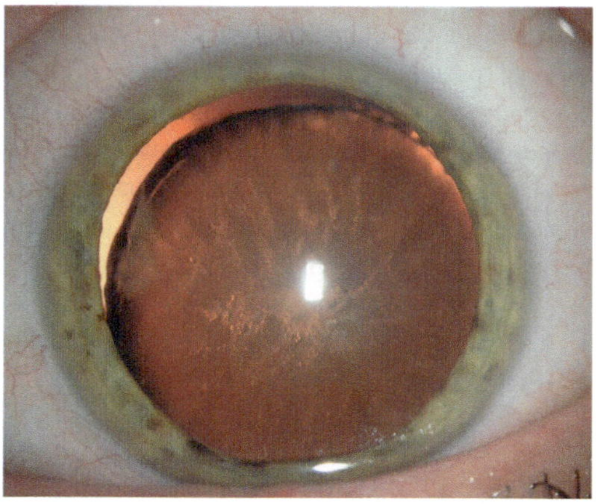

Fig. 6.4 Traumatic subluxated contusive cataract after blunt trauma, involving more than 180° of zonular fibers

Ocular examination should include anterior and posterior segment. Both near and distant distance corrected visual acuity should be determined, keeping in mind that the patient may best see with an aphakic correction if the lens is markedly subluxated. The patient must be examined under full pupil dilatation in the slit lamp before surgery to evaluate the extent of zonular deficiency, since the surgical strategy for the management of subluxation will depend on the number of hours of zonular dehiscence [6] (Figs. 6.4 and 6.5).

The exact degree of zonular loss, location of defect, and presence or absence of vitreous in the anterior chamber should be noted. The position of the crystalline lens at the slit lamp and in the supine position should be compared. Gravity pulls lens downward and the defect is usually noticeable. An inferior subluxation is a sign of extreme zonular weakness and often indicates 360 degrees of zonular insufficiency combined with the effect of gravity [2, 5]. If available, ultrasound biomicroscopy and anterior segment OCT are specially useful for zonular and angle assessment in patients where the pupil fails to dilate, and the UBM has the advantage of being performed in supine position, which is the position during the surgical procedure [7]. Zonular weakness is not always evident at first glance. Of course phacodonesis (Video 6.1), better per-

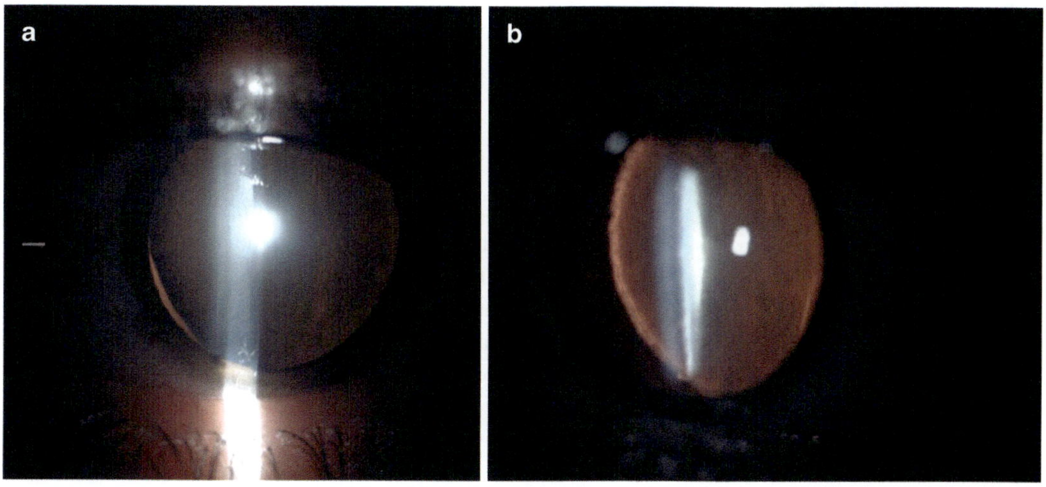

Fig. 6.5 (**a**) Inferonasal zonular deficiency in primary gaze position, involving apparently one quadrant. (**b**) The full extension of zonular dehiscence is better observed in extreme gaze

ceived without dilating the pupil, is the main sign of impaired zonules. Other signs of zonular deficiency include iridodonesis, visibility of lens equator in extreme gaze positions (Fig. 6.5), scalloping of the lens capsule or flattened lens edge (Fig. 6.6), higher space between the iris and the lens, and herniated vitreous. A subtler sign of zonular weakness is the asymmetry in anterior chamber depth; either a shallow or hyperdeep anterior chamber may be caused by zonular dehiscence (Fig. 6.7). Biometry, with the measurement of anterior chamber depth, can confirm anterior chamber depth asymmetry between eyes.

In traumatic cases, any damage of the anterior capsule must be noted and recorded. The density of the cataract should be evaluated, since, together with the extension of zonulopathy and the etiology, it will dictate the surgical strategy. Any vitreous prolapse should be recorded, since vitrectomy will be needed to accomplish the case [6].

Gonioscopy is performed to detect any developmental defects, pseudoexfoliative material, and deformities secondary to trauma or as a sequela of subluxation. The fundus examination is done to look for lattice degeneration, cyclitic membranes, retinal detachment, or posttraumatic pathology. Retinal detachments occur in 10% of eyes with Marfan syndrome, and any evidence of

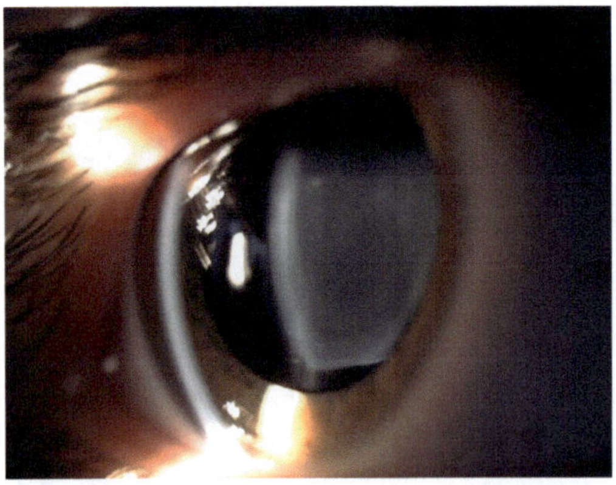

Fig. 6.6 Scalloped or flattened lens edge, which indicates that adjacent remaining zonular fibers should be healthy

retinal tears, breaks, or tufts should be treated prior to performing the elective cataract surgery. If opaque media preclude fundus examination, B-scan ultrasonography is indicated. Also, the presence of uveitis, glaucoma, corneal edema, and amblyopia should be noted. High IOP may be related to pseudoexfoliation, vitreous prolapse, or angle trauma with recession. An endothelial cell count is advisable before surgery since either trauma or vitreous prolapse may damage the endothelium. Traumatic cases may be associated with damages in other structures, recession, iris trauma, or retinal involvement.

Even with a detailed exploration, the full amount of zonular dehiscence may not be detected, or the dehiscence may worsen during surgery (pseudoexfoliation), so the surgeon must be ready to face different scenarios, and the proper instrumentation should be available. The surgeon must be familiar with intraoperative signs that alert about zonular deficiency, in case it has not been detected preoperatively (Fig. 6.8):

- Radial folds when puncturing anterior capsule (Fig. 6.8a).
- Movement of the lens during capsulorhexis (Video 6.2), hydrodissection, or hydrodelineation.
- Difficulty to rotate the nucleus.
- Excessive posterior displacement of the lens when irrigation starts; hyperdeep chamber.
- Ovalization of the capsulorhexis margin.
- Visibility of the capsule equator (Fig. 6.8b) (Video 6.2).
- Vitreous prolapse in the area of dehiscence (Fig. 6.8c) (Video 6.3).

It is of paramount importance to obtain an informed consent from the patient before cataract surgery, considering the risks and complicated nature of surgery, the possibility of changing plans intraoperatively, as well as the need for postoperative monitoring and follow-up.

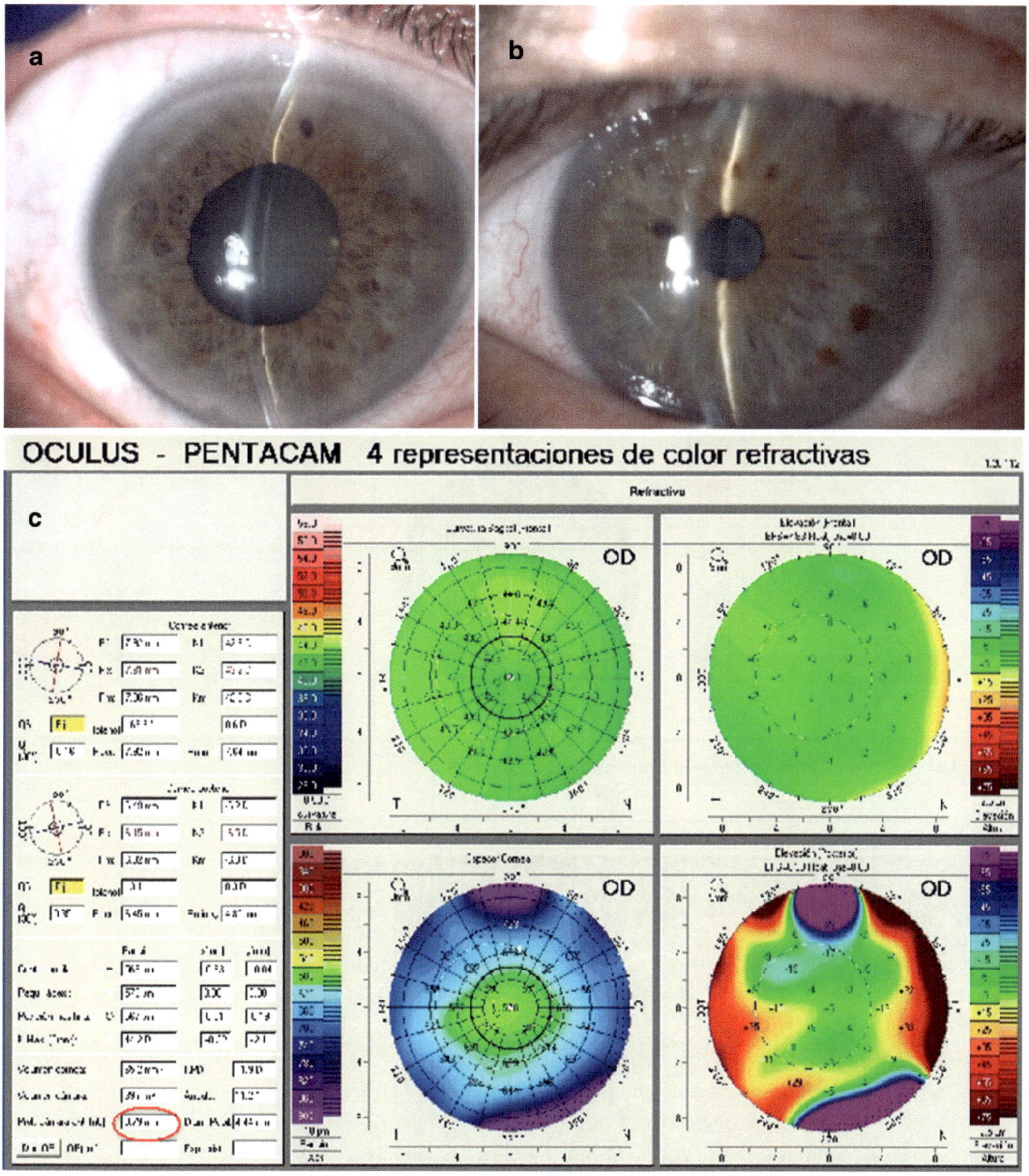

Fig. 6.7 Traumatic cataract, without evident subluxation at first glance. (**a**, **b**) The anterior chamber depth shows asymmetry between eyes, (**c**) measuring 0.75 mm in the right eye and (**d**) 2.04 in the left eye as Pentacam display shows. (**e**, **f**) Scheimpflug images showing the forward displacement of the lens in the right eye as compared to the fellow eye. (**g**) Two Ahmed segments (arrows) combined with a capsular tension ring were necessary to stabilize the capsular bag. **h**) Anterior chamber depth increased to 3.21 mm after surgery

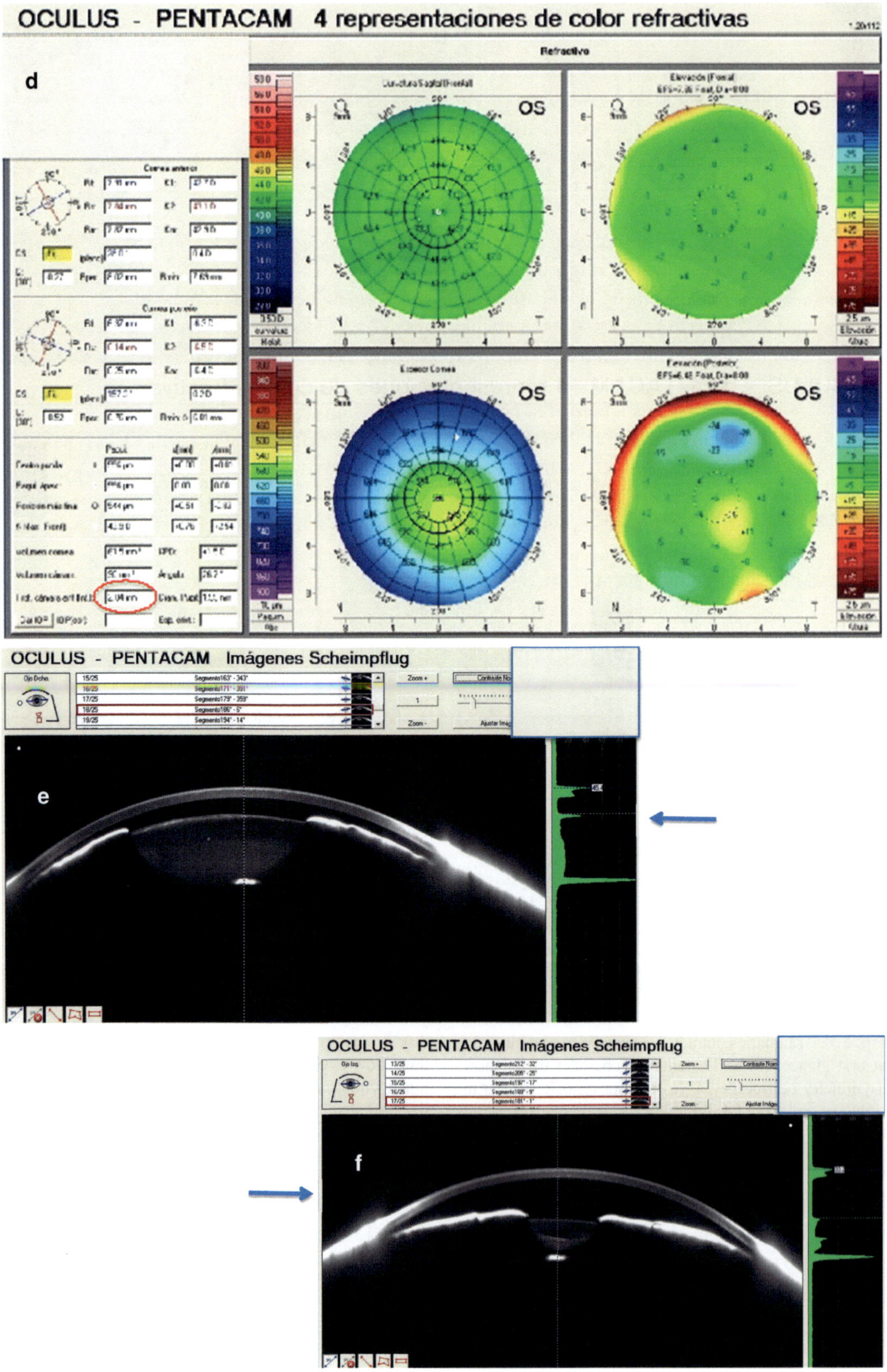

Fig. 6.7 (continued)

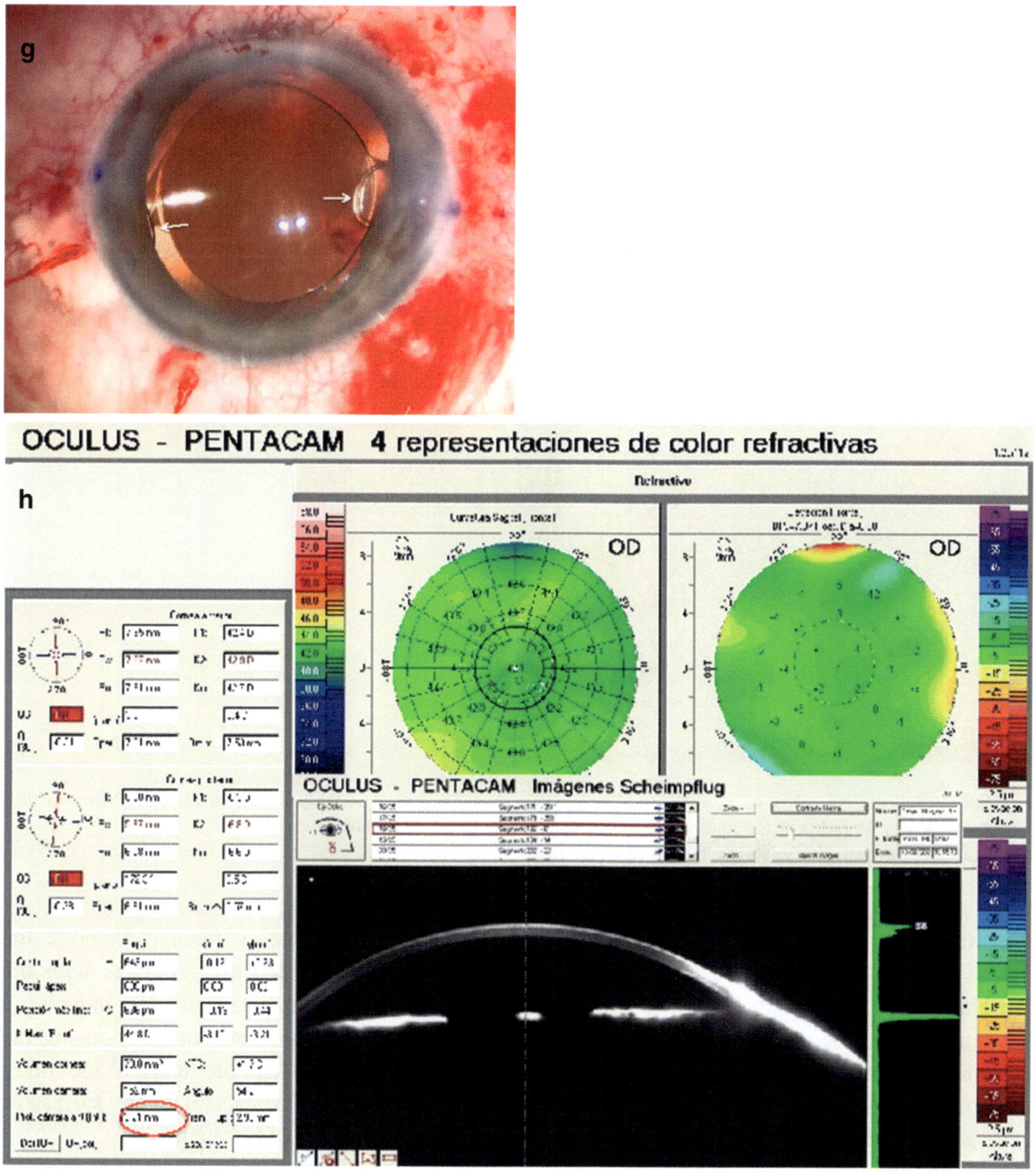

Fig. 6.7 (continued)

Instrumentation

During cataract surgery of subluxated lenses, stabilization of the capsular bag is needed; we need to stabilize the bag in the anterior to posterior axis and also to distend the posterior capsule centrifugally. Depending on the stage of the surgery, we will need one of them or both.

Several devices exist that may help for this two purposes, and the surgeon should know which function each of them serves better in order to utilize them properly. Hooks, capsular tension rings, and related endocapsular devices for scleral fixation have become very useful tools in the armamentarium of cataract surgeons.

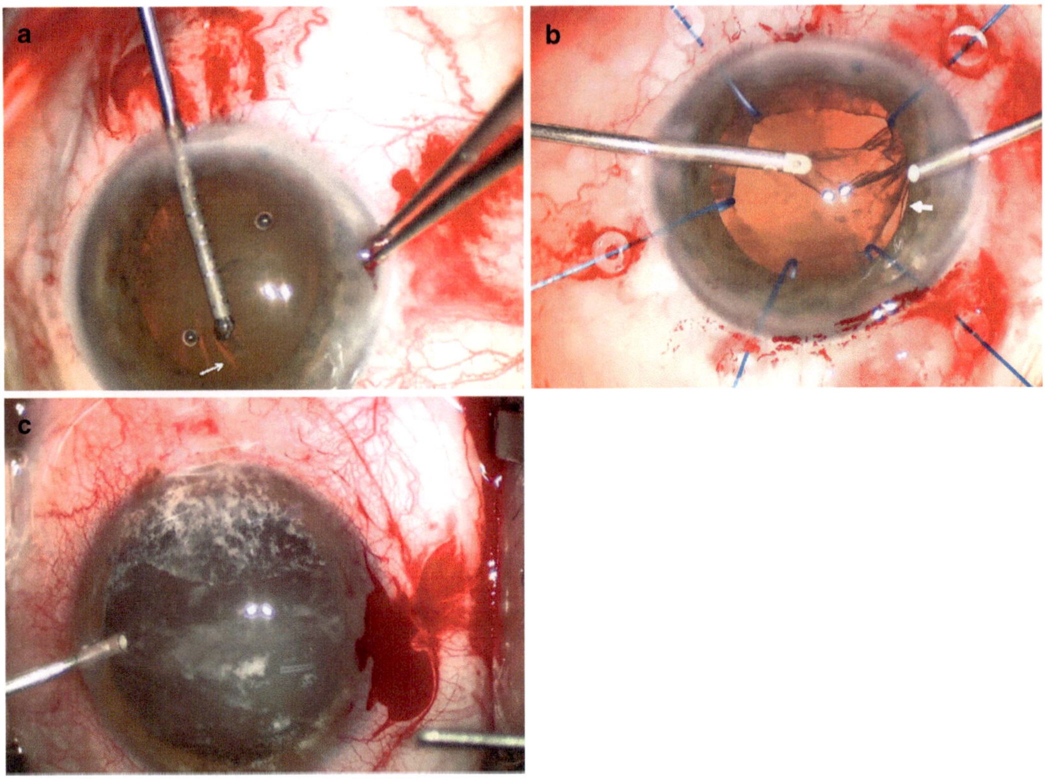

Fig. 6.8 Intraoperative signs of zonular weakness. (**a**) Capsular folds or wrinkles of the anterior capsule during capsulorhexis (arrow). (**b**) Visibility of the capsular bag equator during surgery (white arrow). (**c**) Vitreous prolapse into the anterior chamber

Hooks

Iris Hooks

Iris retractors can be placed at the capsulorhexis edge over the area of zonular weakness to stabilize the loose capsular-zonular complex during surgery.

Flexible iris hooks may stabilize the capsular bag by providing a counterforce to that applied by the surgeon and provide anterior to posterior stabilization of the bag, but they do not expand the capsular fornix. They can be useful as an aid in the completion of the capsulorhexis, hydrodissection, and nuclear rotation. They do not trap the cortex as the capsular tension ring [5, 6, 8, 9] (Fig. 6.9) (Video 6.2).

However, close attention must be paid to the risk of inadvertent dislocation and resultant anterior capsule tear. The capsulorhexis margin must be of adequate size and excessive tension on the hook should be avoided [10].

Sometimes the outer extreme of the hook, the one that is outside the eye, contacts with the blepharostat or the lids, and rotates, inducing a torsion in the capsulorhexis margin, posing the risk of an anterior capsule tear. If the outer extreme of the hook contacts with any surface of the surgical file, it should be cut.

An important point to consider is that if hooks are needed as a counter-traction during capsulorhexis creation, the hooks should be placed at least 2 to 3 clock hours from the leading edge of the capsulorhexis to avoid tractional forces that will cause the leading edge to extend peripherally toward the bag equator [6].

Capsule Hooks

Capsule hooks, in contrast to iris hooks, support the bag by its equator, not the capsule margin, thereby keeping the bag distended and also reducing the likelihood of aspiration of the bag

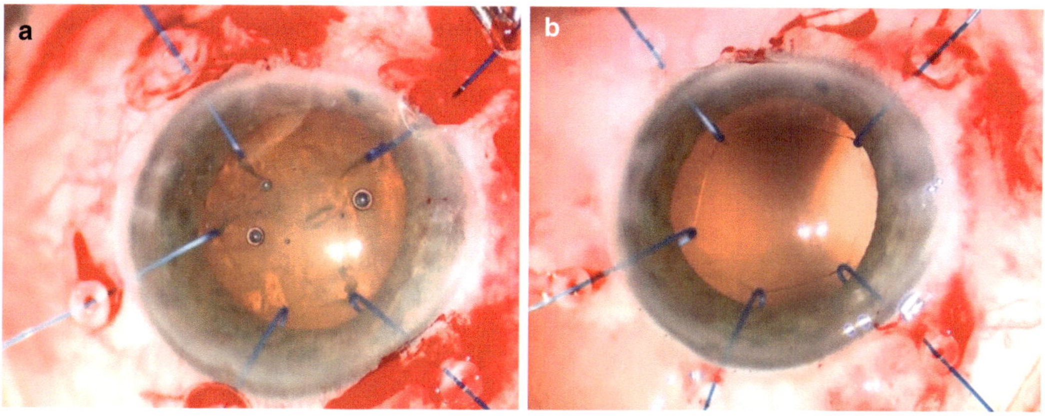

Fig. 6.9 (**a**) Iris hooks can be placed to hold the capsulorhexis edge and provide anterior to posterior support (vertical) during surgery. (**b**) Intraoperative photograph at the end of phacoemulsification and cortical aspiration

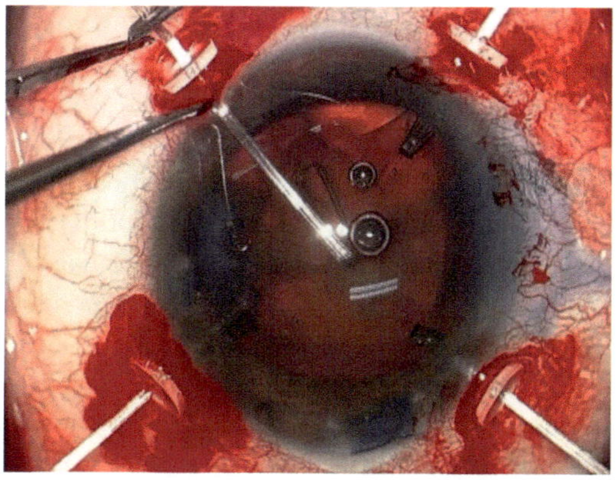

Fig. 6.10 Capsule hooks are another alternative. In contrast to iris hooks, capsular hooks support the bag by its equator, not the capsule margin, thereby keeping the bag distended and also reducing the likelihood of aspiration of the bag equator as the lens material is evacuated. However, they are too large and may interfere with surgical maneuvers, and differently from iris hooks, they cannot hold the iris if it would be necessary

equator as the lens material is evacuated (Fig. 6.10).

A system of titanium or plastic capsule retractors with hooked ends, which are elongated enough to support the peripheral capsular fornix as well as the capsulorhexis, was designed (reusable (Duckworth and Kent Ltd., Hertfordshire, England) or a single use design (Impex, Staten Island, NY), MST capsule retractors (MicroSurgical Technology Inc., Seattle, WA, USA)) [5, 8, 9].

In any case, the tension of the hooks must be enough to stabilize the capsular bag, but one should not try to completely recenter the bag by hooks alone, as they may damage the opposing zonular fibers or place undue stress on the capsulorhexis during phacoemulsification.

In our experience, the length of the capsule hook which is intended to support the bag from the capsule equator is too large and exceeds the capsulorhexis margin, interfering with the maneuvers during phacoemulsification, and thus, it is the author's preference to use flexible iris hooks. The latter can be used to hold the pupillary margin as well if needed.

Capsular Tension Rings

Conventional Capsular Tension Rings

The standard capsular tension ring (CTR) is an open-ring structure made of PMMA. This compressible circular ring has an oval-shaped cross section with two smooth-edge end terminals. The "ski ramp" design of the end terminals aids to avoid entrapment of the capsular equator on insertion and also allows for placement of secondary instrumentation [11, 12] (Fig. 6.11).

The CTR are available in various sizes according to their diameter. The most common, the Morcher ring, has three sizes based on their uncompressed diameter [10]:

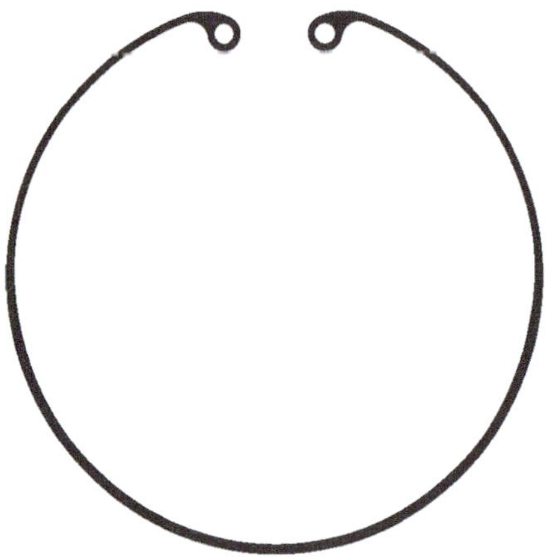

Fig. 6.11 Conventional capsular tension ring

Type	Uncompressed diameter	Compressed diameter
14	12.3 mm	10 mm
14 C	13 mm	11 mm
14 A	14.5 mm	12 mm

The selection of capsular ring size is based on capsular bag dimensions, with larger bags requiring larger CTR. The size of the bag correlates with axial length and corneal diameter, and these two parameters may be used for CTR size selection [13, 14].

However, it is our experience and that of other authors that the use of the larger size of the ring may be chosen since overlap of the end terminals is needed to provide for complete circumferential support, although it may be more challenging to insert. Several studies support the efficacy and safety of CTR in cataract surgery [12].

Because the diameter of the CTR is larger than that of the capsule bag, the centrifugal forces inherent within the ring expand the capsular equator and buttress areas of poor zonular support, providing equal distribution of support from remaining zonules. The CTR re-expands the capsular bag, provides counter-traction, and tautens the posterior capsule intraoperatively. By distending the posterior capsule, the CTR prevents it from being aspirated into the phaco tip or the I/A tip. The CTR also recruits tension from existing zonules and redistributes the forces to the remaining weaker zonules, thereby stabilizing the entire zonular apparatus [5, 6, 9, 11, 12, 15]. The CTR also plays a role in keeping the vitreous in the posterior chamber, because of the seal it creates by the distension of the capsular bag toward the periphery. This added support of the CTR may also help to recenter a mildly subluxed capsular bag to avoid decentration and dislocation. However, they do not provide anterior to posterior support, and standard CTR fail to recenter severely subluxed capsular bags, and do not prevent progressive zonular loss [3, 4]. In these situations, scleral fixated devices like the modified CTR or the capsular tension segment are more appropriate.

The implantation of a CTR is contraindicated if there is an anterior radial or posterior tear of the capsule [5, 6, 9, 11, 12, 15].

There is some controversy about the optimal timing of CTR insertion. Early implantation of the CTR may facilitate phacoemulsification, reducing the risk of aspirating a floppy posterior capsule, since it is stretched by the CTR. However, as a drawback, the entrapment of cortical material by the CTR in the capsular bag fornix may hinder its removal. Also, if a posterior capsule tear or complete zonular dehiscence occurs during lens extraction, the early placed CTR is a risk factor for dislocation into the vitreous cavity. Furthermore, CTR implantation before cataract removal may result in further iatrogenic zonular damage. Ahmed et al. showed, using the Miyake-Apple video camera, that, in terms of minimizing further zonular stress and damage and capsular destabilization, the ideal timing for CTR placement is after lens extraction and decompression of the capsular bag [16].

Insertion and rotation of a CTR in the capsular bag in the presence of crystalline lens is challenging and results in significant zonular stress and capsular bag displacement as confirmed in the Miyake-Apple study, running the risk of intraoperative or postoperative capsular bag dislocation [16]. This risk is likely increased with denser cataracts. Jacob et al. reported on the use of CTR in 21 eyes with mild to moderate zonular dialysis in which the CTR was placed prior to phacoemulsification and found a 9.5% incidence of clinically significant extension of zonular dialysis [17].

One dictum that is followed by many surgeons is to place the CTR "as late as you can, but as soon as you must" (Rosenthal K, Personal communication, circa 2005) [6], or in other words, "as late as safely possible" [6, 8] (Video 6.4).

How to implant a CTR (Fig. 6.12) (Video 6.2)?

Implantation of the CTR may be performed manually (authors' preference) or with an injector [5]. Forceps are necessary in order to use a modified capsular tension ring which has appendages. The injector is only useful for the standard capsular tension ring. The injector delivers the ring in the center of the anterior chamber, avoiding the pressure of the CTR against the capsulorhexis margin.

A complete and intact capsulorhexis is a mandatory prerequisite in order to implant a CTR. The capsular bag must be fully distended with a cohesive ophthalmic viscosurgical device (OVD) [5]. The CTR must be inserted in the direction of the zonular deficiency and with an acute angle, in a tangential direction, to avoid radial pressure from the leading eyelet on the equator. We strongly advise to place a suture in the leading hole of the CTR. The suture has two functions. First, it can be used to retrieve the CTR in case of capsular tear or disinsertion, and second, if a fold at the equator occurs during the dialing of the CTR, pulling the suture through the main incision will help to disengage the CTR from the fold (Video 6.5). A Lester hook may be introduced trough the lateral paracentesis to avoid the contact of the CTR with the capsulorhexis margin and decrease the tension over it while dialing the ring (Video 6.2).

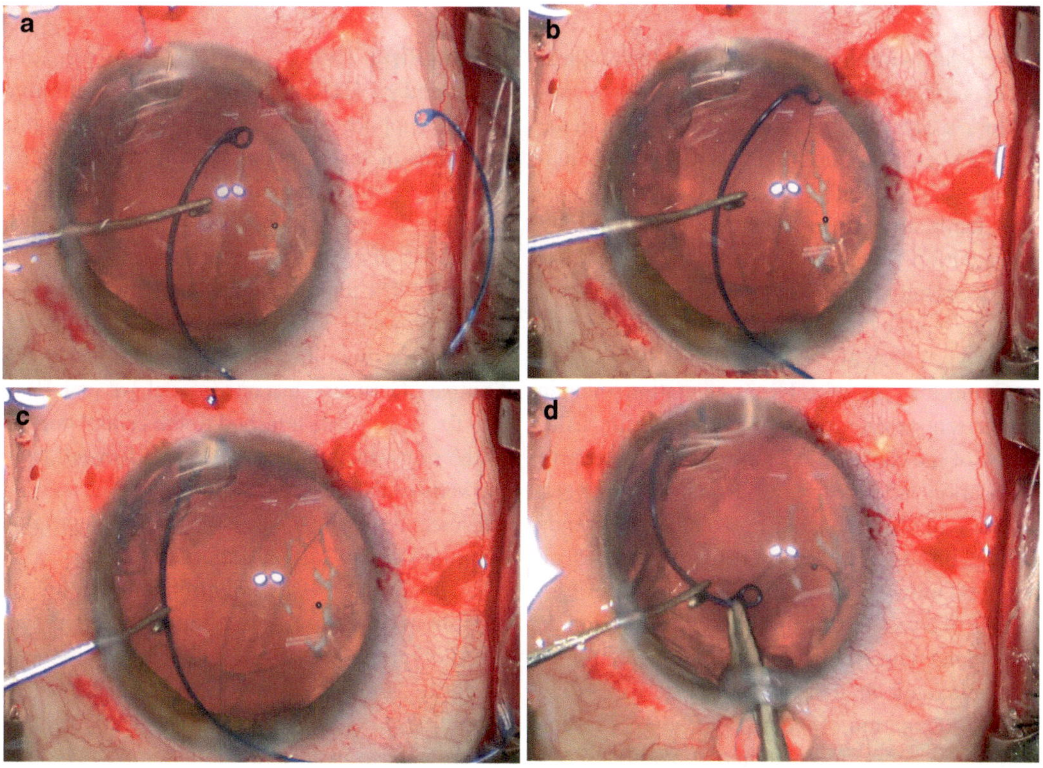

Fig. 6.12 Maneuvers to implant a capsular tension ring. (**a** and **b**) The capsular bag must be fully distended with a cohesive OVD. The CTR must be inserted in the direction of the zonular deficiency and with an acute angle, in a tangential direction, to avoid radial pressure from the leading eyelet on the equator. We strongly advise to place a suture in the leading hole of the CTR. (**c** and **d**) A Lester hook may be introduced through the lateral paracentesis to avoid the contact of the CTR with the capsulorhexis margin and decrease the tension over it while dialing the ring

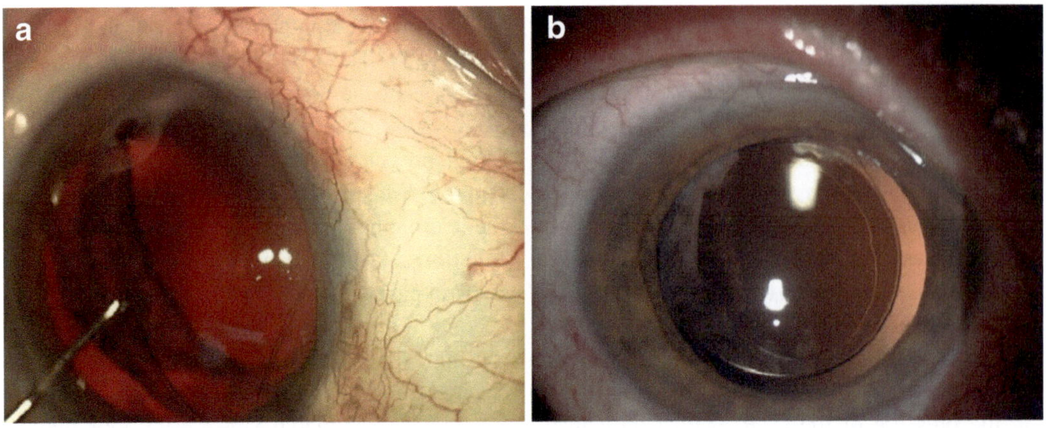

Fig. 6.13 (**a**) During capsular tension ring insertion, an extension of the zonular dehiscence may occur, specially in cases of generalized zonular weakness, as in pseudoexfoliation. In this case of pseudoexfoliation syndrome, an increase in the area of zonular deficiency was noted during insertion. The ring was dialed until this eyelet was adjacent to the area of zonular disinsertion, and the prolene suture that had been threaded through the leading eyelet was used to suture the ring to the scleral wall after creating a Hoffman pocket, without violating the integrity of the capsular bag. (**b**) Postoperative appearance

In order to minimize the stress on the residual zonules in these eyes with already extensive zonule loss, a Sinskey hook may be introduced in the leading eyelet, supporting it away from the equator, in order to avoid stress on the damaged zonules, facilitating the dialing of the CTR during implantation. When more than half of the CTR has been introduced, the eyelet is disengaged from the Sinskey hook. A fishtail technique using a suture has been also described [18, 19].

Complications of CTR implantation include inadvertent anterior capsule tear, posterior dislocation of the capsular tension ring, intraoperative dislocation after early CTR placement, and increase in the extension of zonular deficiency during implantation (Fig. 6.13). Jacob et al. reported intraoperative extension of dialysis in 9.52% of eyes, and in one case, conversion to pars plane vitrectomy to remove nuclear fragments luxated in the vitreous [17]. Regarding tears in the margin of the capsulorhexis, Praveen et al. showed that this prevented implantation of a CTR in two eyes [20].

The implantation of a CTR does not change refractive outcome and modification of IOL power calculation was unnecessary [12].

Cionni Ring

The standard CTR is unable to provide intraoperative support and center the capsular bag in situations of severe zonulolysis (more than 4 h). Alternatives included suturing the standard CTR through the capsule bag (Fig. 6.14) with the added risk of creating a capsular tear [1, 5].

In 1998, Cionni designed the modified CTR which allows the surgeon to suture the CTR to the sclera. The modified CTR (Morcher GmbH, Stuttgart, Germany) has one (model 1-L or 1-R) or two fixation eyelets attached to the central portion of the ring which protrude 0.25 mm forward from the body of the CTR, sitting in front of the anterior capsule, preserving the capsular bag's integrity on suturing [1, 5, 8, 21, 22] (Fig. 6.15a–c).

A double arm 9/10 polypropylene suture on straight needles is pre-placed in the fixation eyelet. Polypropylene 10/0 is not recommended given the risk of hydrolyzation over time with a roughly 5- to 10-year survival time [23]. Another alternative is polytetrafluoroethylene CV-8 suture which is off-label and has cumbersome needles or the use of 9/0 polypropylene. The modified capsular tension ring is injected just under the anterior capsule. The modified CTR is rotated

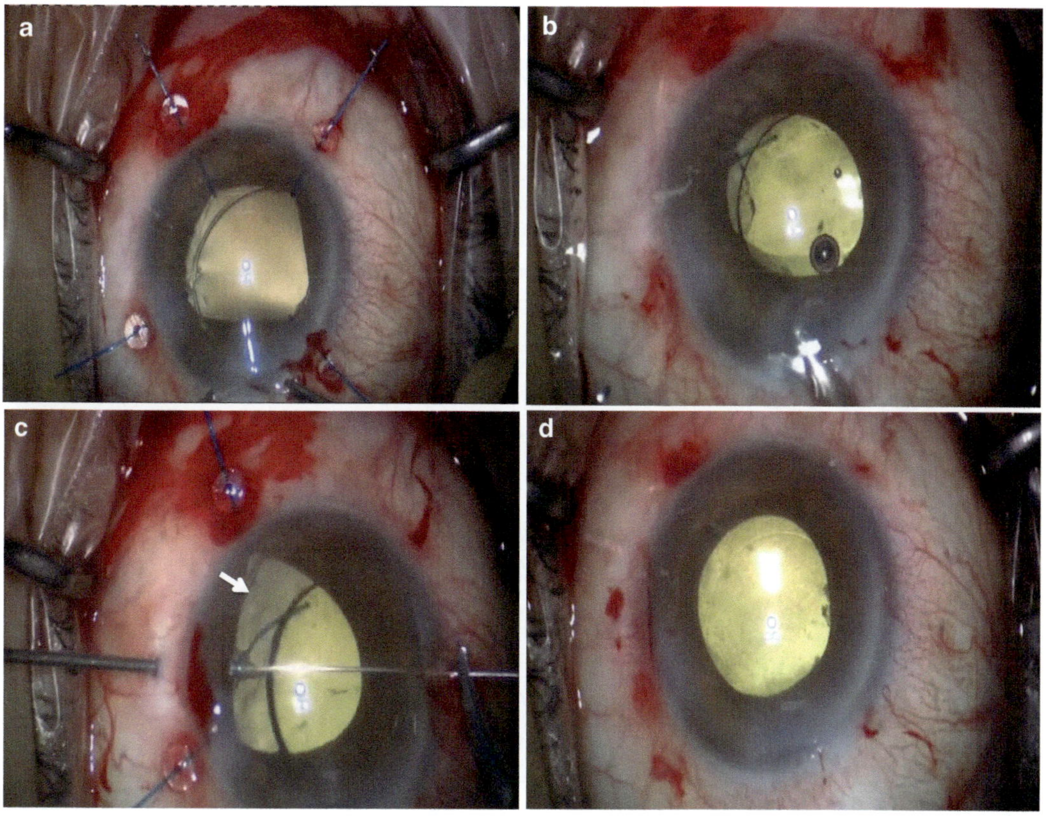

Fig. 6.14 Scleral fixation of a conventional CTR with prolene sutures through a Hoffman pocket. The docking needle punctures the capsular bag, and thus, this maneuver poses the risk of inducing a capsular tear. (**a**) In a case of high myopia and pseudoexfoliation, phacoemulsification had been carried out holding the capsular margin and the iris with iris hooks. A CTR is implanted using the fishtail technique in order to decrease further damage in the zonular apparatus. (**b**) In spite of all these measures, after removing the OVD from the anterior chamber, an inferior zonular dehiscence was evident (arrow indicates the CTR at the equator of capsular bag). (**c**) Using the technique described by Crandall [25], the CTR and the inferior PMMA haptic were sutured to the sclera. (**d**) Intraoperative view at the end of surgery showing a centered IOL (note the good centration of the capsulorhexis margin)

until the eyelet is situated at the area of greatest zonular dehiscence. A scleral flap, Hoffman pocket [24], or scleral groove is created adjacent to the area of dehiscence, and using an *ab externo* technique similar to that described by Ahmed and Crandall [25], the sutures are placed 1.5 mm posterior to the limbus. The suture ends are tied adjusting the tension so that the IOL remains centered (Fig. 6.16) (Video 6.6). An alternative technique using 6/0 polypropylene for sutureless scleral fixation of MCTR has been recently described [26].

Cionni ring either with one or two eyelets has been shown to be useful in the management of severe subluxated traumatic cataracts [15]. Excellent long-term capsule centration and scleral support was reported with this device [22, 27–29].

The most frequent complication of modified CTR is posterior capsule opacification. Other complications include late IOL decentration, elevated intraocular pressure, pigment dispersion, mild iritis, and CME [29].

Malyugin modified Cionni ring so that it could be delivered into the bag using an injector (Morcher GmbH), by moving the fixation element to the very tip of the ring. This makes the device completely retractable into the injector,

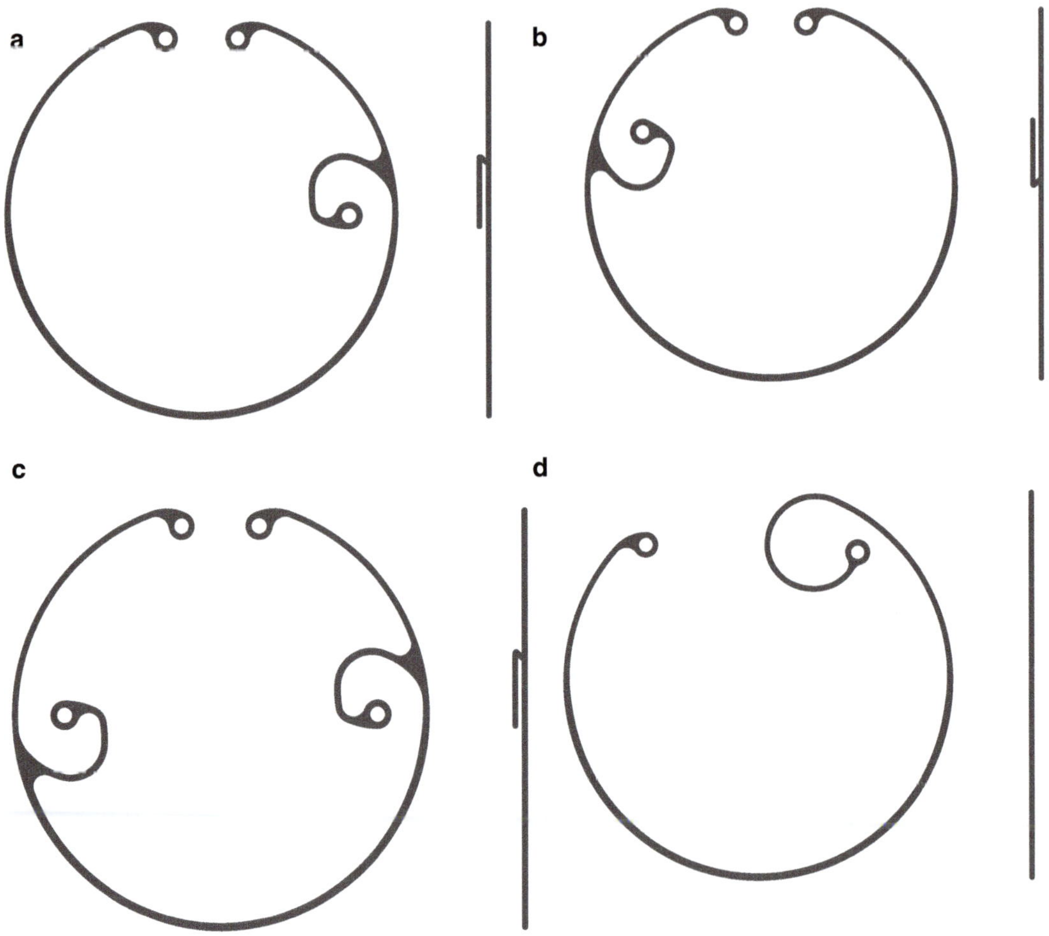

Fig. 6.15 (**a–c**) Cionni modified capsular tension ring with one or two fixation eyelets. (**d**) Malyugin modified capsular tension ring

subsequently allowing it to be inserted into the eye in a very controlled manner [30] (Fig. 6.15d).

Scleral Fixation Devices

The possibility of directly suturing a conventional CTR inserted in the bag to the sclera with a loop of suture around it has been described, but it poses the risk of causing a posterior capsule tear. Currently, different options to perform scleral fixation of the bag are available which respect the bag – apart from the already mentioned modified capsular tension rings – and include the capsular tension segment (CTS), the Assia anchor, and the T-shaped and the endocapsular glued segment.

Ahmed Segment

Designed by Ahmed in 2002, this special device combines the concept of the modified CTR and a capsular retractor. It is a PMMA segment of 120° of arc, with a modified element (appendage with an eyelet) that can be sutured to the sclera if needed, or can be hooked with an iris hook during phacoemulsification. The difference from hooks is that one segment distends 120° of arc of the capsular bag, and at the same time, provides anterior to posterior stabilization (Fig. 6.17) [11, 12].

However, the segment must be complemented with a CTR, since the distension of the bag in 120° is not enough to prevent posterior capsule to be aspirated by the phaco tip.

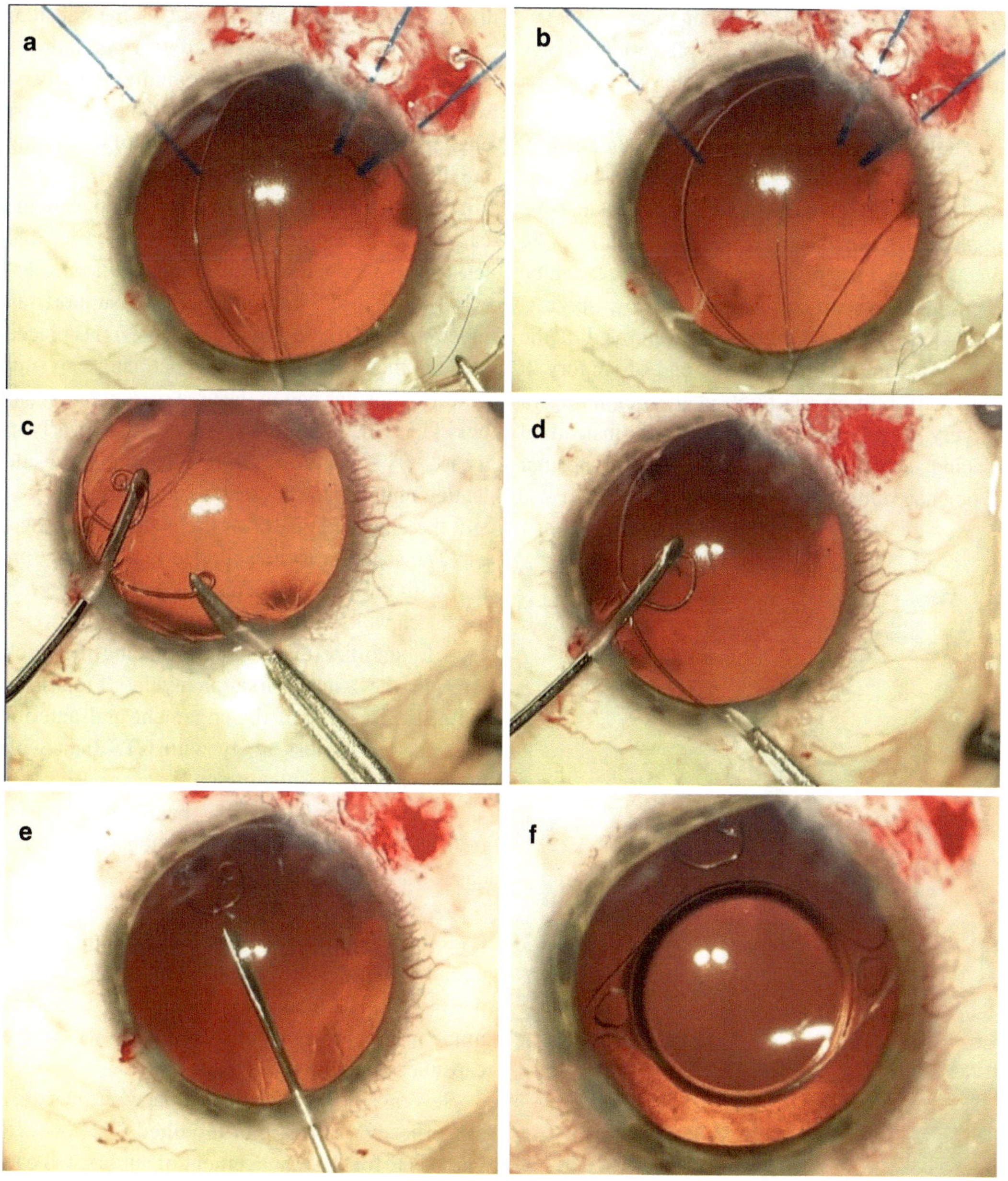

Fig. 6.16 Implantation of Cionni ring. (**a**) Two prolene sutures are placed, one through the leading eyelet and the other through the fixation eyelet. The suture placed on the fixation eyelet must be passed toward the sclera adjacent to the area of zonular dehiscence, before inserting the ring into the anterior chamber. Double needles are inserted into a nesting needle using an *ab externo* technique similar to that described by Crandall [25]. (**b**) The ring is inserted pointing toward the area of dehiscence and dialed until the fixation appendage is in front of the area of zonular deficiency, (**c–e**) taking care that the appendage remains over the capsulorhexis after the implantation. (**f**) Final appearance with good centration of the intraocular lens

Compared to CTR implantation, Miyake-Apple video analysis of CTS placement shows minimal zonular stress on insertion prior to lens extraction (A).

The CTS has several advantages (Videos 6.2, 6.3, 6.7, 6.8, 6.9, and 6.10). Differently from the modified CTR or the Malyugin ring, it can be implanted without sutures, and sutures may be placed later if scleral fixation is needed. It can be used just for vertical support during surgery, instead of hooks, and be easily removed at the end, or it can be sutured at the end of surgery. It is fixated with an iris hook at the beginning of surgery to provide vertical support, instead of placing several iris hooks, in the area of capsular deficiency. Only one hook will be necessary to fixate it, with the added benefit of the capsular tension induced by the 120° arc of ring; and it is possible to place it at the beginning of surgery, when implanting a conventional CTR would be challenging and would pose the risk of increasing the dehiscence. The implantation of the segment, after viscodissection of the space between the capsule and the peripheral cortex, is easier and less risky since a dialing technique is not necessary. When used for intraoperative support, an inverted iris retractor (by a paracentesis) is placed through the eyelet acting as a coat hanger to support the capsular bag in the area of zonular weakness [11, 12]. When the segment is used early in a case, OVD is placed under the anterior capsule leaflet, and a space is created between the cortex and the capsule equator in the quadrant of interest. The segment is then slipped into the bag fornix, with the fixation element remaining anterior to the capsulorhexis. A flexible iris retractor is used to stabilize the segment, placing the hook through the Ahmed fixation eyelet (Fig. 6.18) [11, 12]. The risk of dislodgement and anterior capsular tear is less likely with CTS than with flexible iris or capsule retractors.

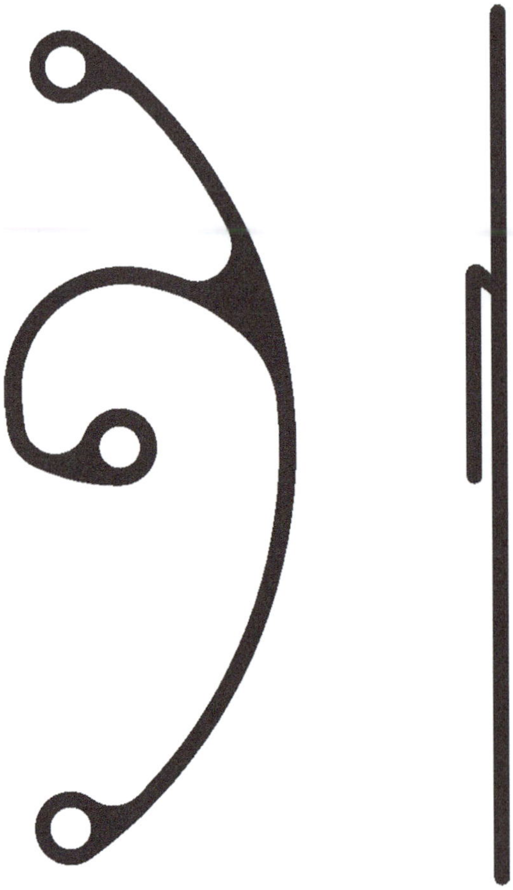

Fig. 6.17 Ahmed segment (CTS)

Multiple CTS devices may be used in a similar fashion, allowing to customize the surgery for cases of severe weakness (Fig. 6.7g) (Video 6.2a), and to address circumferential support, a CTR may be implanted in conjunction with an already positioned CTS which is the author's preference. The CTS provides enough support to implant also an artificial iris implant within the capsular bag (Video 6.10).

Several studies provide evidence of the safety and efficacy of the use of modified CTR or CTS with CTR for the management of subluxated cataract both in adults and pediatric patients [31–33].

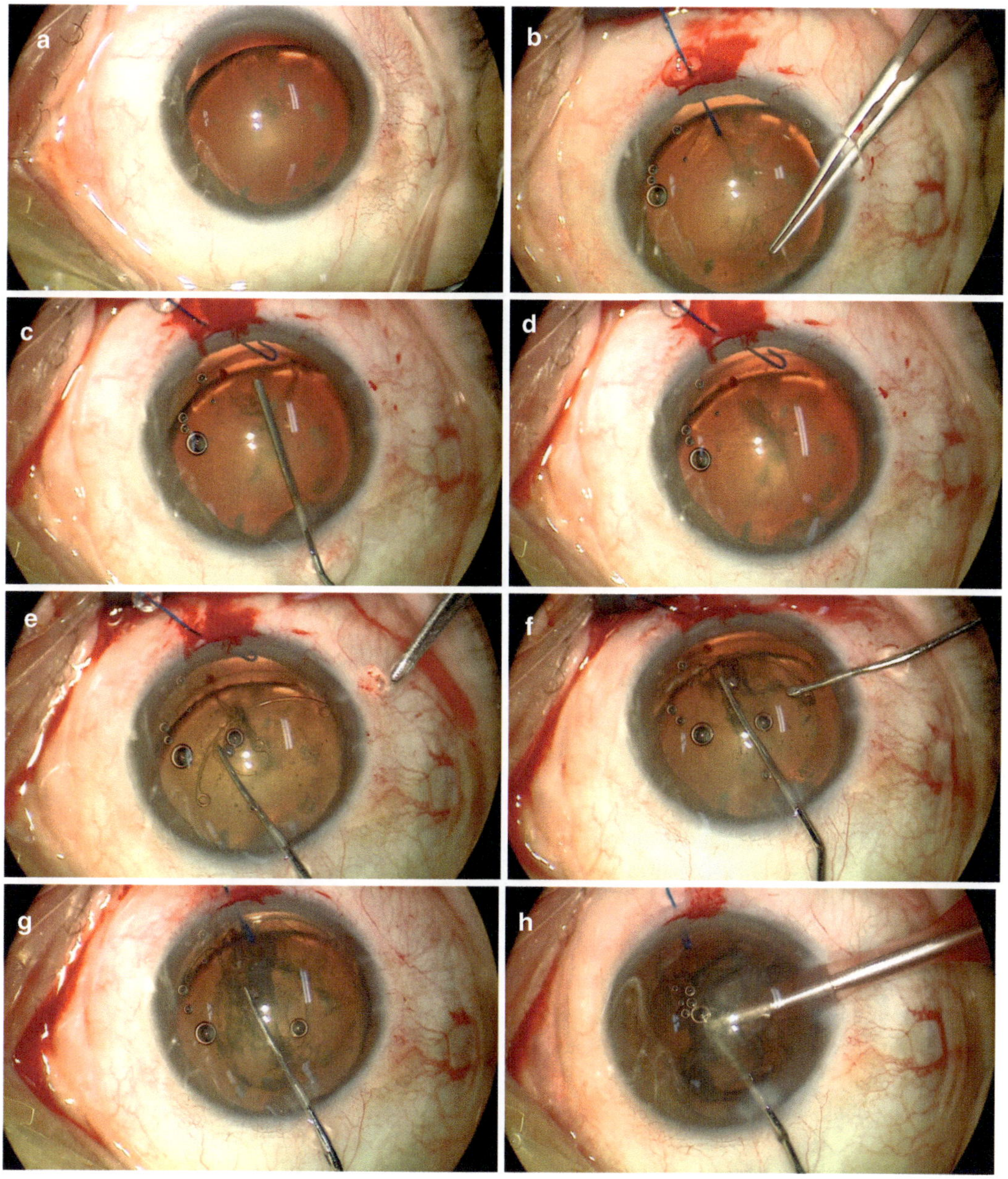

Fig. 6.18 Ahmed segment implantation in a case of traumatic subluxation. (**a**) 180° of zonular dehiscence. (**b**) Capsulorhexis is performed with the aid of an iris hook. (**c, d**) Viscodissection between the capsular bag and the cortical material. (**e, f**) Implantation of the capsular tension segment; the central eyelet must remain anterior to the capsule. Differently to Malyugin or Cionni ring, a dialing technique is not necessary to implant the device. (**g**) An inverted iris retractor is placed through the eyelet acting as a coat hanger. (**h**) Phacoemulsification. (**i**) Insertion of the capsular tension ring. (**j**) The CTS is removed from the capsule equator and is placed vertically in the middle of the anterior chamber. (**k**) The eyelet is threaded with the suture (**l**) creating a loop around it [25]. (**m**) Final appearance

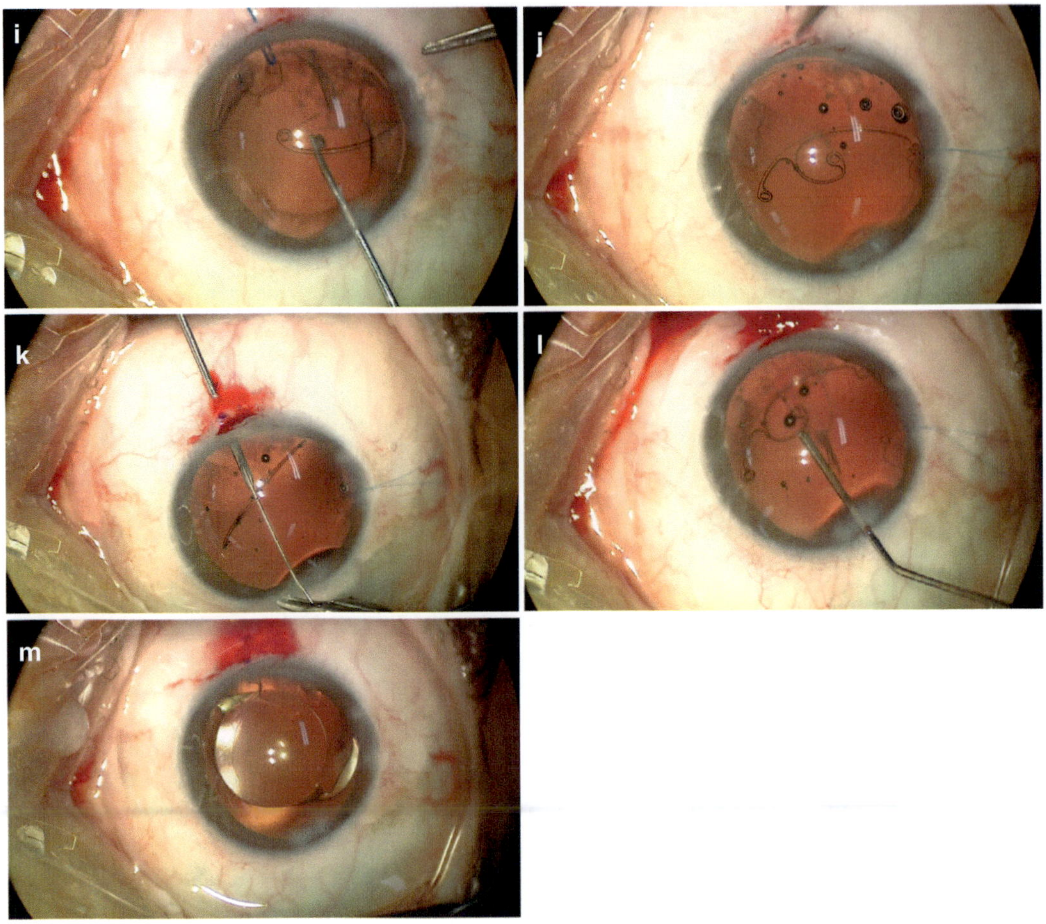

Fig. 6.18 (continued)

Other Devices

Other alternatives to fix the capsular bag and to provide vertical support include the Assia anchor, the Yaguchi hook, and the glued endocapsular tension ring.

The Assia anchor (capsular anchor) is a flat intraocular PMMA implant that consists of a central rod positioned in front of the anterior capsule and two side arms positioned behind the anterior capsule. It is sutured to the sclera [34] (Fig. 6.19).

The T-shaped ending Yaguchi hook is a flexible T-shaped device made of 5–0 polypropylene attached to a curved needle which is sutured to the sclera. The contact portion is bent at 1.25 mm and the end bifurcates in a T configuration to form a 3.75 mm footpad [35].

The glued endocapsular tension ring (Epsilon Eye) is a one-piece device made of polyvinylidene fluoride with three parts: arms on either side to expand the fornix, a Malyugin-type scrolled mechanism to engage the capsulorhexis, and a haptic that goes through the sclerotomy to anchor the device, and thereby the capsular bag, to the sclera by means of fibrin glue-assisted sutureless transscleral fixation of the bag [36].

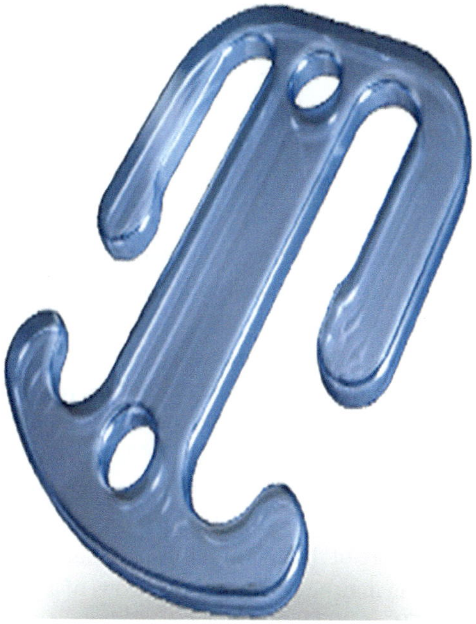

Fig. 6.19 Assia anchor

Either the CTS or any of these devices provide only focal support of the capsular bag, and they neither do not distend the capsular bag equator nor provide circumferential distribution of forces, and thus, they should be combined with conventional of modified CTR.

In order to perform scleral fixation, we use an *ab externo* technique similar to that described by Ahmed and Crandall [25]. Once both sutures are externalized, the IOL is implanted, and with the globe pressurized, suture tension should be titrated to achieve maximal IOL centration. The sutures and knots can be placed under scleral flaps, in a Hoffman pocket [24], into a scleral groove, etc. according to the surgeon's preferences since no system has proven to be superior. A sutureless technique has been reported for the scleral fixation of Ahmed segment using 5/0 prolene [37]. We have used a modified approach to use 6/0 prolene docked into a 30 g ultrathin wall needle (C, D) (Figs. 6.7 and 6.20) (Video 6.2).

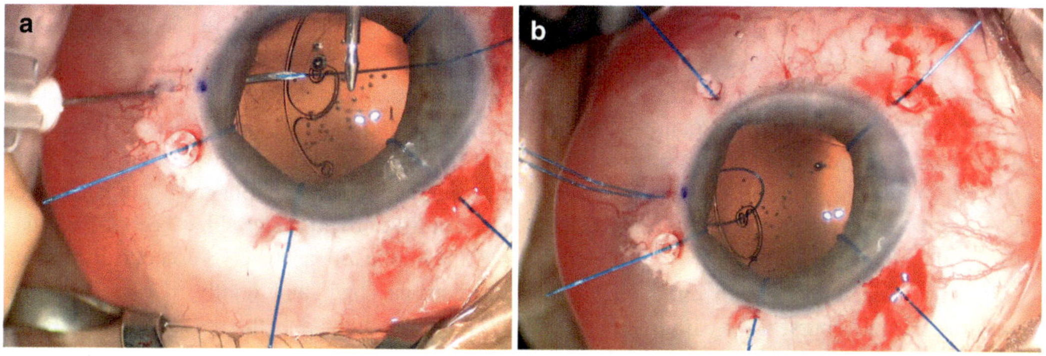

Fig. 6.20 Surgery of a subluxated cataract – preoperative and postoperative details are shown in Fig. 6.7 – with implantation of a CTR and two CTS which were fixated to the sclera using flanged 6/0 prolene without knots. We have used a personal modification of the technique previously published in order to use a 6/0 prolene into a 30 g needle, instead of using 5/0 prolene into a 26 g needle. (**a**) After implanting the CTR, a CTS is inserted into the anterior chamber, and one extreme of 6/0 prolene is threaded through the eyelet and docked into the barrel of a 30 g ultrathin wall needle which has been inserted 2 mm from the limbus. (**b**) After externalizing that extreme of the prolene, the same maneuver is repeated with the other extreme to create a loop around the eyelet. (**c**) The intraocular lens is implanted and another CTS is implanted with the same technique 180° apart from the first one. The appropriate tension is applied to obtain good IOL centration, and the tops of the prolene suture are cut and flanged using a cautery. The flanged tops are buried into the sclera. (**d**) Final appearance

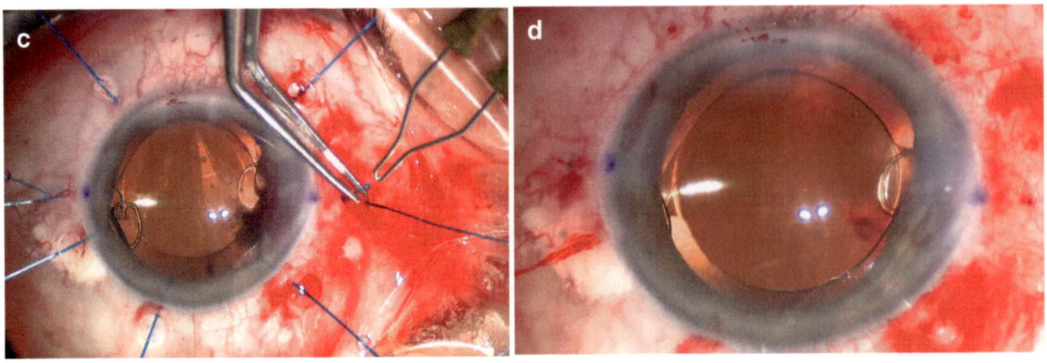

Fig. 6.20 (continued)

Our Surgical Strategy

The surgery of a subluxated lens faces two mechanical challenges. Firstly, the vertical stability of the lens is compromised by the lack of zonular support, and secondly, the distension of the posterior capsule is altered by the lack of zonular fibers.

At the beginning of surgery, the main problem is the vertical support, that is, keeping the lens in the proper horizontal plane, and that is best achieved through the use of iris hooks, or Mackool hooks or CTS implantation. They hold the lens without risking the increase in the zonular deficiency induced by the early placement of a CTR, specially in hard lenses, while dialing the CTR. During hydrodissection, and phacoemulsification, the bag is full and will not collapse until the last phase of phacoemulsification when most of the lens material has been removed. Also, the nuclear fragments themselves can be used to keep the posterior capsule far from the phaco tip [38].

Once the cataract has been emulsified, and depending on the course of hydrodissection, a CTR may be safely implanted to distend the posterior capsule and avoid its aspiration through the phaco tip. At that time, all or almost all of the cortical material must have been removed and in any case, implanting the CTR without the nucleus, induce less stress over the zonules than the implantation before the phacoemulsification, dialing it through the resistance of the bag full of lens content.

Once the CTR is in place, the surgeon must decide whether to fix the bag to the sclera or not. The decision will depend on the extension of the dehiscence (more than 4 hours of deficiency usually will need scleral fixation to get appropriate centration of the bag) and on the progressive or stable nature of the condition. The scleral fixation of the bag may be performed by means of a modified CTR, the CTS, the Assia anchor, etc. according to surgeon's preferences.

Our preference is to use a CTS at the beginning of surgery since its insertion does not pose any risk regarding the increase in the zonular dehiscence, and it provides not only the vertical support but also some distension of the bag in a 120° area. If entrapment of cortical material occurs, it can be disinserted, cortical aspiration can be carried out, and it can be implanted again later. Once most of the cortical material has been aspirated, a CTR is implanted, as the CTS do not fully distend the capsular bag, and finally, if necessary, the CTR will be fixated to the sclera. And additional CTS may be combined if required, depending on the extension of zonular deficiency (see below). The combination of the CTS and CTR allow to address vertical support or bag distension separately, as required, differently from modified CTR (Videos 6.2, 6.3, 6.7, 6.8, 6.9, and 6.10).

Surgical Algorithm

The surgical strategy will depend on the extension of zonular dehiscence and the cause of the deficiency, regarding whether it is progressive or not. Traumatic cases usually have healthy zonules outside the area of the dehiscence, while in congenital cases, as Marfan or adult onset cases such as pseudoexfoliation and retinitis pigmentaria, further damage of the zonules is expected with time.

We use the following algorithm in cases of zonular deficiency [1, 5, 6, 8]:

Extension of zonular dialysis	Management
Mild (<4 h of zonular dehiscence)	One CTR
Moderate (4–8 h of zonular dehiscence)	One CTR Hooks or CTS during surgery Scleral fixation at one point
Severe (>8 h of zonular dehiscence)	Hook or CTS, CTR, scleral fixation at two points

However, this strategy must be adjusted according to the profile of zonular weakness (stable or progressive) and the density of the nucleous.

The surgeon may choose to perform scleral fixation in mild case of Marfan, since it will surely progress. The implantation of a CTR does not halt the progression of zonulopathy in progressive cases; however, it facilitates refixation of the capsular bag IOL complex.

The management of very dangling lenses if they are soft may be accomplished by lensectomy, from a pars plana approach, followed by a secondary implant (Fig. 6.21) (Video 6.11). Severe cases of dehiscence with very hard cataracts may require intracapsular approach, as sometimes happens in pseudoexfoliative patients with important phacodonesis and very hard nucleous (Fig. 6.22).

Even after a detailed preoperative exam, unpredictable surprises may occur during surgery in these cases, so the necessary material must be available and the surgeon must be ready to use

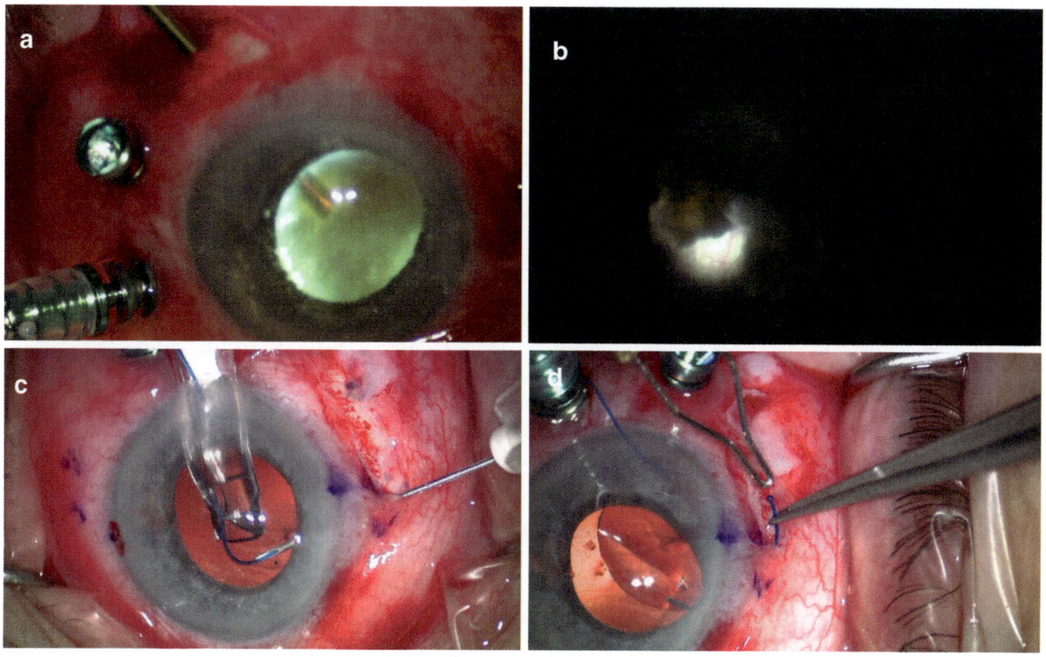

Fig. 6.21 *Pars plana* lensectomy (**a**, **b**) and secondary flanged IOL implantation in a case with severe phacodonesis (**c**–**f**)

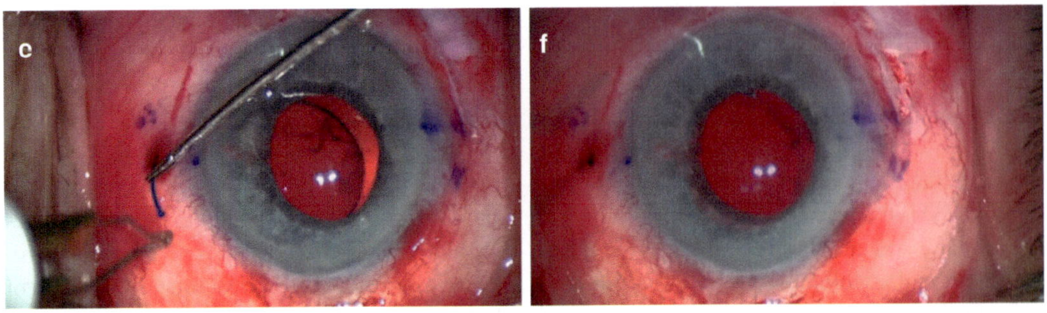

Fig. 6.21 (continued)

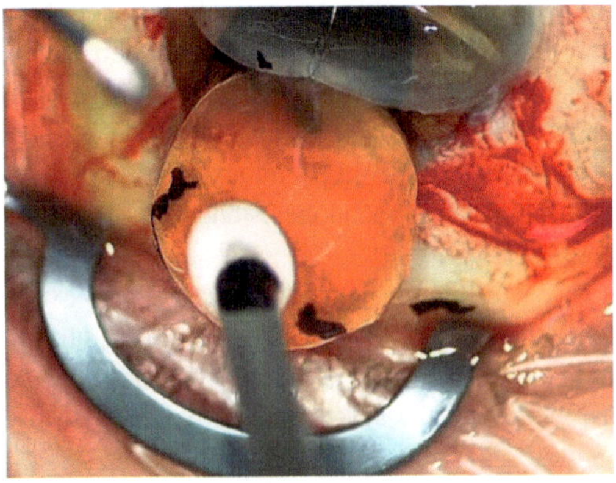

Fig. 6.22 Intracapsular extraction in a case of pseudoexfoliation with severe pseudophacodonesis and dense cataract. After the cataract extraction, a retropupillar iris claw lens was implanted

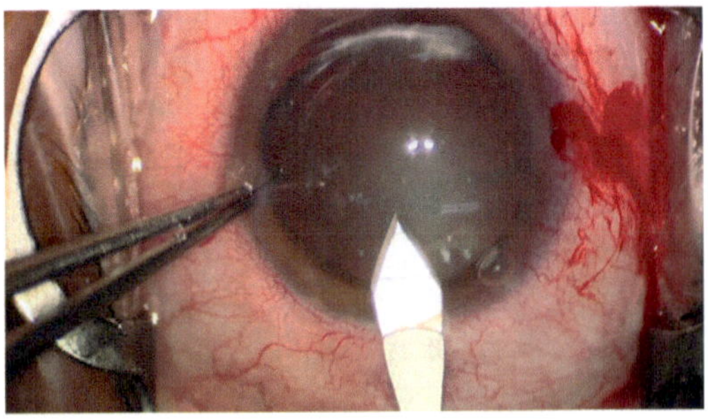

Fig. 6.23 The main incision must be performed in the area opposite the zonular dehiscence

different strategies to face different degrees of zonular weakness (B).

Surgical Technique

Anesthesia

These cases should be performed under peribulbar anesthesia, as additional maneuvers, difficult to perform under topical anesthesia, may be required during surgery and the duration of surgery is usually longer [9].

Incision

The main incision must be performed in the area opposite the zonular dehiscence (Fig. 6.23) (Video 6.3) as long as the surgeon is comfortable, or 90° apart [5, 6, 9]. Whether scleral fixation of a modified CTR or Ahmed segment is planned in advance, the Hoffman pockets, or conjunctival peritomy and scleral flaps, must be performed before the corneal incision. Also, if vitreous is present in the anterior chamber and insertion of a trocar is going to be done in pars plana, it should also be inserted before performing the corneal incision.

Vitrectomy

Vitreous may be present in the anterior chamber, specially in traumatic cases. Anterior vitrectomy must be carried out before capsulorhexis (Fig. 6.24) (Video 6.3) [6, 9]. This procedure may be accomplished from a pars plana approach or form a limbal approach, always using a different incision for the vitrector and for the infusion. Triamcinolone-assisted vitrectomy is performed until no vitreous is identified in the anterior

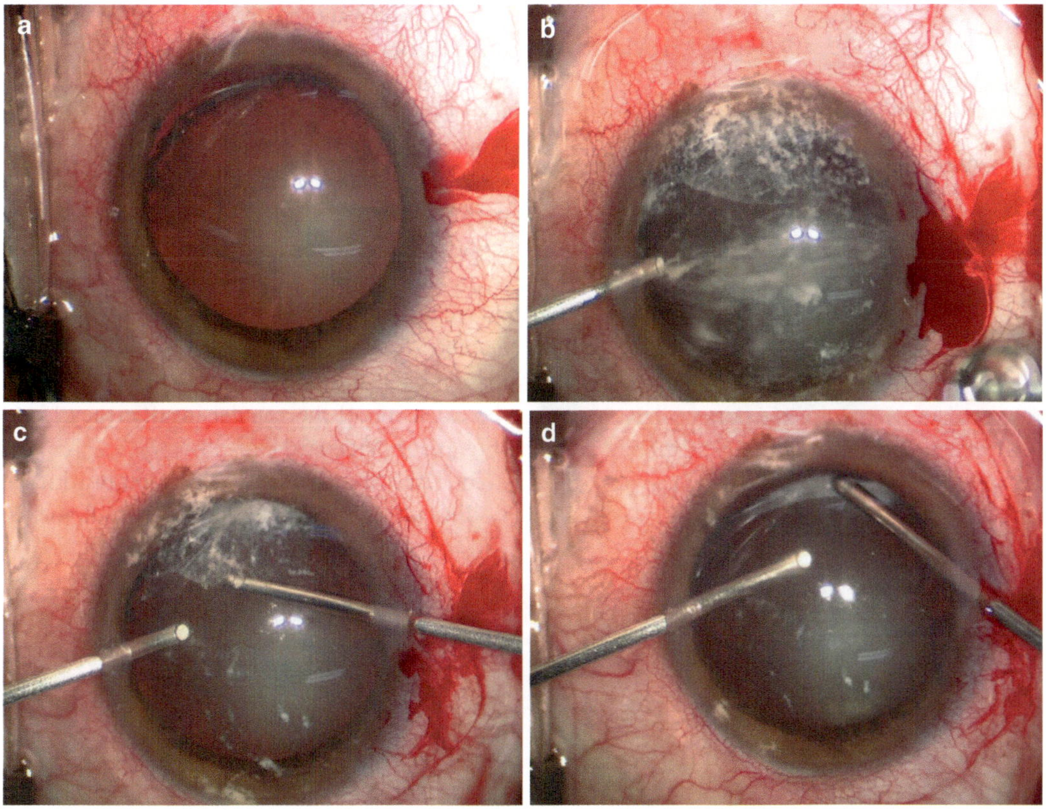

Fig. 6.24 (**a**) Traumatic subluxated cataract. (**b**) If vitreous prolapse is detected in the anterior chamber, a triamcinolone assisted anterior vitrectomy must be performed before capsulorhexis creation (**c**, **d**)

chamber. A dispersive OVD is placed over the area of zonular dehiscence to tamponade the vitreous in the posterior chamber.

In addition, the implantation of a CTR also contributes to control the vitreous prolapse through the area of zonular dehiscence, since it expands the bag and the tension of the CTR together with the use of CTS or iris hooks that lift the bag against the iris, seal the anterior chamber from the vitreous cavity. The creation of this seal between the AC and the vitreous helps to prevent further vitreous prolapse and aqueous misdirection during phacoemulsification [15].

Capsulorhexis

The capsulorhexis is a critical step in any phacoemulsification, and entails facing several difficulties in cases of subluxated cataracts. First, the counterforce produced by the normal zonules is lacking in the area of dehiscence. This is the reason of radial folds and movement of the lens during the capsulorhexis. Second, the lens is decentered, exposing the equator of the lens, while the opposite area of the lens is hidden behind the iris, making it difficult to achieve a centered capsulorhexis.

The use of trypan blue is advisable, not only because it enhances visualization during the capsulorhexis but also to identify the margins of the rhexis during the rest of the surgery. The dye must be applied after the injection of an OVD and under it, to limit the uncontrolled spread of the dye that could reach the area of zonular dehiscence and the vitreous cavity, obscuring the red reflex. In the ultimate soft-shell technique, a viscoadaptive OVD is used to coat the endothelium, and balance salt solution is then injected onto the lens surface below the OVD, creating a low viscosity working space where the trypan blue dye is added [39, 40] (Fig. 6.25) (Videos 6.3 and 6.10).

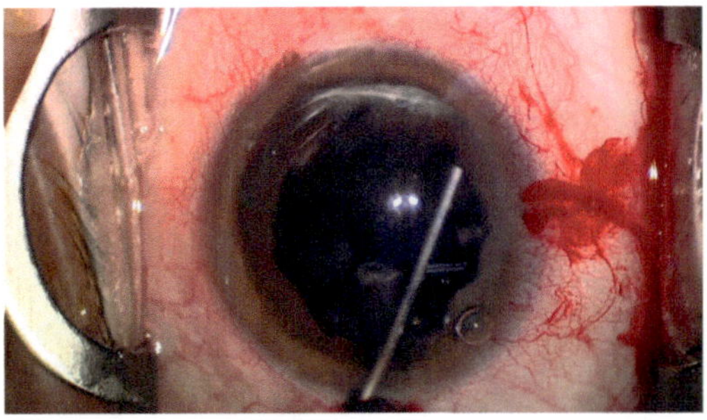

Fig. 6.25 Capsular dye must be applied below using the ultimate soft-shell technique

During capsulorhexis, we find big wrinkles on the quadrant of the zonule weakness, because the zonules cannot readily counteract the pulling force created by capsulorhexis forceps (Video 6.2).

In cases of mild decentration, it is possible to perform a centered capsulorhexis without difficulties. The anterior capsule must be punctured in an area away from the dialysis, and once the flap of the anterior capsule is formed, it is grasped and the tractions are performed in the direction of the dehiscence, not against it, in order to avoid the extension of the zonular insufficiency [5, 6] (Fig. 6.26) (Video 6.2).

In cases of moderate decentration in which it is difficult to obtain a centered capsulorhexis,

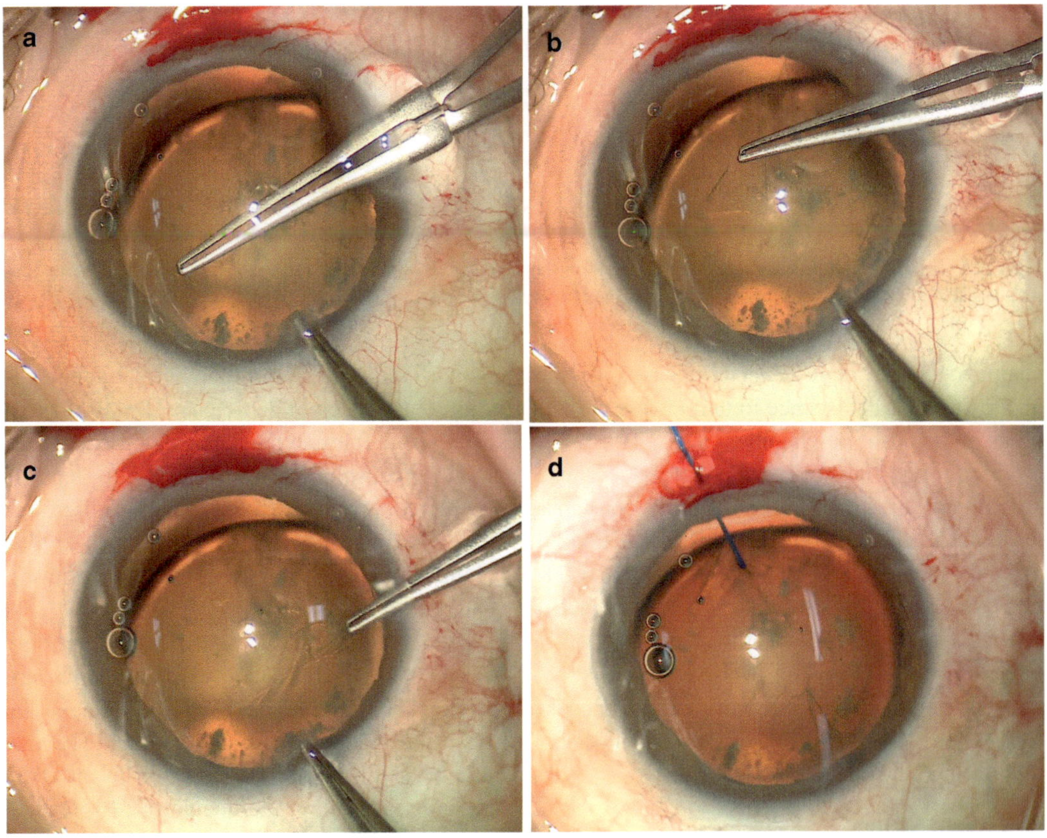

Fig. 6.26 (**a**–**c**) The anterior capsule must be punctured in an area away from the dialysis, and once the flap of the anterior capsule is formed, it is grasped and the tractions are performed in the direction of the dehiscence. (**d**–**f**) The counterforce produced by the normal zonules is lacking in the area of dehiscence. When using hooks as counter-traction during capsulorhexis creation, the hooks should be placed at least 2 to 3 clock hours from the leading edge of the capsulorhexis to avoid tractional forces that will cause the leading edge to extend peripherally toward the bag equator

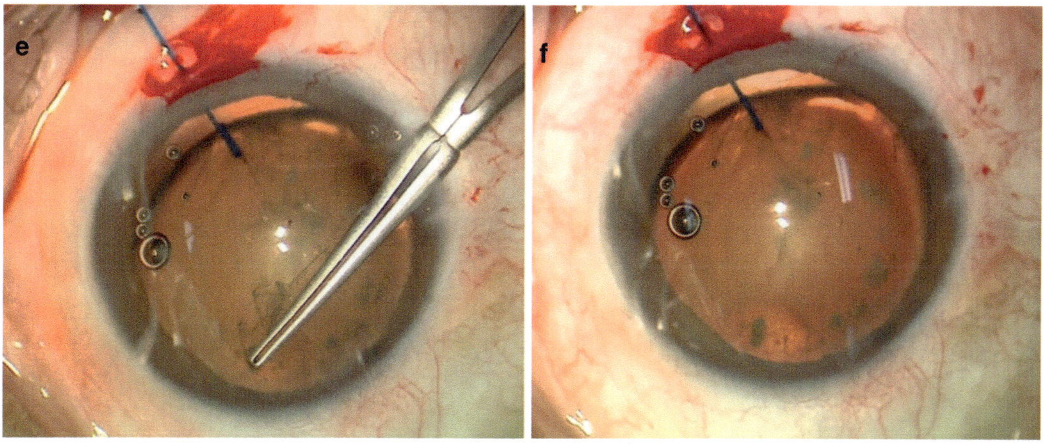

Fig. 6.26 (continued)

once the initial flap is created and part of the capsulorhexis is performed, iris hooks can be placed, which engage the margin of the rhexis, and traction is created to center the lens, so more of the anterior capsule surface is exposed, and better centration for the rhexis is possible. When using hooks as counter-traction during capsulorhexis creation, the hooks should be placed at least 2 to 3 clock hours from the leading edge of the capsulorhexis to avoid tractional forces that will cause the leading edge to extend peripherally toward the bag equator (Fig. 6.26) (Videos 6.2, 6.8, and 6.10). A Lester hook can be used as an alternative to mobilize the subluxated lens [6].

In some cases of very loose zonules, the lack of zonular tension makes it impossible for the needle to penetrate the anterior capsule. In these cases, a bimanual approach must be performed to initiate the rhexis. A coaxial forceps is used to grasp a fold of the anterior capsule, while the needle punctures the anterior capsule near the fold to be able to initiate the flap of the rhexis. In some cases, capsulorhexis must be completed with two micro capsulorhexis forceps to provide counter-traction as required [41] (Fig. 6.27) (Video 6.12).

Capsulorhexis diameter should be between 5 and 6 mm, taking care to keep at least 2 mm from the capsulorhexis margin to the equator, minimal distance required to keep a CRT or segment into the capsular bag.

Hydrodissection and Hydrodelineation

Properly performed hydroprocedures are mandatory to allow the free rotation of the nucleus in the bag, thereby decreasing zonular stress. Multiquadrant cortical cleaving hydrodissection followed by hydrodelineation should be carried out. Also, bimanual rotation of the nucleous is strongly recommended to equally redistribute the stress on the zonules (Video 6.8). The difficulty found during rotation of the nucleous can give us an idea about the extension of the zonulopathy, since the larger the zonulopathy, the more difficult it will be to rotate the nucleous.

Phacoemulsification

Although some authors recommend that soft nucleous be phacoemulsified in the anterior chamber, at a suprascapular level, to decrease stress on the zonules, the maneuver of prolapsing the nucleous through the rhexis toward the anterior chamber poses some stress on the bag, and anterior chamber phacoemulsification may damage the endothelium [1, 6]. Phacoemulsification of soft lenses within the bag does not usually cause significant traction on the zonules. For the remaining cases, direct chop and stop and chop are the nucleofracture techniques that induce less

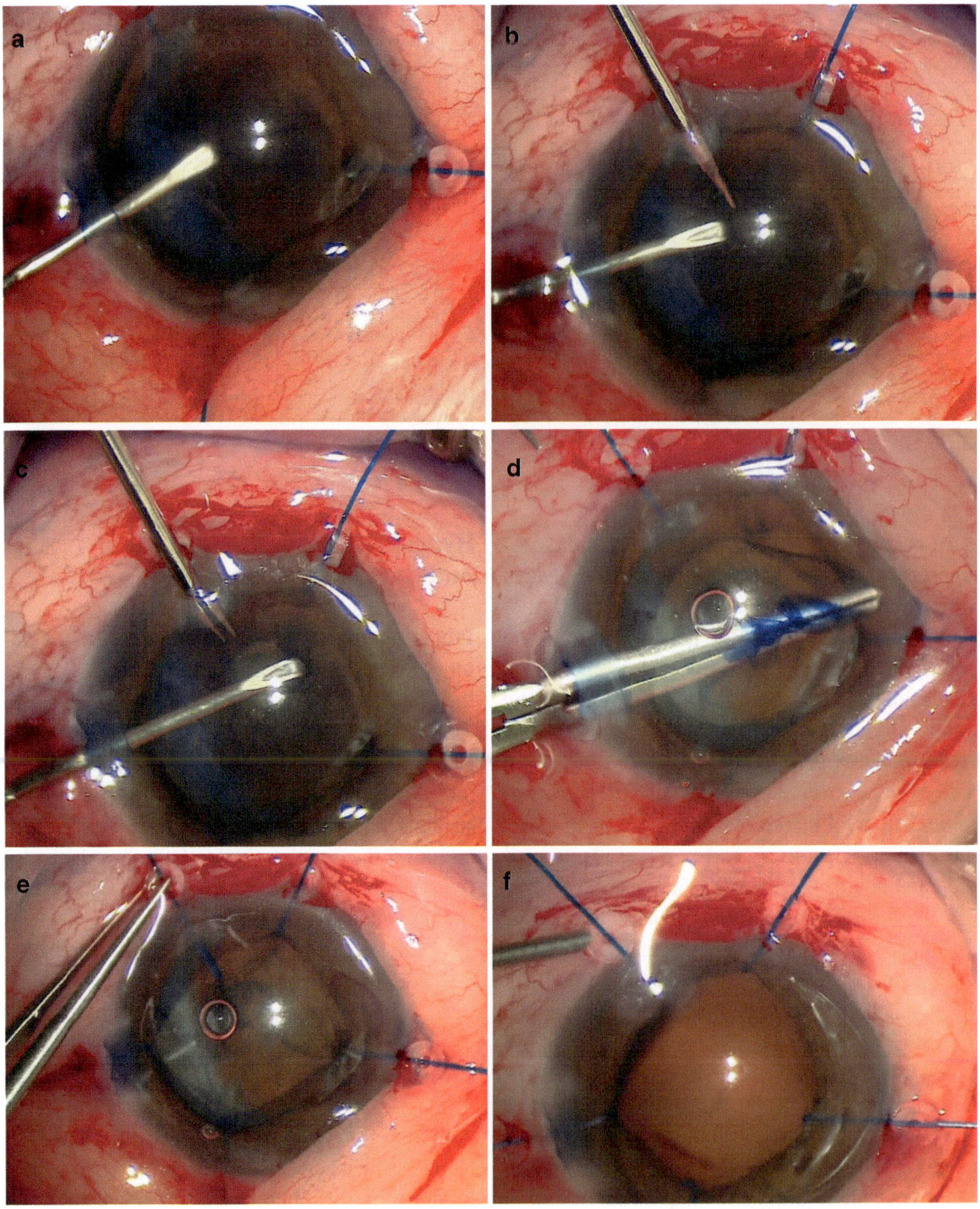

Fig. 6.27 (**a**) Pronounced folds appeared when trying unsuccessfully to puncture the capsule to initiate the rhexis, due to extensive and generalized zonular weakness. (**b**) A capsulorhexis microforceps was used to grasp a fold to create a counter-traction while puncturing the capsule with the needle holder with the other hand, using a bimanual approach. (**c**, **d**) Capsulorhexis was completed. (**e**, **f**) Iris hooks which were already dilating the pupil were transferred to the capsulorhexis margin holding at the same time the iris and the capsular bag and phacoemulsification could be carried out uneventfully

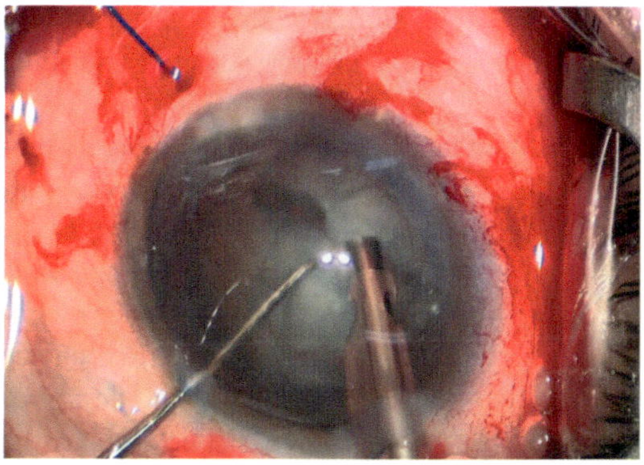

Fig. 6.28 Phaco-chop is the nucleofracture technique that induces less stress on the zonules. The use of slow motion phacoemulsification is highly recommended

stress on the zonules (Fig. 6.28) (Videos 6.2 and 6.3) [9]. Regarding the parameters, the use of slow motion phacoemulsification is highly recommended. In this technique, all the parameters of the equipment, ultrasound energy, aspiration rate, flow rate, and bottle height or pressure are kept to the minimum value with the purpose of decreasing turbulences in the anterior chamber and subsequently, inducing less stress on the zonules [42].

During phacoemulsification, the nuclear fragments themselves can be used as a scaffold to avoid the forward movement of the posterior capsule which is the result of lack of tension because of the absence of counteraction of zonular support [38].

Cortical Aspiration

The greatest amount of traction on the zonules is induced during cortical aspiration.

This step is facilitated by a prior hydrodissection as most of the cortex will be dissected from the capsule during this maneuver. Another recommendation is to perform tangential aspiration with the irrigation/aspiration (I/A) tip, stripping tangentially toward the dehiscence rather than away from it (Fig. 6.29) (Video 6.13). In these

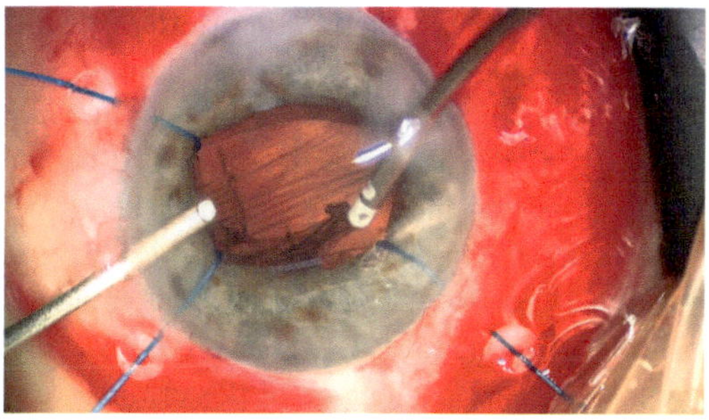

Fig. 6.29 Tangential aspiration of the cortical material using I/A tips toward the dehiscence minimizes traction on the zonules

cases, the use of bimanual I/A tips is highly advisable, since they allow access to any meridian, according to the place where incisions are made. Also, residual recalcitrant cortical material can be mobilized after IOL implantation, when dialing the intraocular lens, and be aspirated afterward. We can also direct the irrigation flow to a point far from the dehiscence to reduce the risk of the BSS penetration toward the vitreous cavity resulting in a misdirection syndrome [1, 5, 6, 9].

The difficulty to perform cortical aspiration varies greatly from one case to another, depending on the extension of zonular dehiscence, and the presence of a CTR inside the bag or not.

If implantation of a CTR was required before cortical aspiration, part of the cortical material will remain entrapped behind the CTR. If the I/A tip aspirates and performs traction of the superior and inferior part of cortical material, it will form a loop around the CTR and it will be impossible to remove it. Instead, traction should be exerted on the material either above or below the CTR, in a tangential fashion.

If no CTR has been implanted, and when performing traction on cortical material, even with a tangential direction, either the lens equator becomes visible or the posterior capsule, which has no tension due to absence of zonular support, tends to come toward the I/A tip; thus, the implantation of a CTR is recommended, since we are running the risk to rupture the posterior capsule. We have to balance the risk of continuing I/A step without the CTR, against the difficulty of removing the cortical material entrapped behind it once it is implanted. Usually, the second scenario is better. One useful procedure is trying to perform viscodissection of cortical material before implanting the CTR. Then it is not surprising that a higher percentage of posterior capsule opacification has been found in cases of implantation of Cionni ring [29].

Injection of dispersive OVD several times may also help to keep backward a floppy posterior capsule; however, we would rather recommend a CTR implantation. Both during phacoemulsification and cortical aspiration, it is of paramount importance to fill the anterior chamber with OVD, before removing the phaco tip or the irrigation from the eye, in order to keep a pressurized anterior chamber; otherwise, we run the risk of facing vitreous prolapse (Videos 6.2 and 6.8).

"While complete cortical removal is a noble and appropriate goal, excessive efforts to remove small strands should not risk capsular or zonular damage" [6].

Intraocular Lens Implantation

If the capsular bag is stable after the completion of I/A aspiration with a CTR, the intraocular lens is implanted within the bag.

If a Cionni or Ahmed segment has been implanted, it is important to implant the lens before tying and adjusting the tension of the suture of the device, since proper centration of the lens will be easier to achieve.

Regarding the type of the intraocular lens, we should consider whether the subluxation is progressive or not. If the subluxation is the result of a trauma, and proper centration of the capsular bag is achieved after surgery, any type of lens could be implanted, including toric and multifocal or EDoF lenses, although with these three types of lenses, we must be very sure that the case fulfills other requisites to implant these lenses.

The use of toric and multifocal lenses will be considered only in very selected and ideal cases [6].

We would recommend to choose a highly biocompatible material and design. With this purpose in mind, a single-piece hydrophobic acrylic intraocular lens with C-shaped haptics and slow unfolding is the best choice. A three-piece hydrophobic acrylic intraocular lens is a good choice also, and some years ago, it was the design of choice since the PMMA haptics could be implanted in the meridian of zonular dehiscence as counter-traction. In recent years, with a CTR in place and scleral fixation if required, a single-piece intraocular lens is adequate, since the centrifugal tension induced by the CTR is enough to keep the capsular bag distended.

Femtosecond Laser Role

Femtosecond laser may be used to perform the capsulorhexis in certain cases of subluxated cataracts [43, 44]. It is able to get a circular rhexis as well as liquefy the lens, perhaps decreasing the risk of further zonular damage, but this theoretical benefit has not been demonstrated. However, it will not be possible to perform the capsulorhexis in very decentered lenses, and excessive tilt of the lens may make a complete rhexis difficult [43, 44].

Take-Home Message

- The approach and algorithm for the management of subluxated cataract will be based on the extension of zonular dehiscence, its etiology – that will determine whether it is progressive or not – and the density of the cataract. An exhaustive preoperative examination is mandatory.
- Stabilization of the capsular bag is needed in two ways: anterior to posterior axis and centrifugal distension. Hooks work providing vertical support,

while the main purpose of conventional CTR is the centrifugal redistribution of forces and distension of the bag.

- CTR should be implanted as late and as safely as possible.
- Scleral fixation is required in cases with more than 4 hours of zonular dehiscence, and it may be advisable in cases with less than 4 hours if the condition that led to subluxation has a progressive profile. Several devices were designed for the purpose of scleral fixation, and some of them provide also 360° or 120° of capsular bag distension (e.g., Cionni ring and CTS segment, respectively).
- The combination of a conventional CTR with a CTS allows to apply the different function of each device according to the step of the surgery, and it has resulted in the best approach in our experience.

References

1. Mendicute J, Ruiz M, López M, Irigoyen C, Sáez de Arregur S. Queratoplastia penetrante a cámara cerrada con cirugía de catarata. In: Lorente R, Mendicute J eds. Cirugía del Cristalino. Ponencia Sociedad Española de Oftalmología. 2008:1039–1055.
2. Kim WS, Kim KH. Challenges in cataract surgery. Berlin Heidelberg: Dislocation of crystalline lens and Marfan's syndrome. Springer-Verlag; 2016. p. 65–71.
3. Lorente BL, de Rojas Silva MV, Moore RL. Intraocular pressure changes before and after surgery for spontaneous in-the-bag intraocular lens dislocation. J Cataract Refract Surg. 2019;45:305–11.
4. Lorente R, de Rojas MV, Vazquez de Parga P, Moreno C, Landaluce ML, Domínguez R, Lorente B. Management of late spontaneous in-the-bag intraocular lens dislocation: a retrospective analysis of 45 cases. J Cataract Refract Surg. 2010;36:1270–82.
5. Buratto L, Brint SF, Caretti L. Cataract surgery in complicated cases. Congenital subluxation of the crystalline lens. SLACK Incorporated. 2013:11–25.
6. Hoffman RS, Snyder ME, Devgan U, Allen QB, Yeoh R, Braga-Mele R, for the ASCRS Cataract Clinical Committee, Challenging/Complicated Cataract Surgery Subcommittee. Management of the subluxated crystalline lens. J Cataract Refract Surg 2013;39:1904–1915.
7. Agarwal T, Saxena R, Vajpayee RB. Ultrasound biomicroscopy in lens "coloboma". Eur J Ophthalmol. 2003;13:390–1.
8. Lorente R, Lorente B, de Rojas MV, Moreno C, de Domingo B, Quiroga E. Desinserción/rotura zonular intraoperatoria. In: Poyales F. Complicaciones en la cirugía del cristalino. Monografías SECOIR Elsevier. Barcelona 2016:233–241.
9. Agarwal T, Sharma N, Vajpayee RB. In: Vajpayee RB, Sharma N, Pandey SK, Titiyal JS, editors. Phacoemulsification in subluxated lenses. Anshan Ltd Kent UK: Phacoemulsification surgery; 2006. p. 319–22.
10. Lee V, Bloom P. Microhook capsule stabilization for phacoemulsification in eyes with pseudoexfoliation-syndrome induced lens instability. J Cataract Refract Surg. 1999;25:1567–70.
11. Hasanee K, Butler M, Ahmed I. Capsular tension rings and related devices. Curr Opin Ophthalmol. 2006;17:31–41.
12. Weber C, Cionni R. All about capsular tension rings. Curr Opin Ophthalmol. 2015;26:10–5.
13. Vass C, Menapace R, Schmetterer K, Findl O, Rainer G, Steinek I. Prediction of pseudophakic capsular bag diameter based on biometric variables. J Cataract Refract Surg. 1999;25:1376–81.
14. Dong EY, Joo CK. Predictability for proper capsular tension ring size and intraocular lens size. Korean J Ophthalmol. 2001;15:22–6.
15. Chee SP, Jap A. Management of traumatic severely subluxated cataracts. Am J Ophthalmol. 2011;151:866–71.
16. Ahmed II, Cionni RJ, Kranemann C, Crandall AS. Optimal timing of capsular tension ring implantation: Miyake-apple video analysis. J Cataract Refract Surg. 2005;31:1809–13.
17. Jacob S, Agarwal A, Agarwal A, Agarwal S, Patel N, Lal V. Efficacy of capsular tension ring for phacoemulsification in eyes with zonular dialysis. J Cataract Refract Surg. 2003;29:315–21.
18. Angunawela RI, Little B. Fish-tail technique for capsular tension ring insertion. J Cataract Refract Surg. 2007;33(5):767–9.
19. Rixen JJ, Oetting TA. Fishtail on a line technique for capsular tension ring insertion. J Cataract Refract Surg. 2014;40:1068–70.
20. Praveen MR, Vasavada AR, Singh R. Phacoemulsification in subluxated cataract. Indian J Ophthalmol. 2003;51:147–54.
21. Cionni RJ, Osher RH. Management of profound zonular dialysis or weakness with a new endocapsular ring designed for scleral fixation. J Cataract Refract Surg. 1998;24:1299–306.
22. Cionni RJ, Osher RH, Marques DM, et al. Modified capsular tension ring for patients with congenital loss of zonular support. J Cataract Refract Surg. 2003;29:1668–73.
23. Price MO, Price FW Jr, Werner L, Berlie C, Mamalis N. Late dislocation of scleral-sutured posterior

chamber intraocular lenses. J Cataract Refract Surg. 2005;31:1320 6.
24. Hoffman RS, Howard F, Packer M. Scleral fixation without conjunctival dissection. J Cataract Refract Surg. 2006;32:1907–12.
25. Ahmed KII, Crandall AS. Ab externo scleral fixation of the Cionni modified capsular tension ring. J Cataract Refract Surg. 2001;27:977–81.
26. Samir A, Ayman M, Elsayed A, Alyan A, Lotfy A. Double-flanged polypropylene suture for scleral fixation of Cionni capsule tension ring. Clin Ophthalmol. 2020;14:1055–8.
27. Hasanee K, Ahmed K II. Capsular tension rings: update on endocapsular support devices. Ophthalmol Clin N Am. 2006;19:507–19.
28. Bahar I, Kaiserman I, Rootman D. Cionni endocapsular ring implantation in Marfan's syndrome. Br J Ophthalmol. 2007;91:1477–80.
29. Moreno-Montan˜e's J, Sainz C, Maldonado MJ. Intraoperative and postoperative complications of Cionni endocapsular ring implantation. J Cataract Refract Surg. 2003;29:492–7.
30. Malyugin B. Surgery of subluxated cataracts: Malyugin modified CTR. In: Chakrabarti A, editor. Cataract surgery in diseased eyes. Jaypee Brothers Medical Publishers (P) LTD New Delhi India; 2014. p. 114–8.
31. Vasavada AR, Praveen MR, Vasavada VA, et al. Cionni ring and in-the-bag intraocular lens implantation for subluxated lenses: a prospective case series. Am J Ophthalmol. 2012;153:1144–53.
32. Buttanri IB, Sevim MS, Esen D, Acar BT, Serin D, Acar S. Modified capsular tension ring implantation in eyes with traumatic cataract and loss of zonular support. J Cataract Refract Surg. 2012;38:431–6.
33. Kim EJ, Berg JP, Weikert MP, Kong L, Hamill MB, Koch DD, Yen KG. Scleral-fixated capsular tension rings and segments for ectopia lentis in children. Am J Ophthalmol. 2014;158:899–904.
34. Assia EI, Ton Y, Michaeli A. Capsule anchor to manage subluxated lenses: initial clinical experience. J Cataract Refract Surg. 2009;35:1372–9.
35. Yaguchi S, Yaguchi S, Asano Y, Kozawa T, Miyawaki T, Negishi K, Tsubota K. Repositioning and scleral fixation of subluxated lenses using a T-shaped capsule stabilization hook. J Cataract Refract Surg. 2011;37:1386–93.
36. Jacob S, Agarwal A, Agarwal A, Sathish K, Prakash G, Kumar DA. Glued endocapsular hemi-ring segment for fibrin glue-assisted sutureless transscleral fixation of the capsular bag in subluxated cataracts and intraocular lenses. J Cataract Refract Surg. 2012;38:193–201.
37. Canabrava S, Canedo AC, Lima D, Arancibia AEL, Dornclas LFB, Ribciro G. Novcl doublc-flangcd tcchnique for managing Marfan syndrome and microspherophakia. J Cataract Refract Surg. 2020;46:333–9.
38. Parkash RO, Mahajan S, Parkash TO, Parkash TO, RAi M. Nuclear scaffold: three dimensional indigenous capsular bag support combined with IOL scaffold and capsular tension ring to prevent posterior capsule rupture in zonulopathy. J Cataract Refract Surg. 2019;45:1696–700.
39. Arshinoff S. Capsule dyes and the USST [letter]. J Cataract Refract Surg. 2005;31:259–60.
40. Arshinoff SA, Norman R. Tri-soft shell technique J Cataract Refract Surg. 2013;39:1196–203.
41. Neuhan TF. Capsulorhexis. In: Steinert RF, editor. Cataract surgery: technique, complications, and management. Philadelphia: WB Saunders Co; 1995. p. 134–420.
42. Osher RH. Slow motion phacoemulsification approach (letter). J Cataract Refract Surg. 1993;19:667.
43. Nagy ZZ, Kranitz K, Takacs A, Filkorn T, Gergely R, Knorz MC. Intraocular femtosecond laser use in traumatic cataracts following penetrating and blunt trauma. J Refract Surg. 2012;28:151–3.
44. Agarwal A, Jacob S. Current and effective advantages of femto phacoemulsification. Curr Opin Ophthalmol. 2017;28:49–57.

Other References

Ahmed IK and coproducers. Capsular hemi-ring: next step in effective Management of Profound Zonular Dialysis, film presented at the ASCRS Symposium on Cataract, IOL and Refractive Surgery, San Francisco, California, USA, April 2003.

De Rojas MV, Álvarez M, Simón P, Zurutuza L, Escofet I. 6/0 polypropylene flanged technique for scleral fixation using 30g ultrathin wall needle. 39th Congress of the ESCRS. Amsterdam, 8–11 October 2021.

De Rojas MV, Álvarez M, Simón P, Zurutuza L, Escofet I. Scleral fixation of a capsular tension segment using 6/0 prolene and a 30g ultrathin wall needle. 36 Congress SECOIR 18–22 May 2021. First Video Award, Lens surgery category.

De Rojas MV, Lorente R, Álvarez M, Simón P, Lorente B, Zurutuza L, Rodríguez S. Zonular weakness, the main challenge of cataract surgery in pseudoexfoliation syndrome. Video. 37th Congress of the ESCRS Paris 14–18 September 2019.

IOL Implantation with Zonulopathy

7

David F. Chang

Top Five Challenges

- Avoid anterior capsule tear out due to capsular pseudoelasticity.
- Avoid zonular dialysis during hydrodissection or phaco.
- Avoid posterior capsular aspiration or tear during cortical cleanup.
- Prevent capsulorrhexis contraction postoperatively.
- Attain long-term IOL centration and stability.

Zonulopathy challenges the cataract surgeon by making virtually every surgical step more difficult, and by creating potential problems with the long-term capsular fixation of IOLs [1–10]. Common risk factors that predispose eyes to zonular weakness include pseudoexfoliation, prior trauma, advanced age, ultrabrunescent cataracts, and prior intraocular surgery, such as pars plana vitrectomy. Less common risk factors would be conditions such as Marfan syndrome, retinopathy of prematurity, retinitis pigmentosa, and myotonic dystrophy. Because of the progressive nature of the associated zonulopathy, it can be argued that cataract surgery in pseudoexfoliation eyes should be performed at the earlier end of the elective surgical window.

Preoperative Signs of Zonulopathy

The presence of a traumatic angle recession, mydriasis, iridodialysis, and vitreous herniation is invariably associated with traumatic zonulopathy. Suspicion should also be high with a history of traumatic hyphema. In the absence of preoperative phacodonesis or visible zonular dialysis, however, the extent of zonular weakness is usually not known until the initiation of surgery. Marques identified subtle signs of zonular weakness that include a wider iridolenticular gap (space between the iris and the anterior lens surface), a decentered nucleus, focal iridodonesis, and visibility of the peripheral lens equator upon lateral gaze [11].

With pseudoexfoliation, the zonulopathy is progressive, and the whitish deposits are found not only on the zonules but also on the posterior iris surface and pupillary margin. Therefore, smaller pupils are often associated with more advanced zonulopathy. Likewise, a brunescent nucleus is frequently accompanied by weak zon-

Supplementary Information The online version contains supplementary material available at [https://doi.org/10.1007/978-3-030-94530-5_7].

D. F. Chang (✉)
University of California, San Francisco,
San Francisco, CA, USA

J. L. Alió et al. (eds.), *Cataract Surgery*, Essentials in Ophthalmology,
https://doi.org/10.1007/978-3-030-94530-5_7

ules. The most ominous sign with pseudoexfoliation, however, is a shallow anterior chamber despite a normal axial length; this invariably indicates extremely weak zonules [4, 9]. One should consider a retrobulbar or peribulbar anesthetic block in cases carrying the higher risk of capsular rupture or dehiscence.

Capsulorrhexis

Performing the capsulorrhexis serves as a zonular stress test and provides the first opportunity to physically assess the presence and degree of zonulopathy [12]. Normal circumferential zonular tension puts the anterior capsule on stretch and provides peripheral counterfixation as the flap is maneuvered. With diffuse zonular laxity, the anterior capsule is not taut and may be difficult to incise with the cystotome, as though the needle was dull (Fig. 7.1). If the needle tip indents rather than incises the central anterior capsule, a halo-shaped light reflex may be seen. The lack of normal centripetal zonular tension may cause anterior capsule wrinkling as the cystotome or forceps advance the flap (Fig. 7.2). With extreme zonular weakness, the entire lens may start to move along with the cystotome or capsule forceps.

The more elastic the capsule is, the more difficult it is to control how it tears because it will first stretch before abruptly splitting radially. This natural elasticity is seen with the thin pediatric anterior capsule or adult posterior capsule. With insufficient, circumferential zonular traction, a capsule that is not taut will exhibit "pseudoelasticity" [12]. This means that although the anterior capsule is of normal adult thickness, it mimics the elastic behavior of a thin, elastic capsule. The lax and pliant peripheral anterior capsule tends to move along with and in the same direction as the flap; the capsular tear is difficult to control and will tend to veer radially. In addition to regrasping the flap more frequently with capsule forceps, the Little capsule tear out rescue technique is frequently necessary to control a tear that wants to escape radially because of weak zonules and pseudoelasticity [13].

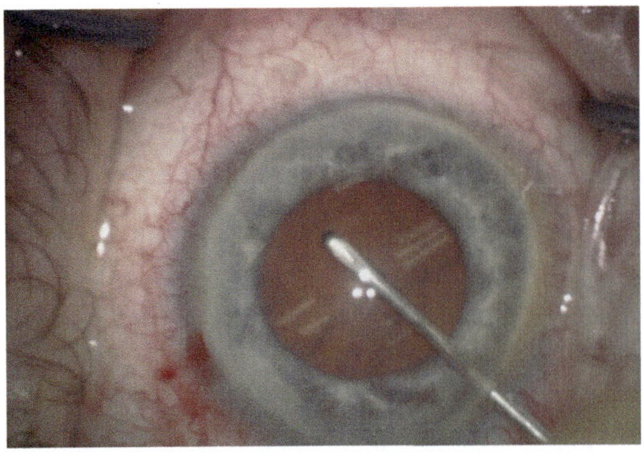

Fig. 7.1 Case with pseudoexfoliation and small pupil. The anterior capsule is lax and the cystotome needle tends to indent rather than incise the capsule

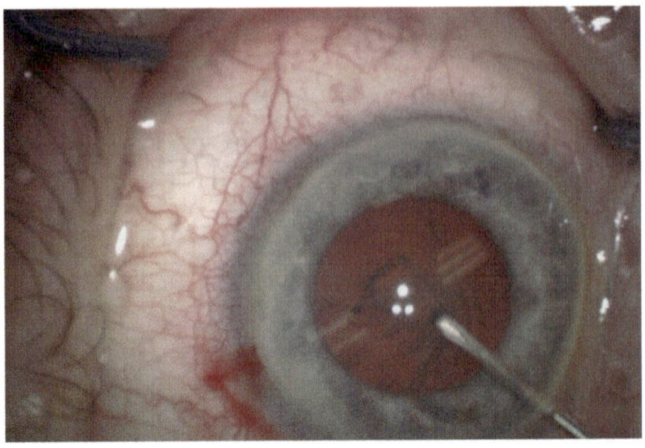

Fig. 7.2 The anterior capsule laxity causes folds to form as the cystotome pulls on the flap

A larger-diameter capsulorrhexis will facilitate nuclear and cortical removal, but it is much harder to control and complete in eyes with capsular pseudoelasticity. With weakened zonules the more peripherally the tear advances, the more it wants to veer radially. By comparison, a smaller-diameter capsulorrhexis is much easier to control and increases the ability to rescue a peripherally escaping tear. Because use of capsular retractors or a capsular tension ring (CTR) requires a continuous curvilinear capsulotomy, the overriding importance of achieving an intact capsulorrhexis dictates erring on the side of a smaller diameter that can be secondarily enlarged after the CTR and IOL have been implanted. Optimal visualization of the peripheral capsular region is important, and small pupils should be mechanically enlarged with retractors or an expansion ring.

Hydrodissection

Upon successful completion of the capsulorrhexis, loose zonules still pose multiple problems for the phacoemulsification and cortical aspiration steps. The nucleus is more difficult to rotate if zonular counterfixation of the capsular bag is deficient. One should always suspect significant circumferential zonular weakness if, despite proper hydrodissection, the nucleus does not spin easily [12]. With pseudoexfoliation, overly forceful attempts to rotate a brunescent nucleus may shear the zonules and cause a large zonular dialysis.

Although one can attempt to employ two instruments to bimanually rotate the nucleus, the safest strategy is to insert capsule retractors to facilitate nuclear rotation in the face of significant diffuse zonulopathy (Figs. 7.3, 7.4, and 7.5). By fixating the capsular bag to the eye wall, capsule retractors provide the necessary counterfixation and limit further zonular stress during nuclear rotation and disassembly.

Capsular Tension Rings

PMMA capsular tension rings partially compensate for a weakened zonular apparatus in several ways [14–26]. Using forceps or an injector, the ring can be inserted at any stage following completion of the capsulorrhexis [27, 28] (Fig. 7.9).

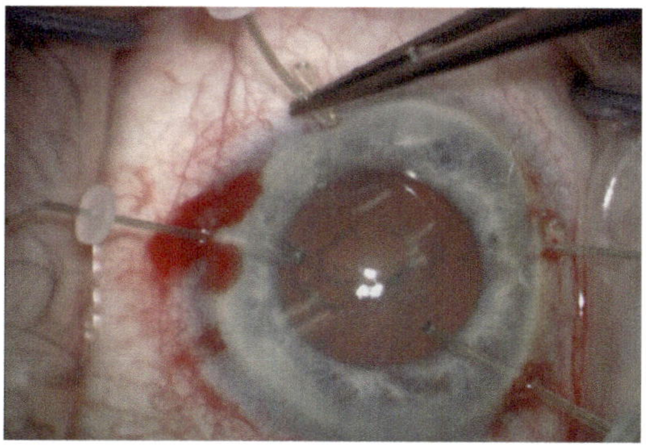

Fig. 7.3 Double-stranded capsule retractors (Chang Modification, Microsurgical Technologies, Redmond, Washington) are inserted through paracentesis incisions in four quadrants to support the capsular bag

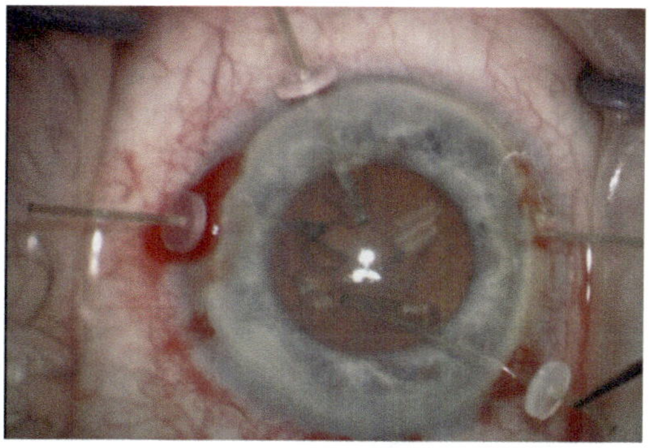

Fig. 7.4 The capsule retractors hook the capsulorrhexis edge without excessive tension. The rounded tip will not perforate through the capsular fornix and will not allow a CTR to pass through the terminal loop

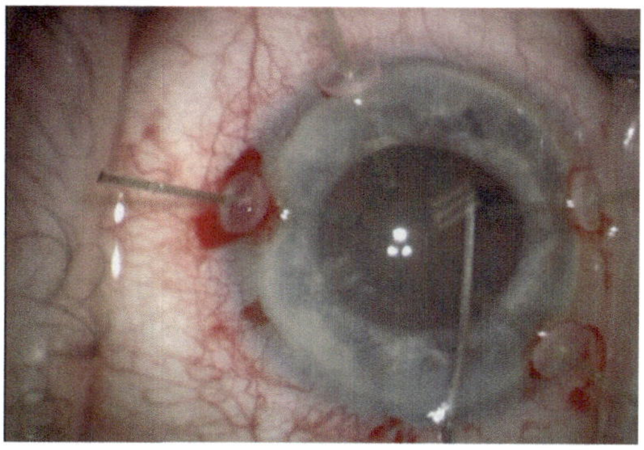

Fig. 7.5 Nuclear rotation is performed after inserting the capsular retractors

If there is a focal zonular dehiscence or weakness, the ring can redistribute mechanical forces, such as those of nuclear sculpting or IOL insertion, to areas of stronger zonular support. However, this benefit is lost if there is diffuse entire circumferential zonulopathy.

A second advantage is that centrifugal internal pressure applied by the ring makes the flaccid capsular bag tauter. This can reduce redundant capsule folds, forward trampolining of the posterior capsule, and inward collapsing of the capsular fornices toward any aspirating instrument tip. In the absence of a CTR, the stiff PMMA haptics of a three-piece foldable IOL can provide some of the same benefits during cortical aspiration. In addition, the IOL optic can block a floppy posterior capsule from vaulting toward the IA tip in the subincisional area.

The final benefit of a CTR is to mechanically counter progressive postoperative capsular contraction. Normally, centrifugal zonular tension resists capsulorrhexis shrinkage as the capsular bag contracts, but severe zonulopathy can lead to capsulophimosis. Excessive or asymmetric capsular contracture can decenter the IOL and further weaken the remaining zonules. This is a likely contributing factor in spontaneous late dislocation of the entire capsular bag with pseudoexfoliation [10, 29].

CTRs pose two potential disadvantages. Significant compression is required to implant the ring into the capsular bag. By deforming or displacing the bag CTR insertion may further weaken or shear remaining zonules. CTRs should never be inserted in the presence of an anterior or posterior capsule tear because of this compressive force. Compared to manual methods, using a CTR injector can reduce decentering capsular forces as the ring is implanted [27] (Fig. 7.10). CTRs may also impede cortical aspiration by pinning and trapping cortex in the capsular fornix. CTR insertion can be delayed until after the cortex has been removed by using capsule retractors to stabilize the bag during phaco. The Henderson modified CTR has a scalloped contour that facilitates cortical removal following placement and can be considered when a CTR must be implanted prior to cortical aspiration [30].

Capsule Retractors

In addition to enlarging a small pupil, flexible iris retractors can be used to support the capsular bag in the presence of severe zonulopathy [31–34]. Merriam first described using self-retaining iris retractors through paracentesis openings to hook and fixate the capsulorrhexis [31]. However, because the hooked ends are very short and flexible, iris retractors will tend to slip off of the anterior capsulotomy edge during phaco and will not support the equator of the capsular bag.

Richard Mackool designed the "Capsular Support System" (Impex, FCI Ophthalmics, Inc., Marshfield Hills, MA) with capsular hooks that are elongated enough to support the peripheral capsular fornix and not just the capsulorrhexis edge [35]. In this way, the retractors function as artificial zonules to stabilize the entire bag during phaco and cortical cleanup. Unlike capsular tension rings, capsule retractors provide support for the bag in the anterior-posterior direction and do not trap or ensnare the cortex. MicroSurgical Technology's (MST; Redmond, WA) disposable nylon capsular retractors are a newer alternative to the Mackool design. They feature a double-stranded design that creates a loop at the tip, which will not puncture through the equatorial capsule.

Capsule retractors can be inserted through limbal stab incisions at any stage including midway through the capsulorrhexis step (Fig. 7.3). Anywhere from one to four retractors may be deployed, depending on the extent and location of zonular weakness. By anchoring the bag to the limbus, the improved anteroposterior support and rotational stability facilitate hydrodissection and nuclear rotation. The self-retaining capsule retractors are also strong enough to center and immobilize a capsular bag that is partially subluxated due to a zonular dialysis. They also restrain the peripheral anterior and equatorial capsule from being accidentally aspirated and dehisced by the phaco or IA tip.

As a single strategy for preventing capsular complications due to severe zonular deficiency, capsule retractors are significantly more effective than a CTR [12]. The CTR redistributes instrument and mechanical forces across the strongest and intact zonules. Therefore, the greater the zonular defect or deficiency is, the less effective a CTR is at stabilizing the bag. If, after first inserting capsule retractors, the unsupported equatorial regions of the capsular bag tend to collapse inward toward the phaco tip, a CTR can be inserted to distend the equator of the bag to its proper anatomic configuration.

Although the tip of the capsule retractor is dull, it is possible for the hooks to tear the capsulorrhexis margin during surgery. A key objective is to support the capsular bag without excessive tension and stretching of the capsulorrhexis (Fig. 7.4). There is a tendency to overtighten the capsular retractors because their tension is initially adjusted with a soft eye. Inserting the phaco tip with irrigation suddenly displaces the nucleus and capsular bag posteriorly, which effectively tightens the retractors further. After inserting the phaco tip, it is therefore important to momentarily assess whether the capsule retractors have become so taut that they tent the capsulorrhexis edge. If so, they should be loosened slightly so that the anterior capsular rim does not tear during phacoemulsification.

Nuclear Emulsification

Fragile zonules are very prone to further damage during nuclear disassembly and emulsification. In addition, poor capsular bag stability increases the risk of capsular rupture. Surgeons must therefore avoid causing excessive nuclear movement with sculpting, chopping, or rotation. Phaco chop significantly reduces the stress placed on the zonules and capsule by replacing sculpting and cracking maneuvers with the mechanical force of the chopper instrument pushing centripetally against the phaco tip [12]. Because of the centrally directed instrument forces, horizontal chopping is particularly effective at avoiding nuclear tilt or displacement (Fig. 7.6). After initially bisecting the nucleus, one should attempt to elevate each hemi-nucleus out of the capsular bag where it can be further fragmented or emulsified within the supracapsular space.

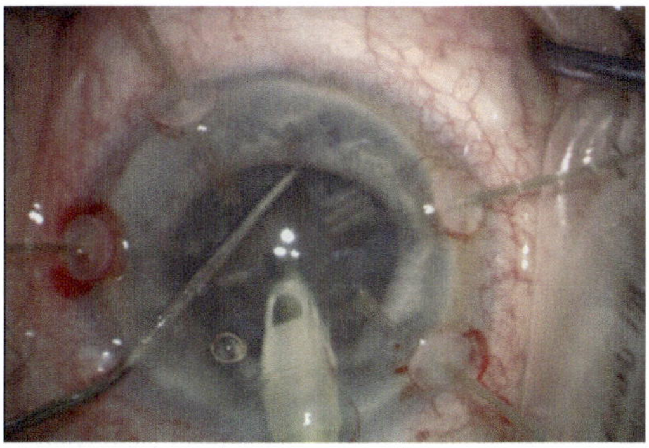

Fig. 7.6 Horizontal phaco chop bisects the nucleus with minimal capsular stress

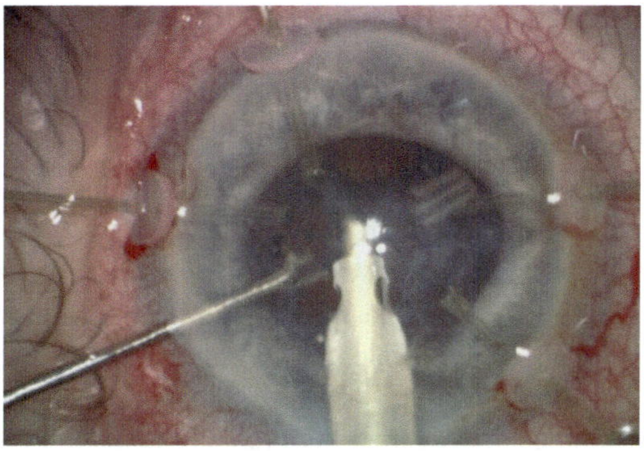

Fig. 7.7 Capsule retractors restrain the peripheral capsular fornix from being aspirated by the phaco tip. The vacuum setting is lowered for the epinucleus due to greater capsular laxity caused by insufficient centrifugal zonular stretch

During nuclear fragment emulsification and cortical cleanup, one should anticipate that deficient centrifugal zonular tension will result in greater posterior capsule laxity than normal. The flaccid posterior capsule will tend to trampoline toward any aspirating tip as the last nuclear fragments, epinucleus, and cortex are removed. Because the nuclear bulk will initially mask this situation, one must be more vigilant as increasingly more nucleus is removed. A preprogrammed vacuum setting that usually avoids post-occlusion surge with routine cases may not be safe with a lax posterior capsule that is lacking normal centrifugal zonular tension. Therefore, consider decreasing the vacuum to lower than normal levels to prevent trampolining of the capsule (Fig. 7.7). Finally, repeatedly inflating the capsular bag with a dispersive OVD will stretch and tense a flaccid posterior capsule to prevent it from vaulting toward the aspirating instrument as the final fragments and epinucleus are aspirated [12]. Guarding the phaco tip by placing the horizontal chopper tip beneath it is another strategy. These safety measures are especially important if there is little or no epinuclear shell present.

Cortical Cleanup

Safely aspirating and stripping cortex from its capsular attachments requires that the posterior capsule be taut. With deficient circumferential zonular tension, the lax posterior capsule tends to cling to epinucleus and cortex that is being aspirated. Inadvertently aspirating the more pliant anterior capsule may cause a zonular dialysis. Redundant capsular folds can be easily ensnared by the aspirating instrument or snagged by a capsule polisher. Effective hydrodissection is critical because the more easily lens material separates from a floppy capsule, the less likely it is for the capsular folds to be aspirated. Stripping the cortex tangentially rather than radially helps to distribute the tractional forces across as large an area of zonules as possible (Fig. 7.8).

Continually reinflating the capsular bag with a dispersive OVD is an excellent strategy for removing cortex from a floppy bag. This will place both anterior and posterior capsules on stretch and prevent a pliant posterior capsule from trampolining toward the aspiration port. In this situation, cortical aspiration can be performed either with or without irrigation (dry technique). Dispersive agents are preferable to cohesive viscoelastics because they better resist aspiration.

Bimanual IA instrumentation provides several advantages in the presence of weak zonules. The ability to alternate between two aspirating ports improves access to the subincisional cortex, which is especially challenging to remove if the capsulorrhexis diameter is small and the posterior capsule is lax. A dual port system also means that the aspirating port can be kept facing the cornea rather than toward the equator of the capsular bag. Without a constraining infusion sleeve, the surgeon is better able to reach across to the opposite equatorial quadrants where the aspirating port can be safely blocked with cortex before vacuum builds. Finally, in the presence of a zonular dialysis, the ability to dissociate the irrigating and aspirating tips can help to prevent misdirection of irrigating fluid through the zonular defect.

If possible, CTR insertion should be delayed until the cortex has been removed [12, 27]. Fully expanding the capsular bag with OVD prevents the leading CTR tip from snagging or perforating posterior capsular folds during its insertion. Brian Little has described the fish tail method of reducing zonular stress when inserting a ring without an injector [28]. As mentioned earlier, using an injector has the advantage of introducing the CTR into the capsular bag without excessively stretching the capsulorrhexis [27]. One can either load the ring manually with a reusable metal injector or use a pre-loaded, disposable plastic injector (Morcher) (Fig. 7.9). The injector tip should be positioned as far peripherally within the bag as possible in order to minimize lateral displacement of the capsular bag as the ring emerges (Fig. 7.10). If used, capsular retractors should be left in place to stabilize the bag and counter the lateral decentering forces of the CTR as it is injected [36]. The retractors can then be removed prior to IOL implantation (Fig. 7.11).

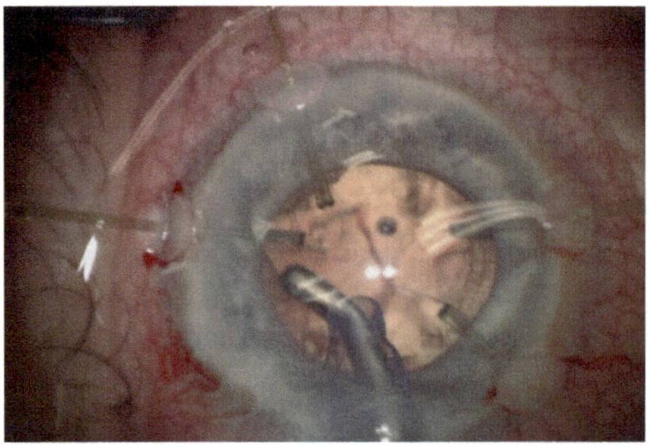

Fig. 7.8 Unlike a CTR, capsule retractors do not trap the cortex. Tangential stripping motions are employed with abnormal counterfixation caused by focal or diffuse zonulopathy

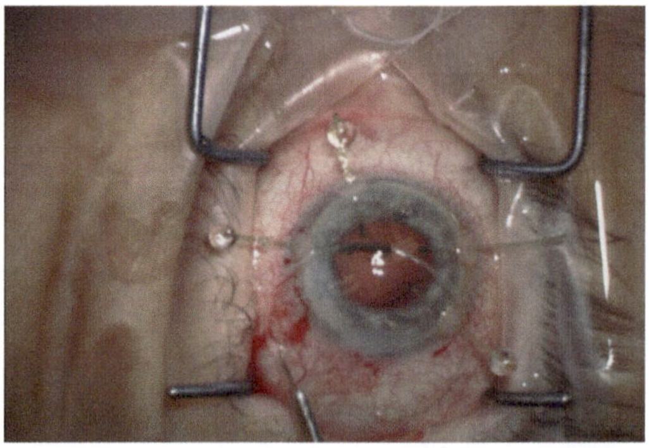

Fig. 7.9 The CTR is loaded with an injector and placement is delayed until after cortical removal

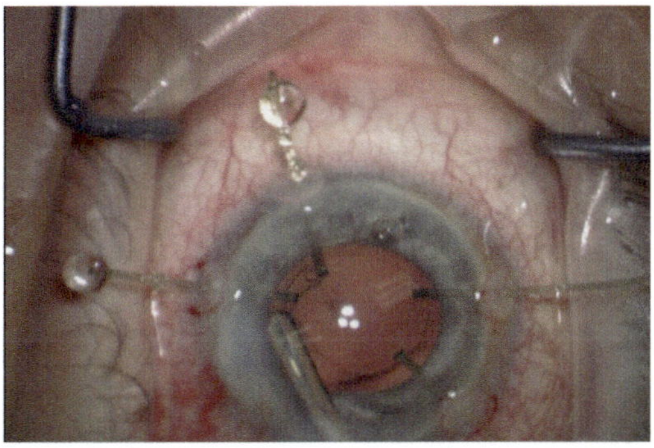

Fig. 7.10 The CTR is inserted with the injector tip aimed toward the peripheral bag to minimize lateral bag displacement with the expansion of the ring. The capsule retractors further stabilize the bag against the decentering forces of the CTR implantation

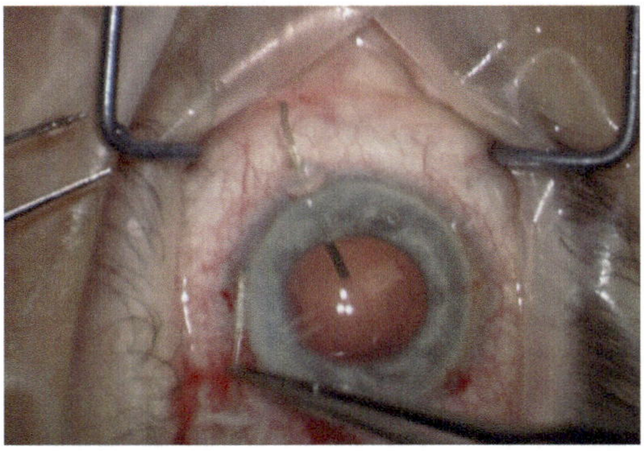

Fig. 7.11 The capsule retractors are removed prior to IOL implantation

IOL Selection and Implantation

With any significant zonulopathy, intracapsular IOL implantation should be combined with a CTR. The objective is to prevent capsulophimosis, reduce progressive centripetal zonular stress caused by capsulorrhexis contraction, and prevent IOL decentration caused by asymmetric capsular fibrosis [9, 10, 37]. With pseudoexfoliation even mild evidence of zonulopathy should warrant CTR placement because of the likelihood of progressive zonulopathy. Although a CTR alone may not prevent late bag-IOL dislocation, it affords the surgical option of suture fixating the ring to the sclera should bag subluxation occur in the future [38–43]. With a zonular dialysis or severe zonulopathy, a variety of intracapsular devices can be sutured to the sclera to enhance long-term capsular bag support. These include the Cionni and Malyugin CTR modifications (Morcher), the Ahmed capsular tension segment (Morcher GmbH, Stuttgart, Germany), the Assia Anchor, and others [44–48]. Scleral suture fixation is more surgically demanding and requires that the device be available in the operating room.

An underutilized alternative to implanting these devices is to place a three-piece foldable IOL in the ciliary sulcus [37](Figs. 7.12, 7.13, 7.14, 7.15, and 7.16). The haptics will abut against the ciliary body and provide supplemental two-point fixation that is independent of the zonular complex. This will stabilize the bag against inertial IOL displacement forces generated by lateral saccadic eye movements. These forces would otherwise be born solely by the abnormal zonular complex. If sulcus IOL placement is elected because of severe zonular weakness, a CTR should still be implanted to prevent capsulorrhexis contraction with progressive zonular dehiscence postoperatively. While both haptics remain in the sulcus, capsulorrhexis-optic capture will also prevent capsulophimosis, IOL decentration (if the capsulotomy is centered), and late rotation of the haptics through an occult zonular defect. In addition, the same IOL power selected for intracapsular fixation can be used. However, capsulorrhexis-optic capture will often trap OVD behind the optic. The distended capsular bag may produce a myopic shift due to the more anterior axial optic location, requiring a

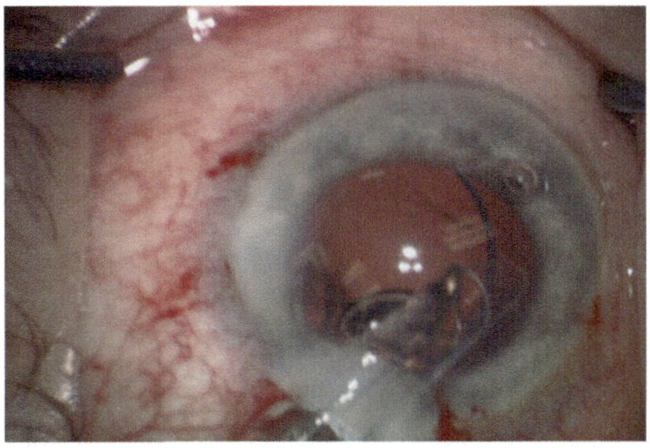

Fig. 7.12 A three-piece hydrophobic acrylic IOL (Sensar AR40, J&J Surgical) is implanted into the sulcus because of severe diffuse zonulopathy

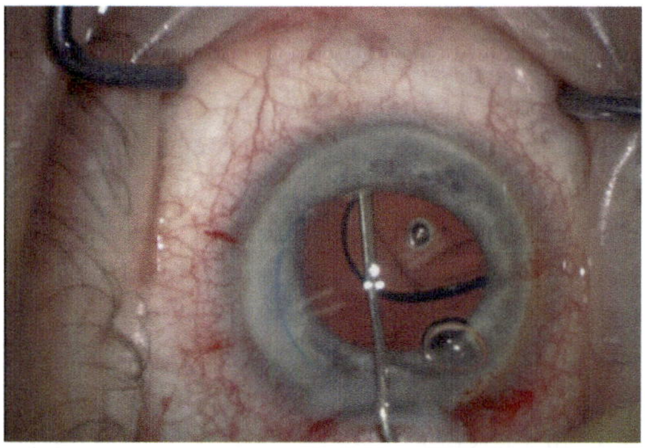

Fig. 7.13 The trailing haptic is dialed into the ciliary sulcus

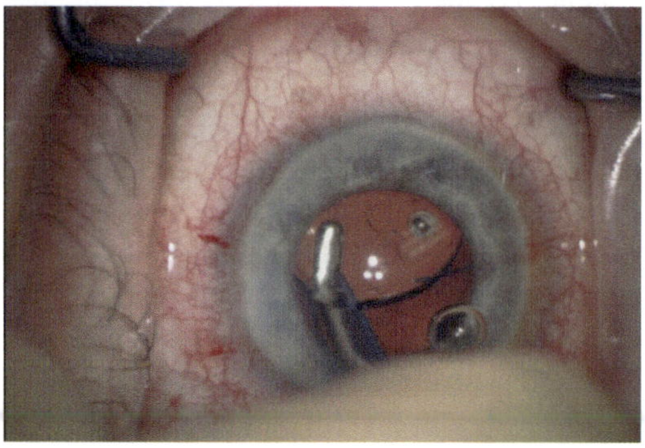

Fig. 7.14 OVD behind the optic is removed with the IA tip, prior to capsulorrhexis-optic capture

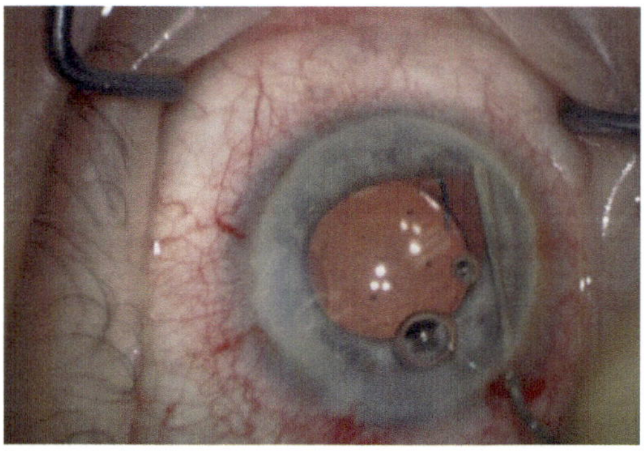

Fig. 7.15 The haptics are rotated so that they abut against the nasal and temporal ciliary body prior to capturing the optic with the capsulorrhexis

Nd:YAG posterior capsulotomy to empty the distended capsular compartment. To prevent this, after the IOL haptics are positioned in the sulcus, the IA instrument tip should displace the optic laterally in order to evacuate most of the OVD from within the capsular bag (Fig. 7.14). If possible, the IOL is then rotated so that the haptics are aligned along the 180-degree axis, prior to capturing the optic with the capsulorrhexis (Fig. 7.15). This allows the haptics to stabilize the capsular bag from lateral saccadic decentering forces. Single-piece foldable IOLs should not be placed in the sulcus, and the haptics are too short to provide supplemental two-point fixation.

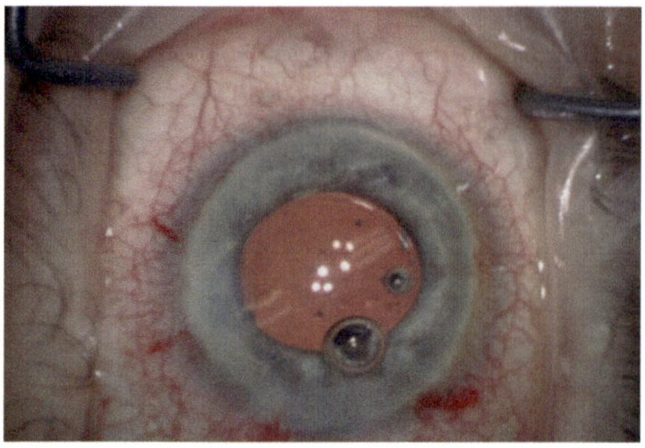

Fig. 7.16 The haptics remain in the ciliary sulcus, while the optic is captured with the capsulorrhexis

Take-Home Notes

- Use capsule retractors to support capsular bag.
- Horizontal phaco chop reduces zonular stress; try elevating heminuclei out of the capsular bag.
- Expand capsular bag with dispersive OVD to prevent trampolining.
- Delay CTR implantation until after cortical removal.
- Implant three-piece IOL in sulcus if there is diffuse zonulopathy.

References

1. Fine IH, Hoffman RS. Phacoemulsification in the presence of pseudoexfoliation: challenges and options. J Cataract Refract Surg. 1997;23:160–5.
2. Avramides S, Traianidis P, Sakkias G. Cataract surgery and lens implantation in eyes with exfoliation syndrome. J Cataract Refract Surg. 1997;23:583–7.

3. Kuchle M, Viestenz A, Martus P, et al. Anterior chamber depth and complications during cataract surgery in eyes with pseudoexfoliation syndrome. Am J Ophthalmol. 2000;129:281–185.
4. Shingleton BJ, Heltzer J, O'Donoghue MW. Outcomes of phacoemulsification in patients with and without pseudoexfoliation syndrome. J Cataract Refract Surg. 2003;29:1080–6.
5. Blecher MH, Kirk MR. Surgical strategies for the management of zonular compromise. Curr Opin Ophthalmol. 2008;19:31–5. Review
6. Shingleton BJ, Crandall AS, Ahmed K. Pseudoexfoliation and the cataract surgeon: preoperative, intraoperative, and postoperative issues related to intraocular pressure, cataract, and intraocular lenses. J Cataract Refract Surg. 2009;35:1101–20.
7. Belovay GW, Varma DK, Ahmed II. Cataract surgery in pseudoexfoliation syndrome. Curr Opin Ophthalmol. 2010;21:25–34. Review
8. Shingleton BJ, Marvin AC, Heier JS, O'Donoghue MW, Laul A, Wolff B, Rowland A. Pseudoexfoliation: High risk factors for zonule weakness and concurrent vitrectomy during phacoemulsification. J Cataract Refract Surg. 2010;36:1261–9.
9. Fontana L, Coassin M, Iovieno A, Moramarco A, Cimino L. Cataract surgery in patients with pseudoexfoliation syndrome: current updates. Clin Ophthalmol. 2017;11:1377–83.
10. Jahan FS, Mamalis N, Crandall AS. Spontaneous late dislocation of intraocular lens within the capsular bag in pseudoexfoliation patients. Ophthalmology. 2001;108:1727–31.
11. Marques DMV, Marquess FF, Osher RH. Subtle signs of zonular damage. J Cataract Refract Surg. 2004;30:1295–9.
12. Chang DF. Chapter 23: Strategies for weak zonules. In: Chang DF, editor. Phaco Chop and advanced Phaco techniques. Slack; 2013.
13. Little BC, Smith JH, Packer M. Little capsulorhexis tear-out rescue. J Cataract Refract Surg. 2006;32:1420–2.
14. Nagamato T, Bissen-Miyajima H. A ring to support the capsular bag after continuous curvilinear capsulorhexis. J Cataract Refract Surg. 1994;20:417–20.
15. Legler UFC, Witschel BM. The capsular ring: a new device for complicated cataract surgery. Ger J Ophthalmol. 1994;3:265.
16. Cionni RJ, Osher RH. Endocapsular ring approach to the subluxed cataractous lens. J Cataract Refract Surg. 1995;21:245–9.
17. Gimbel HV, Sun R, Heston JP. Management of zonular dialysis in phacoemulsification and IOL implantation using the capsular tension ring. Ophthalmic Surg Lasers. 1997;28:273–81.
18. Menapace R, Findl O, Georgopoulos M, Rainer G, Vass C, Schmetterer K. The capsular tension ring: designs, applications, and techniques. J Cataract Refract Surg. 2000;26:898–912.
19. Bayraktar S, Altan T, Küçüksümer Y, Yılmaz ÖF. Capsular tension ring implantation after capsulorhexis in phacoemulsification of cataracts associated with pseudoexfoliation syndrome; intraoperative complications and early postoperative findings. J Cataract Refract Surg. 2001;27:1620–8.
20. Gimbel HV, Sun R. Clinical applications of capsular tension rings in cataract surgery. Ophthalmic Surg Lasers. 2002;33:44–53.
21. Lee D-H, Shin S-C, Joo C-K. Effect of a capsular tension ring on intraocular lens decentration and tilting after cataract surgery. J Cataract Refract Surg. 2002;28:843–6. (reduces tilt and decentration).
22. Jacob S, Agarwal A, Agarwal A, Agarwal S, Patel N, Lal V. Efficacy of a capsular tension ring for phacoemulsification in eyes with zonular dialysis. J Cataract Refract Surg. 2003;29:315–21.
23. Price FW Jr, Mackool RJ, Miller KM, Koch P, Oetting TA, Johnson AT. Interim results of the United States investigational device study of the Ophtec capsular tension ring. Ophthalmology. 2005;112:460–5.
24. Hasanee K, Butler M, Ahmed II. Capsular tension rings and related devices: current concepts. Curr Opin Ophthalmol. 2006;17:31–41. Review
25. Hasanee K, Ahmed II. Capsular tension rings: update on endocapsular support devices. Ophthalmol Clin N Am. 2006;19:507–19. Review
26. Boomer JA, Jackson DW. Anatomic evaluation of the Morcher capsular tension ring by ultrasound biomicroscopy. J Cataract Refract Surg. 2006;32:846–8.
27. Ahmed IIK, Cionn RJ, Kranemann C, Crandall AS. Optimal timing of capsular tension ring implantation: Miyake-Apple video analysis. J Cataract Refract Surg. 2005;31:1809–13.
28. Angunawela RI, Little B. Fish-tail technique for capsular tension ring insertion. J Cataract Refract Surg. 2007;33:767–9.
29. Chang DF. Prevention of bag-fixated IOL dislocation in Pseudoexfoliation (letter). Ophthalmology. 2002;109:5–6.
30. Henderson BA, Kim JY. Modified capsular tension ring for cortical removal after implantation. J Cataract Refract Surg. 2007;33:1688–90.
31. Merriam JC, Zheng L. Iris hooks for phacoemulsification of the subluxated lens. J Cataract Refract Surg. 1997;23:1295–7.
32. Lee V, Bloom P. Microhook capsule stabilization for phacoemulsification in eyes with pseudoexfoliation-syndrome-induced lens instability. J Cataract Refract Surg. 1999;25:1567–70.
33. Santoro S, Sannace C, Cascella MC, Lavermicocca N. Subluxated lens: phacoemulsification with iris hooks. J Cataract Refract Surg. 2003;29:2269–73.
34. Sethi HS, Sinha A, Pal N, Saxena R. Modified flexible iris retractor to retract superior iris and support inferior capsule in eyes with iris coloboma and inferior zonular deficiency. J Cataract Refract Surg. 2006;32:715–6.
35. Mackool RJ. Capsule stabilization for phacoemulsification (letter). J Cataract Refract Surg. 2000;26:629.
36. Grove K, Condon G, Erny BC, Chang DF, Kim T. Complication from combined use of capsule retrac-

tors and capsular tension rings in zonular dehiscence. J Cataract Refract Surg. 2015;41:2576–9.
37. Chang DF. Chapter 13: Step-wise IOL fixation strategies for varying severity of zonulopathy. In: Chang DF, editor. Advanced IOL fixation techniques. Slack; 2019.
38. Ahmed II, Chen SH, Kranemann C, Wong DT. Surgical repositioning of dislocated capsular tension rings. Ophthalmology. 2005;112:1725–33.
39. Gross JG, Kikame GT, Weinberg DV. In-the-bag intraocular lens dislocation: the dislocated in-the-bag lens study group. Am J Ophthalmol. 2004;137(4):630–5.
40. Gimbel HV, Condon GP, Kohnen T, et al. Late in-the-bag intraocular lens dislocation: incidence, prevention, and management. J Cataract Refract Surg. 2005;31:2193–204.
41. Davis D, Brubaker J, Espandar L, et al. Late in-the-bag spontaneous intraocular lens dislocation: evaluation of 86 consecutive cases. Ophthalmology. 2009;116:664–70.
42. Lorente R, de Rojas V, Vazquez de Parga P, et al. Management of late spontaneous in-the-bag intraocular lens dislocation: retrospective analysis of 45 cases. J Cataract Refract Surg. 2010;36:1270–82.
43. Werner L, Zaugg B, Neuhann T, Burrow M, Tetz M. In-the-bag capsular tension ring and intraocular lens subluxation or dislocation: a series of 23 cases. Ophthalmology. 2012;119:266–71.
44. Cionni RJ, Osher RH, Marques DMV, et al. Modified capsular tension ring for patients with congenital loss of zonular support. J Cataract Refract Surg. 2003;29:1668–73.
45. Moreno-Montañés J, Sainz C, Maldonado MJ. Intraoperative and postoperative complications of Cionni endocapsular ring implantation. J Cataract Refract Surg. 2003;29:492–7.
46. Assia EI, Ton Y, Michaeli A. Capsule anchor to manage subluxated lenses: initial clinical experience. J Cataract Refract Surg. 2009;35:1372–9.
47. Vasavada AR, Praveen MR, Vasavada VA, Yeh RY, Srivastava S, Koul A, Trivedi RH. Cionni ring and in-the-bag intraocular lens implantation for subluxated lenses: a prospective case series. Am J Ophthalmol. 2012;153:1144–53.
48. Buttanri IB, Sevim MS, Esen D, Acar BT, Serin D, Acar S. Modified capsular tension ring implantation in eyes with traumatic cataract and loss of zonular support. J Cataract Refract Surg. 2012;38:431–6.

Cataract Surgery in Eyes with Ocular Surface Problems and Severe Dry Eye

8

Christoph Holtmann and Gerd Geerling

Top Five Bullet Points

- Dry eye disease (DED) and cataracts are often comorbid conditions. Severe ocular surface disease (OSD) can be associated with inflammatory conditions such as graft-versus-host disease (GvHD) or mucous membrane pemphigoid (MMP). These are often treated with steroids, which in turn are cataractogenic.
- The decision to perform cataract surgery in patients with severe DED has to balance the functional impairment due to cataract-induced loss of vision against the risk of preoperative (e.g., challenging biometry), intraoperative, or postoperative complications.
- Intraoperative considerations have to address, e.g., reduced intraocular visibility, with associated risk of complications, measures to avoid additional ocular surface damage such as from mechanical manipulation, or light- and medication-associated toxicity.
- Postoperatively, frequent application of unpreserved lubricants, avoidance of epitheliotoxic topical NSAIDs, and intensive follow-up to diagnose and treat complications early are recommended.
- With proactive management and intense perioperative therapy, a good outcome with improved visual acuity can be achieved also in comorbid cataract in patients with severe DED.

Supplementary Information The online version contains supplementary material available at [https://doi.org/10.1007/978-3-030-94530-5_8].

C. Holtmann · G. Geerling (✉)
Department of Ophthalmology, University Hospital Duesseldorf, Duesseldorf, Germany
e-mail: Christoph.Holtmann@med.uni-duesseldorf.de; g.geerling@med.uni-duesseldorf.de

Part 1

Definition of DED and Epidemiology

Dry eye disease (DED) is a very frequent diagnosis in ophthalmological practice and often impacts patients' quality of life. It is accompanied by instability and increased osmolarity of the tear film and inflammation of the ocular surface [1]. According to the Tear Film & Ocular Surface Society (TFOS), DED is defined as a "multifactorial disease of the ocular surface characterized by a loss of homeostasis of the tear film, and accompanied by ocular symptoms, in which tear film instability and hyper-osmolarity, ocular surface inflammation and damage, and

J. L. Alió et al. (eds.), *Cataract Surgery*, Essentials in Ophthalmology,
https://doi.org/10.1007/978-3-030-94530-5_8

neuro-sensory abnormalities play etiological roles" [2]. DED has a rising prevalence of up to 75% in some populations. Its risk factors include age, female gender, Sjögren's syndrome, contact lens wear, Meibomian gland dysfunction (MGD), ethnicity, and other genetic factors [3]. Likewise, cataract is an age-associated leading cause of vision loss. In the USA, it alone is responsible for about 60% of all Medicare costs related to vision [4]. The effect of age-related cataract and DED can be expected to grow in aging populations. Given the overlapping demographics, it comes as no surprise that dry eye and cataracts are often comorbid conditions [5].

Causes of Ocular Surface Problems/ Severe Dry Eye

Severe DED is often caused by systemic conditions. Primary Sjögren's syndrome or a secondary cause such as rheumatoid arthritis, systemic lupus erythematosus, granulomatosis with polyangiitis, as well as sarcoid or graft-versus-host diseases (GvHD) can lead to ocular surface problems [2]. Non-Sjögren tear deficiencies can be caused by trachoma, cicatricial mucous membrane pemphigoid with ocular involvement, neurotrophic keratopathy, or long-term contact lens use.

Causes of Cataract in DED

As these chronic diseases progress, patients are often treated long term with systemic and topical steroids. With increased longevity, those patients are more likely to suffer from chronic inflammation and encounter late therapy-associated side effects, such as clinically significant cataract [6]. De Melo Franco et al. found that in chronic GvHD patients, posterior subcapsular cataract was the most common type of cataract, reflecting the high incidence of systemic corticosteroid use in these patients [6]. Additional reasons for the development of cataracts in severe DED patients can be associated chronic intraocular inflammation or previous surgery such as penetrating keratoplasty.

Impact of Cataract Surgery on DED

Many patients who have undergone cataract surgery complain of dry eye and symptoms of irritation postoperatively [7, 8]. These surgery-related symptoms have multiple causes: reduced tear breakup time (TBUT), squamous metaplasia of conjunctiva, phototoxic damage caused by microscope light, epithelial damage caused by frequent irrigation, decreased corneal sensitivity, as well as elevated inflammatory cytokines in tears [7, 9, 10]. The ocular surface is prone to damage from exposure and dryness during the surgery as well as intra- and postoperative application of preservative containing eye drops, inducing corneal epithelial toxicity [11–13]. A reduction in conjunctival goblet cell density as well as an impairment of Meibomian gland function due to inflammation, bacterial colonization, and/or preservative-containing postoperative medication are also present after cataract surgery [5, 14]. Corneal incisions as well as limbal relaxing incisions induce localized damage to the corneal nerves with subsequent reduced corneal sensation [15]. Phacoemulsification itself can affect or interrupt the neurogenic response of the ocular surface and decrease tear secretion volume [8]. Ophthalmologists should be mindful of the numerous detrimental intraoperative effects of cataract surgery on the ocular surface [3, 16].

Impact of DED on Cataract Surgery

Preoperatively

The decision to perform cataract surgery in patients with severe DED has to balance the functional impairment due to cataract-induced against OSD-related loss of vision against the risk of intraoperative or postoperative complications [17]. Visual function of patients with severe DED becomes abnormal due to an expanded interblink interval (e.g., with reduced blinking reflex), resulting in epithelial irregularity and even corneal scars, all generating higher-order optical aberrations and loss of contrast sensitivity leading to significant visual impairment [18, 19]. Therefore, it is crucial to determine whether the visual acuity is reduced because of severe DED or due to cataract preoperatively. While visual acuity usually fluctuates in DED, vision loss due to cataract is slowly progressing, but not fluctuating. When taking the patient's history, this should be addressed. In patients with Sjögren's syndrome, for example, surface asymmetry index, mean astigmatism, and potential visual acuity improve after instillation of artificial tears [20]. Other measures to improve visual acuity include the use of rigid gas permeable contact lenses [21]. Limbal or scleral contact lenses in particular allow for tear exchange under the contact lens and improve the patients' visual acuity in addition to reducing symptoms related to severe DED by decreasing tear evaporation [21–23].

If the ocular surface is not stable prior to surgery, intensive topical as well as systemic therapy may be necessary. Besides lubricants, anti-inflammatory agents play a major role in the treatment of moderate-to-severe DED because of the critical role of inflammation in the pathogenesis of OSD [15]. The most beneficial effect of steroids is the rapid onset of action and making them first choice in circumstances that immediate response is intended [12]. There is evidence that the addition of cyclosporine drops is beneficial and may be a useful adjunct in patients with pre-existing DED, sparing steroids in the long term, but being associated with a sometimes strong initial burning sensation [3, 24]. Autologous serum functions as a biological tear substitute and is able to stabilize the ocular tear film and ocular surface [25–28]. The concept of temporary or permanent occlusion of one or both puncta to retain tears on the ocular surface by blocking their drainage is another option [29]. With present Meibomian gland dysfunction, treatment regimens include the regular use of warm compressors, lid margin hygiene, treatment of demodex, and the use of systemic tetracycline antibiotics as well as topical azithromycin [3, 29]. The use of food/nutritional supplements in this context is seen controversial: While some studies report improved dry eye symptoms and ocular surface conditions (e.g., after vitamin D supplements [30]), scientific evidence is not strong enough to recommend the supplementation of omega-3 and omega-6 fatty acids in the treatment of severe DED [31–33].

Preoperative treatment of Meibomian gland dysfunction with vectored thermal pulsation before cataract surgery prevents the decline of TBUT postoperatively [34]. Surgical treatment for severe DED includes amniotic membrane transplantation in the presence of a persistent epithelial defect and, if needed, an oral mucosa graft for fornix reconstruction [3]. Severe diseases such as ocular cicatricial pemphigoid should be controlled for a minimum of 1 year before proceeding to cataract surgery [15, 17].

Lens Power Calculation

Even in healthy corneas, tear film surface regularity and corneal power readings change significantly following the addition of eye drops, such as sodium fluorescein [35]. Preoperative planning is even more difficult in severe DED since the precision of biometry varies in this patient group. There is more variability in average K readings and anterior corneal astigmatism in DED patients with a hyperosmolar tear film resulting in significant differences in intraocular lens (IOL) power calculations [36]. Osmolarity in the hyperosmolar group was 327.8 +/− 10.5 (mOsml/I.) versus 301.1 +/− 4.9 (mOsml/I.) in the normal group. In the hyperosmolar group, 10% had a difference of calculated IOL power of more than 0.5 diopters, the highest difference being 5.5 diopters, while the difference in the normal group was less than 0.5 diopters in all cases. Intensive preoperative hourly preservative-free topical lubricant therapy as well as an ointment overnight with the goal of improving the corneal staining to obtain accurate preoperative diagnostic imaging improves biometric IOL power calculation [37, 38]. Especially in cases of suspected or obvious DED, repeat IOL power calculations are advisable to ensure a stable biometry. Placement of a self-retaining cryopreserved amniotic membrane (PROKERA; Bio-Tissue, Miami, FL, USA) for 1 week has been advocated in more severe DED for the same purpose. Optical biometry should then be performed within 24 hours of amniotic membrane removal [37, 39].

Choice of IOL

The corneal tear film is the major refractive plane of the eye, and therefore its integrity is very important when choosing a lens implant. The choice of the intraocular lens (IOL) regarding its functionality (monofocal, multifocal, EDOF) will depend on the severity of tear film and ocular surface alterations as well as the patient's desires. Foldable preloaded monofocal aspheric IOLs will be the standard choice. However, adjustments need to be taken in complicated cases, e.g., posterior capsular rupture, anterior vitrectomy, and instable anterior capsulorhexis edge. As astigmatism is more prone to fluctuate in DED, toric IOLs or multifocal intraocular lens implantation is not recommended [40]. While there is no clear definition of when to avoid toric or multifocal IOLs, it seems sensible not to implant IOLs with advanced features, as patient expectations should be guarded in severe DED, e.g., persistent punctate keratopathy with 2 to 3+ staining according to the Oxford grading [41]. In the unlikely case that spectacle independence is demanded by the individual patient, despite severe burden of DED, the surgeon should clearly highlight the limitations of and advise against such lens implants.

Dysphotopsia and loss of contrast sensitivity are an issue with multifocal, less so with enhanced depth of focus (EDOF) IOLs even in the absence of chronic and severe ocular surface disease [42, 43]. The data on this topic is limited; however, ocular comorbidities such as severe DED limit reaching target refraction of multifocal or EDOF IOL implantation and increase patient dissatisfaction due to blurry or foggy vision both for distance and near, as well as complaints attributed to residual refractive error (57%) and exacerbation of DED postoperatively [41]. In a larger cohort of 399 patients with DED, only 3.36% of implanted IOLs were aspheric multifocal, 2 (0.48%) aspheric toric, and 2 (0.48%) aspheric toric-multifocal IOLs [44].

Timing of Surgery

The timing of surgery must also be chosen carefully. Postponing cataract surgery due to anticipated intraoperative complications is likely to make things more difficult. Progressive lens density will require more use of ultrasound energy with an increased risk of damaging the corneal endothelium. Also the OSD may progress and further reduce intraocular visibility, thus further raising the risk for complications or making phacoemulsification impossible [45, 46]. Hence, we favor earlier intervention, when accommodation is no longer substantial, DED chronic and potentially worsening as in patients with ocular involvement of mucous membrane pemphigoid (MMP) [17]. However, cataract surgery may also carry the risk of exacerbating any underlying disease, as in MMP. Therefore, a careful surgical plan considering grade of cataract and severity of DED is paramount. Kato et al. recommend that patients with severe DED, e.g., Sjögren's syndrome or GvHD, should not undergo cataract surgery during the winter because the cold and dry environmental conditions may increase DED [47].

Intraoperatively

Anesthesia

Preoperative frequent application of anesthetics and mydriatics eye drops may further reduce intraocular visibility in eyes with DED and should be avoided. Intracameral mydriatics and anesthetics are now available and should be preferred. Their use has been found to also improve postoperative results, as they are associated with a reduction of DED symptoms at 8 and 30 days postoperatively [11, 48]. Although in mild disease topical anesthesia is an option, in more severe cases, care should be taken to minimize risks with a para- or retrobulbar block to ensure anesthesia and akinesia. General anesthesia is usually preferable in the most complex cases with poor intraocular visibility and a history of previous intraocular surgery. This also avoids any toxicity from topically applied anesthetics and preserves epithelial health as best as possible.

Surgical Preparations

To ensure preoperative antisepsis, the application of povidone–iodine 5–10% to the cornea, conjunctival sac, as well as periocular surface for a

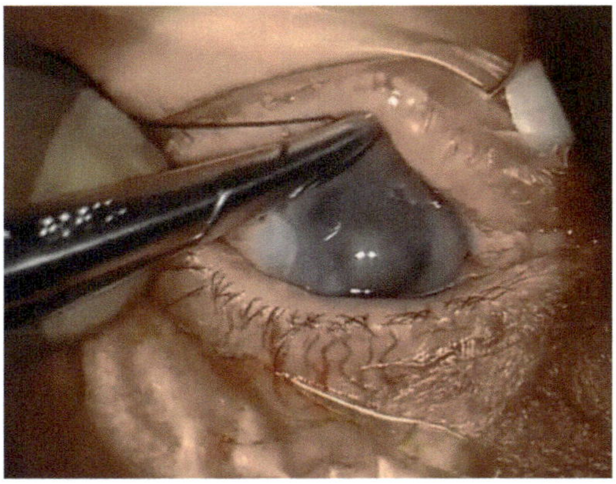

Fig. 8.1 Placement of lid everting transpalpebral 4.0 silk sutures instead of using a speculum in a patient with severe shortened conjunctival fornices

minimum of 3 min is recommended [49]. Shortened conjunctival fornices can make the placement of a speculum complicated or even impossible. To overcome this, we use lid everting transpalpebral 4.0 silk sutures (see Fig. 8.1) [17]. If a corneal pannus or superficial scar reduces intraocular visibility, a superficial keratectomy may be required, but this should be balanced against the risk of inducing a persistent epithelial defect with the risk of corneal ulceration.

Incision

When placing the incisions, minimal conjunctival handling is paramount, especially in patients with underlying conjunctival inflammation at risk of exacerbation such as MMP [17]. Whenever possible corneal or limbal incisions are preferred, while scleral incisions, requiring conjunctival recession, should be limited for cases with expected necessity for a large intraocular access, either for lens removal via manual excision or special, large diameter (i.e., nonfoldable) implants. For the choice between temporal and superior access, we prefer to place the clear corneal incision under the upper lid, as this is protected by the eyelid and has a lower impact on postoperative corneal sensitivity, i.e., reduces the risk of postoperative neurotrophic keratopathy [50]. Nonetheless, the pattern and density of the regenerated corneal nerves are rarely restored completely, as the subepithelial nerve fiber plexus is reduced and nerve fiber regeneration is inhibited due to the absence of Bowman's layer and to several vacuoles in the superficial stroma [51]. Main nerve density and nerve branches density continue to be significantly lower compared with normal corneas at least 10 years postoperatively [52].

Adjunctive Measures

Intraoperatively, the use of methylcellulose on the corneal surface minimizes epithelial trauma. The tear film parameters and ocular surface health benefitted from this adjunctive measure especially in patients with dry eye, male sex, and if surgery was prolonged [53]. Trypan blue dye staining of the anterior lens capsule can help to better visualize the anterior capsule especially in cases with corneal opacifications or very dense cataracts (see Fig. 8.2) [44, 54].

Exposure to light from the operating microscope should be limited as it is also associated with postoperative dry eye [55]. The production of reactive oxygen species due to phototoxic effects of operating microscope may lead to devitalization of corneal and conjunctival epithelial cells and squamous metaplasia of the conjunctival epithelium and results in a decrease in conjunctival goblet cell density [56]. A decreased aqueous tear production, a decreased expression

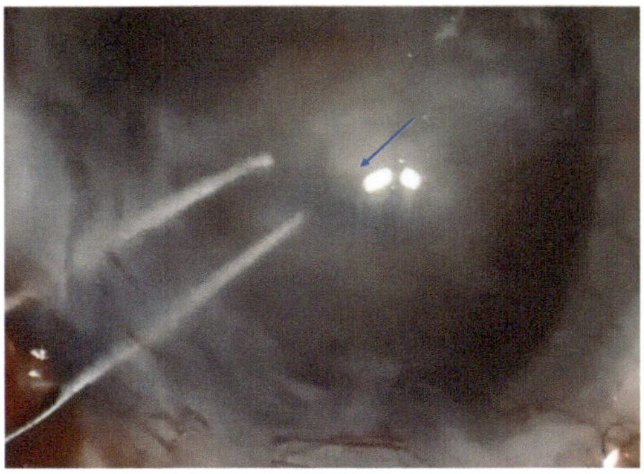

Fig. 8.2 Trypan blue dye staining of the anterior lens capsule helps to better visualize the anterior capsular edge (blue arrow) during capsulorhexis especially in cases with corneal opacifications or very dense cataracts

of mucin, as well as an increased interleukin 1-beta expression in tears were found in an animal model (rabbit) which supports a phototoxic effects on the ocular surface and tear film [57]. To further improve visualization in severe corneal opacifications, different types of illumination have been described: transcorneal oblique, chandelier anterior chamber endoillumination, chandelier retroillumination, or intracameral dynamic spotlight illumination [58]. Endoillumination can be used in eyes with moderate-to-severe keratopathy for capsulorhexis but also during phacoemulsification, posterior capsule polishing, and visualization of the IOL [44, 59]. Basically, the surgeon should be familiar with and prepared to try various approaches, when needed.

Lens Removal

During phacoemulsification, the cumulative dissipated energy should be kept as low as possible, as DED parameters decline with higher energy as well as with an increase in operating microscope light exposure time [60]. The use of more ultrasound energy leads to damage not only of the corneal endothelium, but subsequently with bullous keratopathy also of the stromal keratocytes and epithelium, as well as the nerve plexuses leading to signs of dry eye. Sahu et al. reported in a cohort of 100 consecutive patients without a control group that the use of more ultrasound energy was associated with a reduction of Schirmer test results from 17.46 mm preop to 12.30 mm 2 months postop ($p < 0.001$) and BUT from 16.11 seconds to 11.48 seconds $p < 0.001$) [60]. In general, phacoemulsification is reserved for patients' *removal* with adequate media clarity and good pupillary dilatation. Manual small-incision cataract surgery (MSICS) and extracapsular cataract extraction (ECCE) are back-up techniques for eyes with significant corneal opacity or hard cataract. The combination of cataract surgery with other measures (e.g., bandage contact lenses, punctum plugs) may be necessary in severe DED to prevent early and late complications, such as superficial punctate keratopathy, (persistent) epithelial defect, conjunctivalization, neovascularization, opacification, and keratinization, symblepharon formation, as well as eyelid complications (e.g., trichiasis) [22, 61]. Ideally, surgery should be performed by an experienced surgeon, who is not only skilled in a variety of different cataract procedures (phacoemulsification with endoillumination, MSICS, or ECCE) but also able to address the ocular surface (e.g., AMT, tarsorrhaphy). In case of intraoperative complications (e.g., a dropped nucleus), a nearby vitreoretinal surgeon is required.

The role of the femtosecond laser-assisted cataract surgery (FLACS) in severe dry eye is poorly investigated. While it may be possible that the applied vacuum in an aspirating speculum (in order to apply suction to the eye for subsequent stabilization) damages conjunctival goblet cells, overall objective dry eye parameters (such as OSDI, corneal fluorescein staining, breakup time, and tear meniscus height) remain unchanged 3 months after FLACS [62, 63]. However, Yu et al. found that patients with preexisting DED who had FLACS had more severe ocular surface staining than those having conventional surgery [64]. The use of an aspirating speculum as in FLACS aggravates DED after *removal* cataract surgery [65]. Furthermore, corneal opacifications in DED may prevent optical coherence tomography (OCT) analysis and cause the laser beam to be disturbed leading to an incomplete capsulotomy as well as to unpredictable corneal access and nucleus fragmentation [66, 67]. Given the absence of any benefit and the additional costs of FLACS compared with conventional phacoemulsification in large randomized controlled trials, this new technique cannot be advocated in severe DED with poor visualization [68].

IOL Placement

IOL fixation depends on the severity of the case. Capsular bag placement is intended in most cases. However, due to a higher incidence of other previous intraocular interventions or intraoperative complications (e.g., due to limited visibility), the surgical plan may have to be adjusted and special IOL fixation may be necessary. Hence, the availability of the correct power of iris fixated or scleral sutured IOLs must be ensured before embarking on cataract surgery in such cases.

Postoperatively

The risk of potentially sight-threatening complication following cataract surgery such as persisting epithelial defect/erosion leading to a corneal ulceration and perforation is much higher in severe DED [69]. The incidence of postoperative corneal melts in a GvHD cohort undergoing cataract surgery can be up to 1/3 of the cases [70, 71]. In preexisting inflammation (e.g., in ocular MMP), it is important to maximally suppress inflammation preoperatively, given that inflammation typically increases after surgery [15] resulting in a prolonged use of postoperative medications. Topical NSAIDs are associated with a higher incidence of corneal complications such as corneal ulceration or perforation and should thus be prescribed judiciously in patients with severe DED [69]. However, only six cases of sterile corneal melt with perforation following cataract surgery are reported in the literature so far, and all showed additional risk factors such as rheumatoid arthritis, Sjögren's syndrome, and DED [69]. Topical NSAIDs should be minimized or even avoided completely in patients with severe DED [11, 15], although they may be required to treat cystoid macular edema (CME) [47], which was reported to be the most common postoperative complication in a GvHD cohort undergoing cataract surgery [6].

Postoperative Routine Management

Postoperative routine management should consist of the preoperative DED therapy regiment [11] plus preservative-free, topical antibiotics and steroids [13]. All patients should be advised that even after successful cataract surgery, visual acuity may fluctuate due to DED. Additional support might be necessary to gain best postoperative visual acuity and reduce glare by using cut-off filter spectacles or gas permeable scleral lenses [21].

Complications

In general, the risk of complications of cataract surgery in severe DED is increased. Using a multivariable analysis, ocular comorbidities such as DED were a significant risk factor for a poor outcome after cataract surgery [72]. Ocular surface disease and systemic immunosuppression are major, often associated, risk factors for the development of acute postoperative endophthalmitis, as is poor personal hygiene [49]. This is likely to be due to an increased microbial load on the ocular surface [73]. Besides preoperative adequate treatment of DED, an increased frequency of postop follow-up visits is recommended to promptly diagnose and treat possible complications such as infectious endophthalmitis [15, 74].

Secondary cataract, although not reported in the literature with an increased rate in DED, remains a postoperative frequent problem, since ND:YAG capsulotomy will be more challenging again due to reduced visibility. Surgical posterior capsulotomy, conducted either before IOL implantation or later using a 25 vitrector via a pars plana port, can be performed alternatively.

Even though corneal ulceration with a perforation is a rare complication, this scenario can present even 1 year after successful cataract surgery and may require amniotic membrane transplantation and an emergency keratoplasty, e.g., in combination with tarsorrhaphies or other measures [6]. As complications can occur even several months after cataract surgery, DED patients need a longer duration of follow-up [11].

Conclusion

Cataract surgery in the face of DED remains challenging. As comorbid DED is very frequent in the age group seeking cataract surgery, a basic assessment of DED for all patients may be considered and is recommended by some authors [3, 11]. However, with special attention to intraoperative adjustments as well as proactive pre- and postoperative management and intense therapy, a good outcome with improved visual acuity and associated quality of life even in the group of patients who are suffering substantially from severe DED can be ensured [11].

Part 2

Recommendations

Preoperatively

1. Take a proper patient history.
2. Diagnose DED with OSDI, Schirmer test, Meibomian gland expression, corneal sensitivity, corneal +/− conjunctival staining at the slit lamp, and probing and flushing the lacrimal drainage system and check for lid abnormalities.
3. Treat DED according to the severity of the diseases.

   Medically: preservative-free lubricants, anti-inflammatory agents (topical steroid and cyclosporine), autologous serum, bandage contact lens, punctum occlusion, use of warm compressors, lid margin hygiene, and treatment of demodex, topical azithromycin, and systemic tetracycline antibiotics if needed.

   Surgically: correct lid malposition, tarsorrhaphy, AMT, reconstruct fornices using oral mucosa.
4. Stable disease prior to surgery.
5. Educate patients about the importance of therapy adherence, frequent follow-up visits after surgery, and limited visual prognosis due to DED and possible exacerbation of DED after surgery.
6. Intensify the use of lubricants prior to IOL calculation.
7. Choose a foldable preloaded monofocal aspheric IOL; be prepared to change the choice of IOL intraoperatively.

Intraoperatively

1. Choose para- or retrobulbar block or general anesthesia if available/needed.
2. Apply povidone–iodine 5–10% to the cornea, conjunctival sac, as well as periocular surface for a minimum of 3 min.
3. Limit the microscope light exposure during surgery and consider endoillumination.
4. Do not use an aspirating speculum/femtosecond laser.
5. Place larger corneal incisions under the upper lid.
6. Use methylcellulose on the corneal surface to minimize epithelial trauma.
7. Use trypan blue dye to better visualize the anterior capsule.
8. Keep cumulative dissipated energy during phacoemulsification low.
9. Be able to convert to MSICS or ECCE as needed.

Postoperatively

1. Avoid the use of topical NSAIDs as a single agent.
2. Continue preoperative preservative-free DED therapy.
3. Reduce follow-up intervals to diagnose complications early.
4. Add cut-off filter spectacles or gas permeable scleral lenses to improve best-corrected visual acuity.

Part 3

Case and Video

A 61-year-old male patient presented to the Department of Ophthalmology for cataract surgery on the left eye. His past medical history included GVHD after bone marrow transplantation due to a mantle cell lymphoma. During the course of his systemic treatment, he had received long-term immunosuppression with methylprednisolone and cyclosporine. His severe ocular surface disease including recurrent epithelial defects was managed with repeated AMT, symblepharolysis, and allogenic limbal stem cell transplantation. To prevent an immunoreaction, he was on systemic steroids and mycophenolate mofetil. Preoperatively, his best-corrected visual acuity was 0.2 (dec) in his right and 0.02 (dec) in his left eye with a left corticonuclear cataract. The ocular surface prior to surgery was intensively treated with topical dexamethasone, 0.1% ciclosporine, as well as autologous serum eye drops and protected with a soft bandage contact lens. The lower puncta were occluded with silicone plugs and the upper puncta by cautery.

Intraoperatively, due to persistent fornix shortening and symblephara, a speculum could not be placed, and lid everting sutures (silk 6–0) in combination with limited symblepharolysis were used (see Video 8.1, 0:03 sec.). The main corneal incision was placed under the upper lid at the 2 o'clock position (0:48 sec.). Intracameral trypan blue dye was used to improve the anterior lens capsule visualization through the opaque cornea (0:54 sec.). Capsulorhexis was performed using a cystotome and forceps under high magnification with reduced light exposure (1:01 sec.). Further surgery included hydrodissection (1:32 sec.), phacoemulsification using a horizontal chop technique with a cumulative dissipated energy of 9%s (1:36 sec.), and bimanual irrigation and aspiration of cortex (2:54 sec.). To protect the corneal surface, methylcellulose was applied repetitively (3:28 sec.). Due to suspected posterior capsular rupture, intracameral triamcinolone was administered (3:33 sec.) to enhance visualization during anterior vitrectomy (3:45 sec.) and a three-piece IOL implanted in the ciliary sulcus (3:52 sec.) (4:14 sec.). Finally, any intracameral ophthalmic viscosurgical device (OVD) was removed with bimanual irrigation and aspiration (4:38 sec.), the corneal incisions secured with a 10–0 nylon interrupted suture (4:40 sec.), and the lid everting sutures removed at the end of surgery (4:57 sec.). Postoperatively, the visual acuity increased to 0.05 only, but he reported a much-improved visual field. Postoperative topical therapy included dexamethasone 2x/d, 0.1% ciclosporine 1x/d, ofloxacin 3x/d, autologous serum 8x/d, and systemic mycophenolate mofetil 500 mg 2x/d.

This case illustrates the challenging nature of cataract surgery in the face of severe DED with resulting limitations of intraocular visibility and the measures available to overcome these and manage intraocular complications.

Take-Home Notes

- Prior to cataract surgery, diagnose and treat dry eye disease (DED) according to the severity of the disease and be mindful of the effects of DED on biometry.
- Educate patients about the importance of therapy adherence, frequent follow-up visits after surgery, and limited visual prognosis due to DED and possible exacerbation of DED after surgery.
- Intraoperatively, limit the microscope light exposure during surgery and consider endoillumination.
- Place larger corneal incisions under the upper lid and use methylcellulose on the corneal surface to minimize epithelial trauma.
- Avoid the use of topical NSAIDs as a single agent and continue preoperative preservative-free DED therapy.

References

1. Siffel C, Hennies N, Joseph C, et al. Burden of dry eye disease in Germany: a retrospective observational study using German claims data. Acta Ophthalmol. 2020;98:e504–12. https://doi.org/10.1111/aos.14300.
2. Craig JP, Nichols KK, Akpek EK, et al. TFOS DEWS II definition and classification report. Ocul Surf. 2017;15:276–83. https://doi.org/10.1016/j.jtos.2017.05.008.
3. Naderi K, Gormley J, O'Brart D. Cataract surgery and dry eye disease: a review. Eur J Ophthalmol. 2020; https://doi.org/10.1177/1120672120929958.
4. Congdon N. Prevalence of cataract and Pseudophakia/Aphakia among adults in the United States. Arch Ophthalmol. 2004;122:487–94. https://doi.org/10.1001/archopht.122.4.487.
5. Sutu C, Fukuoka H, Afshari NA. Mechanisms and management of dry eye in cataract surgery patients. Curr Opin Ophthalmol. 2016;27:24–30. https://doi.org/10.1097/ICU.0000000000000227.
6. de Melo Franco R, Kron-Gray M, MD P, et al (2015) Outcomes of cataract surgery in graft-versus-host disease. Cornea 34:506–511.
7. Choi YJ, Park SY, Jun I, et al. Perioperative ocular parameters associated with persistent dry eye symptoms after cataract surgery. Cornea. 2018;37:734–9.

8. Kasetsuwan N, Satitpitakul V, Changul T, Jariyakosol S. Incidence and pattern of dry eye after cataract surgery. PLoS One. 2013;8:1–6. https://doi.org/10.1371/journal.pone.0078657.
9. Elksnis Ē, Lāce I, Laganovska G, Erts R. Tear osmolarity after cataract surgery. J Curr Ophthalmol. 2019;31:31–5. https://doi.org/10.1016/j.joco.2018.08.006.
10. Cung LX, Nga NTT, Nga DM, et al. Cataract surgery destabilises temporary the tear film of the ocular surface. Klin Monatsbl Augenheilkd. 2020; https://doi.org/10.1055/a-1179-0373.
11. Labetoulle M, Rousseau A, Baudouin C. Management of dry eye disease to optimize cataract surgery outcomes: two tables for a daily clinical practice. J Fr Ophtalmol. 2019;42:907–12. https://doi.org/10.1016/j.jfo.2019.03.032.
12. Afsharkhamseh N, Movahedan A, Motahari H, Djalilian AR. Cataract surgery in patients with ocular surface disease: an update in clinical diagnosis and treatment. Saudi J Ophthalmol. 2014;28:164–7. https://doi.org/10.1016/j.sjopt.2014.06.013.
13. Baudouin C, Labbé A, Liang H, et al. Preservatives in eyedrops: the good, the bad and the ugly. Prog Retin Eye Res. 2010;29:312–34. https://doi.org/10.1016/j.preteyeres.2010.03.001.
14. El Ameen A, Majzoub S, Vandermeer G, Pisella PJ. Influence of cataract surgery on Meibomian gland dysfunction. J Fr Ophtalmol. 2018;41:e173–80. https://doi.org/10.1016/j.jfo.2018.03.001.
15. Movahedan A, Djalilian AR. Cataract surgery in the face of ocular surface disease. Curr Opin Ophthalmol. 2012;23:68–72. https://doi.org/10.1097/ICU.0b013e32834d90b7.
16. Cung LX, Nga NTT, Nga DM, et al. Cataract surgery destabilises temporary the tear film of the ocular surface. Klin Monatsbl Augenheilkd. 2021;238:282–7. https://doi.org/10.1055/a-1179-0373.
17. Geerling G, Dart JKG. Management and outcome of cataract surgery in ocular cicatricial pemphigoid. Graefes Arch Clin Exp Ophthalmol. 2000;238:112–8. https://doi.org/10.1007/PL00007877.
18. Villarreal-Gonzalez AJ, Jocelyn Rivera-Alvarado I, Rodriguez-Gutierrez LA, Rodriguez-Garcia A. Analysis of ocular surface damage and visual impact in patients with primary and secondary Sjögren syndrome. Rheumatol Int. 2020;40:1249–57. https://doi.org/10.1007/s00296-020-04568-7.
19. Goto E, Yagi Y, Matsumoto Y, Tsubota K. Impaired functional visual acuity of dry eye patients. Am J Ophthalmol. 2002;133:181–6. https://doi.org/10.1016/s0002-9394(01)01365-4.
20. Iskeleli G, Kizilkaya M, Arslan OS, Ozkan S. The effect of artificial tears on corneal surface regularity in patients with Sjögren syndrome. Ophthalmologica. 2002;216:118–22. https://doi.org/10.1159/000048310.
21. Hänisch KT, Neppert B, Geerling G. Gasdurchlässige sklerallinsen als konservative therapiealternative bei extremen hornhautektasien und schwerem tränenmangel. Ophthalmologe. 2005;102:387–92. https://doi.org/10.1007/s00347-004-1101-6.
22. Sotozono C, Ueta M, Yokoi N. Special issue severe dry eye with combined mechanisms is involved in the ocular sequelae of SJS/TEN at the chronic stage. 2018; https://doi.org/10.1167/iovs.18-24019.
23. Magro L, Gauthier J, Richet M, et al. Scleral lenses for severe chronic GvHD-related keratoconjunctivitis sicca: a retrospective study by the SFGM-TC. Nat Publ Gr. 2017;52:878–82. https://doi.org/10.1038/bmt.2017.9.
24. Thulasi P, Djalilian A Update in current diagnostics and therapeutics of dry eye disease. https://doi.org/10.1016/j.ophtha.2017.07.022
25. Poon AC, Geerling G, Dart JKG, et al. Autologous serum eyedrops for dry eyes and epithelial defects: clinical and in vitro toxicity studies. Br J Ophthalmol. 2001;85:1188–97. https://doi.org/10.1136/bjo.85.10.1188.
26. Geerling G, Unterlauft JD, Kasper K, et al. Eigenserum und alternative blutprodukte zur behandlung von augenoberflächenerkrankungen. Ophthalmologe. 2008;105:623–31. https://doi.org/10.1007/s00347-008-1750-y.
27. Geerling G, Hartwig D. Autologe serum-augentropfen zur therapie der augenoberfläche. Eine übersicht zur wirksamkeit und empfehlungen zur anwendung. Ophthalmologe. 2002;99:949–59. https://doi.org/10.1007/s00347-002-0661-6.
28. Geerling G, Mac Lennan S, Hartwig D. Autologous serum eye drops for ocular surface disorders. Br J Ophthalmol. 2004;88:1467–74. https://doi.org/10.1136/bjo.2004.044347.
29. Jones L, Downie LE, Korb D, et al. TFOS DEWS II management and therapy report. Ocul Surf. 2017;15:575–628. https://doi.org/10.1016/j.jtos.2017.05.006.
30. Yang C-H, Albietz J, Harkin DG, et al. Impact of oral vitamin D supplementation on the ocular surface in people with dry eye and/or low serum vitamin D. Cont Lens Anterior Eye. 2018;41:69–76. https://doi.org/10.1016/j.clae.2017.09.007.
31. Gatell-Tortajada J. Oral supplementation with a nutraceutical formulation containing omega-3 fatty acids, vitamins, minerals, and antioxidants in a large series of patients with dry eye symptoms: results of a prospective study. Clin Interv Aging. 2016;11:571–8. https://doi.org/10.2147/CIA.S98102.
32. Asbell PA, Maguire MG, Pistilli M, et al. N-3 fatty acid supplementation for the treatment of dry eye disease. N Engl J Med. 2018;378:1681–90. https://doi.org/10.1056/NEJMoa1709691.
33. Molina-Leyva I, Molina-Leyva A, Bueno-Cavanillas A. Efficacy of nutritional supplementation with omega-3 and omega-6 fatty acids in dry eye syndrome: a systematic review of randomized clinical trials. Acta Ophthalmol. 2017;95:e677–85. https://doi.org/10.1111/aos.13428.
34. Zhao Y, Li J, Xue K, et al. Preoperative management of MGD with vectored thermal pulsation before cata-

ract surgery: a prospective, controlled clinical trial. Semin Ophthalmol. 2021;36:2–8. https://doi.org/10.1080/08820538.2021.1881567.
35. Mulder JA, van Tilborg MM, Huntjens B. The effect of sodium fluorescein on anterior eye surface measurements. Cont Lens Anterior Eye. 2020;43:402–7. https://doi.org/10.1016/j.clae.2020.02.016.
36. Epitropoulos AT, Matossian C, Berdy GJ, et al. Effect of tear osmolarity on repeatability of keratometry for cataract surgery planning. J Cataract Refract Surg. 2015;41:1672.
37. Yeu E, Cuozzo S. Matching the patient to the intraocular lens: preoperative considerations to optimize surgical outcomes. Ophthalmology. 2020; https://doi.org/10.1016/j.ophtha.2020.08.025.
38. Röggla V, Leydolt C, Schartmüller D, et al. Influence of artificial tears on keratometric measurements in cataract patients. Am J Ophthalmol. 2021;221:1–8. https://doi.org/10.1016/j.ajo.2020.08.024.
39. Cheng AMS, Zhao D, Chen R, et al. Accelerated restoration of ocular surface health in dry eye disease by self-retained cryopreserved amniotic membrane. Ocul Surf. 2016;14:56–63. https://doi.org/10.1016/j.jtos.2015.07.003.
40. Alio JL, Plaza-Puche AB, Fе́rnandez-Buenaga R, et al. Multifocal intraocular lenses: an overview. Surv Ophthalmol. 2017;62:611–34. https://doi.org/10.1016/j.survophthal.2017.03.005.
41. Gibbons A, Ali TK, Waren DP, Donaldson KE. Causes and correction of dissatisfaction after implantation of presbyopia-correcting intraocular lenses. Clin Ophthalmol. 2016;10:1965–70. https://doi.org/10.2147/OPTH.S114890.
42. Buckhurst PJ, Naroo SA, Davies LN, et al. Assessment of dysphotopsia in pseudophakic subjects with multifocal intraocular lenses. BMJ Open Ophthalmol. 2017;1:1–8. https://doi.org/10.1136/bmjophth-2016-000064.
43. Liu J, Dong Y, Wang Y. Efficacy and safety of extended depth of focus intraocular lenses in cataract surgery: a systematic review and meta-analysis. BMC Ophthalmol. 2019;19:1–10. https://doi.org/10.1186/s12886-019-1204-0.
44. Donthineni PR, Das AV, Shanbhag SS, Basu S. Cataract surgery in dry eye disease: visual outcomes and complications. Front Med. 2020;7:1–8. https://doi.org/10.3389/fmed.2020.575834.
45. Narang P, Mohamed A, Mittal V, Sangwan VS. Cataract surgery in chronic Stevens-Johnson syndrome: aspects and outcomes. Br J Ophthalmol. 2016;100:1542–6. https://doi.org/10.1136/bjophthalmol-2015-308041.
46. Sangwan VS, Gupta S, Das S. Cataract surgery in ocular surface diseases: clinical challenges and outcomes. Curr Opin Ophthalmol. 2018;29:81–7. https://doi.org/10.1097/ICU.0000000000000441.
47. Kato K, Miyake K, Hirano K, Kondo M. Management of postoperative inflammation and dry eye after cataract surgery. Cornea. 2019;38:S25–33. https://doi.org/10.1097/ICO.0000000000002125.
48. Labetoulle M, Findl O, Malecaze F, et al. Evaluation of the efficacy and safety of a standardised intracameral combination of mydriatics and anaesthetics for cataract surgery. Br J Ophthalmol. 2016;100:976–85. https://doi.org/10.1136/bjophthalmol-2015-307587.
49. Tranos P, Dervenis N, Vakalis AN, et al. Current perspectives of prophylaxis and management of acute infective endophthalmitis. Adv Ther. 2016;33:727–46. https://doi.org/10.1007/s12325-016-0307-8.
50. Kohlhaas M. Corneal sensation after cataract and refractive surgery. J Cataract Refract Surg. 1998;24:1399–409. https://doi.org/10.1016/S0886-3350(98)80237-X.
51. Kohlhaas M. Corneal sensation after cataract and refractive surgery. J Cataract Refract Surg. 1998;24:1399–409.
52. Garcia-Gonzalez M, Cañadas P, Gros-Otero J, et al. Long-term corneal subbasal nerve plexus regeneration after laser in situ keratomileusis. J Cataract Refract Surg. 2019;45:966–71. https://doi.org/10.1016/j.jcrs.2019.02.019.
53. He Y, Li J, Zhu J, et al. The improvement of dry eye after cataract surgery by intraoperative using ophthalmic viscosurgical devices on the surface of cornea: The results of a consort-compliant randomized controlled trial. Medicine (United States). 2017;96:e8940. https://doi.org/10.1097/MD.0000000000008940.
54. Bhartiya P, Sharma N, Ray M, et al. Trypan blue assisted phacoemulsification in corneal opacities. Br J Ophthalmol. 2002;86:857–9. https://doi.org/10.1136/bjo.86.8.857.
55. Cho YK, Kim MS. Dry eye after cataract surgery and associated intraoperative risk factors. Korean J Ophthalmol. 2009;23:65–73. https://doi.org/10.3341/kjo.2009.23.2.65.
56. Kohli P, Arya SK, Raj A, Handa U. Changes in ocular surface status after phacoemulsification in patients with senile cataract. Int Ophthalmol. 2019;39:1345–53. https://doi.org/10.1007/s10792-018-0953-8.
57. Bin HH, Kim HS. Phototoxic effects of an operating microscope on the ocular surface and tear film. Cornea. 2014;33:82–90. https://doi.org/10.1097/ICO.0000000000000001.
58. Yuksel E. Intracameral endoilluminator-assisted phacoemulsification surgery in patients with severe corneal opacity. J Cataract Refract Surg. 2020;46:168–73. https://doi.org/10.1097/j.jcrs.0000000000000050.
59. Moon H, Lee JH, Lee JY, et al. Intracameral dynamic spotlight-assisted cataract surgery in eyes with corneal opacity, small pupil or advanced cataract. Acta Ophthalmol. 2015;93:388–90. https://doi.org/10.1111/aos.12428.
60. Sahu PK, Das GK, Malik A, Biakthangi L. Dry eye following phacoemulsification surgery and its relation to associated intraoperative risk factors. Middle East Afr J Ophthalmol. 2015;22:472–7. https://doi.org/10.4103/0974-9233.151871.
61. Wu X, Ma Y, Chen X, et al. Efficacy of bandage contact lens for the management of dry eye disease after

cataract surgery. Int Ophthalmol. 2021;41:1403–13. https://doi.org/10.1007/s10792-021-01692-6.
62. Shao D, Zhu X, Sun WEI, et al. Effects of femtosecond laser-assisted cataract surgery on dry eye. Exp Ther Med. 2018;16:5073–8. https://doi.org/10.3892/etm.2018.6862.
63. Schargus M, Ivanova S, Stute G, et al. Comparable effects on tear film parameters after femtosecond laser-assisted and conventional cataract surgery. Int Ophthalmol. 2020;40:3097. https://doi.org/10.1007/s10792-020-01532-z.
64. Yu Y, Hua H, Wu M, et al. Evaluation of dry eye after femtosecond laser-assisted cataract surgery. J Cataract Refract Surg. 2015;41:2614–23. https://doi.org/10.1016/j.jcrs.2015.06.036.
65. Moon H, Yoon JH, Hyun SH, Kim KH. Short-term influence of aspirating speculum use on dry eye after cataract surgery: a prospective study. Cornea. 2014;33:373–5. https://doi.org/10.1097/ICO.0000000000000072.
66. Roberts TV, Lawless M, Sutton G, Hodge C. Clinical ophthalmology Dovepress update and clinical utility of the LenSx femtosecond laser in cataract surgery. Clin Ophthalmol. 2016:10–2021. https://doi.org/10.2147/OPTH.S94306.
67. Huang PW, Huang WH, Tai YC, Sun CC. Femtosecond laser-assisted cataract surgery in a patient with traumatic cataract and corneal opacity after LASIK: a case report. BMC Ophthalmol. 2020;20:1–4. https://doi.org/10.1186/s12886-020-01491-0.
68. Schweitzer C, Brezin A, Cochener B, et al. Femtosecond laser-assisted versus phacoemulsification cataract surgery (FEMCAT): a multicentre participant-masked randomised superiority and cost-effectiveness trial. Lancet. 2020;395:212–24. https://doi.org/10.1016/S0140-6736(19)32481-X.
69. Ting DSJ, Ghosh S. Acute corneal perforation 1 week following uncomplicated cataract surgery: the implication of undiagnosed dry eye disease and topical NSAIDs. Ther Adv Ophthalmol. 2019;11:251584141986950. https://doi.org/10.1177/2515841419869508.
70. Shah A, Santhiago MR, Espana EM. Cataract surgery in patients with chronic severe graft-versus-host disease. J Cataract Refract Surg. 2016;42:833–9. https://doi.org/10.1016/j.jcrs.2016.02.046.
71. Yang HK, Kline OR Jr. Corneal melting with intraocular lenses. Arch Ophthalmol. 1982;100:1272–4. https://doi.org/10.1001/archopht.1982.01030040250008.
72. Khanna Id RC, Rathi VM, Guizie E, et al. Factors associated with visual outcomes after cataract surgery: a cross-sectional or retrospective study in Liberia. 2020; https://doi.org/10.1371/journal.pone.0233118.
73. Yu CQ, Ta CN. Prevention of postcataract endophthalmitis: evidence-based medicine. Curr Opin Ophthalmol. 2012;23:19.
74. Galor A, Goldhardt R, Wellik SR, et al. Management strategies to reduce risk of postoperative infections. Curr Ophthalmol Rep. 2013;1 https://doi.org/10.1007/s40135-013 0021-5.

Cataract Surgery in Stevens-Johnson Syndrome and Pemphigoid Diseases

9

Volkan Tahmaz, Philipp Steven,
and Claus Cursiefen

Bullet Points
This chapter will discuss how cicatricial diseases of the ocular surface impact cataract surgery with regard to:

- Which diseases cause scarring of the ocular surface and adnexae
- To what extent medical and/or surgical therapy might be necessary in preparation for cataract surgery
- How pre- and perioperative care need to be adjusted
- Which intraoperative strategies can be employed to increase safety and optimize outcomes
- How aftercare should be arranged to minimize risk of postoperative complications

V. Tahmaz (✉) · P. Steven
Department of Ophthalmology, University of Cologne, Faculty of Medicine and University Hospital Cologne, Cologne, Germany

Division for Dry-Eye and Ocular GVHD, Department of Ophthalmology, University of Cologne, Faculty of Medicine and University Hospital Cologne, Cologne, Germany
e-mail: Volkan.tahmaz@uk-koeln.de

C. Cursiefen
Department of Ophthalmology, University of Cologne, Faculty of Medicine and University Hospital Cologne, Cologne, Germany

Division for Dry-Eye and Ocular GVHD, Department of Ophthalmology, University of Cologne, Faculty of Medicine and University Hospital Cologne, Cologne, Germany

Center for Molecular Medicine Cologne (CMMC), University of Cologne, Cologne, Germany

Cicatricial diseases of the eye constitute a group of mostly complex immune-mediated entities that can induce severe changes to the ocular surface including (recurring) conjunctivitis, corneal epithelial defects, ulceration, corneal scarring, formation of symblepharon, ankyloblepharon, and keratinization of the cornea [1, 2]. These changes to the ocular surface can – besides a reduction in visual acuity – lead to especially challenging conditions for cataract surgery and require adaptation of appropriate techniques and strategies. Additionally, proper calculation of the intraocular lens to be implanted can be challenging due to severe (irregular) astigmatism and severe dry eye.

To find the most suitable approach to each of these conditions, one must first understand the similarities and especially differences of different cicatrizing eye diseases and their individual characteristics. The first group can be summarized as blistering skin diseases with either autoimmune or drug-induced etiology, the latter including

J. L. Alió et al. (eds.), *Cataract Surgery*, Essentials in Ophthalmology,
https://doi.org/10.1007/978-3-030-94530-5_9

Stevens-Johnson syndrome (SJS) and toxic epidermal necrolysis (TEN). Both are considered to be entities of the same spectrum and resemble severe epidermolytic adverse drug reactions of the skin that differ only by the amount of body surface affected and both initially present with a cutaneous rash, erythema, and erosions, typically at the trunk, face, palms, and soles. Involvement of the oral, ocular, and genital mucosa occurs in over 90% of cases [3]. The second phase is characterized by large epidermal detachments that can be fatal depending on extent. Late stages can show hypo- or hyperpigmentations of the skin, nail dystrophies, or Sjögren-like syndromes. Drugs that have been associated with SJS and TEN include allopurinol, carbamazepine, sulfamethoxazole, lamotrigine, and NSAID of oxicam-type. The exact underlying mechanism is not fully understood; however, histopathological examination of affected skin shows apoptosis of keratinocytes followed by necrosis [4]. From an ophthalmologist's perspective, SJS and TEN can be seen as acute diseases that may inflict significant damage and scarring to the ocular surface (Fig. 9.1), but come to a halt after the active phase and are not expected to show further progression afterward. Still, the acute phase can inflict devastating damage to the ocular surface and adnexae, leading to a cascade of complications needing surgical intervention. Figure 9.2 shows a case of severe SJS, in which conjunctival scarring and chafing of the eyelashes had, despite multiple surgical corrections of the eyelids and amniotic membrane transplantation, lead to recurring corneal erosions and subsequently terminal damage to the cornea with extensive vascularization. In such a high-risk setting with vascularization of the cornea and impaired ocular surface integrity, keratoplasty bears little chance of functional and anatomical success. Ultimately, the eye had to be supplied with a keratoprosthesis (Boston KPro).

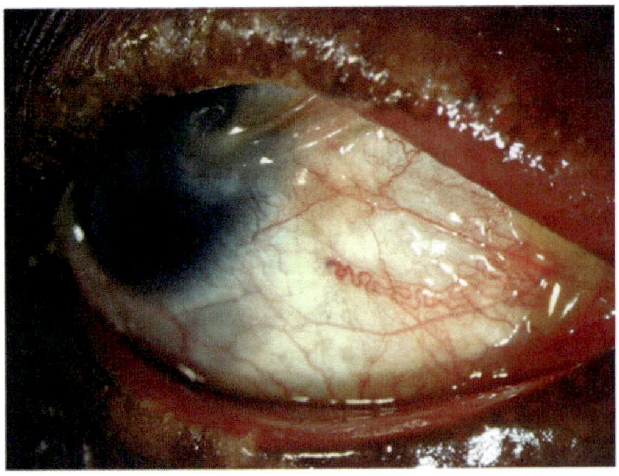

Fig. 9.1 Right eye of a 51-year-old female patient with severe symblepharon due to Stevens-Johnson syndrome. The condition manifested itself 6 years prior to this picture as a suspected reaction to azithromycin or sulfonamide-type antibiotics

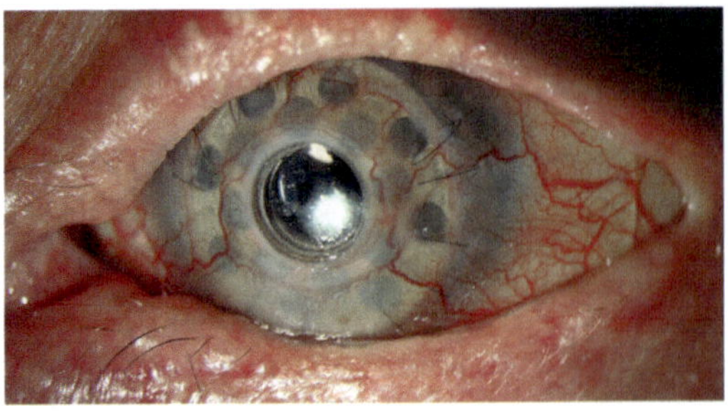

Fig. 9.2 Left eye of a 64-year-old male patient with Boston keratoprosthesis after severe Stevens-Johnson syndrome and consecutive scarring of the ocular surface and eyelids

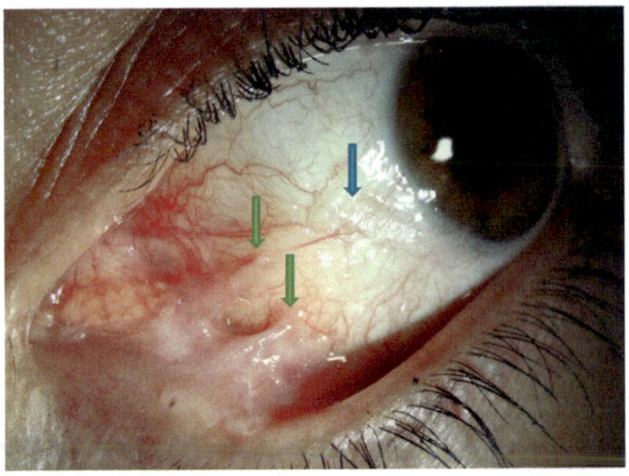

Fig. 9.3 Left eye of a 33-year-old female patient with ocular cicatricial pemphigoid. Besides the conjunctival scarring (green arrows), a significant keratinization of the conjunctiva (blue arrow) can be seen. These pathological changes to the ocular surface are typical of both OCP and SJS and demonstrate that severe diseases of the ocular surface usually include a keratoconjunctivitis sicca

On the other side of blistering skin diseases, the ocular cicatricial pemphigoid (OCP, Fig. 9.3) is the most prominent representative of autoimmune-mediated entities. It is regarded as a subset of the systemic autoimmune disease benign mucous membrane pemphigoid (MMP), in which the primary manifestation affects the ocular mucosa. The underlying mechanism is characterized by deposition of IgG, IgA, and C3 in the epithelial basement membrane with consecutive inflammation and subepithelial blistering; however, there is a wide array of antigens that have been identified and linked to bullous pemphigoid and other pemphigoid diseases [2, 5]. In contrast to SJS and TEN, OCP needs to be regarded as a chronic progressive disease (Fig. 9.4) that may very well show a spike in activity after mechanical trauma like surgery.

Apart from blistering skin diseases, cicatricial changes to the ocular surface can also be signs of rosacea or decade-long eye drop use ("pseudopemphigoid") [6], long-term complication of thermal or chemical burns [7], or a manifestation of chronic ocular graft-versus-host disease (GvHD, Fig. 9.5) [8, 9]. When examining a patient with scarring of the ocular surface prior to cataract surgery, these diagnoses need to be kept in mind, and the exact etiology of scarring needs to be specified before operating on the eye. Inquiry about patient history is the first step to narrow down the possible causes. For example, most patients will be able to recall if they ever experienced a violent adverse drug reaction or

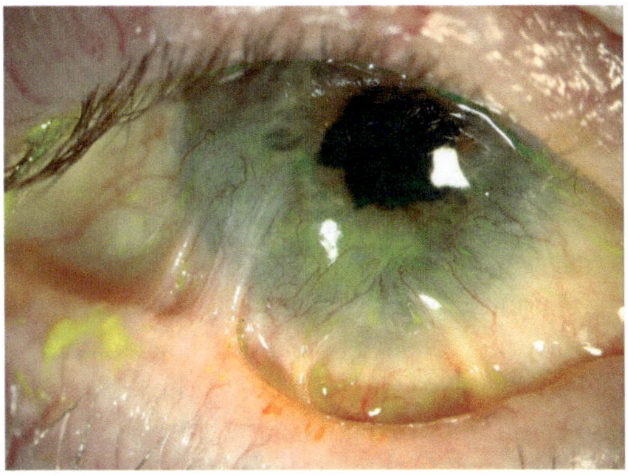

Fig. 9.4 Right eye of an 87-year-old male patient with ocular cicatricial pemphigoid (OCP). If existing symblepharon spare the visual axis, cataract surgery may be performed without manipulating the scar tissue in order to prevent a "rebound effect" by triggering scarring through mechanical manipulation

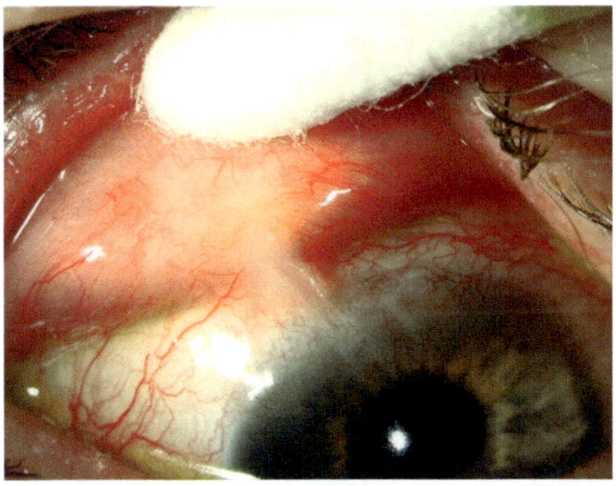

Fig. 9.5 Right eye of a 49-year-old male patient with conjunctival scarring due to chronic ocular graft-versus-host disease after hematopoietic stem cell transplantation

underwent allogeneic stem cell transplantation, which would lead to the probable diagnosis of SJS/TEN or GvHD, respectively. Rosacea can usually be diagnosed by clinical examination through an ophthalmologist specialized in the field of ocular surface disease or by a dermatologist. Establishing the diagnosis of OCP, however, is usually not possible based on clinical features alone, making serology and direct immunofluorescence microscopy and follow-up eye exams to detect progression necessary [5], at least prior to establishing a systemic immunosuppressive therapy. For monitoring ocular disease course, regular measurements of fornix depth in upper and lower eyelids at three locations (nasal, temporal, and middle part) using a fornix scale or standardized slit-lamp pictures every 3–6 months are highly recommended, as in particular reduction of upper fornix depth cannot be detected unless is has progressed extensively.

A precise etiologic classification is not only essential for the general therapy of the underlying disease but also to precondition the eye, as soon as cataract surgery becomes necessary. A sufficient medical therapy preceding and following cataract surgery is as essential as optimal surgical performance despite more challenging conditions. This often includes a separate surgical pretreatment to enable access to the eye or to reduce corneal opacities using Excimer PTK (Fig. 9.6) or lamellar keratoplasty.

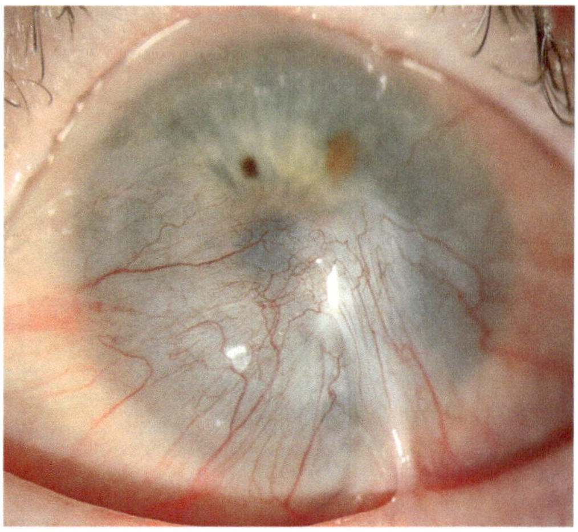

Fig. 9.6 Left eye of the patient in Fig. 9.3. If the visual axis is compromised by conjunctival scarring, the corneal surface has to be restored surgically, before cataract surgery can be planned. Usually, the most sensible approach is to perform either lamellar keratectomy alone or combined with lamellar keratoplasty (deep anterior lamellar keratoplasty, DALK)

Regarding cataract surgery in patients suffering from cicatricial diseases of the eye, there is little published evidence to rely on due to rarity of the underlying diseases. However, the most reasonable surgical approach for all aforementioned diseases can be broken down into three general principles with some additional recommendations for each individual disease.

As soon as cataract surgery is indicated, the *first step is to rigorously prepare the ocular surface for cataract extraction*, in terms of anatomical conditions, ocular surface inflammation, and tear film stabilization. The latter is also very relevant if optical methods for IOL calculation shall be used [10]. This may require previous eyelid surgery to correct misalignment of eyelid margins or chafing of the eyelashes and, if necessary, treatment of ankyloblepharon or lagophthalmos beforehand. In the presence of corneal scarring, surgical or laser therapy might be advisable before any intraocular surgery. Conjunctival surgery may be necessary, if extensive scarring impairs access to the cornea and hinders safe cataract surgery (Fig. 9.7). For patients with an underlying systemic autoimmune disease, especially OCP, stable systemic immunosuppressive therapy must have been established before planning ocular surgery. In our clinic, these patients must present with a history of stable disease for at least 6 months, documented by fornix measurements (e.g., using a fornix ruler; see Fig. 9.8), before being cleared for surgery. Naturally, emergency indications present an exception to this rule. In most severe cases with corneal thinning and significant risk of perforation, tectonic repair via (preferably lamellar) keratoplasty might be necessary while keeping in mind that corneal surgery inherently bears higher risk in patients with cicatricial diseases [11]. Should penetrating keratoplasty become necessary, a triple procedure might be the most sensible approach in order to spare the patient two separate surgical procedures. In patients with presumed aggressive ocular surface disease and consecutive corneal and conjunctival epitheliopathy and barrier dysfunction, preoperative treatment with autologous serum eye drops might be beneficial in order to reduce ocular surface inflammation and improve wound healing, which has been proven beneficial in ocular surface diseases like GvHD [12], although robust evidence for this approach in blistering skin diseases is limited [13]. Additionally, aggressive lubrication using preservative-free artificial tears and intensive anti-inflammatory therapy with topical steroids and/or cyclosporine eye drops is recommended preoperatively.

The *second principle of cataract surgery in cicatricial eye diseases applies to the intraoperative approach*: due to possible resurgence of ocular surface inflammation following surgery, it is imperative to inflict as little mechanical trauma to the cornea as feasible while altogether sparing the conjunctiva, if possible. This can be achieved by favoring clear corneal over sclerocorneal incisions, utilizing a minimally invasive technique and optimizing machine settings in order to reduce the duration of nuclear fragmentation and fragment removal. Often, a normal lid speculum cannot be used due to symblepharon, so that the lids have to be retracted surgically, e.g., using silk 5-0 sutures. In general, duration of

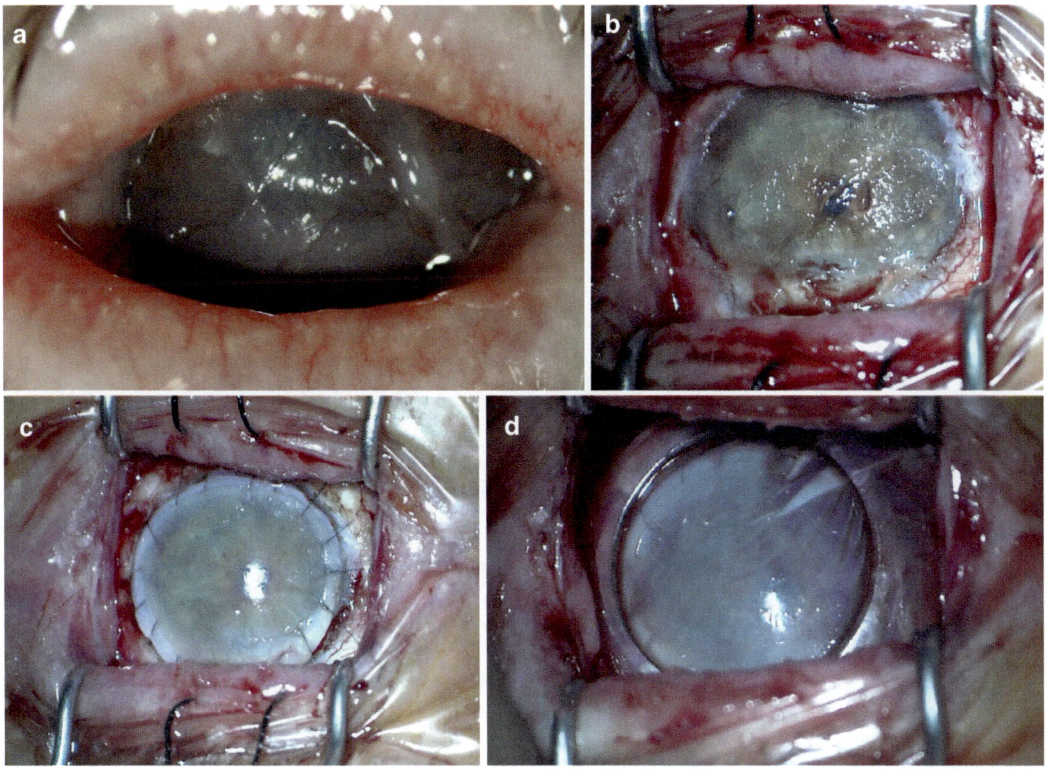

Fig. 9.7 (**a**) 89-year-old female patient with ocular cicatricial pemphigoid (OCP). If there is insufficient corneal insight, the first step is to reconstruct the corneal surface by removing corneal scarring (**b**), perform lamellar keratoplasty (**c**), and put a placeholder with an amniotic membrane on the eye to prevent further scarring (**d**). Cataract surgery can now be planned as a separate procedure

surgery should be as short as possible to prevent further desiccating stress to the ocular surface, as our experience shows higher rates of corneal complications with longer surgical procedures. This can primarily be achieved by assigning experienced surgeons to these cases. To reduce the inherently increased risk of postoperative infection, sutures may be placed in all paracenteses, especially if surface traction due to residual symblepharon still exists. In addition, temporary placement of a soft bandage contact lens under antibiotic coverage may speed epithelial healing if epithelial defects occurred [14]. When lid and surface preparation are combined with cataract surgery, general anesthesia may be preferred over topical anesthesia. In all eyes with significantly reduced visibility, trypan blue or equivalent staining dyes should be used to increase safety. Irrespective of possible sutures to all paracenteses as mentioned above, clear corneal incisions should always be sutured with traction to the ocular surface in these cases to reduce the risk of postoperative endophthalmitis.

The *third general principle applies to postoperative management*, where patients with cicatricial diseases should receive glucocorticoid eye drops in higher frequency compared to normal eyes and depending on preoperative disease activity. Depending on ocular surface inflammation activity, even preoperative application of topical steroids might be considered, especially in ocular GvHD. A temporary pretreatment with topical steroids for 4 weeks has been shown to significantly reduce the risk for dry eye disease induced by desiccating stress (e.g., cataract surgery) in normal eyes [15]. Systemic immunosuppressive therapy should be intensified, if necessary, and patients should be more closely

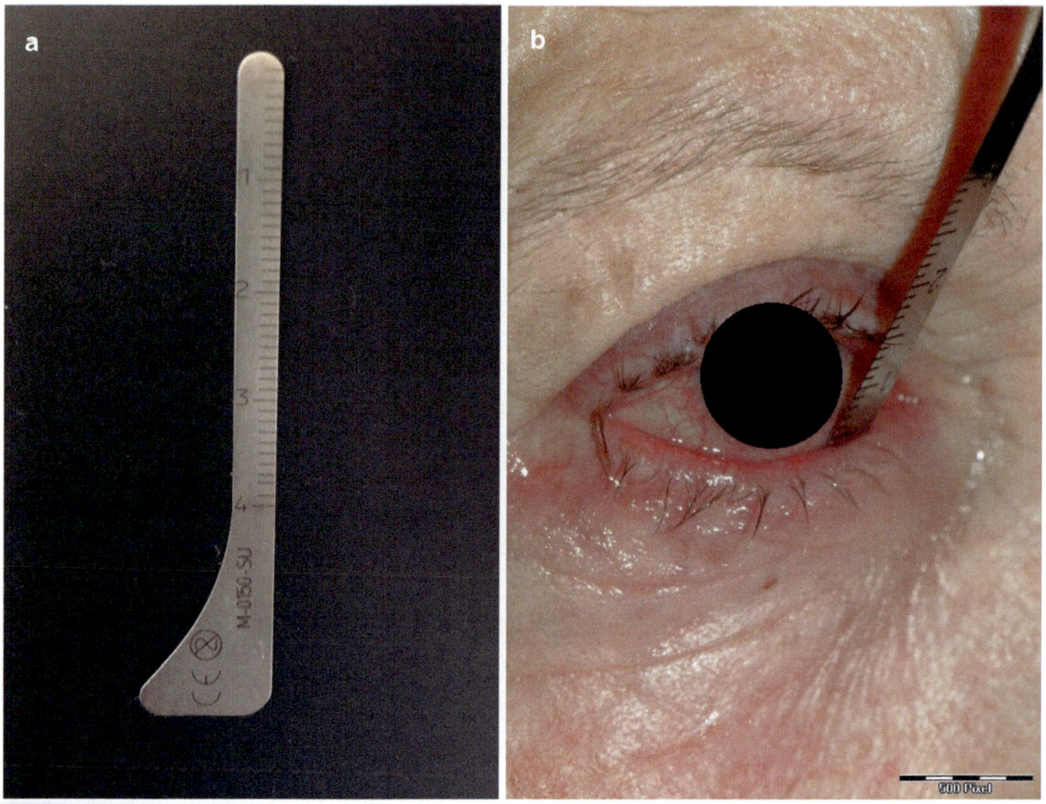

Fig. 9.8 (**a**) Fornix ruler for exact measurement of fornix changes in cicatricial diseases ("Messschablone nach Prof. Steven," Si Us Instruments GmbH, Berlin, Germany), (**b**) Application

monitored in order to detect and treat inflammation peaks and conjunctival scarring early on. Aggressive lubricating therapy with preservative-free eye drops is mandatory in all these eyes, ideally for a prolonged period. Systemic antibiotics such as doxycycline can be given in eyes with severe blepharitis (preoperatively, if necessary).

In addition to these general principles, some specific recommendations apply to singular entities in the spectrum of cicatricial eye diseases. In patients status post SJS or TEN, the active disease has usually ceased at time of cataract surgery, and reactivation of the underlying process is not to be expected (postoperative worsening in these cases is usually caused by decompensation of ocular surface disease and not reappearance of the actual immunological process that caused the disease in the first place). OCP, on the other hand, needs to be regarded as chronically present and can actually be triggered by mechanical trauma like surgery. In these cases, we strongly recommend not to perform surgery before a period of at least 6 months without progression in fornix measurements. If there is progression, systemic immunosuppressive therapy should be revised by a dermatologist or rheumatologist and escalated, if necessary. In GvHD, which also shows chronically progressive features, disease activity should be monitored via corneal fluorescein staining, and surgery should be planned, when staining has improved or stabilized.

Postoperatively, patients with preexisting conditions of the ocular surface require more intensive and more frequent care with regard to higher risk of complications such as delayed-onset epithelial defects, intraocular or surface-level infections, wound leakage, or spikes in inflammatory activity. These complications need to be diagnosed as early as possible and treated aggressively. Especially the potentially devastating complication of endophthalmitis is more likely in patients with ocular surface disease and needs to be anticipated [16].

As a general consideration for patients with cicatricial diseases, the necessity for cataract surgery should be evaluated more critically than in regular eyes because of the mentioned complicating factors that put the patient at higher risk of limited vision gain or even vision loss after surgery. Only if the cataract affects the patient's visual quality of life and a significant benefit is to be expected from surgery, the procedure should be planned. The patient should be well informed about the planned procedure and the risks linked to the individual case and give informed consent beforehand. However, despite the high-risk setting and surgically challenging nature of these cases, no patient should be withheld cataract surgery if he can be expected to gain visual function and quality of life.

Take-Home Notes

- The presence of cicatricial changes to the ocular surface greatly impacts timing, planning, execution, and aftercare of cataract surgery.
- Accurate identification of the causative disease is essential prior to surgery in order to anticipate whether the procedure may trigger a disease reactivation.
- In cases with extensive scarring, it may be necessary to perform reconstructive eyelid, conjunctival, and/or corneal surgery first to enable safe cataract surgery as a second-step procedure.
- Chronic inflammatory diseases responsible for ocular surface scarring must be sufficiently suppressed prior to cataract surgery.
- Postoperative follow-up must be adequately frequent to detect and treat complications as early as possible (these occur more often after normal cataract surgery).

Support DFG FOR 2240 (www.for2240.de); EU COST ANIRIDIA (www.aniridia-net.eu); EU Arrest Blindness (www.arrest-blindness.eu)

Literature

1. Saeed HN, Chodosh J. Ocular manifestations of Stevens-Johnson syndrome and their management. Curr Opin Ophthalmol. 2016;27(6):522–9.
2. Wang KSG, Gonzales JA. Ocular cicatricial pemphigoid. Curr Opin Ophthalmol. 2018;29:543–51.
3. Harr T, French LE. Stevens-Johnson syndrome and toxic epidermal necrolysis. Chem Immunol Allergy. 2012;97:149–66.
4. Harr T, French LE. Toxic epidermal necrolysis and Stevens-Johnson syndrome. Orphanet J Rare Dis. 2010;5(39):1–11.
5. Schmidt E, Zillikens D. Pemphigoid diseases. Lancet. 2013;381:320–32.
6. Geerling G, Roth M. Pseudopemphigoid induced by topical glaucoma medications. Klin Monatsbl Augenheilk. 2019;236(6):762–6.
7. Chen LB, Zhang S, Yan CX, Yao QK, Shao CY, Fu Y. Evaluation of chronic ocular sequelae in patients with symblepharon caused by ocular burn. Int J Ophthalmol. 2020;13(7):1066–73.
8. Tung CI. Graft versus host disease: what should the oculoplastic surgeon know? Curr Opin Ophthalmol. 2017;28:499–504.
9. Steven P, Sauerbier L, Siebelmann S, Gehlsen U, Tahmaz V, Wittig S, Scheid C, Cursiefen C. Therapy for ocular graft-vs-host disease. Klin Monatsbl Augenheilk. 2015;232:658–63.
10. Chuang J, Shih K, Chan T, Wan KH, Jhanjii V, Tong L. Preoperative optimization of ocular surface disease before cataract surgery. J Cataract Refract Surg. 2017;43(12):1596–607.
11. Tugal-Tutkun I, Akova AY, Foster CS. Penetrating keratoplasty in cicatrizing conjunctival diseases. Ophthalmology. 1994;102(4):576–85.
12. Tahmaz V, Gehlsen U, Sauerbier L, Holtick U, Engel L, Radojska S, Petrescu-Jipa VM, Scheid C, Hallek M, Gathof B, Cursiefen C, Steven P. Treatment of severe chronic ocular graft-versus-host disease using 100% autologous serum eye drops from a sealed manufacturing system: a retrospective cohort study. Br J Ophthalmol. 2016. Published Online First on June 6, 2016: p. 1–5.
13. Alvarado Valero MC, Martinez Toldos JJ, Borras Blasco J, Alminana Alminana A, Perez Ramos JM. Treatment of persistent epithelial defects using autologous serum application. Arch Soc Esp Oftalmol. 2004;79(11):537–42.
14. Chen D, Lian Y, Li J, Ma Y, Shen M, Lu F. Monitor corneal epithelial healing under bandage contact lens using ultrahigh-resolution optical coherence tomography after pterygium surgery. Eye Contact Lens. 2014;40(3):175–80.

15. Pinto-Fraga J, et al. Topical fluorometholone protects the ocular surface of dry eye patients from desiccating stress: a randomized controlled clinical trial. Ophthalmology. 2016;123(1):141–53.
16. Barry P, Cordoved L, Gardner S. ESCRS Guidelines for prevention and treatment of endophthalmitis following cataract surgery: data. Dilemmas and Conclusions. 2013.

Cataract Surgery in Keratoconus

10

Jorge L. Alió and Francesco D'Oria

Bullet Points

- How to evaluate visual impairment due to cataract in a keratoconus patient?
- Which IOL power calculation formula is superior in eyes with steep and irregular corneas?
- How to avoid intraoperative surgical problems with the correct preoperative planning?
- Which type of IOL should be implanted in a keratoconic eye?

Supplementary Information The online version contains supplementary material available at [https://doi.org/10.1007/978-3-030-94530-5_10].

J. L. Alió (✉)
Division of Ophthalmology, School of Medicine, Miguel Hernandez University, Alicante, Spain

Cornea, Refractive and Cataract Surgery Unit, Vissum Miranza Alicante, Alicante, Spain
e-mail: jlalio@vissum.com

F. D'Oria
Vissum Miranza Alicante, Alicante, Spain

Division of Ophthalmology, Universidad Miguel Hernández, Alicante, Spain

Section of Ophthalmology, Department of Basic Medical Science, Neuroscience and Sense Organs, University of Bari, Bari, Italy

Introduction

Keratoconus (KCN) is an ectatic corneal disease that leads to decreased vision due to progressive corneal thinning with the consequent alterations in corneal geometry and biomechanics and a reported annual incidence of approximately 1:7500 or 13.3 new cases per 100,000 [1].

It has been described that KCN patients are more prone to develop cataract compared with non-KCN patients and at a younger age than the general cataract populations, due to association with atopy and use of some medications [2]; nuclear cataract is the most common variant [2, 3]. Therefore, as these patients age, cataract becomes a more probable etiology for their low vision, and cataract surgery may be necessary.

In this chapter preoperative, intraoperative, and postoperative problems that surgeons may encounter when treating a KCN patient requiring cataract surgery will be discussed.

Preoperative Evaluation: How to Evaluate the Postop Vision and How Relevant Is the Cataract for the Vision of the Patient?

Despite numerous advances in cataract surgery regarding lens calculation, lens design, as well as phacoemulsification procedures and techniques, one of the main problems of clinicians is attributing

J. L. Alió et al. (eds.), *Cataract Surgery*, Essentials in Ophthalmology,
https://doi.org/10.1007/978-3-030-94530-5_10

Table 10.1 Clinical findings in a sample of patients with different degrees of keratoconus (defined by the level of visual limitation)

Sex/ age	Sim-Km	Internal astigmatism (diopters)	RMS coma-like (μm)	Q_{8mm}	Pachymetry	CDVA (estimated)	Grade	CDVA (real)
M/32	49.82	4.3	4.37	−1.07	458	0.4–0.6	**III**	0.5
F/16	47.24	2.94	3.49	−0.53	478	0.6–0.9	**II**	0.8
M/17	44.82	0.96	2.07	−0.31	497	>0.9	**I**	0.98
M/19	61.79	6.1	5.6	−1.87	410	<0.2	**IV plus**	0.15
F/25	49.5	3.58	3.7	−1.05	469	0.4–0.6	**III**	0.5
F/21	44.65	1.07	1.74	−0.17	493	>0.9	**I**	1
F/31	48.34	3.03	2.85	−0.71	482	0.6–0.9	**II**	0.86
M/53	45.7	1.54	2.06	−0.34	507	>0.9	**I**	1
F/26	52.53	3.71	4.35	−0.85	463	0.4–0.6	**III**	0.54
M/52	56.08	4.72	4.58	−1.4	441	0.2–0.4	**IV**	0.38

Abbreviations: *CDVA* corrected distance visual acuity, *Sim-Km* mean corneal power in the 3.0 mm zone, Q_{8mm} mean asphericity in an 8.0-mm-diameter corneal area, *RMS* root mean square

what is the real influence of the cataract on the visual acuity of KCN patient. It is difficult to assess how much the corneal ectasia on one hand and the evolution of the cataract on the other affect the visual acuity, to be able to provide the patient with the best possible preoperative information and to estimate the postoperative visual recovery.

In 2011, Alio et al. [4] developed a new classification system based on characterization of almost 800 cases of KCN in which visual, refractive, topographic, aberrometric, and biomechanical parameters were evaluated. By integrating the different data, four groups were formed, each representing a different degree of visual limitation, as follows: Group 1, corrected distance visual acuity (CDVA) better than 0.05 logMAR; Group 2, CDVA between 0.05 and 0.19; Group 3, CDVA between 0.19 and 0.40; and Group 4, CDVA worse or equal to 0.40.

They have demonstrated that visual deterioration in KCN patients can be consistently explained by biomechanical and corneal topographic alterations, as CDVA is significantly correlated with changes in keratometric values, corneal hysteresis and corneal resistance factors, as well as aberrometric measures, and these parameters significantly differ between groups. Therefore, starting from the knowledge of the topographical, biomechanical, and aberrometric corneal parameters, it is possible to determine the degree of visual impairment and therefore estimate the postoperative visual recovery. Table 10.1 shows a sample of KCN patients where the degree of visual limitation can be derived from the topographic, biomechanical, and aberrometric parameters and thus corresponds to the real level of CDVA.

Nevertheless, periodic evaluations to check the progression of the KCN (measured by changes in K values, astigmatism, pachymetry, corneal hysteresis, or visual acuity) and the cataract are strongly recommended before making any surgical decision, to confirm the stabilization of the disease before to proceed with the cataract surgery.

Planification of the Surgical Technique and Preventing Surgical Problems in the OR

Cataract surgery in KCN can be technically challenging depending on the degree of the disease: early stages can be handled like normal surgery, while advanced stages of the disease require special precautions. The wound creation, although now irrelevant in healthy corneas especially with the novel micro-incisional cataract surgery (MICS), can cause an effect that is difficult to predict in ectatic and thin corneas, with the consequent increase in the surgically induced astigmatism and the changes in corneal shape. The choice of the main incision should be made preoperatively, according to the peripheral corneal thickness and the astigmatism axis. In the common case of infero-temporal cone, the main incision should be placed superiorly or supero-temporal. Vice versa, in those rare cases with a superior steep cone, the main incision should be placed temporally [5]. The incision should also be made as close as possible to the limbus to avoid areas of corneal thinning [6]. In advanced KCN eyes with very thinned corneas, less prone to resist to surgical trauma, a well-constructed two-step sclerocorneal wound is advisable to reduce the risk of postoperative wound leak and to induce less change in corneal shape [5].

Additionally, clear corneal wounds are more prone to leak after surgery due to the different biomechanical behavior of these corneas: one suggestion is to suture the clear corneal incisions to ensure wound apposition [7]. A further problem is represented by poor intraoperative visualization, secondary to high astigmatism or stromal scarring in more advanced cases. The subsequent intraocular image distortion and the lack of visual perspective are the main problems during capsulorhexis, phacoemulsification, and I/A. To improve visibility, considering that the diffuse light source employed by the surgical microscope provides the surgeon with a worse view compared with the slit-lamp examination, it can be useful to spread ophthalmic viscoelastic device on the corneal surface: however, in advanced cases, it may not be uniformly dispersed on the cornea. For that purpose, Oie et al. [8] recommend the use of rigid gas-permeable (RGP) contact lens to maximize intraoperative vision. In corneas with advanced disease and very poor transparency, a combined DALK-cataract surgery is advisable. In this scenario, surgical planning is imperative, to decide if performing or not the corneal graft surgery at the same setting of the cataract surgery: the sequential approach to DALK and cataract surgery in a two-step procedure might be beneficial to avoid endothelial damage [9, 10]. The use of capsular staining dye is also recommended to enhance capsular visualization during continuous curvilinear capsulorhexis in cases of poor red reflex.

We report the case of a 51-year-old keratoconus patient who had implantation of intrastromal corneal ring segment (ICRS) to reduce the corneal astigmatism followed by implantation of a phakic posterior chamber IOL (pc-IOL) to correct the residual refractive error. One year after pc-IOL implantation, she developed an anterior subcapsular cataract that required a bilesenctomy (Fig. 10.1). Her CDVA prior to the cataract surgery was 0.42, despite an estimated CDVA according to the RETICS classification between 0.6 and 0.9. We performed a bilesenctomy with pc-IOL extraction followed by MICS and monofocal toric IOL implantation (see Video 10.1 illustrating the surgery). The IOL power was calculated using the Barrett Toric calculator. Extreme caution was taken during the surgery to implant the toric IOL in the correct axis and to avoid the risk of postoperative wound leakage (given the instability of the ectatic cornea) by suturing the corneal wound: the suture was eventually removed after 2 weeks. Her final CDVA after the cataract surgery was 0.7, in agreement with the topographic and aberrometric condition of the cornea.

Intraocular Lens Calculation Targeting the Right Power

The peculiar optical structure of KCN explains the interest that this condition has in clinical practice as regards the calculation of the IOL power. This measurement in patients with KCN has a significant variability of refractive results due to the optical properties of the cornea, the inhomogeneity in the depth of the anterior chamber, and the lower accuracy in the detection of the axial length. These limits are partially reduced by the ongoing development of technology and data science that can improve the accuracy of IOL selection.

Hashemi et al. [11] examined the repeatability of keratometry measurements with five different

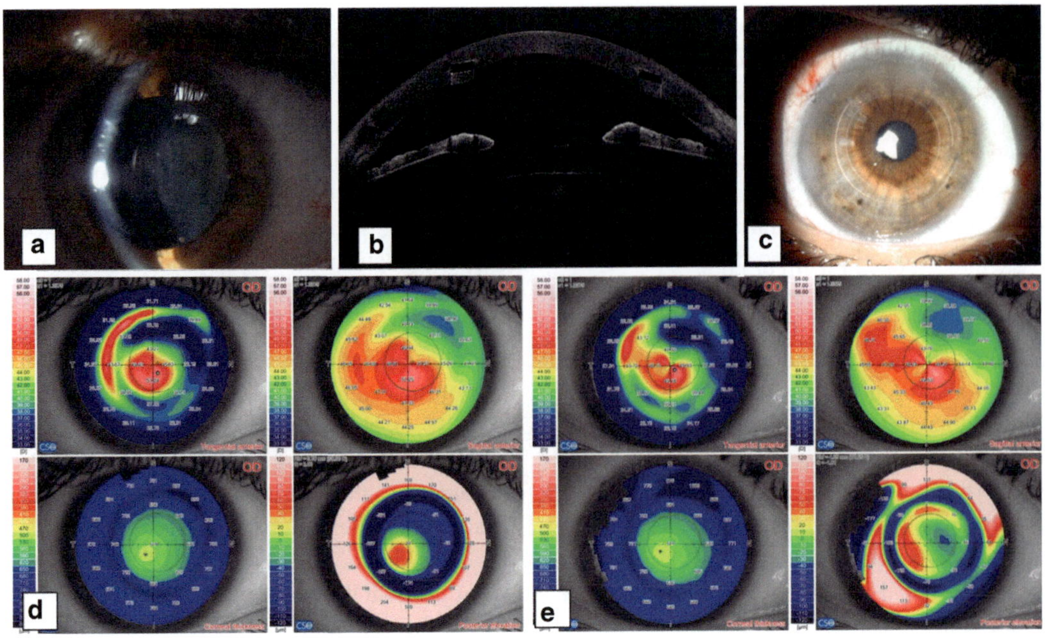

Fig. 10.1 A 51-year-old female keratoconus patient. (**a**) Preoperative slit-lamp image showing the anterior subcapsular cataract following the phakic posterior chamber IOL implantation. (**b**) Anterior segment OCT image showing the intrastromal corneal ring segment placement and an anterior opacity in the crystalline lens. (**c**) Postoperative appearance of the eye. (**d**) Corneal topography showing a paracentral cone with posterior elevation and reduction in the corneal thickness. (**e**) Early postoperative corneal topography showing the increased astigmatism in the supero-temporal meridian related to the corneal suture at the site of the main incision

devices based on five different measurement techniques (Pentacam, Eyesys, Orbscan, IOLMaster, Javal manual keratometer) in 78 eyes with different grades of KCN. The study found that in patients with K values, up to 55.0 D keratometry readings had good repeatability among all the devices and Pentacam had the highest repeatability, while Orbscan had the lowest. In Group 3 ($K > 55$D), all five devices had low repeatability. The same authors found that the lowest mean absolute error was obtained with the SRK/T formula in patients with mild to moderate KCN and SRK/T and SRK II formulas in patients with severe KCN [11].

Vergence formulas use up to six biometry parameters, introducing a series of modifications to know how IOL power changes with the varying corneal curvatures and axial lengths of the eye [12]. Recently, Savini et al. [13], comparing five different formulas, showed that SRK/T is the most accurate formula, yielding an acceptable percentage of patients with a prediction error within ±0.5 D, which reached a rate of 61.90% in eyes with a grade I KCN. The outcomes reported by the authors were even worst in eyes with more advanced degrees of the disease, suggesting caution when targeting any refractive outcome in eyes with preoperative K value higher than 48 D [13]. This finding agrees with what has been observed by our research group in a previous study that showed a higher refractive accuracy when the SRK/T formula was used [14] and probably depends on the fact that the SRK/T tends to overestimate the IOL power in eyes with steep corneas [15]. Such overestimation can be useful in eyes with keratoconus since it counterbalances the average trend toward hyperopic refraction observed with most formulas. Moreover, the axial length (AL) was, on average, relatively high, and it was longer than 26.0 mm in 34.1% of eyes. This might be another factor contributing to the good performance of the SRK/T because this formula has been shown to be one of the most accurate in long eyes [16]. Alio et al. [14] showed that the axial length had a stronger correlation with the final spherical equivalent than the preoperative keratometry in ten KCN patients who had MICS with toric IOL implantation.

Reitblat et al. [17] analyzed the performance of commonly used IOL power calculation formulas in a subgroup of eyes with steep corneal geometry ($K > 46$D). They found that IOL power calculations for eyes with an average K value greater than 46.00 D yielded myopic prediction errors with the SRK/T and Hill-RBF formulas and hyperopic errors with Haigis and Olsen-C formulas. Compared with all other formulas, the SRK/T showed a higher systemic error. The authors described then a new regression formula for K value adjustment to be used with the SRK/T formula (optimized $K = -1.91 + 1.05$ x measured K), in order to reduce the refractive error using the SRK/T formula for IOL power calculation in eyes with extreme corneal measurements ($K > 46$ D).

The Barrett Universal II is becoming accepted as one of the most accurate IOL formulas in use today, contributing to its increasing popularity among surgeons. The formula is based on a theoretical model eye and retains the positive correlation of AL and keratometry to ACD. Importantly, the Barrett Universal II is able to maintain its accuracy across a wide range of ALs and ACD [15].

Newer methodologies are being applied to IOL calculation with promises of improved accuracy. As opposed to vergence-based equations, the Olsen formula uses both exact and paraxial ray tracings of optical light through the refractive media in the eye, including the specific optics of a particular IOL, to derive the postoperative position of that lens [18]. In the Olsen formula, the lens constant is no longer related to AL and corneal power but to the characteristic of the crystalline lens and the dimension of the anterior chamber. In the 2020 study of 10,930 eyes, the Barrett Universal II had larger overall mean absolute errors compared with the Olsen formula and Hill-RBF (2.0 version) calculator and was comparable with the AL-adjusted Holladay 2 formula. However, when analyzed by different categories of AL, the Barrett had less error than Olsen and Hill-RBF 2.0 in long eyes (AL >26.0 mm) and is equivalent to the Olsen for medium eyes (22.0–26.0 mm) [19].

We should expect a poor refractive result with a higher hyperopic shift in eyes with advanced KCN (stage II or III), based on three major motivating reasons [13]. First, calculating the corneal power with the standard keratometric index (n = 13,375) can lead to erroneous results. This fictitious index can be correctly used to achieve the refractive power of the whole cornea based on just the anterior corneal curvature, but only on the condition that the ratio between the anterior and posterior corneal curvature is within normal limits: in KCN eyes, the standard keratometric index overestimates corneal power [20, 21]. Second, keratometers and corneal topographers provide measurements of corneal curvature that might be inaccurate because of asymmetry of corneal curvature. Every keratometer, in fact, assumes that the corneal curvature is constant along a given meridian, but this is not the case in most keratoconic eyes [13]. Third, keratoconus can alter the usual relationship between corneal curvature, anterior chamber depth, and IOL position, thus reducing the accuracy of any formula in predicting the effective lens position.

Intraocular Lens Choice

A very important moment in the intraoperative planning is the choice of the IOL to be implanted. Whenever planning cataract surgery in a KCN eye, the surgeon will have to decide whether a toric IOL is more suitable than a monofocal IOL.

Hashemi et al. [22] reported the results using an AcrySof toric IOL in 23 eyes of 17 patients with KCN and cataract. They showed that toric IOLs improved vision and refraction in all types of KCN including mild, moderate, and even severe KCN; however, in case of severe KCN, the refractive outcomes had less predictability. Similarly, Nanavaty et al. [23] showed that the use of pseudophakic toric IOL in KCN cataract patients was effective and resulted in an acceptable and stable vision in patients with mild and moderate KCN. Alio et al. [14] retrospectively evaluated 17 keratoconic eyes of 10 patients who underwent MICS and reported a significant improvement in UDVA, CDVA, and cylinder but not in the sphere.

When considering the lower predictability and outcomes in severe KCN, one should take into account that being the astigmatism of those corneas more irregular, this aspect might affect the final visual outcomes. Another explication is the possible increased postoperative rotation. Zhu et al. [24] reported that postoperative toric IOL rotation was positively correlated with axial length myopia and capsular bag size. We suggest capsular tension ring placement whenever a toric IOL is to be implanted in a keratoconic eye; optic capture might represent an option. Another relevant consideration is the asphericity of the IOL. As many KCN eyes have a steep cornea with a large negative preoperative anterior surface Q value, adding an IOL with a zero or even positive Q value may have a better visual outcome [25].

In case of progression and/or keratoplasty, mixed implant techniques like power split approaches are an alternative option: the surgeon may implant an initial non-toric, monofocal IOL to correct the majority of the refractive error and then utilize a subsequent procedure, such as a secondary sulcus-supported IOL (piggyback IOL), to correct the residual refractive error [26]. In cases of eyes with keratoconus, piggyback IOLs may rotate significantly, and in these cases, a sulcus suture might be utilized to improve stability [27]. Also, multicomponent IOL (MCIOL) technologies are available having a basic power and a toric IOL attached like the new Precisight IOL (InfiniteVision Optics, Strasbourg, France): this compact IOL is composed of a hydrophobic base lens that serves as a docking station and an exchangeable hydrophilic front lens that is connected to the base lens by bilateral bridge openings [28]. Moreover, in situations like potential progression, expected corneal decompensation or need for keratoplasty is recommended to implant a "space holder" in the bag like a capsular bending ring in order to ease IOL exchange.

Other interesting commercially available IOLs are coming onto the market, which might be good options/alternatives given the potential deviation from target refraction in KCN patients. A small-aperture IOL (IC-8, AcuFocus, Inc.) is one of such alternatives that improves vision in eyes with severe corneal irregularities (e.g., due to advanced keratoconus) using the pinhole effect [29]. Selected cases of keratoconus could be treated by a new intraocular pinhole device (XtraFocus, Morcher), which can be safely implanted either in the sulcus or in the bag [30, 31]. Finally, light adjustable lens (RxSight Inc., Aliso Viejo, California, USA) is a foldable, posterior chamber three-piece silicone lens that has been explored as a potential advancement in improving postoperative visual outcomes after cataract surgery, being able to adjust spherical power from −2.00 to +2.00 D and cylindrical power from −0.75 to −2.00 D by 0.25 D increments [32].

KCN patients, even with a forme fruste KCN, represent an important contraindication to multifocal IOL, given the high amount of high-order aberration (especially coma) and the consequent poor visual outcomes if an IOL with an advanced multifocal optic is implanted.

Postoperative Complications: Management of Postoperative Residual Astigmatism

Patients should be aware of the possible inaccuracies in IOL measurements because of KCN and understand that a subsequent medical or surgical treatment may be necessary because of poor postoperative refractive outcomes and postoperative residual astigmatism.

Irregular astigmatism of the cornea obviously persists, or sometimes even worsen, after surgery: many patients might require RGP or scleral contact lens in order to correct the residual astigmatism and thus achieve the best visual and refractive outcome. A deep evaluation and fitting of the contact lens is recommended after surgery, as the corneal surface may have changed [6, 8].

ICRS is a refractive technology that flattens the central cornea by an arc-shortening effect on the corneal lamellae structure which improves the optical quality of the cornea and the visual acuity [33]. ICRS have been extensively used in the management of ectatic corneal conditions, such as KCN, pellucid marginal degeneration, and post-laser in situ keratomileusis corneal ectasia [34, 35], and might represent an effective issue in the correction of postoperative astigmatism in cataract KCN patients. Another use of this device is represented by the sequential ICRS first and IOL implantation thereafter: Alfonso et al. [36] reported it to be a safe and effective procedure with good visual and refractive outcomes in the treatment of patients with KCN and cataract. IOL calculation in KCN corneas with ICRS in place can be difficult with a more variable refractive outcome. We reported an interesting difficult case of a 61-year-old high-myopic patient with a grade IV KCN (assessed according to the visual impairment [4]) who has been implanted with an ICRS (Fig. 10.2) to reduce the corneal astigmatism and had developed cataract. His CDVA was limited to 0.3 (−22, −3.50 @175°). After using the ASSORT software to evaluate the residual ocular astigmatism and thus help in the surgical planning, we implanted a Rainer RayOne -10D IOL, using the SRK/T formula, aiming to a myopic target. CDVA after surgery was 0.36 (+5, −4 @ 165°) with a further improvement in BCVA up to 0.8 with a rigid gas-permeable contact lens.

Finally, refractive surprises following cataract surgery in KCN eyes can be managed by performing a photorefractive keratectomy (PRK) [37]; nevertheless, to be performed with safety, PRK should be advised only in stable cases of KCN, without progression over the last 2 years, and with a maximum grade I/II of the disease [38]. PRK is recommended to be customized for coma, to reduce corneal high-order aberrations and possibly improve postoperative CDVA [39]; alternative choices would be piggyback with iris-fixated PIOL or sulcus-fixated PIOL. When choosing between keratorefractive procedure and intraocular option, one should consider that the eye is reopened maybe with a wide incision.

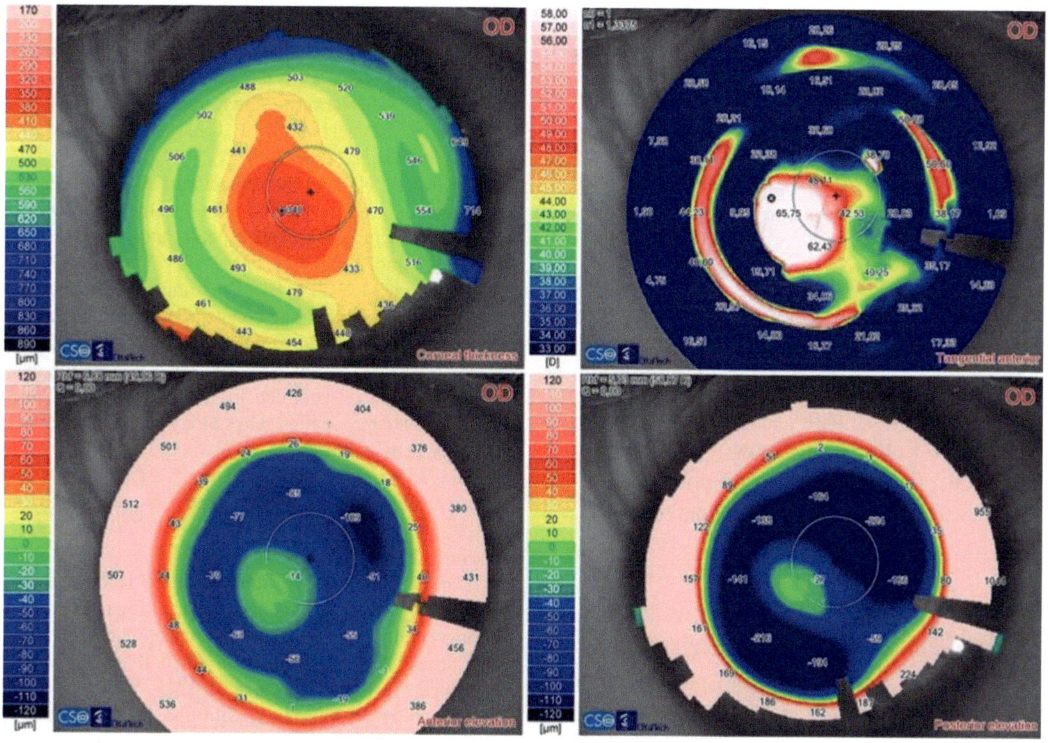

Fig. 10.2 Corneal topography showed an infero-temporal paracentral corneal steepening in the right eye, with a Kmax of 67.98 D and a corneal thinning point of 370 µm

Conclusion

Cataract surgery in KCN requires extensive preoperative evaluation to obtain the best visual result for the patient. Ophthalmologists must know the exceptional difficulties related to the peculiar characteristics of these eyes, so that they can choose the best IOL of adequate power, to be able to deal with any intraoperative complications, and to be able to correct without difficulty any residual postoperative refractive error. In conclusion, the preoperative evaluation of the patient represents the fundamental moment: it is necessary to evaluate the real incidence of the cataract in the visual impairment of the patient, referring to the theoretical functional limit of the eye considering the topographical and aberrometric conditions of the cornea. The IOL power should be calculated using those formulas that have a greater accuracy. Intraoperatively, the corneal incision should be made as close as possible to the limbus and in the steepest meridian, implanting a toric IOL, if suitable, to correct the high astigmatism. The suture of the corneal wound may be required in advanced cases, given the higher risk of postoperative leakage in ectatic corneas.

Take-Home Messages

- Assessment of the possible progression of keratoconus is required before planning surgery.
- Biomechanical and topographical changes of the ectatic cornea can estimate the component of visual impairment due to keratoconus and in what percentage it is affected by cataract.
- SRK/T formula is recommended for IOL power calculation, possibly corrected according to keratometry readings in very steep corneas.
- It is recommended to perform corneal incision in the steep axis, as close as possible to the limbus, eventually suturing the incision to avoid postoperative corneal leakage.
- Multifocal IOLs are not recommended due to the presence of corneal high-order aberrations.
- If available and possible, toric IOLs are recommended to correct corneal astigmatism.

Financial Support This study has been financed in part by the Network for Cooperative Research in Health "OFTARED," Nodo Dioptrio Ocular, Biobanco Iberia (Reference: RD16/0008/0012.), *funded by Instituto de Salud Carlos III, and co-funded by the European Regional Development Fund (ERDF), Project "A way to make Europe."*

References

1. Godefrooij DA, de Wit GA, Uiterwaal CS, Imhof SM, Wisse RPL. Age-specific incidence and prevalence of keratoconus: a nationwide registration study. Am J Ophthalmol. 2017;175:169–72.
2. Thebpatiphat N, Hammersmith KM, Rapuano CJ, et al. Cataract surgery in keratoconus. Eye Contact Lens. 2007;33:244–6.
3. Bozorg S, Pineda R. Cataract and keratoconus: minimizing complications in intraocular lens calculations. Semin Ophthalmol. 2014;29(5–6):376e379.
4. Alio JL, Pinero DP, Aleson A, et al. Keratoconus-integrated characterization considering anterior corneal aberrations, internal astigmatism, and corneal biomechanics. J Cataract Refract Surg. 2011;37(3):552–68.
5. Aiello F, Nasser QJ, Nucci C, Angunawela RI, Gatzioufas Z, Maurino V. Cataract surgery in patients with keratoconus: pearls and pitfalls. Open Ophthalmol J. 2017;11:194–200.
6. Moshirfar M, Walker BD, Birdsong OC. Cataract surgery in eyes with keratoconus: a review of the current literature. Curr Opin Ophthalmol. 2018;29(1):75–80.
7. Bourges JL. Cataract surgery in keratoconus with irregular astigmatism. In: Goggin M, editor. Astigmatism – optics, physiology and management. Rijeka: InTech; 2012.
8. Oie Y, Kamei M, Matsumura N, et al. Rigid gas-permeable contact lens-assisted cataract surgery in patients with severe keratoconus. J Cataract Refract Surg. 2014;40:345–8.
9. Den S, Shimmura S, Shimazaki J. Cataract surgery after deep anterior lamellar keratoplasty and penetrating keratoplasty in age- and disease-matched eyes. J Cataract Refract Surg. 2018;44(4):496–503. https://doi.org/10.1016/j.jcrs.2018.01.024.
10. Shimmura S, Ohashi Y, Shiroma H, Shimazaki J, Tsubota K. Corneal opacity and cataract: triple

procedure versus secondary approach. Cornea. 2003;22:234–8.
11. Hashemi H, Yekta A, Khabazkhoob M. Effect of keratoconus grades on repeatability of keratometry readings: comparison of 5 devices. J Cataract Refract Surg. 2015;41:1065–72.
12. Xia T, Martinez C, Tsai L. Update on intraocular lens formulas and calculations. Asia Pac J Ophthalmol (Phila). 2020;9:186–93.
13. Savini G, Abbate R, Hoffer KJ, et al. Intraocular lens power calculation in eyes with keratoconus. J Cataract Refract Surg. 2019;45(5):576–81.
14. Alió JL, Peña-García P, Abdulla Guliyeva F, Soria FA, Zein G, Abu-Mustafa SK. MICS with toric intraocular lenses in keratoconus outcomes and predictability analysis of postoperative refraction. Br J Ophthalmol. 2014;98:365–70.
15. Melles RB, Holladay JT, Chang WJ. Accuracy of intraocular lens calculation formulas. Ophthalmology. 2018;125:169–78.
16. Hoffer KJ. The Hoffer Q formula: a comparison of theoretic and regression formulas. J Cataract Refract Surg. 1993;19:700–12; errata, 1994; 20:677; 2007; 33: 2–3
17. Reitblat O, Levy A, Kleinmann G, Lerman TT, Assia EI. Intraocular lens power calculation for eyes with high and low average keratometry readings: comparison between various formulas. J Cataract Refract Surg. 2017;43(9):1149–56. https://doi.org/10.1016/j.jcrs.2017.06.036.
18. Olsen T, Funding M. Ray-tracing analysis of intraocular lens power in situ. J Cataract Refract Surg. 2012;38:641–7.
19. Darcy K, Gunn D, Tavassoli S, Sparrow J, Kane JX. Assessment of the accuracy of new and updated intraocular lens power calculation formulas in 10 930 eyes from the UK National Health Service. J Cataract Refract Surg. 2020;46:2–7.
20. Pinero DP, Camps VJ, Caravaca-Arens E, Perez-Cambrodi RJ, Artola A. Estimation of the central corneal power in keratoconus: theoretical and clinical assessment of the error of the keratometric approach. Cornea. 2014;33:274–9.
21. Kamiya K, Kono Y, Takahashi M, Shoji N. Comparison of simulated keratometry and total refractive power for keratoconus according to the stage of Amsler-Krumeich classification. Sci Rep. 2018;8:12436.
22. Hashemi H, Heidarian S, Seyedian MA, et al. Evaluation of the results of using toric IOL in the cataract surgery of keratoconus patients. Eye Contact Lens. 2015;41:354–8.
23. Nanavaty MA, Lake DB, Daya SM. Outcomes of pseudophakic toric intraocular lens implantation in keratoconic eyes with cataract. J Refract Surg. 2012;28:884–9.
24. Zhu X, He W, Zhang K, Lu Y. Factors influencing 1-year rotational stability of AcrySof Toric intraocular lenses. Br J Ophthalmol. 2016;100:263–8.
25. Savini G, Hoffer KJ, Barboni P. Influence of corneal asphericity on the refractive outcome of intraocular lens implantation in cataract surgery. J Cataract Refract Surg. 2015;41(4):785–9. https://doi.org/10.1016/j.jcrs.2014.07.035.
26. Meyer JJ, McGhee CN. Supplementary, sulcus-fixated intraocular lens in the treatment of spherical and astigmatic refractive errors in pseudophakic eyes after keratoplasty. Cornea. 2015;34(9):1052–6. https://doi.org/10.1097/ICO.0000000000000506.
27. Meyer JJ, Kim BZ, Ziaei M, McGhee CN. Postoperative rotation of supplementary sulcus-supported toric intraocular lenses. J Cataract Refract Surg. 2017;43(2):285–8. https://doi.org/10.1016/j.jcrs.2016.12.014.
28. Uy HS, Tesone-Coelho C, Ginis H. Enhancement-procedure outcomes in patients implanted with the Precisight multicomponent intraocular lens. Clin Ophthalmol. 2019;13:107–14. https://doi.org/10.2147/OPTH.S188383.
29. Shajari M, Mackert MJ, Langer J, et al. Safety and efficacy of a small-aperture capsular bag-fixated intraocular lens in eyes with severe corneal irregularities. J Cataract Refract Surg. 2020;46(2):188–92. https://doi.org/10.1097/j.jcrs.0000000000000045.
30. Trindade BLC, Trindade FC, Trindade CLC. Toric intraocular lens combined with a supplementary pinhole implant to treat irregular corneal astigmatism [published online ahead of print, 2020 Jul 28]. J Cataract Refract Surg. 2020. https://doi.org/10.1097/j.jcrs.0000000000000356.
31. Trindade BLC, Trindade FC, Werner L, Trindade CLC. Long-term safety of in-the-bag implantation of a supplementary intraocular pinhole. J Cataract Refract Surg. 2020;46(6):888–92. https://doi.org/10.1097/j.jcrs.0000000000000163.
32. Moshirfar M, Wagner WD, Linn SH, et al. Astigmatic correction with implantation of a light adjustable vs monofocal lens: a single site analysis of a randomized controlled trial. Int J Ophthalmol. 2019;12(7):1101–7. https://doi.org/10.18240/ijo.2019.07.08.
33. Fleming JF, Wan WL, Schanzlin DJ. The theory of corneal curvature change with the intrastromal corneal ring. CLAO J. 1989;15(2):146–50.
34. Alio JL, Salem T, Artola A, Osman AA. Intracorneal rings to correct corneal ectasia after laser in situ keratomileusis. J Cataract Refract Surg. 2002;28(9):1568–74.
35. Vega-Estrada A, Alio JL, Brenner LF, et al. Outcome analysis of intracorneal ring segments for the treatment of keratoconus based on visual, refractive, and aberrometric impairment. Am J Ophthalmol. 2013;155(3):575–84.
36. Alfonso JF, Lisa C, Fernandez L, et al. Sequential intrastromal corneal ring segment and monofocal intraocular lens implantation for keratoconus and cataract: long-term follow-up. J Cataract Refract Surg. 2017;43:246–54.
37. Roszkowska AM, Urso M, Signorino GA, Spadea L, Aragona P. Photorefractive keratectomy after cataract surgery in uncommon cases: long-term results.

Int J Ophthalmol. 2018;11(4):612–5. https://doi.org/10.18240/ijo.2018.04.12.

38. Khakshoor H, Razavi F, Eslampour A, Omdtabrizi A. Photorefractive keratectomy in mild to moderate keratoconus: outcomes in over 40-year-old patients. Indian J Ophthalmol. 2015;63(2):157–61. https://doi.org/10.4103/0301-4738.154400.

39. Jun I, Kang DSY, Arba-Mosquera S, et al. Comparison between wavefront-optimized and corneal wavefront-guided transepithelial photorefractive keratectomy in moderate to high astigmatism. BMC Ophthalmol. 2018;18(1):154. https://doi.org/10.1186/s12886-018-0827-x.

11 Cataract in Cases with Previous Corneal Graft Surgery; High Astigmatism

Mitchell Weikert and Anirudh Mukhopadhyay

Top Five Issues with Cataract Surgery in Eyes with Corneal Graft Surgery and High Astigmatism

- Should cataract surgery be performed at the time of or subsequent to corneal transplantation?
- What specific issues accompany biometry and intraocular lens calculations in patients with corneal transplants?
- How must cataract surgery technique be modified for eyes that require or have undergone corneal transplantation?
- What techniques are available for managing astigmatism in patients with corneal grafts?
- What is the best choice for astigmatism correction in eyes that have undergone corneal transplantation?

Introduction

Cataract formation is often associated with ocular conditions that necessitate corneal transplantation. Sometimes the underlying pathology that caused corneal opacification or decompensation also causes opacification of the crystalline lens, such as with severe and/or prolonged infectious keratitis or chronic uveitis. In other instances, cataract development follows corneal transplantation and may be related to the utilization of intracameral gas or other iatrogenic traumas. As such, cataract surgery in the setting of corneal transplantation, whether sequential or concurrent, presents a variety of challenges, one of which is the management of astigmatism. While several of these considerations are common to all corneal transplantation techniques, many are specific to the type of corneal transplantation. As such, this discussion will address the pre-, intra-, and postoperative factors to consider in these patients and will be organized around the major varieties of corneal transplantation: conventional penetrating, anterior lamellar, and endothelial keratoplasty.

M. Weikert (✉) · A. Mukhopadhyay
Baylor College of Medicine, Houston, TX, USA
e-mail: mweikert@bcm.edu

Conventional Penetrating Keratoplasty (PKP) and Cataract Surgery

The choice of transplantation technique is directly related to the corneal pathology and its visual impact. While penetrating keratoplasty (PKP) was the mainstay for many decades, the advent of improved anterior and posterior lamellar techniques has led to a substantial reduction in its use [1]. While still common, today PKP is typically reserved for corneal pathologies that

J. L. Alió et al. (eds.), *Cataract Surgery*, Essentials in Ophthalmology,
https://doi.org/10.1007/978-3-030-94530-5_11

involve the full thickness of the cornea, compromising both the stroma and endothelium, or conditions where a lamellar technique cannot be successfully performed, e.g., advanced keratoconus with a history of hydrops. When a cataract is present and the patient has elected to proceed with a PKP, the surgeon's next decision is whether to perform each procedure concurrently or sequentially.

Concurrent PKP and Cataract Surgery

Full-thickness corneal transplantation combined with cataract removal and intraocular lens (IOL) implantation is often called a "triple procedure." A triple procedure can be quite successful and carries the single-surgery benefits of reduced anesthesia, a single exposure to infectious risk, faster visual rehabilitation, lower cost, etc. However, these benefits are accompanied by other significant surgical challenges.

Due to limited visibility, the cataract is often removed "open sky" after the host cornea is excised. This open anterior chamber creates an unequal pressure gradient with unopposed vitreous pressure. The excessive posterior pressure behind the crystalline lens increases the risk for capsulorhexis loss, posterior capsule rupture, or even expulsive hemorrhage [2]. Even with successful capsulorhexis creation and extracapsular delivery of the lens, the typically convex posterior capsule can make cortical removal and lens implantation more difficult. A small capsulorhexis aided by trypan blue staining is recommended, along with implantation of a three-piece IOL. Yokokur et al. described the use of retrolenticular illumination with a chandelier to facilitate capsulorhexis creation in a closed anterior chamber prior to corneal trephination [3]. Their rate of successful capsulorhexis was 86% in the chandelier group vs. 30% in the non-chandelier group. Core vitrectomy prior to a triple procedure has also been shown to increase the success of IOL implantation with reduced risk of vitreous prolapse and reduced operative time [4, 5].

One major challenge associated with simultaneous PKP and cataract surgery is the choice of IOL power. The refractive power of the cornea following PKP is extremely unpredictable, which can translate into high postoperative refractive prediction errors (RPE) [6, 7]. Since the refractive power of the donor cornea and the true effect of the corneal sutures are unknown, the surgeon is left to estimate the corneal power in the IOL calculations. Choices include using the average corneal power of the fellow eye or the selection of a fixed value based on prior experience. Either method is inherently subject to significant error. In addition, since the donor cornea is sutured in place, there is substantial risk of high postoperative astigmatism that may also be irregular. This unpredictability can also result in a high level of anisometropia following suture removal. Shimomura et al. found less than 50% of eyes to have RPEs within ±2 diopters (D) following a triple procedure, as compared to 91% when cataract surgery followed PKP [4]. For these reasons, whenever possible we prefer to perform cataract surgery after PKP once the graft is adequately healed and all the sutures have been removed.

Sequential PKP and Cataract Surgery

While sequential PKP and cataract surgery has the disadvantages of slower visual rehabilitation, additional surgical exposure, higher cost, and the potential for endothelial damage, in our opinion, these are far outweighed by its increased safety and improved refractive outcomes. Since PKP sutures can have major effects on corneal refractive power and astigmatism levels, it is recommended to perform cataract surgery after all of the corneal sutures have been removed [6, 7]. If this is not possible, the patient should be carefully counseled on the potential for future refractive unpredictability.

Cataract surgical technique typically requires minimal alteration due to the presence of the transplant, but some points are worth noting. Care should be taken when constructing surgical incisions to avoid the graft-host junction (GHJ). This often results in "shorter" incisions that are more prone to leaking and are at higher risk for iris prolapse. In addition, the biomechanical forces associated with the GHJ may also reduce the ability of incisions to self-seal. Therefore, it is recommended that incisions be sutured if there is any question of their integrity. A scleral tunnel may be considered in eyes with a large diameter graft. The corneal transplant may also produce some optical distortion, typically in the mid-periphery near the GHJ. This slight compromise in visualization may be offset by the use of trypan blue capsular stain, even in the presence of an adequate red reflex. A dispersive ocular viscosurgical device (OVD) is preferred over the cohesive variety, as it will be better retained during the cataract surgery to protect the corneal endothelium. Den et al. found an average endothelial cell loss of 31% 1 year following cataract removal, with a steady decline through the first 6 months after surgery [8]. Finally, these eyes are often associated with additional ocular pathology, such as posterior synechiae, glaucoma, zonular loss, and mature cataracts, and are more likely to need additional tools and instrumentation, such as trypan blue, capsule support devices, and pupillary expansion devices.

Astigmatism Management

As noted previously, posttransplant corneas (more commonly post-PKP or ALK) often require management of high levels of astigmatism, which may also be irregular. This is due to several factors, including wound healing, vascularization, suturing technique, graft size, and donor tissue characteristics [6, 9–12]. While several options are available to manage astigmatism, it is crucial to accurately set patient expectations prior to surgery so that they understand they will most likely require additional measures to achieve their best postoperative vision.

Selective suture removal is one technique to adjust astigmatism [13, 14]. Once the cornea has adequately healed, corneal topography or tomography can be used to guide suture removal along the steep corneal meridians. If regular astigmatism is achieved and total astigmatism is reduced to a level that is correctable with glasses that are tolerated by the patient, suture removal may be halted. However, the patient should be counseled that their sutures may degrade with time and their astigmatism may change with subsequent removal. Posttransplant patients frequently tolerate spectacle correction of higher astigmatism levels, especially if they have bilateral grafts. Eyeglasses also carry the additional benefit of eye protection, which is especially important following PKP or DALK, due to the unavoidable weakness of the GHJ.

Contact lenses are a mainstay of refractive correction, both for astigmatism and ametropia, following corneal transplantation. If the astigmatism is regular and relatively low, toric soft contact lenses may be sufficient to achieve functional vision. However, if the corneal astigmatism is of high magnitude and/or irregular, rigid gas-permeable (RGP) lenses may be required. Unfortunately, RGP contact lenses are often difficult to fit and poorly tolerated by patients, due to discomfort or difficulty with insertion/removal [15]. Scleral contact lens technology has advanced significantly in the last several years [16]. Scleral lenses have several advantages when compared to RGP lenses: they are typically more comfortable since they vault over the cornea, they contribute to ocular surface health by maintaining constant lubrication, and they can be fit over highly irregular corneas with substantial improvement in visual acuity and quality (Fig. 11.1).

Irregular astigmatism and contact lens intolerance are quite common in this patient population, often limiting practical improvement in their visual function. Small aperture optics is a relatively new approach to management of irregular astigmatism. By blocking nonparaxial light rays, pinhole apertures reduce the effect of corneal aberrations and increase depth of focus. The XtraFocus pinhole intraocular implant (Morcher, GmbH) is an opaque, black, round-edged device with a 1.3-mm central aperture designed for placement in the ciliary sulcus in a piggyback fashion [17]. The device has a 6-mm optic, a total length of 14 mm, and is transparent to infrared light. While the device prevents indirect ophthalmoscopy, infrared-based examinations such as optical coherence tomography or laser scanning

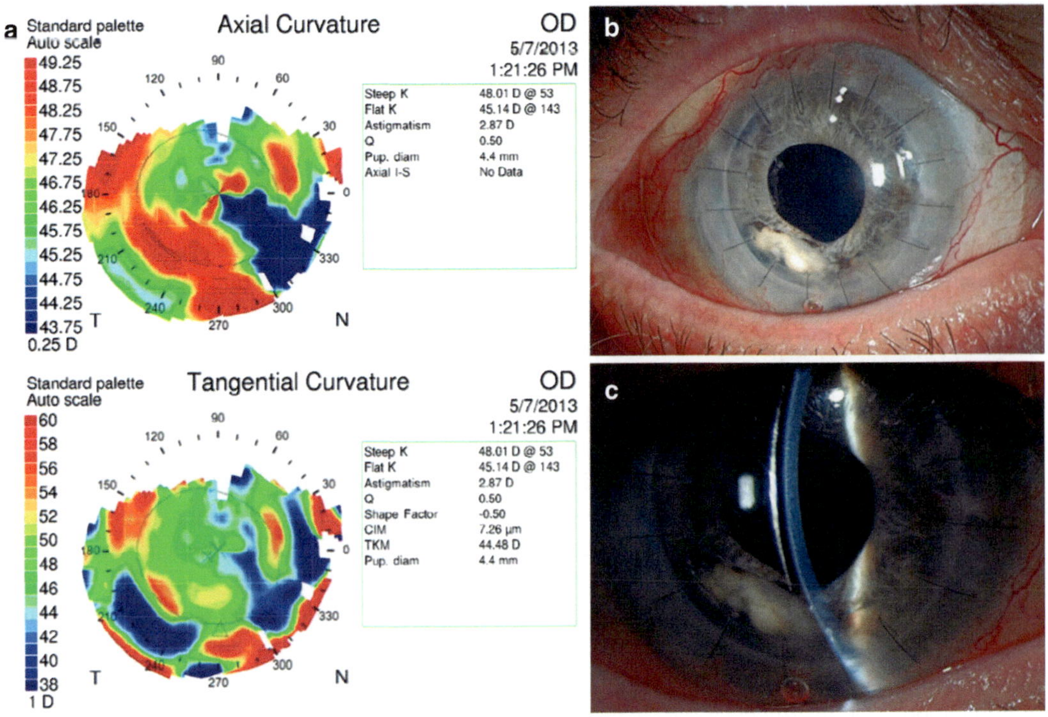

Fig. 11.1 Management of astigmatism and surface irregularity post-PKP with a scleral lens. The Placido-based topographic image (**a** – left) demonstrates irregular oblique astigmatism. The slit-lamp images show the scleral lens (**b** – top right) and its vault over the corneal surface (**c** – bottom right)

ophthalmoscopy are still possible permitting postoperative retinal examination. Although the device is not currently available in the United States, it has been shown to significantly improve both objective and subjective distance and near visual acuities in patients with irregular astigmatism following PKP, without associated complications, such as uveitis-glaucoma-hyphema syndrome.

Arcuate keratotomy (AK) or corneal relaxing incisions (CRI) can also be used to reduce corneal astigmatism during or after cataract surgery (Fig. 11.2). Incisions can be placed manually along the steep corneal meridian using a calibrated diamond blade or femtosecond laser [18–23]. They can be single or paired and are typically made to a depth of 90% in the cornea stroma. The incisions flatten the cornea along the meridian of the incision and steepen the cornea 90 degrees away, otherwise known as coupling. Their effect is dependent on many factors, including length and depth. Published nomograms are available and are clinically applicable in eyes that have undergone DSAEK or DMEK. However, uncertain force vectors associated with the GHJ following DALK or PKP create unpredictable results that do not obey these nomograms. Because of this, we recommend a conservative approach starting with small, paired incisions of approximately 45 degrees. If adequate reduction is not achieved, they can be enlarged by 10–20 degrees over two to three intervals until the desired effect is achieved or the incision length reaches 90 degrees. While generally safe, CRIs can be subject to gape and should be avoided in patients who have undergone keratoplasty to treat ectatic corneal degeneration, such as keratoconus.

Laser refractive surgery is another option for treating astigmatism in eyes following corneal transplantation and cataract surgery and has the additional benefit of treating any associated ametropia. Laser in situ keratomileusis (LASIK), laser-assisted subepithelial keratectomy (LASEK), and photorefractive keratectomy

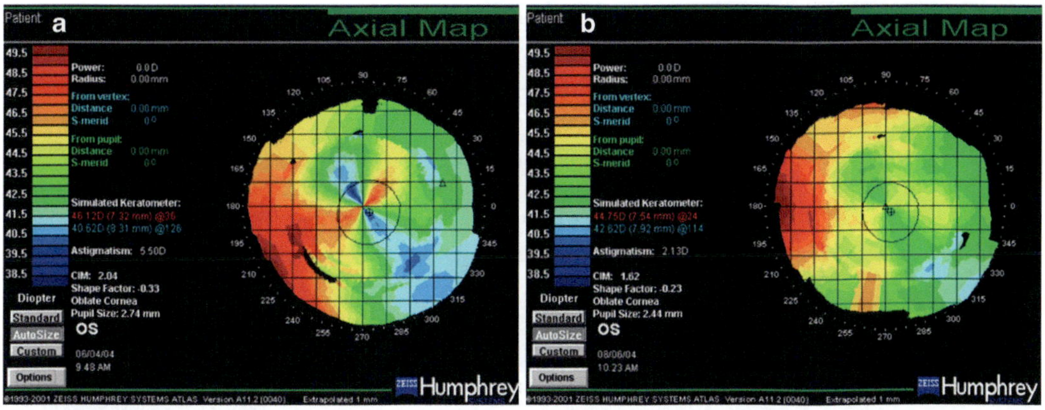

Fig. 11.2 Placido-based topographic image of a cornea post-PKP before (**a** – left) and after (**b** – right) arcuate keratometry. Paired incisions (60 degrees in length, 600 μm in depth) were placed just anterior to the GHJ. Note the reduction in astigmatism from 5.50D to 2.13D

(PRK) have all been used for this application [24–28]. PRK and LASEK are more commonly employed since they do not require the creation of a flap. The use of mitomycin C is recommended to reduce the risk of haze formation, and success has been seen with conventional, wavefront-guided, and topography-guided treatments. LASIK can also be used to treat refractive errors and can be performed in one or two steps. Concurrent flap creation and excimer ablation (one step) carry a decreased risk of complications such as epithelial ingrowth but is associated with decreased refractive predictability. Conversely, flap creation followed by laser ablation (two steps) produces better refractive results since the patient's refractive error is allowed to stabilize after flap creation. However, the two-step method does carry a higher risk of flap complications. If corrective laser surgery is considered, an acceptable improvement in visual acuity should be demonstrable with refraction prior to treatment.

Toric IOLs can be implanted to manage corneal astigmatism following transplant surgery in certain circumstances (Fig. 11.3). If the corneal astigmatism seen on corneal topography/tomography after PKP or ALK is regular, the patient accepts the astigmatic correction in their refraction (despite the presence of the cataract), and the corneal endothelial cell count is at least 1500–2000 cells/mm^2, then toric IOL implantation is a reasonable consideration. If the astigmatism is irregular or there is a chance that the patient will need a repeat keratoplasty in the future, a non-toric IOL is preferred. If contact lens correction is still needed following cataract surgery, it will be much more difficult to properly fit the patient if a toric IOL was implanted, as a toric RGP or scleral lens would be required. If the corneal astigmatism exceeds the maximum level currently available in toric IOLs (6.0 D at the IOL plane, approximately 4.0 D at the corneal plane), then corneal relaxing incisions can be used to supplement the correction.

Anterior Lamellar Keratoplasty (ALK) and Cataract Surgery

Anterior lamellar keratoplasty (ALK) refers to the corneal transplantation technique where some portion of the anterior corneal stroma is removed and replaced. The primary advantage of ALK is preservation of the host endothelium with the associated elimination of endothelial rejection, the most common type of corneal graft rejection. ALK comes in several varieties: manual dissection via blade, femtosecond laser-assisted, manual shearing along a collagen lamella ("grip and rip"), and the big bubble technique of Anwar and Teichmann [29, 30]. The challenges pertaining to cataract surgery in this patient population are very similar to those seen with PKP.

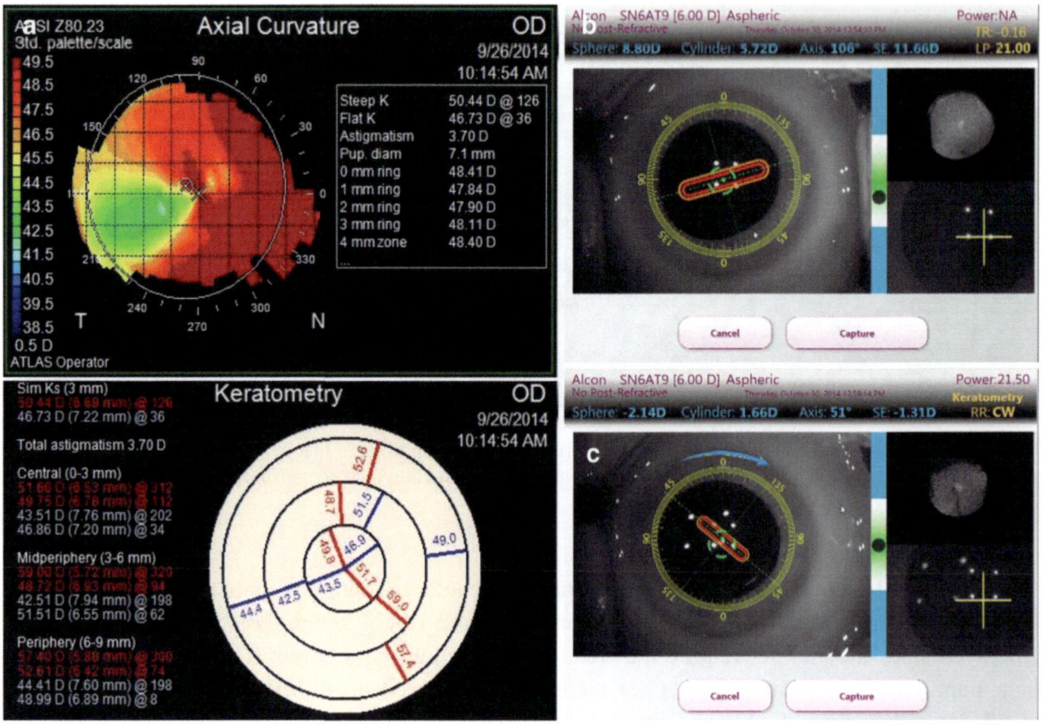

Fig. 11.3 Toric IOL implantation in cataract surgery following PKP. The Placido-based topographic image (**a** – left) demonstrates somewhat irregular astigmatism. Sim-K measurements underestimate astigmatism when compared to the central 3-mm zone (3.70D vs. 5.55D). Intraoperative aberrometry before (**b** – top right) and after (**c** – bottom right) toric IOL implantation demonstrates the reduction in refractive astigmatism. The postoperative uncorrected visual acuity was 20/25

Concurrent ALK and Cataract Surgery

ALK is performed in eyes where corneal pathology has produced some level of opacification and irregularity, compromising the view for cataract surgery. Authors have described concurrent cataract surgery following removal of the anterior cornea with the big bubble technique and before placement of the donor graft [31–33]. While achievement of a big bubble can be challenging, Zaki and colleagues found that cataract surgery can be safely performed if a type 1 bubble is obtained with preservation of Dua's layer. If only Descemet's membrane remains following lamellar dissection, they found the risk of rupture during cataract removal to be excessively high. Even with successful concurrent ALK and cataract surgery, the surgeon and patient are still faced with uncertain postoperative corneal power and astigmatism, leading to a significant risk of high refractive prediction errors. For these reasons which are similar to those of PKP, we prefer sequential cataract surgery in patients who've undergone ALK.

Sequential ALK and Cataract Surgery

Cataract surgery in patients with prior ALK is essentially identical to cataract surgery in post-PKP eyes. The technical challenges relating to the view, IOL selection, and the need for additional tools are the same (as described previously). One area where they may differ is in the risk of endothelial cell loss. Acar et al. found greater endothelial cell loss following cataract surgery in post-PKP eyes as compared to post-DALK eyes (44% vs. 11%) at 1 year following cataract surgery [34]. Of note, the rate of endothelial cell loss in the DALK eyes was the same as that seen in eyes with no history of keratoplasty. Den et al. also found a lower rate of endothelial cell loss in post-DALK vs. post-PKP eyes (11% vs. 31%) at 1 year after cataract removal. They found that endothelial cell loss in the DALK group stabilized at 1 month, while the PKP group continued to experience cell loss in the first 6 months following cataract removal.

The options available for astigmatism management during or following cataract surgery in patients with a history of ALK are the same as with PKP and include eyeglasses, contact lenses, selective suture removal, arcuate keratometry, laser refractive, and toric IOLs. Please refer to the prior discussion.

Endothelial Keratoplasty (EK) and Cataract Surgery

The most common modern endothelial keratoplasty (EK) techniques include Descemet stripping automated endothelial keratoplasty (DSAEK) and Descemet membrane endothelial keratoplasty (DMEK). These techniques are reserved for patients with corneal pathologies that only involve the endothelium and Descemet's membrane, such as Fuchs' endothelial dystrophy or bullous keratopathy. They have multiple advantages when compared to PKP, including reduced rejection risk, smaller incisions, fewer sutures, and quicker visual rehabilitation. And since both procedures result in minimal alteration to the corneal surface, they produce significantly lower levels of surgically induced astigmatism. As with PKP and ALK, EK is known to increase the risk of cataract progression [35–37]. The risk of needing cataract surgery following EK increases with age, with a rate of 55% for those older than 50 and 7% for younger patients. Thus, cataracts are commonly seen in patients who need or have already undergone DSAEK or DMEK and present unique issues worth addressing.

Concurrent EK and Cataract Surgery

Out of all the keratoplasty techniques available, DSAEK and DMEK are most amenable to concurrent cataract surgery. In contrast to PKP and DALK, standard cataract surgery can be performed immediately prior to EK, with a closed anterior chamber and normal fluidics. In cases of Fuchs' dystrophy or mild corneal decompensation, the surgeon will experience little to no compromise of their surgical view. A few alterations in surgical technique will facilitate performance of the subsequent EK.

The paracenteses and main surgical incision should be shorter as to avoid contact with the donor cornea post insertion. This permits the surgeon to easily enter with their cannulas to manage the gas fill and gas-fluid exchange. A cohesive OVD is recommended for the cataract surgery since it can be easily removed prior to donor implantation. Retained OVD can be trapped in the interface between the donor and host corneas, increasing the risk of detachment. The anterior chamber often shallows during EK, purposefully in the case of DMEK, so a smaller capsulorhexis is recommended to decrease the risk of the IOL prolapsing out of the capsule. A miotic agent should be used to constrict the pupil after OVD removal to minimize donor contact with the IOL, which can damage the donor endothelium. An inferior peripheral iridotomy (PI) is recommended to minimize the risk of postoperative intraocular pressure spikes due to pupillary block by the gas bubble. If a preoperative laser PI was not performed, a PI should be created following pupil constriction with a vitrector, needle, or blade using the surgeon's preferred technique. An intraoperative PI does increase the risk of bleeding and hyphema, but this does not appear to adversely affect surgical outcomes [38]. However, anticoagulant discontinuation prior to surgery is still recommended when medically possible.

Hyperopic shifts in corneal refractive power are seen with both DSAEK and DMEK. DSAEK grafts are thinner in the center relative to the periphery and act as a "minus lens." [39, 40] While DMEK grafts are very thin (approximately 15 μm) and uniform in thickness, patients still experience a hyperopic shift. This shift is lower in magnitude as compared to DSAEK. It is assumed that, preoperatively, the cornea is more edematous centrally so that when the edema clears, the cornea thins more centrally relative to the periphery causing the hyperopic shift (Fig. 11.4). Due to these shifts, a refractive target of −0.75 to −1.25 D is recommended for cataract surgery in DSAEK and − 0.5 to −1.0 D in DMEK [41–44]. Finally, hydrophilic acrylic IOLs should be avoided in these cases since they are prone to opacification/calcification following exposure to intracameral gas, including air, SF_6, or C_3F_8 [45–47].

Sequential EK and Cataract Surgery

In cases of severe endothelial dysfunction, corneal edema may preclude an adequately clear view for cataract surgery. In these cases, EK can be performed first with cataract surgery to follow once healing is complete. In addition to improving the surgical view, it should also be easier to obtain accurate keratometry following EK. While a myopic refractive target is still required for sequential cataract surgery in DSAEK eyes, no such target is needed in DMEK eyes. Since the thin DMEK graft is uniform in thickness, once the postoperative edema clears, keratometry measurements will accurately reflect the refractive power of the cornea.

Astigmatism Management

As with the other forms of keratoplasty, the same options are available to manage astigmatism in DMEK or DSAEK eyes. However, toric IOL implantation following DMEK or DSAEK deserves additional consideration. While DMEK corneas may experience changes in astigmatism early in the postoperative period, once the graft attaches and any edema clears, corneal power can be accurately measured, and the risk of irregular astigmatism induction is very low. Repeat DMEK would also be expected to have minimal effect on long-term astigmatism levels. Thus, toric IOLs are a reasonable consideration in this population. If concurrent DMEK and cataract surgery are considered, it is best to restrict the use of toric IOLs to patients with more than 1.75 D of regular astigmatism due to poor refractive predictability in milder cases [48, 49].

While the risk of irregular astigmatism with DSAEK corneas is generally low, it can occur

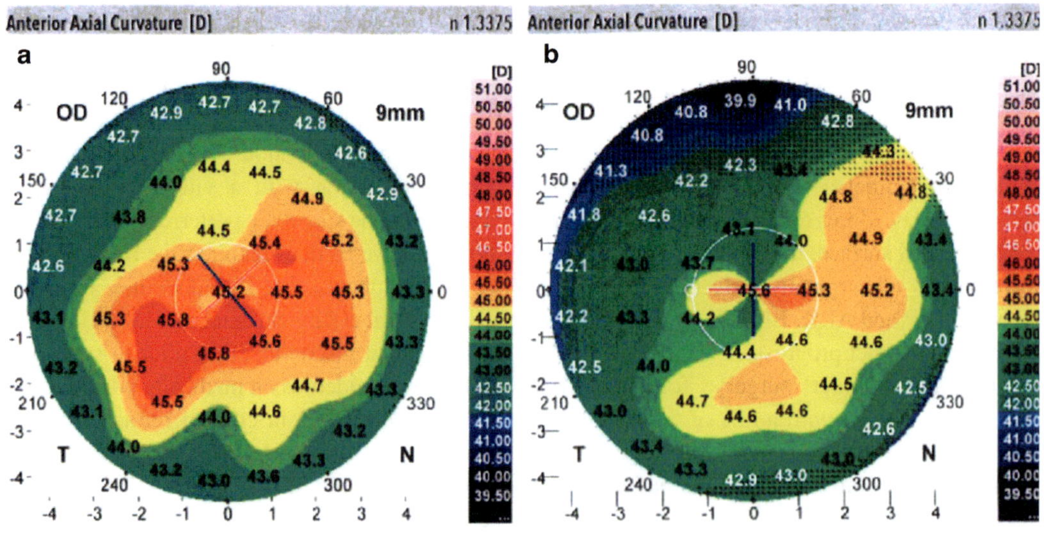

Fig. 11.4 Placido-based topographic image of a cornea pre- (**a** – left) and post-DMEK (**b** – right). The topography demonstrates improved astigmatism regularity with a change in the location of the steep meridian

with thicker grafts, irregular trephinations, and decentered graft placement. Accurate measurement of total corneal astigmatism following DSAEK can also be more challenging since the posterior corneal curvature is altered by the lamellar transplant. Since intraoperative aberrometry measures total ocular astigmatism including the posterior cornea's contribution, it may provide some benefits in toric IOL selection in this patient population. Finally, if the patient undergoes a repeat DSAEK, astigmatism measurements can change significantly. For these reasons, toric IOL use in conjunction with DSAEK surgery should be employed with caution.

Conclusion

Cataract surgery in conjunction with or following keratoplasty can be quite successful. The surgical approach will vary depending on the type of keratoplasty, as will the decision to perform the procedures concurrently or sequentially. As each approach carries certain advantages and disadvantages, the surgeon and patient will both benefit from careful assessment and surgical planning. Keratoplasty is often associated with postoperative astigmatism, and multiple options are available for its management. Thorough counseling before and after keratoplasty is essential to optimize patient understanding and satisfaction.

Take-Home Points

- Cataract surgery should follow penetrating keratoplasty whenever possible, due to increased procedure safety and improved accuracy of IOL power calculations.
- Cataract surgery in the setting of concurrent or prior corneal transplantation can be aided by adjuvant devices, such as trypan blue capsular stain, dispersive OVD for endothelial protection, pupil expanders, and suturing of incisions.
- Scleral contact lenses are often well-tolerated in patients with corneal grafts and high astigmatism who have been unsuccessful with soft or rigid gas-permeable contact lenses.
- Endothelial keratoplasty techniques are more amenable to concurrent cataract surgery, but adjustments need to be made in the refractive target to account for the hyperopic effect of the corneal graft.
- Toric IOLs should be used with caution in patients with corneal transplants and should be considered only when the graft is healthy with an acceptable endothelial cell count, the astigmatism is regular, and astigmatism correction is accepted in the preoperative refraction.

References

1. Tan DT, Dart JK, Holland EJ, Kinoshita S. Corneal transplantation. Lancet. 2012;379:1749–61.
2. Inoue Y. Corneal triple procedure. Semin Ophthalmol. 2001;16:113–8.
3. Yokokura S, Hariya T, Uematsu M, et al. Efficacy of chandelier illumination for && combined cataract operation and penetrating keratoplasty. Cornea. 2015;34:275–8.
4. Shimomura Y, Hosotani H, Kiritoshi A, et al. Core vitrectomy preceding triple corneal procedure in patients at high risk for increased posterior chamber pressure. Jpn J Ophthalmol. 1997;41:251–4.
5. Higaki S, Fukuda M, Matsumoto C, Shimomura Y. Results of penetrating keratoplasty triple procedure with 25-gauge core vitrectomy. Cornea. 2012;31:730–3.
6. Riddle HK Jr, Parker DA, Price FW Jr. Management of postkeratoplasty astigmatism. Curr Opin Ophthalmol. 1998;9:15–28.
7. Touzeau O, Borderie VM, Allouch C, et al. Effects of penetrating keratoplasty suture removal on corneal topography and refraction. Cornea. 1999;18:638–44.
8. Den S, Shimmura S, Shimazaki J. Cataract surgery after deep anterior lamellar keratoplasty and penetrating keratoplasty in age- and disease-matched eyes. J Cataract Refract Surg. 2018;44:496–503.
9. Fares U, Sarhan AR, Dua HS. Management of post-keratoplasty astigmatism. J Cataract Refract Surg. 2012;38:2029–39.
10. Landau D, Siganos CS, Mechoulam H, et al. Astigmatism after Mersilene and nylon suture use for penetrating keratoplasty. Cornea. 2006;25:691–4.

11. Sarhan AR, Fares U, Al-Aqaba MA, et al. Rapid suture management of postkeratoplasty astigmatism. Eye. 2010;24:540–6.
12. Alio JL, Abdou AA, Abdelghany AA, et al. Refractive surgery following corneal graft. Curr Opin Ophthalmol. 2015;26:278–87.
13. Karabatsas CH, Cook SD, Figueiredo FC, et al. Combined interrupted and continuous versus single continuous adjustable suturing in penetrating keratoplasty: a prospective, randomized study of induced astigmatism during the first postoperative year. Ophthalmology. 1998;105:1991–8.
14. Fares U, Mokashi AA, Elalfy MS, Dua HS. Sequential selective same-day suture removal in the management of postkeratoplasty astigmatism. Eye. 2013;27:1032–7.
15. Szczotka LB, Lindsay RG. Contact lens fitting following corneal graft surgery. Clin Exp Optom. 2003;86:244–9.
16. Severinsky B, Behrman S, Frucht-Pery J, Solomon A. Scleral contact lenses for visual rehabilitation after penetrating keratoplasty: long term outcomes. Contact Lens Anterior Eye. 2014;37:196–202.
17. Trindade CC, Trindade BC, Trindade FC, et al. New pinhole sulcus implant for the correction of irregular corneal astigmatism. J Cataract Refract Surg. 2017;43:1297–306.
18. Viswanathan D, Kumar NL. Bilateral femtosecond laser enabled intrastromal astigmatic keratotomy to correct high postpenetrating keratoplasty astigmatism. J Cataract Refract Surg. 2013;39:1916–20.
19. Cleary C, Tang M, Ahmed H, et al. Beveled femtosecond laser astigmatic keratotomy for the treatment of high astigmatism postpenetrating keratoplasty. Cornea. 2013;32:54–62.
20. Hoffart L, Touzeau O, Borderie V, Laroche L. Mechanized astigmatic arcuate keratotomy with the Hanna arcitome for astigmatism after keratoplasty. J Cataract Refract Surg. 2007;33:862–8.
21. Wilkins MR, Mehta JS, Larkin DF. Standardized arcuate keratotomy for postkeratoplasty astigmatism. J Cataract Refract Surg. 2005;31:297–301.
22. Kumar NL, Kaiserman I, Shehadeh-Mashor R, et al. IntraLase-enabled astigmatic keratotomy for postkeratoplasty astigmatism: on-axis vector analysis. Ophthalmology. 2010;117(1228–1235):e1221.
23. Ho Wang Yin G, Hoffart L. Postkeratoplasty astigmatism management by relaxing incisions: a systematic review. Eye Vis. 2017;4(29)
24. Afshari NA, Schirra F, Rapoza PA, et al. Laser in situ keratomileusis outcomes following radial keratotomy, astigmatic keratotomy, photorefractive keratectomy, and penetrating keratoplasty. J Cataract Refract Surg. 2005;31:2093–100.
25. Camellin M, Arba MS. Simultaneous aspheric wavefront-guided transepithelial photorefractive keratectomy and phototherapeutic keratectomy to correct aberrations and refractive errors after corneal surgery. J Cataract Refract Surg. 2010;36:1173–80.
26. Bilgihan K, Ozdek SC, Akata F, Hasanreisoglu B. Photorefractive keratectomy for postpenetrating keratoplasty myopia and astigmatism. J Cataract Refract Surg. 2000;26:1590–5.
27. Prince J, Chuck RS. Refractive surgery after Descemet's stripping endothelial keratoplasty. Curr Opin Ophthalmol. 2012;23:242–5.
28. Rajan MS, O'Brart DP, Patel P, et al. Topography-guided customized laser- assisted subepithelial keratectomy for the treatment of postkeratoplasty astigmatism. J Cataract Refract Surg. 2006;32:949–57.
29. Anwar M, Teichmann KD. Big-bubble technique to bare Descemet's membrane in anterior lamellar keratoplasty. J Cataract Refract Surg. 2002;28:398–403.
30. Vital MC. Grip and rip ALK for Ectasia and stromal opacity: a big bubble alternative. Eyetube 2016. https://eyetube.net/videos/grip-and-rip-alk-for-ectasia-and-stromal-opacity-a-big-bubble-alternative%2D%2Dumumu.
31. Zaki AA, Elalfy MS, Said DG, Dua HS. Deep anterior lamellar keratoplasty triple procedure: a useful clinical application of the pre-Descemet's layer (Dua's layer). Eye. 2015;29:323–6.
32. Panda A, Sethi HS, Jain M, et al. Deep anterior lamellar keratoplasty with phacoemulsification. J Cataract Refract Surg. 2011;37:122–6.
33. Coelho RP, Messias A. Phacoemulsification with big-bubble deep anterior lamellar keratoplasty: variant of the triple procedure. J Cataract Refract Surg. 2019;45:1064–6.
34. Acar BT, Utine CA, Acar S, et al. Endothelial cell loss after phacoemulsification in eyes with previous penetrating keratoplasty, previous deep anterior lamellar keratoplasty, or no previous surgery. J Cataract Refract Surg. 2011;37:2013–7.
35. Price MO, Price DA, Fairchild KM, Price FW. Rate and risk factors for cataract formation and extraction after Descemet stripping endothelial keratoplasty. Br J Ophthalmol. 2010;94:1468–71.
36. Burkhart ZN, Feng MT, Price FW, Price MO. One-year outcomes in eyes remaining phakic after Descemet membrane endothelial keratoplasty. J Cataract Refract Surg. 2014;40:430–4.
37. Musa FU, Cabrerizo J, Quilendrino R, et al. Outcomes of phacoemulsification after Descemet membrane endothelial keratoplasty. J Cataract Refract Surg. 2013;39:836–40.
38. Crews JW, Price MO, Lautert J, et al. Intraoperative hyphema in Descemet & membrane endothelial keratoplasty alone or combined with phacoemulsification. J Cataract Refract Surg. 2018;44:198–201.
39. Dupps WJ Jr, Qian Y, Meisler DM. Multivariate model of refractive shift in Descemet-stripping automated endothelial keratoplasty. J Cataract Refract Surg. 2008;34:578–84.
40. Hwang RY, Gauthier DJ, Wallace D, et al. Refractive changes after Descemet stripping endothelial keratoplasty: a simplified mathematical model. Invest Ophthalmol Vis Sci. 2011;52:1043–54.

41. Terry MA, Shamie N, Chen ES, et al. Endothelial keratoplasty for Fuchs' dystrophy with cataract: complications and clinical results with the new triple procedure. Ophthalmology. 2009;116:631–9.
42. van Dijk K, Rodriguez-Calvo-de-Mora M, van Esch H, et al. Two-year refractive outcomes after descemet membrane endothelial keratoplasty. Cornea. 2016;35:1548–55.
43. Alnawaiseh M, Rosentreter A, Eter N, Zumhagen L. Changes in corneal refractive power for patients with fuchs endothelial dystrophy after DMEK. Cornea. 2016;35:1073–7.
44. Ham L, Dapena I, Moutsouris K, et al. Refractive change and stability after Descemet membrane endothelial keratoplasty. Effect of corneal dehydration- induced hyperopic shift on intraocular lens power calculation. J Cataract Refract Surg. 2011;37:1455–64.
45. Neuhann IM, Neuhann TF, Rohrbach JM. Intraocular lens calcification after keratoplasty. Cornea. 2013;32:e6–e10.
46. Werner L, Wilbanks G, Nieuwendaal CP, et al. Localized opacification of hydrophilic acrylic intraocular lenses after procedures using intracameral injection of air or gas. J Cataract Refract Surg. 2015;41:199–207.
47. Nieuwendaal CP, van der Meulen IJ, Patryn EK, et al. Opacification of the intraocular lens after Descemet stripping endothelial keratoplasty. Cornea. 2015;34:1375–7.
48. Schoenberg ED, Price FW Jr, Miller J, et al. Refractive outcomes of Descemet membrane endothelial keratoplasty triple procedures (combined with cataract surgery). J Cataract Refract Surg. 2015;41:1182–9.
49. Yokogawa H, Sanchez PF, Mayko ZM, et al. Astigmatism correction with toric intraocular lenses in descemet membrane endothelial keratoplasty triple procedures. Cornea. 2017;36:269–74.

Cataract Surgery in Eyes with Fuchs Endothelial Corneal Dystrophy

12

Theofilos Tourtas, Julia M. Weller, and Friedrich E. Kruse

Key Issues

- Take always a closer look at the endothelium when planning a cataract surgery in order to avoid inferior results after surgery
- Strategy for decision-making regarding cataract surgery only or combined with endothelial keratoplasty in eyes with FECD
- Challenges in IOL calculation in combined cataract surgery with endothelial keratoplasty
- The role of femtosecond laser-assisted cataract surgery in eyes with FECD
- What complications to expect and how to deal with them when performing cataract surgery in eyes with FECD

Introduction

Clinical evaluation of the corneal endothelium is of high importance when screening patients for cataract surgery. Slit-lamp examinations should be accompanied by endothelial microscopy to exclude endothélial pathologies. Corneal guttae are the most common endothelial disorder in candidate cataract patients. The clinical significance of corneal guttae without edema is often underestimated. The quality of vision in early stages of Fuchs endothelial corneal dystrophy (FECD) with corneal guttae is impaired way before development of corneal edema. The first symptoms are glare, reduced contrast sensitivity, and color vision, mainly when the lighting conditions are bad. Several studies have confirmed that corneal guttae cause an additional decrease in contrast sensitivity, as well as an additional increase in stray light in cataract patients [1–3]. These parameters are not routinely tested in cataract patients. It is therefore crucial to inform patients before cataract surgery about the presence of corneal guttae, which may lead to inferior results after surgery.

T. Tourtas · J. M. Weller · F. E. Kruse (✉)
Department of Ophthalmology, Friedrich-Alexander-University of Erlangen-Nürnberg, Erlangen, Germany
e-mail: friedrich.kruse@uk-erlangen.de

Cataract Surgery in Eyes with FECD: When to Do It and How

The decision when to perform cataract surgery only, combined cataract surgery with keratoplasty, or a staged procedure (first cataract surgery or first keratoplasty) in eyes with FECD can be challenging even for experienced corneal surgeons.

Among the various types of keratoplasty, lamellar corneal surgery is used in patients with FECD because endothelial keratoplasty (EK) allows for a layer specific correction of

J. L. Alió et al. (eds.), *Cataract Surgery*, Essentials in Ophthalmology,
https://doi.org/10.1007/978-3-030-94530-5_12

the corneal pathology. There are two forms of EK a corneal surgeon can choose from: In Descemet stripping automated endothelial keratoplasty (DSAEK), a thin lamella of posterior corneal stroma is transplanted along with Descemet membrane and endothelial layer, while in Descemet membrane endothelial keratoplasty (DMEK), only Descemet membrane and endothelium are exchanged. Due to the better visual results, DMEK is generally preferred over DSAEK.

In case of moderate cataract and confluent guttae with corneal edema, it is mandatory to perform cataract surgery combined with EK. Otherwise, endothelial decompensation with bullous keratopathy can be provoked by cataract surgery alone.

The following three scenarios can be encountered:

1. Moderate cataract with mild corneal guttae

Phacoemulsification is known to affect the corneal endothelium, and corneal decompensation can occur postoperatively even if the guttae appear to be relatively mild prior to surgery. This can be explained by the pathophysiology of FECD, in which not only the (clinically visible) guttae occur but endothelial cells are reduced in number, have an altered metabolism, and are reduced in viability. Preoperative biomicroscopy of corneal endothelial cells is mandatory in these cases to quantify the endothelial cell density, since values vary greatly in eyes with mild guttae (Fig. 12.1). There is no cutoff value for the prediction of postoperative corneal decompensation. Preoperatively the surgeon has to estimate the risk of corneal decompensation on the basis of nuclear opacity (and presumed necessary duration of phacoemulsification) in relation to the number and morphology of existing endothelial cells. The patient has to be informed that in case of a corneal decompensation after cataract sur-

OS

Patient ID: 1004711563
Name :
Sex :
Birthday :

Exam Date : 06.03.2019 14:06:08
Exam Comments :

Doctor :

Auto

Number	21	
CD	1761	/mm2
AVG	568	um2
CCT	522 um	

SD	256	um2
CV	45	%
Max	1062	um2
Min	236	um2

Area (Polymegathism)

000-100	um2	0 %
100-200	um2	0 %
200-300	um2	14 %
300-400	um2	19 %
400-500	um2	14 %
500-600	um2	14 %
600-700	um2	14 %
700-800	um2	5 %
800-900	um2	5 %
900-	um2	14 %

Apex (Pleomorphism)

3	0 %
4	13 %
5	13 %
6A	0 %
7	50 %
8	0 %
9	13 %
10-	13 %

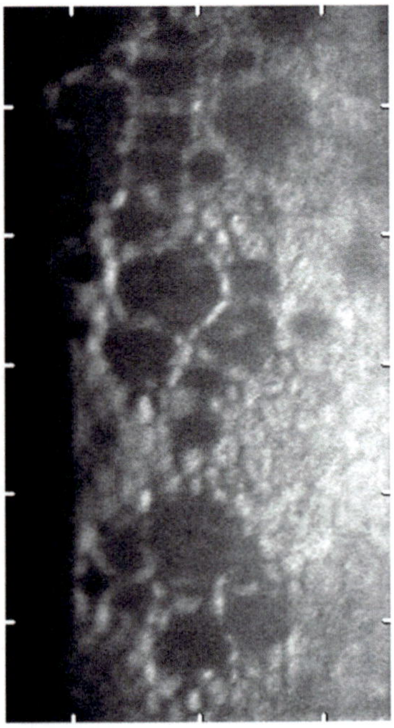

Fig. 12.1 Endothelial microscopy picture of a patient with mild corneal guttae. In this patient, cataract surgery without endothelial keratoplasty would be a viable option

gery, an EK procedure might be necessary. In case of confluent central guttae without visible endothelial cells in the biomicroscopy scan, a combined cataract surgery with EK is usually recommended.

Decision-making based on central corneal thickness can be misleading since a thicker cornea does not necessarily implicate corneal edema, while subclinical edema can occur in corneas with normal thickness [4, 5]. Pentacam Scheimpflug tomography is a helpful tool to detect subclinical edema in FECD patients who will benefit from EK. By assessment of three structural parameters with the Pentacam, the risk for FECD eyes to require endothelial keratoplasty after cataract surgery has been estimated [5]. To our knowledge, this is the only evidence-based approach guiding the decision-making process of a combined surgery. Corneal thickness alone is not a useful tool in the decision when to perform cataract surgery only or combined surgery. Thus, there is no consensus about a cutoff value for corneal thickness, e.g., 650 μm, beyond which a combined surgery should be performed. Instead, in cases without clinically visible corneal edema, the surgeon should take into consideration the structural parameters mentioned above, the extent of corneal guttae, as well as the guttae-specific symptoms of glare and reduced contrast sensitivity. As a rule of thumb, we suggest to perform a combined surgery in cases in which guttae are dense and confluent (Figs. 12.2 and 12.3).

In case of corneal guttae limited to the central 4–5 mm of the cornea, descemetorhexis only (without keratoplasty) (DSO) might be a promising option in the future [6]. This procedure can be combined with cataract surgery, as well. The supporting effect of Rho kinase inhibitors on the endothelial wound healing currently is investigated in randomized clinical trials.

L OS

Patient ID: 1015593322
Name :
Sex :
Birthday :

Exam Date : 06.05.2021 07:56:20
Exam Comments :
Doctor :

Auto

Number	16	
CD	751	/mm2
AVG	1332	um2
CCT	572 um	

SD	1459	um2
CV	110	%
Max	5866	um2
Min	364	um2

Area (Polymegathism)

000-100	um2	0 %
100-200	um2	0 %
200-300	um2	0 %
300-400	um2	6 %
400-500	um2	25 %
500-600	um2	6 %
600-700	um2	0 %
700-800	um2	13 %
800-900	um2	0 %
900-	um2	50 %

Apex (Pleomorphism)

3	0 %
4	14 %
5	0 %
6A	29 %
7	14 %
8	14 %
9	14 %
10-	14 %

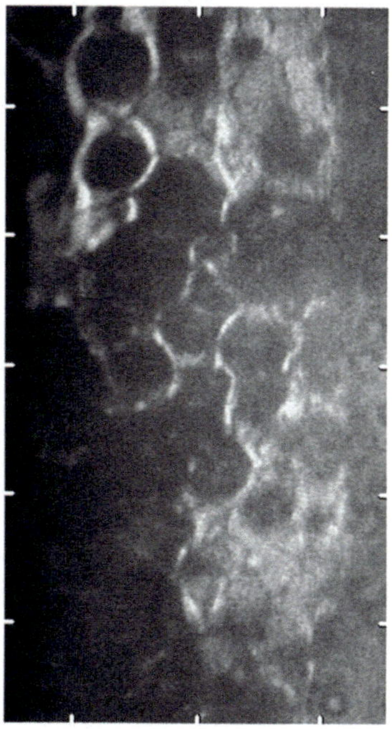

Fig. 12.2 Endothelial microscopy picture of a patient with dense and confluent corneal guttae. In this patient, cataract surgery with endothelial keratoplasty would be recommended

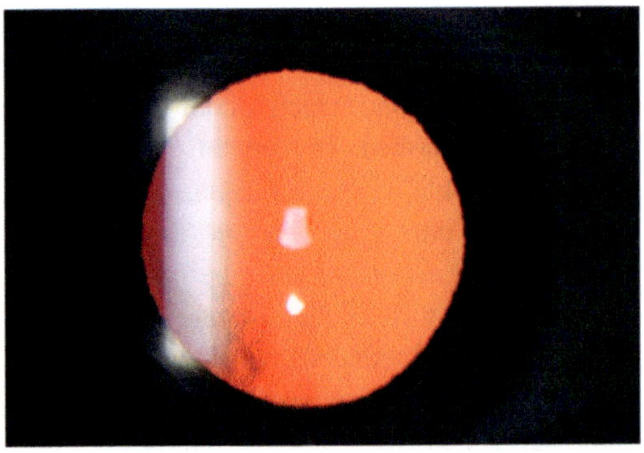

Fig. 12.3 Retroillumination slit-lamp picture of a patient with dense and confluent corneal guttae

2. Mild cataract with moderate corneal guttae

In phakic eyes with clinically significant guttae, EK can be performed with or without simultaneous cataract surgery. Patient's age and the remaining ability for accommodation of the eye are important factors for decision-making.

In patients above the age of 60, DMEK is usually combined with cataract surgery even if the cataract is only mild to avoid the second (cataract) surgery shortly after EK [7]. In young patients under the age of 50, EK only is often the preferred choice. If DMEK only is preferred, the cataract-inducing effect of the steroid treatment after keratoplasty leading to a second surgery months or years after DMEK has to be discussed with the patient. In a recent study investigating the incidence of cataract after DMEK in phakic eyes, only 13% (35/261) developed cataract during a follow-up of 10 years after DMEK [8]. The average interval between DMEK and phacoemulsification was 18 ± 13 months. Mean loss of endothelial cell density was as high as 11% in the first 6 months after phacoemulsification, which is acceptable, but higher than the natural decrease of endothelial cells after DMEK without additional subsequent surgery. The main advantage of DMEK only is the much higher accuracy of IOL calculation in a patient with postponed cataract surgery as compared to IOL calculation in a combined procedure.

Also, the morphology of the anterior chamber should be taken into consideration when the decision to perform a combined or staged procedure is made. If the anterior chamber depth is less than 2 mm, e.g., in high hyperopia, or the likelihood of vitreous pressure is high, a combined cataract surgery with DMEK is preferable even if the lens is clear in order to facilitate graft manipulation and unfolding of the graft.

3. FECD patients with bullous keratopathy or focal central edema

Eyes with extensive corneal edema and cataract may benefit from a staged procedure. In these cases, the cornea is quite cloudy and does not allow for a safe cataract surgery even after removal of the corneal epithelium. In order not to jeopardize the success of the cataract surgery, EK should be performed first. In general, cornea will reach a stable condition for an accurate IOL calculation 3 months after EK, and a cataract surgery can be safely performed.

Some eyes with FECD may develop a central or paracentral focal edema instead of diffuse corneal decompensation (Fig. 12.4). IOL calculation is difficult in these eyes which makes the refractive outcome unpredictable. Although EK and cataract surgery might be indicated clinically, a staged procedure (EK first, cataract surgery second) can be reasonable in these cases, as well. However, the potential to harm the corneal endothelium due to the phacoemulsification under the graft has to be weighed against the advantage of a precise IOL calculation.

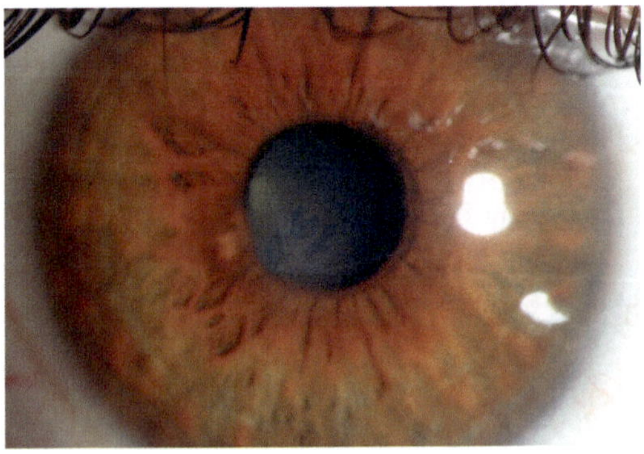

Fig. 12.4 Slit-lamp picture of a FECD patient with significant paracentral focal edema. IOL calculation is difficult in this case which makes a staged procedure (endothelial keratoplasty first, cataract surgery second) reasonable

Combined Cataract Surgery with Endothelial Keratoplasty and IOL Implantation: Technical Aspects and IOL Calculation

When EK is combined with cataract surgery, phacoemulsification and IOL implantation are performed prior to insertion of the EK graft. The same primary incision site is used for delivery of the IOL and the graft. Special care should be taken to use highly cohesive viscoelastic for cataract surgery in order to allow for complete removal of the entire viscoelastic prior to proceeding with graft insertion. An overuse of mydriatics before surgery should be avoided in order to allow best possible constriction of the pupil prior to EK. Intracameral acetylcholine chloride is used for this purpose after implantation of the IOL.

Many surgeons prefer to use hydrophobic IOLs to prevent postoperative calcification of the IOL associated with the intracameral air or gas, although the incidence of calcification of hydrophilic IOLs after EK is very low [9]. There is no standard suggestion as to the lens design used during combined procedure. We suggest using a plate haptic to ensure maximum stability of the iris-lens diaphragm and to prevent displacement of the IOL during the presence of air in the anterior chamber.

The biggest challenge when performing an EK combined with cataract surgery is the IOL calculation to avoid refractive surprises after surgery. Even though EK is a suture-less technique, several studies have shown that combined procedures are not neutral concerning the effect on postoperative refraction but cause a hyperopic shift. Furthermore, the refractive shift seems to be quite unpredictable. The effect is higher for Descemet stripping endothelial keratoplasty (DSEK) than for Descemet membrane endothelial keratoplasty (DMEK) but has still a wide range.

The hyperopic refractive shift has been quantified for both DSEK [ranged from +0.31 D (± 2.03 D) to +1.26 D (± 0.53 D)] and DMEK [ranged from −1.14 D (± 1.7 D) to +0.90 D (± 1.5 D)] [10]. Changes of the posterior corneal curvature seem to have an influence on the refractive shift. In a fellow eye comparison, a good predictability was found for the second eye when the refractive outcome of the first eye was used as a reference [11]. The refractive shift of the second eye seems to follow that of the first eye. We tend to set a myopic refractive target of about −0.75 to −1.5 D dependent on the curvature of the posterior cornea. Nevertheless, the patient needs to be informed properly about the poor predictability of the IOL calculation in case of a combined surgery.

Technical Aspects of Cataract Surgery Only in Eyes with Corneal Guttae/FECD

1. Conventional phacoemulsification

   When performing a cataract surgery in eyes with corneal guttae, it is advisable to use a highly dispersive viscoelastic during surgery in order to provide the best possible protection of the diseased endothelium.

2. Femtosecond laser-assisted cataract surgery

   The role of a femtosecond laser-assisted cataract surgery (FLACS) in eyes with FECD remains controversial. The hypothesis is that the use of the femtosecond laser allows for reduction of the duration of the exposure of the endothelium to ultrasound and therefore reduces the amount of ultrasonic energy when compared to conventional cataract surgery. This allows for a more gentle handling of the endothelium. In a retrospective analysis of 207 eyes with FECD, which focused on postoperative corneal decompensation, FLACS did not decrease the rate of clinically significant corneal decompensation compared with conventional phacoemulsification [12]. In contrast, another retrospective study of 140 eyes with FECD reported reduced endothelial cell loss after FLACS compared to conventional phacoemulsification [13]. In a small prospective study of 31 eyes with FECD evaluating endothelial cell density and central corneal thickness, the outcomes were slightly in favor of the FLACS group compared to conventional phacoemulsification [14]. Larger prospective randomized studies evaluating the role of FLACS in FECD are necessary to confirm the positive effect of FLACS in eyes with FECD.

Complication Management During Cataract Surgery in Eyes with Corneal Guttae/FECD

Posterior Capsule Rupture

Complications regarding the capsular bag during cataract surgery can be managed well by different options of extracapsular IOL positioning. However, eyes with FECD undergoing cataract surgery need special consideration in anticipation of a required endothelial keratoplasty in the future.

Although sulcus fixation of the IOL is often the preferred option for eyes with capsular complications, it can affect the feasibility of the DMEK surgery: The air or gas bubble in the anterior chamber, which is necessary for graft adherence, leads to a retropulsion of the IOL with possible dislocation of the IOL into the vitreous cavity. In case of sulcus fixation of the IOL due to a damaged capsular bag, IOL revision with implantation of an iris-fixated or scleral-sutured posterior chamber IOL is recommended.

The exact position of the IOL should be documented because it is of high importance for the corneal surgeon especially in cases with pseudophakic bullous keratopathy following a complicated cataract surgery. Difficulties in IOL positioning should be communicated clearly to the corneal surgeon to make an adequate procedure planning possible. Vitreous prolapse into the anterior chamber does significantly complicate EK. Anterior vitrectomy must be performed thoroughly in this case. However, extensive vitrectomy should be avoided, since EK is more difficult in vitrectomized eyes.

In aphakic eyes, a secondary posterior chamber IOL implantation is necessary. Otherwise, a tight DMEK roll could fall through the pupil into the vitreous cavity which has been described for DSAEK grafts in aphakic eyes [15]. The probability to lose the graft through the pupil in aphakic eyes is even more probable in DMEK compared to DSAEK since the graft is thinner and forms a tight roll with a diameter which is smaller than the constricted pupil. Furthermore, the air or gas bubble has no barrier to the posterior segment in aphakic eyes and tends to move behind the iris in the early postoperative period after DMEK. This situation can lead to an angle closure but most important to a dislocation of the graft since there is no support of the air or gas bubble. DMEK has been tried in aphakic eyes by some surgeons, but with discouraging results: Graft detachment occurred in 67%, and graft failures occurred in 88% [16]. A temporary suture fixation of the graft in aphakic eyes as described in DSAEK is not possible in DMEK because of the fragility of the thin graft [17]. In eyes with anterior chamber IOLs, we recommend a two-step procedure: removal of the anterior chamber IOL and implantation of an IOL in the posterior chamber (iris fixation or scleral-sutured fixation) [18]. DMEK has been performed successfully in eyes with retained anterior chamber IOLs by some surgeons [19, 20]. However, the compromising effect of anterior chamber IOLs on the endothelium of the graft should be considered. Graft survival is lower in eyes with retained anterior chamber IOLs compared to secondary posterior chamber IOLs [21].

Cystoid Macular Edema

Cystoid macular edema (CME) has been shown to occur in 2–13% of eyes after DMEK [22–26]. Combination of DMEK with simultaneous cataract surgery or DMEK as staged procedure during the first 6 months after phacoemulsification does not increase the incidence of CME [24].

Inoda et al. even found a decreased risk of CME in eyes with a staged procedure (DMEK 1 month after cataract surgery) compared to DMEK alone, possibly because the eyes were on treatment with steroids and nonsteroidal anti-inflammatory eye drops between cataract surgery and DMEK [25]. Iris damage should be avoided during cataract surgery in eyes undergoing DMEK since it is a risk factor for the development of CME [25]. An intensified topical steroid regimen (hourly during the first week after DMEK with phaco) has been shown to reduce the incidence of postoperative CME significantly [26].

IOL Calcification

Calcification of the IOL is a rare long-term complication after DMEK in pseudophakic eyes. The presumed mechanism of IOL calcification is contact of the air/gas bubble with the surface of the IOL. The number of air injections is associated with the occurrence of IOL opacification [9]. This complication has been reported in hydrophilic acrylic IOLs first but can occur in hydrophobic material as well [9].

The management of IOL calcifications depends on the individual visual impairment. Although visibility of the fundus can be diminished by the calcifications, the patient might be impaired only mildly, and vice versa. The only option to treat IOL calcification consists of IOL removal/exchange. The possible use of IOL exchange has to be weighed against the risk of endothelial graft damage by the secondary surgical procedure. High-resolution optical coherence tomography might be a tool for prediction of stray light and visual disturbance by IOL opacifications [27].

Take-Home Messages

- Corneal guttae have a significant impact on vision quality.
- Inform your patient thoroughly about the presence of corneal guttae and how this condition can affect the postoperative course.
- When corneal edema is present or the likelihood of corneal decompensation is high, it is advisable to perform a combined cataract surgery with endothelial keratoplasty.
- When the cornea is too cloudy, consider to perform endothelial keratoplasty first in order to perform later a safe cataract surgery with a more accurate IOL calculation.
- The hyperopic shift in combined cataract surgery with endothelial keratoplasty should be taken into account in IOL calculation.
- If a posterior capsular rupture occurs during cataract surgery, try to reconstitute a stable iris-lens diaphragm in order to allow for a successful endothelial keratoplasty in the future.

References

1. Augustin VA, Weller JM, Kruse FE, Tourtas T. Influence of corneal guttae and nuclear cataract on contrast sensitivity. Br J Ophthalmol. 2020: bjophthalmol-2019-315206. Epub ahead of print.
2. Watanabe S, Oie Y, Fujimoto H, Soma T, Koh S, Tsujikawa M, Maeda N, Nishida K. Relationship between corneal Guttae and quality of vision in patients with mild Fuchs' endothelial corneal dystrophy. Ophthalmology. 2015;122(10):2103–9.
3. Viberg A, Liv P, Behndig A, Lundström M, Byström B. The impact of corneal guttata on the results of cataract surgery. J Cataract Refract Surg. 2019;45(6):803–9.
4. Sun SY, Wacker K, Baratz KH, Patel SV. Determining subclinical edema in Fuchs endothelial corneal dystrophy: revised classification using Scheimpflug tomography for preoperative assessment. Ophthalmology. 2019;126(2):195–204.
5. Patel SV, Hodge DO, Treichel EJ, Spiegel MR, Baratz KH. Predicting the prognosis of Fuchs endothelial corneal dystrophy by using Scheimpflug tomography. Ophthalmology. 2020;127(3):315–23.
6. Macsai MS, Shiloach M. Use of topical rho kinase inhibitors in the treatment of Fuchs dystrophy after descemet stripping only. Cornea. 2019;38(5):529–34.
7. Sarnicola C, Sarnicola E, Panico E, Panico C, Sarnicola V. Cataract surgery in corneal transplantation. Curr Opin Ophthalmol. 2020;31(1):23–7.
8. Vasiliauskaitė I, Dhubhghaill SN, Ham L, Van Dijk K, Oellerich S, Melles GRJ. Phacoemulsification after descemet membrane endothelial keratoplasty: incidence and influence on endothelial cell density. J Refract Surg. 2021;37(2):119–25.
9. Schrittenlocher S, Penier M, Schaub F, Bock F, Cursiefen C, Bachmann B. Intraocular lens calcifica-

tions after (triple-) descemet membrane endothelial keratoplasty. Am J Ophthalmol. 2017;179:129–36.
10. Augustin VA, Weller JM, Kruse FE, Tourtas T. Can we predict the refractive outcome after triple descemet membrane endothelial keratoplasty? Eur J Ophthalmol. 2019;29(2):165–70.
11. Augustin VA, Weller JM, Kruse FE, Tourtas T. Refractive outcomes after descemet membrane endothelial keratoplasty + cataract/intraocular lens triple procedure: a fellow eye comparison. Cornea. 2020; Epub ahead of print
12. Zhu DC, Shah P, Feuer WJ, Shi W, Koo EH. Outcomes of conventional phacoemulsification versus femtosecond laser-assisted cataract surgery in eyes with Fuchs endothelial corneal dystrophy. J Cataract Refract Surg. 2018;44(5):534–40.
13. Yong WWD, Chai HC, Shen L, Manotosh R, Anna Tan WT. Comparing outcomes of phacoemulsification with femtosecond laser-assisted cataract surgery in patients with Fuchs endothelial dystrophy. Am J Ophthalmol. 2018;196:173–80.
14. Fan W, Yan H, Zhang G. Femtosecond laser-assisted cataract surgery in Fuchs endothelial corneal dystrophy: long-term outcomes. J Cataract Refract Surg. 2018;44(7):864–70.
15. Afshari NA, Gorovoy MS, Yoo SH, et al. Dislocation of the donor graft to the posterior segment in Descemet stripping automated endothelial keratoplasty. Am J Ophthalmol. 2012;153:638–42.
16. Santaella G, Sorkin N, Mimouni M, Trinh T, Cohen E, Chan CC, Rootman DS. Outcomes of descemet membrane endothelial keratoplasty in aphakic and aniridic patients. Cornea. 2020;39(11):1389–93.
17. Patel AK, Luccarelli S, Ponzin D, et al. Transcorneal suture fixation of posterior lamellar grafts in eyes with minimal or absent iris-lens diaphragm. Am J Ophthalmol. 2011;151:460–4.
18. Weller JM, Tourtas T, Kruse FE. Feasibility and outcome of descemet membrane endothelial keratoplasty in complex anterior segment and vitreous disease. Cornea. 2015;34(11):1351–7.
19. Droutsas K, Lazaridis A, Kymionis G, Chatzistefanou K, Papaconstantinou D, Sekundo W, Koutsandrea C. Endothelial keratoplasty in eyes with a retained angle-supported intraocular lens. Int Ophthalmol. 2019;39(5):1027–35. https://doi.org/10.1007/s10792-018-0899-x. Epub 2018 Apr 4. PMID: 29619650.
20. Liarakos VS, Ham L, Dapena I, Tong CM, Quilendrino R, Yeh RY, Melles GR. Endothelial keratoplasty for bullous keratopathy in eyes with an anterior chamber intraocular lens. J Cataract Refract Surg. 2013;39(12):1835–45. https://doi.org/10.1016/j.jcrs.2013.05.045. PMID: 24286840.
21. Woo JH, Arundhati A, Chee SP, Tong W, Li L, Ti SE, Htoon HM, Choo JQH, Tan D, Mehta JS. Endothelial keratoplasty with anterior chamber intraocular lens versus secondary posterior chamber intraocular lens. Br J Ophthalmol. 2020:bjophthalmol-2020-316711. Epub ahead of print.
22. Ching G, Covello AT, Bae SS, Holland S, McCarthy M, Ritenour R, Iovieno A, Yeung SN. Incidence and outcomes of cystoid macular edema after Descemet Membrane Endothelial Keratoplasty (DMEK) and DMEK combined with cataract surgery. Curr Eye Res. 2020;9:1–5. Epub ahead of print
23. Heinzelmann S, Maier P, Böhringer D, Hüther S, Eberwein P, Reinhard T. Cystoid macular oedema following descemet membrane endothelial keratoplasty. Br J Ophthalmol. 2015;99(1):98–102.
24. Flanary WE, Vislisel JM, Wagoner MD, Raecker ME, Aldrich BT, Zimmerman MB, Goins KM, Greiner MA. Incidence of cystoid macular edema after descemet membrane endothelial keratoplasty as a staged and solitary procedure. Cornea. 2016;35(8):1040–4.
25. Inoda S, Hayashi T, Takahashi H, Oyakawa I, Yokogawa H, Kobayashi A, Kato N, Kawashima H. Risk factors for cystoid macular edema after descemet membrane endothelial keratoplasty. Cornea. 2019;38(7):820–4.
26. Hoerster R, Stanzel TP, Bachmann BO, Siebelmann S, Felsch M, Cursiefen C. Intensified topical steroids as prophylaxis for macular edema after posterior lamellar keratoplasty combined with cataract surgery. Am J Ophthalmol. 2016;163:174–9.
27. Yildirim TM, Łabuz G, Hammer M, Son HS, Schickhardt SK, Auffarth GU, Khoramnia R. A novel approach for assessing visual impairment caused by intraocular lens opacification: high-resolution optical coherence tomography: Straylight prediction in locally opacified IOLs. Am J Ophthalmol. 2021:S0002–9394(21)00063–5. Epub ahead of print.

The Posterior Polar Cataract

13

Robert H. Osher

- Avoid overpressurizing the anterior chamber with excessive OVD.
- Hydrodelineation is preferred to hydrodissection.
- Slow-motion phaco reduces turbulence.
- The escape route concept is helpful for atraumatic loosening of the epinucleus.
- Maintain the chamber with OVD before withdrawing the phaco and I&A tip.
- IOL implantation should avoid any pressure on the capsular bag.

When I entered ophthalmology as a resident, the standard of care was to follow the posterior polar cataract by conservative observation. Patients were told that they had this cataract their entire life and to wait until it became mature at which time surgical intervention would be justified. This approach seemed counterintuitive because the associated glare was often incapacitating. I joined my father's practice in 1980 and eventually accumulated more than a dozen patients with posterior polar cataracts for whom I had performed phacoemulsification with posterior chamber lens implantation. I collaborated with Douglas Koch, MD, in Houston, a very close friend who shared the same opinion, and we combined our patients publishing the first surgical series in 1990 [1]. While our frequency of an open posterior capsule (either congenital or iatrogenic) was quite high in a range of 26%, the patients were genuinely ecstatic with the improvement in their vision, especially with the reduction of glare.

A number of surgical principles have evolved which have markedly reduced the incidence of posterior capsule rupture. This brief chapter will review the surgical principles which have allowed us to enjoy a highly successful visual outcome following contemporary small incision cataract surgery in the patient with a posterior polar cataract.

The Patient Discussion

It is necessary to invest the time to explain that the normal "wrapping" or "envelope" around the back of the lens is usually 3 or 4 microns thick. I like to explain that this type of cataract has a much thinner wrapping which is more fragile and may even be incomplete due to flawed development before birth. It should be emphasized that this type of cataract is more challenging to remove and often associated with complications that may alter the type and location of the

Supplementary Information The online version contains supplementary material available at [https://doi.org/10.1007/978-3-030-94530-5_13].

R. H. Osher (✉)
Cincinnati Eye Institute, University of Cincinnati, Cincinnati, OH, USA
e-mail: rhosher@cvphealth.com

J. L. Alió et al. (eds.), *Cataract Surgery*, Essentials in Ophthalmology,
https://doi.org/10.1007/978-3-030-94530-5_13

intraocular lens to be implanted. This discussion should be documented in the medical record.

Preoperative Testing and Biomicroscopy

Some surgeons have recommended anterior segment OCT to see if a break in the posterior capsule can be identified [2–6]. While I do not routinely order this study, I am very careful to confirm that the patient actually has a posterior polar cataract rather than a posterior subcapsular cataract, based upon the location and thickness of the circular opacity which extends anteriorly into the posterior cortex. Moreover, I try to observe the continuity of the posterior capsule which may reveal a preexisting opening. Finally, I look for tiny opacities or "oil droplets" in the anterior vitreous which suggest that an opening in the posterior capsule may be present.

The Surgical Procedure: Filling the Anterior Chamber with OVD

While it is necessary to inject OVD into the anterior chamber in order to perform a safe manual capsulorhexis, it is important not to overfill which can raise the IOP. Excessive pressure in the anterior chamber can actually propel the lens contents through a thin or defective posterior capsule into the vitreous.

Capsulorhexis

The surgeon should be as meticulous as possible in centering and sizing the capsulorhexis. The reason for this precision is that optic capture may be necessary for lens fixation.

Hydrodissection or Hydrodelineation

A traditional hydrodissection is contraindicated because the fluid wave may dissect around the lens and "blow out" the posterior capsule. For this same reason, visco-dissection is not recommended. Dr. Abhay Vasavada from India has advocated hydrodelamination which is performed by placing the cannula more centrally so the stream of fluid will separate the nucleus from the epinucleus [7]. More central injections can separate the fetal from the adult nucleus. By creating a trench with the phacoemulsification needle, the surgeon may also use "inside out" hydrodelineation where the fluid wave is started in the troth which will also delineate the different nuclear layers [8]. The key concept is to keep the delamination within the lens rather than allow a stream to generate pressure on the weakened or open posterior capsule. Dr. Vasavada has also introduced the technique of femtodelineation in which three nuclear cylinders are created within the lens surrounded by an outermost epinucleus [9, 10].

Phacoemulsification

Many surgeons have published their preferences for removing the nucleus by phacoemulsification [11–14]. Most agree that the surgeon should remove the more central nucleus which has been delineated and an in situ approach is preferable rather than rotating or decentering the lens. Slow-motion phacoemulsification utilizing lower parameters is preferable in order to prevent turbulence and a more volatile chamber [15].

The Escape Route

I am enthusiastic about a new concept which I call the escape route. Once the fetal and adult nuclear layers have been emulsified, there is inevitably an epinucleus that is "stuck" because we have avoided hydrodissection. The strategy for mobilizing this epinucleus is both novel and effective (Video 13.1). With the phaco tip, the surgeon borrows into the epinucleus opposite the incision. It is usually soft because these patients are typically quite young and therefore can often be aspirated by the phaco needle. Then the adjacent cortex opposite the incision is also aspirated, which provides the escape route. Now it is safe to hydrodissect under the capsule with either a straight cannula or a curved reverse cannula to loosen the epinucleus, especially the sub-incisional epinucleus. Because the fluid wave can easily escape through the escape route, the remaining epinucleus can be safely mobilized and then emulsified without placing stress on the posterior capsule.

Cortical Removal

The surgeon may elect to use either a coaxial, bimanual, or dry technique to remove the cortex. I favor the silicone tip for micro-coaxial I/A. Starting with the most difficult sub-incisional cortex is ideal because the capsular bag is held open by the cortical bowl. The stubborn cortex has been reported to be removed by careful and gentle visco-dissection [16].

Central Plaque Management

After the cortex has been removed, there is often an axial opacity. Under normal circumstances, the opacity would be removed by polishing, vacuuming, or dissecting the plaque off the posterior capsule. But given the fragile nature of the central capsule, it is probably safest to perform a Nd:YAG laser in the postoperative period. Alternatively, a minimum aspiration technique can be performed by tapping on the footswitch to create vacuum by the re-expansion of the tubing. Yet if the posterior capsule tears, the surgeon should be prepared to perform a posterior capsulorhexis, excising the abnormal central plague and then performing either traditional optic capture, reverse optic capture, or a variant where the IOL is prolapsed through the posterior capsulorhexis into Berger's space [17].

Maintaining the Chamber

Before withdrawing the phaco or the I&A tip, the OVD should be injected through the stab incision in order to maintain a deep chamber. Otherwise, when the instrument is withdrawn, the chamber will shallow, and the anterior hyaloid may rupture allowing vitreous to prolapse forward.

IOL Insertion

It is a natural tendency to take a deep breath and lower one's guard after the cataract has been removed. However, the surgeon must remain vigilant. Any pressure against the capsular bag by the leading haptic may cause a severe tear in either the intact or open posterior capsule. One strategy to prevent unwanted contact is to use a retentive OVD like Healon 5 which keeps the haptics of a single-piece IOL folded over the optic as the IOL is being maneuvered into the capsular bag. After it is oriented, the haptics can be gently unfolded with an instrument or the I&A tip. The surgeon has the option of implanting a single-piece lens into the capsular bag, even if the central posterior capsule is open, as long as there is still sufficient peripheral support where the capsule is normal. Although difficult, it is advantageous to convert a posterior capsular tear to a posterior capsulorhexis. If the capsular support is in question, the surgeon may either prolapse the optic forward achieving reverse optic capture or simply implant a three-piece lens into the ciliary sulcus displacing the optic posteriorly through the capsulorhexis opening achieving traditional optic capture. Other viable options include sutured iris or scleral fixation as well as intrascleral fixation.

Final Maneuvers

Hydration of the incision is recommended before the OVD is removed from behind the optic and then from in front of the optic. Again, before withdrawing the I&A tip, the chamber should be maintained by injecting balanced salt solution through the stab incision. Acetylcholine can be used when the surgeon prefers to constrict the pupil. If the anterior hyaloid face is open and the surgeon is trying to keep the vitreous back, an air bubble may be injected and subsequently exchanged in small aliquots for either balanced salt solution or acetylcholine. The incision is hydrated for a final time and its water tightness is confirmed.

Conclusion

The posterior polar cataract remains a surgical challenge because the central posterior capsule is extremely thin and fragile. Multiple techniques, like creating an escape route, will offer the surgeon the best chance of achieving a successful outcome.

References

1. Osher RH, Yu BC-Y, Koch DD. Posterior polar cataracts: a predisposition to intraoperative posterior capsule rupture. J Cataract Refract Surg. 1990;16:157–62.
2. Kymionis GD, Diakonis VF, Liakopoulos DA, Tsoulnaras KI, Klados NE, Pallikaris IG. Anterior segment optical coherence tomography for demonstrating posterior capsular rent in posterior polar cataract. Clin Ophthalmol. 2014;8:215–7.
3. Chan TCY, Li EYM, Yau JCY. Application of anterior segment optical coherence tomography to identify eyes with posterior polar cataract at high risk for posterior capsule rupture. J Cataract Refract Surg. 2014;40:2076–81.
4. Pavan Kumar G, Krishnamurthy P, Nath M, Baskaran P, Janai M, Venkatesh R. Can preoperative anterior segment optical coherence tomography predict posterior capsule rupture during phacoemulsification in patients with posterior polar cataract? J Cataract Refract Surg. 2018;44:1441–5.
5. Pujari A, Yadav S, Sharma N, Khokhar S, Sinha R, Agarwal T, Titiyal JS, Sharma P. Study 1: evaluation of the signs of deficient posterior capsule in posterior polar cataracts using anterior segment optical coherence tomography. J Cataract Refract Surg. 2020;46:1260–5.
6. Titiyal JS, Kaur M, Shaikh F, Rani D, Bageshwar, Lalit MS. Elucidating intraoperative dynamics and safety in posterior polar cataract with intraoperative OCT-guided phacoemulsification. J Cataract Refract Surg. 2020;46:1266–72.
7. Vasavada A, Singh R. Phacoemulsification in eyes with posterior polar cataract. J Cataract Refract Surg. 1999;25:238–45.
8. Vasavada AR, Raj SM. Inside-out delineation. J Cataract Refract Surg. 2004;30:1167–9.
9. Vasavada AR, Vasavada V, Vasavada S, Srivastava S, Vasavada V, Raj S. Femtodelineation to enhance safety in posterior polar cataracts. J Cataract Refract Surg. 2015;41:702–7.
10. Titiyal JS, Kaur M, Sharma N. Femtosecond laser-assisted cataract surgery technique to enhance safety in posterior polar cataract. J Refract Surg. 2015;31:826–8.
11. Fine IH, Packer M, Hoffman RS. Management of posterior polar cataract. J Cataract Refract Surg. 2003;29:16–9.
12. Hayashi K, Hayashi H, Nakao F, Hayashi F. Outcomes of surgery for posterior polar cataract. J Cataract Refract Surg. 2003;29:45–9.
13. Haripriya A, Aravind S, Vadi K, Natchiar G. Bimanual microphaco for posterior polar cataracts. J Cataract Refract Surg. 2006;32:914–7.
14. Chee S-P. Management of the hard posterior polar cataract. J Cataract Refract Surg. 2007;33:1509–14.
15. Osher RH. Slow motion phacoemulsification approach. [Letter.]. J Cataract Refract Surg. 1993;19(5):667. https://doi.org/10.1016/S0886-3350(13)80025-9.
16. Allen D, Wood C. Minimizing risk to the capsule during surgery for posterior polar cataract. J Cataract Refract Surg. 2002;28:742–4.
17. Foster GJL, Ayers B, Fram N, Hoffman RS, Khandewal S, Ogawa G, MacDonald SM, Snyder ME, Vasavada A. Phacoemulsification of posterior polar cataracts. J Cataract Refract Surg. 2019;45:228–35.

14 Cataract Surgery in the Edematous, Partially Opaque Cornea and After Corneal Graft

Ahmed A. Abdelghany, Jorge Alió del Barrio, Ahmed M. Khalafallah, and Jorge L. Alió

Introduction

Corneal pathology is a relatively common situation when facing cataract surgery in older patients [1]. In this scenario, we should take into account that visual loss is not only due to the cataract itself but also due to the abnormal cornea. Potential visual gain after cataract removal should be estimated, so patients can have realistic expectations regarding the surgery [2].

Cataract surgery in patients with corneal pathologies can be demanding not only because of difficulties with intraoperative visualization under the surgical microscope during surgery but mainly due to difficulties with intraocular lens (IOL) power calculation and prediction of the refractive outcome preoperatively. Adequate and careful preoperative assessment is essential in these patients, and a correct acquisition and understanding of diagnostic tools such as corneal topography and aberrometry are of critical importance [3].

Modern cataract surgery techniques, IOL technologies, and advanced methods for IOL power calculation allow most cataract patients to obtain an adequate visual and refractive outcome, even in the presence of corneal abnormalities [3]. In this chapter, we will discuss cataract surgery in the presence of some types of corneal pathologies such as lack of adequate corneal transparency, low endothelial cell count, and eyes with a previous corneal graft and the management of such cases to try to achieve the best results possible.

Cataract Surgery in Eyes with Corneal Opacity

Corneal opacities may be due to corneal dystrophies or corneal scars from previous trauma, infection, or inflammation of corneal tissues [4]. Corneal scars may preclude a proper intraoperative visualization of the intraocular structures, and limit the postoperative visual outcome, to a degree depending on their location, density, and capacity to induce irregular astigmatism [5]. Peripheral corneal opacities might not interfere with intraoperative visualization during cataract surgery, but may influence the refractive outcome by inducing astigmatism, which should be

Supplementary Information The online version contains supplementary material available at [https://doi.org/10.1007/978-3-030-94530-5_14].

A. A. Abdelghany · A. M. Khalafallah
Ophthalmology Department, Faculty of Medicine, Minia University, Minia, Egypt

J. Alió del Barrio · J. L. Alió (✉)
Cornea, Refractive and Cataract Surgery Unit, Vissum Miranza Alicante, Alicante, Spain

Division of Ophthalmology, School of Medicine, Miguel Hernandez University, Alicante, Spain
e-mail: jlalio@vissum.com

J. L. Alió et al. (eds.), *Cataract Surgery*, Essentials in Ophthalmology,
https://doi.org/10.1007/978-3-030-94530-5_14

addressed preoperatively with corneal topography [5]. When facing scars due to previous trauma, surgeons should examine the eye carefully before surgery to look for potential capsular or zonular damage [3].

In a similar fashion as previously discussed, the first thing to do when facing a cataract in a patient with a partially opaque cornea is to estimate the potential visual gain with cataract surgery and so determine if the corneal opacity requires prior management in the form of laser ablation (PTK), manual keratectomy, or keratoplasty. Corneal anterior segment optical coherence tomography (AS-OCT) is critical for such purpose as it allows a precise measurement of the opacity depth and location and so assists in the choice of the optimal surgical approach to the opacity.

However, corneal opacities may impact the visual function not only because of the loss of transparency itself but also because of the potential induction of irregular astigmatism, and so, corneal topography becomes an essential tool in the preoperative assessment regarding corneal ectasias. Severely aberrated corneas may be better considered for simultaneous corneal graft procedure and cataract surgery rather than for cataract surgery alone [3]. Nevertheless, simultaneous corneal graft (either penetrating or lamellar) and phacoemulsification may be necessary not only to enhance the visual outcome but also to allow the cataract surgery itself by allowing sufficient intraoperative visualization of the intraocular structures [4, 6, 7].

On the other hand, simultaneous keratoplasty and cataract surgery has many serious preoperative (poor expected graft survival, no available corneal tissue, etc.), intraoperative (expulsive choroidal hemorrhage), and postoperative (delayed visual rehabilitation, rejection risk which is increased in vascularized opacities, etc.) drawbacks.

To overcome these drawbacks, phacoemulsification can be assisted and visualization improved by the use of endoscopic lights such as the chandelier light used for vitreoretinal surgery as a retroillumination-assisted torsional oscillation technique, chandelier anterior chamber endoillumination-assisted phacoemulsification, intracameral dynamic spotlight-assisted phacoemulsification, and endoscope-assisted cataract surgery or by transcorneal oblique illumination (which does not provide as high-quality images as the endoilluminators). Thus, corneal reflection and scattering are diminished, and better visualization is provided [8–14].

As an example of intracameral endoilluminator-assisted phacoemulsification in these patients, Yuksel E. used a 23-gauge Shielded Widefield Endoilluminator (Shielded Widefield Endoillumination; Bausch & Lomb, Inc.) which was inserted intracamerally through a 0.6 mm limbal paracentesis. This has advantages over the chandelier retroilluminator in that it does not need additional vitrectomy tools and carries no increased risk of retinal detachment. In addition, the chandelier system is not shielded, so the light spreads in both anterior and posterior directions, and in this way, the anterior spread impairs the view with the scattering of light from the cornea. In contrast to other intracameral manipulators, this shielded illuminator has no more risk than a chopper in terms of Descemet tear during its usage which did not occur in this study [15].

Our surgical recommendations:

- Preoperative meticulous evaluation of the site and density of the corneal opacity using slit-lamp examination, corneal topography, and anterior segment optical coherence tomography (AS-OCT).
- If corneal opacity is superficial, it can be managed preoperatively using phototherapeutic keratectomy before proceeding to cataract surgery.
- Noncentral dense corneal opacities should be considered as a main astigmatic issue especially if paracentral, and if so, preoperative counseling with toric intraocular lenses should be considered with no or little effect on visualization during cataract surgery which can be bypassed by avoiding the area under the corneal opacity, looking through a clear window to initiate capsulorhexis, and then completing it with a constant tethered force under the opaque area.

- In central corneal opacities of moderate density, the Shielded Widefield Endoilluminator and other previously mentioned endoillumination techniques should be considered. Also, other techniques may be helpful such as using 2% hydroxypropyl methylcellulose (HPMC) to coat the cornea, red reflex enhancement, or capsular stain and moving the eye around to look through clear corneal parts.
- If corneal opacity is dense and central with a depth reaching or exceeding posterior stroma, penetrating keratoplasty (PKP) or deep anterior lamellar keratoplasty (DALK) should be considered as a triple procedure in cases of dense significant cataracts or as a primary management of corneal opacity in cases of insignificant cataracts.

Cataract Surgery in Eyes with Low Endothelial Cell Count and Fuchs' Endothelial Dystrophy

The most common type of endothelial dystrophy is Fuchs' endothelial corneal dystrophy (FECD), but low endothelial cell density (ECD) may also be present in patients with a previous history of corneal and/or intraocular inflammation or trauma [16], advanced age, diabetes mellitus [17], renal impairment [18], and pulmonary diseases [19]. Preoperative low endothelial cell count is one of the most common causes for developing pseudophakic bullous keratopathy (PBK) after cataract surgery. Incidence of PBK increases from about 1 to 2 percent after conventional cataract surgery in normal corneas and up to 11–24 percent in corneas with endothelial cell count below 1000 cells/mm^2 [16].

In the presence of cataracts, deciding whether a patient with FECD can expect improved vision after cataract surgery alone remains a challenge. Firstly, blurred vision, glare, and loss of contrast sensitivity may be caused by corneal deterioration, but these can also be simply signs of a cataract. Secondly, phacoemulsification may trigger corneal deterioration in FECD if the number of remaining endothelial cells drops below the critical threshold necessary to provide sufficient pumping activity (1500 cells/mm^2). Central corneal thickness (CCT) or corneal backscatter correlates with disease severity and has been proposed to help identify risk of corneal decompensation after cataract surgery in FECD [20, 21].

The recently updated American Academy of Ophthalmology's Preferred Practice Pattern identifies slit-lamp biomicroscopic microcystic edema or stromal thickening, low central ECD, and a CCT greater than 640 microns as risk factors for decompensation following cataract surgery [22]. However, the predictive value of these data has not been completely satisfactory [23, 24]. In this scenario, novel scoring systems based on easily available preoperative Scheimpflug data have been suggested to demonstrate good accuracy in estimating the risk of corneal decompensation after cataract surgery in FECD patients [25]. Arnalich et al. assessed cases preoperatively using multiple data including preoperative best spectacle-corrected visual acuity (BSCVA), a modified Krachmer scale for grading of Fuchs' dystrophy, Scheimpflug photography (measuring corneal thickness (apical, pupillary, and thinnest), relative pachymetry, central corneal light backscatter: data are provided on four annular zones centered on the apex (0–2, 2–6, 6–10, and 10–12 mm in diameter) from the anterior (AL backscatter, the anterior 120 mm), central (CL backscatter, from the previous point up to 60 micrometers above the posterior surface), and posterior layers (PL backscatter, the deepest 60 micrometers) and anterior chamber depth), specular microscopy, ultrasound CCT, and cataract grading using the Lens Opacities Classification System III (LOCS III). The Pentacam estimates for CCT are around 10 micrometers higher than with ultrasound, so the results of these systems are not interchangeable. Relative pachymetry performed the best of all the pachymetry-related parameters. A central increase greater than 7.8% above the normal database provides better sensitivity (85%) than any CCT for 95% of specificity. AL backscatter at 0–2 mm zone using Pentacam has good sensitivity (89%) and high specificity (95%). Using IVCM (in vivo confocal microscopy) to assess corneal backscatter has lower sensitivity for 95% specificity [26]. In addition, the Pentacam module easily assesses the entire cornea, and scattering provides better image brightness than specular reflection. ECD measurements were significant but did not provide much more information for risk assessment.

Therefore, a formula was suggested with 96% sensitivity and 95% specificity by using the relative increase in corneal thickness at the central cornea with respect to normal corneal thickness (relative pachymetry) and the central corneal backscatter at 0–2 mm zone [25]. A positive score value on this formula signifies that a given patient will progress to DMEK after cataract surgery. Such scoring systems ensure that patients can be fully informed of their predictive risk as well as the treatment options and allow surgeons to optimize perioperative care and organize the logistics for a second surgery.

In order to plan for cataract surgery in eyes with low corneal endothelial cell count, other risk factors of developing postoperative PBK should be considered such as shallow anterior chamber, dense cataracts, and previous intraocular surgeries [4]. During surgery, careful phacoemulsification technique using repeated dispersive ocular viscoelastic devices (OVD) and injection and ultrasound-sparing techniques such as phaco chop or femtosecond laser-assisted cataract surgery are recommended in order to preserve the diseased corneal endothelium [27].

For cataract patients when the risk of postoperative PBK is considered very high, severe symptoms associated with corneal guttata are already present, or some degree of corneal edema already exists, the surgeon may perform the cataract surgery just before the endothelial keratoplasty (EK) or simultaneously by performing a triple procedure (EK and phacoemulsification with IOL implantation) [28]. An unintended hyperopic result following such triple procedures has been reported, occasionally inducing a significant deviation from target. In DSEK (Descemet stripping endothelial keratoplasty) triple procedures, the difference in thickness between the center and periphery of the DSEK graft induces a change in posterior corneal curvature, resulting in a hyperopic shift that remains in the range of +0.75/+1.5D approximately, and this fact should be taken into account when selecting the IOL power [29]. When performing a DMEK (Descemet membrane endothelial keratoplasty) triple procedure, this hyperopic shift might not be expected, as a DMEK graft is homogeneous in its thickness without a negative lenticule effect as this does occur with DSEK. However, some hyperopic shift still occurs (although to a lesser degree, in the range of +0.5/+1D approximately), and it is thought to be the result of a reversal of a preceding myopic shift induced by the stromal swelling [30]. Stromal swelling in endothelial disease induces flattening of the posterior cornea (considering that the posterior cornea produces negative power) which increases the net power of the cornea preoperatively. Postoperatively, the cornea returns to normal hydration status resulting in increased posterior corneal curvature which produces more negative corneal power and an unintended hyperopic result. Nevertheless, several authors have proven only a weak correlation between preoperative flattening of the posterior corneal curvature and unintended hyperopic results [31, 32]. In order to avoid such unintended hyperopic results, it is recommended that surgeons target for more myopia in DMEK triple procedures ranging from −0.5 to −1.0 D. However, the important variability in the severity of the corneal disease at the time of surgery makes these adjustments probably not suitable for all eyes. A recent study reported that Hoffer Q, SRK/T, Holladay I, and Barrett Universal II formulas resulted in mean hyperopic errors after DMEK triple procedures, while Haigis formula was the only one that resulted in a slight myopic error [33]. In agreement with previous authors, they also found that a flatter posterior corneal curvature was weakly associated with hyperopic shifts, indicating a poor predictive value to guide surgical planning.

Performing femtosecond laser-assisted cataract surgery without DMEK in CCT less than 630 micrometer and endothelial cell count exceeding 1500 cells/mm^2 has better results than conventional phacoemulsification cataract surgery [34]. The CCT remained thicker than the preoperative thickness 12 months after surgery. In recent studies, the femtosecond cases had a thinner CCT and less endothelial cell loss than the phacoemulsification cases postoperatively [35]. The role of femtosecond laser-assisted cataract surgery in these patients remains poorly defined [36]. The benefits of femtosecond laser-assisted cataract surgery include lower endothelial cell loss due to low total ultrasound time and perfect centration of the capsulotomy which allows multifocal IOL implantation if needed. The major disadvantages of femtosecond laser-assisted cataract surgery are the high cost and intraoperative miosis which can be lessened by preoperative topical NSAID (nonsteroidal anti-inflammatory drugs) [37].

Cataract surgery in such cases should be performed before the cataract turns critically dense because dense cataracts increase the risk of posterior capsule rupture which in turn increases the risk of future corneal transplantation even in normal corneas [38]. The negative effect of low endothelial count on visual acuity persists at least 3 months postoperatively but was most obvious during the first 3 weeks [39].

Preoperative, Surgical, and Postoperative Recommendations

- Patient should be counseled about the importance of performing cataract surgery in soft cataracts rather than dense ones, delayed postoperative recovery, and possibility of corneal decompensation (the presence of stromal thickening, low endothelial cell count (less than 1000 cells/mm^2), and microcystic edema).
- Due to the expected hyperopic shift mentioned before, the IOL power is recommended to be calculated with a target postoperative refraction range of between −1 and − 1.5D.
- The choice of surgical technique depends on the cataract density, the status of cornea, and the surgeon's experience with each technique. Femtosecond laser-assisted cataract surgery is recommended if available and applicable in such cases.
- The soft shell technique of OVD is mandatory, and OVD should be periodically reinjected with complete removal of OVD at the end of the surgery to prevent acute postoperative rise in intraocular pressure.
- Balanced salt solution (BSS) is recommended to be used or other solutions containing glutathione, glucose, and sodium bicarbonate with low-flow parameters, and staying away from the corneal endothelium will decrease endothelial cell loss.
- A new phaco tip should be used, and longitudinal phacoemulsification should be combined with lateral phacoemulsification (transverse or torsional).
- If there is a posterior capsular tear, meticulous automated anterior vitrectomy is mandatory as well as avoidance of an anterior chamber IOL.
- A suture would be better than excessive stromal hydration.
- Postoperative frequent steroids and hypertonic saline and regular follow-up visits are recommended.

Cataract Surgery in Eyes with Previous Keratoplasty

One of the common reasons that causes impaired visual acuity after keratoplasty is cataract. This could be present before or developed after the keratoplasty. There are several reasons which cause postoperative cataract such as steroid-induced cataract, corneal graft rejection, or acceleration of a preexisting cataract [40].

There are *three dominant types of keratoplasty* [41]: penetrating keratoplasty (PK), deep anterior lamellar keratoplasty (DALK), and endothelial keratoplasty (either DSEK or DMEK).

In Cases with Previous PK or DALK

There are three main problems:

1. Preoperative astigmatism.
2. The condition of the existing corneal endothelium.

Stability of the Corneal Scar at the Graft-Host Junction

Preoperative Astigmatism

The underlying factors for post-PK/DALK astigmatism are multiple and may be preoperative factors (either in the donor or the host tissue), intraoperative factors (like the suturing technique), or postoperative related to corneal wound healing [42]. To overcome the problem of post-graft astigmatism, different procedures can be done such as performing astigmatic keratotomies (AK) (either manual or femtosecond laser-assisted) [43, 44] or implanting a toric IOL [45]. Intracorneal ring segment implantation is also an alternative approach for the management of post-PK/DALK high astigmatism [46]. Corneal procedures are not recommended to be performed at the moment of cataract surgery because they are affected by a high variability of the refractive outcome, and thus such procedures must be done at least 3 months in advance in order to obtain stable keratometry readings. Toric spherical IOLs are an alternative approach to correct residual corneal astigmatism at the moment of cataract surgery [45]. However, they should be used with caution, as an eventual failure of the graft (either due to a loss of transparency in the context of endothelial failure or due to a morphological failure in the context of an ectasia recurrence) and its replacement by a repeat PK/DLAK graft will completely change the refractive status of the cornea, and so any previous toric IOL will interfere with the postoperative visual recovery of the patient by the underlying IOL within the bag with a wrong toricity [47]. Because of this, toric IOLs should be only considered to be used within the capsular bag when the risk of repeat keratoplasty is marginal (PK with good endothelial cell density in aged patients with low risk of rejection, long-standing DALKs with low risk of ectasia recurrence, etc.). High astigmatism (over 5D) or high levels of irregular astigmatism should be managed in advance with corneal procedures (as seen above) before considering the implantation of any toric IOL. Multifocal IOLs are not indicated for such cases [48].

Nowadays, a large number of failed PK of DALK grafts are rescued with EK techniques [49]. Due to this, hydrophobic IOL materials are recommended since hydrophilic IOLs have been associated with IOL calcification and opacification risk after EK with gas injections.

The Condition of the Existing Corneal Endothelium

According to the endothelium, cataract surgery-related endothelial cell loss of the graft is usually markedly higher in transplanted corneas than in normal virgin eyes, and the rate of endothelial cell loss after cataract surgery increases up to 44.9% at 1 year and 58% at 2 years postop, as reported by Kim et al. [50].

Endothelial damage can be minimized by decreasing the amount of ultrasound energy used and by protecting the endothelium with repeat injections of dispersive viscoelastic during surgery [51–53]. For cases with very hard cataracts, extracapsular cataract extraction might be considered in order to cause less endothelial damage than phacoemulsification [54].

No clinically relevant loss in endothelial cell density has been found after phacoemulsification in eyes that developed *cataracts after DALK* [52, 55].

Stability of the Corneal Scar at the Graft-Host Junction

Wound healing at the graft-host junction is markedly delayed due to the avascularity of the cornea and the long-term use of topical corticosteroids, so the tensile strength of a corneal wound is never comparable to that of normal corneal tissue [56], and there is a risk of graft-host junction dehiscence during cataract surgery. Phacoemulsification is generally recommended after suture removal is completed, and any potential high or irregular astigmatism has been managed by corneal procedures, so a stable keratometry that could allow a precise IOL power calculation is obtained. However, stability of the graft-host junction should be confirmed by slit-lamp examination before surgery, especially in elderly patients or those with long-term use of high-dose topical steroids. If possible, phacoemulsification surgery should be performed 1–3 months after topical steroids have been discontinued or tapered to a minimal maintenance dose.

Cataract Surgery in Cases with Previous Endothelial Keratoplasty

Cataract surgery in cases with previous endothelial keratoplasty has some advantages but also some potential serious complications. Advantages include easy IOL calculation and predictability of the postoperative refractive outcome without risk of hyperopic shift because corneal curvature values are stable and definitive [57, 58]. Potential complications include graft dislodgement, endothelial trauma, and graft failure [59]. Therefore, if there is some degree of significant phacosclerosis in the presence of endothelial dysfunction, it is always better to perform the cataract surgery in advance or simultaneously to the EK (endothelial keratoplasty) procedure in order to avoid such risks. However, in young patients with no cataracts, particularly if accommodation is preserved, EK surgery should be performed without adjuvant lensectomy, even in the knowledge that the surgery itself, and the postoperative use of topical steroids, might induce the appearance of an early cataract.

When cataract surgery is necessary in the presence of a healthy EK graft, endothelial damage should be minimized by decreasing the amount of ultrasound energy used and by protecting the endothelium with repeat injections of dispersive viscoelastic during surgery. DMEK has been reported to have a low risk of graft dislocation associated with cataract surgery due to strong adherences of its Descemet membrane to the recipient posterior stroma [60]. When a DSEK graft is present, graft dislocation at the inner lip of the entry incision must be avoided [61].

The Table 14.1 below shows some results from two studies on cataract surgery after the main corneal transplants:

Table 14.1 Results of cataract surgery after the main corneal transplants

	PKP [62]		DALK [62]		DMEK [63]	
	Preoperative	Postoperative (12 months)	Preoperative	Postoperative (12 months)	Preoperative	Postoperative (about 12 months)
Main endothelial cell density (cells/mm2 ± SD	1833 ± 835	1257 ± 634	1694 ± 835	1505 ± 796	1535 ± 195	1158 ± 520
CDVA	0.1 ± 3.9	0.5 ± 1.9	0.1 ± 3.4	0.5 ± 1.7		
Mean refraction	−5.5 ± 2.0	−2.0 ± 1.0	−4.7 ± 5.7	−1.6 ± 2.1		± 0.5 diopter of predicted emmetropia

PKP penetrating keratoplasty, *SD* standard deviation, *DALK* deep anterior lamellar keratoplasty, *CDVA* corrected distance visual acuity, *DMEK* Descemet membrane endothelial keratoplasty

Take-Home Messages

- In this chapter, we discussed different situations of cataract surgeries with different situations of abnormal corneas. As these cases are not uncommon and are considered challenging cases for cataract surgeons, we have aimed to describe some of the most troublesome corneal problems and their appropriate management techniques.
- Simultaneous partial- or full-thickness keratoplasty and cataract surgery is still indicated in eyes with visually significant central corneal opacities for successful visual outcome but with significant drawbacks. To overcome these drawbacks, phacoemulsification can be assisted and visualization improved by the use of endoscopic lights such as the chandelier light and others.
- In eyes with a low corneal endothelial cell count, manual small incision cataract surgery or extracapsular cataract extraction should be considered; also femtosecond laser-assisted cataract surgery using dispersive OVD is a recommended choice. The optimal cutoff point is 630 μm for CCT, and exceeding that point requires the triple procedure (keratoplasty (DMEK) + cataract removal + IOL implantation).
- In an eye with a previous penetrating keratoplasty, implantation of a toric spherical IOL is recommended. Multifocal IOLs are not indicated.
- No clinically significant loss in endothelial cell density was found after phacoemulsification in eyes that developed cataract after DALK (deep anterior lamellar keratoplasty), but it was relevant after penetrating keratoplasty and DMEK (Descemet membrane endothelial keratoplasty).

References

1. Den S, Shimmura S, Shimazaki J. Cataract surgery after deep anterior lamellar keratoplasty and penetrating keratoplasty in age- and disease-matched eyes. J Cataract Refract Surg. 2018;44(4):496–503.
2. Eghrari AO, Daoud YJ, Gottsch JD. Cataract surgery in Fuchs corneal dystrophy. Curr Opin Ophthalmol. 2010;21(1):15–9.
3. Alio JL, Abdelghany AA, Maldonado MJ. Cataract surgery in cases with previous corneal surgery Expert Rev. Ophthalmol. 2014. Early online, 1–11.
4. Greene JB, Mian SI. Cataract surgery in patients with corneal disease. Curr Opin Ophthalmol. 2013;24(1):9–14.
5. Alio JL, Abdelghany AA, Abbouda A. Cataract surgery in eyes after corneal surgery. In: Chakrabati A, editor. Cataract surgery in diseased eyes. Jaypee Brothers Medical Publisher; 2014. p. 35–51.
6. Lee D, Kim JH, Oh SH, et al. Femtosecond laser lamellar keratoplasty to aid visualization for cataract surgery. J Refract Surg. 2009;25(10):902–4.
7. Panda A, Sethi HS, Jain M, et al. Deep anterior lamellar keratoplasty with phacoemulsification. J Cataract Refract Surg. 2011;37(1):122–6.
8. Farjo AA, Meyer RF, Faryo QA. Phacoemulsification in eyes with corneal opacification. J Cataract Refract Surg. 2003;29:242–2453.
9. Nishimura A, Kobayashi A, Segawa Y, Sugiyama K. Endoilluminationassisted cataract surgery in a patient with corneal opacity. J Cataract Refract Surg. 2003;29:2277–2280 4.
10. Oshima Y, Shima C, Maeda N, Tano Y. Chandelier retroillumination-assisted torsional oscillation for cataract surgery in patients with severe corneal opacity. J Cataract Refract Surg. 2007;33:2018–22.
11. Srinivasan S, Kiire C, Lyall D. Chandelier anterior chamber endoilluminationassisted phacoemulsification in eyes with corneal opacities. Clin Exp Ophthalmol. 2013;41:515–7.
12. Al Sabti K, Raizada S, Al Abduljalil T. Cataract surgery assisted by anterior endoscopy. Br J Ophthalmol. 2009;93:531–4.
13. Moon H, Lee JH, Lee JY, Kim KH, Lee DY, Nam DH. Intracameral dynamic spotlight-assisted cataract surgery in eyes with corneal opacity, small pupil or advanced cataract. Acta Ophthalmol. 2015;93:388–90.
14. Uka J, Minamoto A, Hirayama T, Adachi T, Yamane K, Mishima HK. Endoscope aided cataract surgery in corneal opacity associated with aniridia. J Cataract Refract Surg. 2005;31:1455–6.
15. Yuksel E. Intracameral endoilluminator-assisted phacoemulsification surgery in patients with severe corneal opacity. J Cataract Refract Surg. 2020;46(2):168–73.
16. Hayashi K, Yoshida M, Manabe S, Hirata A. Cataract surgery in eyes with low corneal endothelial cell density. J Cataract Refract Surg. 2011;37:1419–25.

17. Shenoy R, Khandekar R, Bialasiewicz A, et al. Corneal endothelium in patients with diabetes mellitus: a historical cohort study. Eur J Ophthalmol. 2009;19:369–75.
18. Diaz-Couchoud P, Bordas FD, Garcia JR, et al. Corneal disease in patients with chronic renal insufficiency undergoing hemodialysis. Cornea. 2001;20:695–702.
19. Soler N, Romero-Aroca P, Gris O, et al. Corneal endothelial changes in patients with chronic obstructive pulmonary disease and corneal vulnerability to cataract surgery. J Cataract Refract Surg. 2015;41:313–9.
20. Van Cleynenbreugel H, Remeijer L, Hillenaar T. Cataract surgery in patients with Fuchs' endothelial corneal dystrophy: when to consider a triple procedure. Ophthalmology. 2014;121(2):445–53.
21. Seitzman GD, Gottsch JD, Stark WJ. Cataract surgery in patients with Fuchs' corneal dystrophy. Ophthalmology. 2005;112(3):441–6.
22. Olson RJ, Braga-Mele R, Chen SH, et al. Cataract in the adult eye preferred practice pattern®. Ophthalmology 2017;124(2):P1-P119.
23. Van Cleynenbreugel H, Remeijer L, Hillenaar T. Cataract surgery in patients with Fuchs' endothelial corneal dystrophy: when to consider a triple procedure. Ophthalmology. 2014;121(2):445–53.
24. Seitzman GD, Gottsch JD, Stark WJ. Cataract surgery in patients with Fuchs' corneal dystrophy. Ophthalmology. 2005;112(3):441–6.
25. Arnalich-Montiel F, Mingo-Botín D, De Arriba-Palomero P. Preoperative risk assessment for progression to Descemet membrane endothelial keratoplasty following cataract surgery in Fuchs endothelial corneal dystrophy. Am J Ophthalmol. 2019;208:76–86. https://doi.org/10.1016/j.ajo.2019.07.012.
26. McLaren JW, Wacker K, Kane KM, Patel SV. Measuring corneal haze by using Scheimpflug photography and confocal microscopy. Invest Ophthalmol Vis Sci. 2016;57(1):227–35.
27. Conrad-Hengerer I, Al Juburi M, Schultz T, et al. Corneal endothelial cell loss and corneal thickness in conventional compared with femtosecond laser-assisted cataract surgery: three-month follow-up. J Cataract Refract Surg. 2013;39:1307.
28. Laaser K, Bachmann BO, Horn FK, Cursiefen C, Kruse FE. Descemet membrane endothelial keratoplasty combined with phacoemulsification and intraocular lens implantation: advanced triple procedure. Am J Ophthalmol. 2012;154(1):47–55.e2.
29. Scorcia V, Matteoni S, Scorcia GB, Scorcia G, Busin M. Pentacam assessment of posterior lamellar grafts to explain hyperopization after Descemet's stripping automated endothelial keratoplasty. Ophthalmology. 2009;116(9):1651–5.
30. Ham L, Dapena I, Moutsouris K, et al. Refractive change and stability after Descemet membrane endothelial keratoplasty. Effect of corneal dehydration-induced hyperopic shift on intraocular lens power calculation. J Cataract Refract Surg. 2011;37(8):1455–64.
31. Augustin VA, Weller JM, Kruse FE, Tourtas T. Can we predict the refractive outcome after triple Descemet membrane endothelial keratoplasty? Eur J Ophthalmol. 2019;29(2):165–70.
32. Fritz M, Grewing V, Böhringer D, et al. Avoiding hyperopic surprises after Descemet membrane endothelial keratoplasty in Fuchs' dystrophy eyes by assessing corneal shape. Am J Ophthalmol. 2019;197:1–6.
33. Campbell JA, Ladas JG, Wang K, Woreta F, Srikumaran D. Refractive accuracy in eyes undergoing combined cataract extraction and Descemet membrane endothelial keratoplasty. Br J Ophthalmol 2021 (published online ahead of print).
34. Zhu DC, Shah P, Feuer WJ, Shi W, Koo EH. Outcomes of conventional phacoemulsification versus femtosecond laser–assisted cataract surgery in eyes with Fuchs endothelial corneal dystrophy. J Cataract Refract Surg. 2018;44(5):534–40.
35. Fan W, Yan H, Zhang G. Femtosecond laser–assisted cataract surgery in Fuchs endothelial corneal dystrophy: long-term outcomes. J Cataract Refract Surg. 2018;44(7):864–70.
36. Koo EH. Femtosecond laser-assisted cataract surgery: does it improve outcomes in Fuchs endothelial corneal dystrophy? Cornea. 2021;40(4):405–7.
37. Kanclerz P, Alio JL. The benefits and drawbacks of femtosecond laser-assisted cataract surgery. Eur J Ophthalmol. 2020;7:1120672120922448.
38. Viberg A, Byström B. Incidence of corneal transplantation after challenging cataract surgery in patients with and without corneal guttata. J Cataract Refract Surg. 2021;47(3):358–65.
39. Viberg A, Liv P, Behndig A, Lundström M, Byström B. The impact of corneal guttata on the results of cataract surgery. J Cataract Refract Surg. 2019;45(6):803–9.
40. Rathi VM, Krishnamachary M, Gupta S. Cataract formation after penetrating keratoplasty. J Cataract Refract Surg. 1997;23(4):562–4. (23)
41. Reinhart WJ, Musch DC, Jacobs DS, et al. Deep anterior lamellar keratoplasty as an alternative to penetrating keratoplasty; a report by the American Academy of Ophthalmology (Ophthalmic Technology Assessment). Ophthalmology. 2011;118(1):209–18.
42. Fares U, Sarhan AR, Dua HS. Management of post-keratoplasty astigmatism. J Cataract Refract Surg. 2012;38(11):2029–39.
43. Abbey A, Ide T, Kymionis GD, Yoo SH. Femtosecond laser-assisted astigmatic keratotomy in naturally occurring high astigmatism. Br J Ophthalmol. 2009;93(12):1566–9.
44. Nubile M, Carpineto P, Lanzini M, et al. Femtosecond laser arcuate keratotomy for the correction of high astigmatism after keratoplasty. Ophthalmology. 2009;116(6):1083–92.
45. Allard K, Zetterberg M. Toric IOL implantation in a patient with keratoconus and previous penetrating keratoplasty: a case report and review of literature. BMC Ophthalmol. 2018;18(1):215.

46. Lisa C, Garcı'a-Ferna'ndez M, Madrid-Costa D, et al. Femtosecond laser-assisted intrastromal corneal ring segment implantation for high astigmatism correction after penetrating keratoplasty. J Cataract Refract Surg. 2013;39(11):1660–7.
47. Alió Del Barrio JL, Bhogal M, Ang M, et al. Corneal transplantation after failed grafts: options and outcomes. Surv Ophthalmol. 2020. https://doi.org/10.1016/j.survophthal.2020.10.003 [published online ahead of print].
48. Alio JL, Plaza-Puch AB, Javaloy J, et al. Comparison of a new refractive multifocal intraocular lens with an inferior segment near add and a diffractive multifocal intraocular lens. Ophthalmology. 2012;119(3):555–63.
49. Alió Del Barrio JL, Bhogal M, Ang M, et al. Corneal transplantation after failed grafts: options and outcomes. Surv Ophthalmol. 2020. https://doi.org/10.1016/j.survophthal.2020.10.003 [published online ahead of print].
50. Kim EC, Kim MS. A comparison of endothelial cell loss after phacoemulsification in penetrating keratoplasty patients and normal patients. Cornea. 2010;29(5):510–5.
51. Storr-Paulsen A, Nørregaard JC, Farik G, Tarnhøj J. The influence of viscoelastic substances on the corneal endothelial cell population during cataract surgery: a prospective study of cohesive and dispersive viscoelastics. Acta Ophthalmol Scand. 2007;85(2):183–7.
52. Den S, Shimmura S, Shimazaki J. Cataract surgery after deep anterior lamellar keratoplasty and penetrating keratoplasty in age-and disease-matched eyes. J Cataract Refract Surg. 2018;44(4):496–503.
53. Cung LX, Thuy DT, Hang NXH, Do Quyet TVT, Nga NDBVT. Evaluation of phacoemulsification cataract surgery outcomes after penetrating keratoplasty. Open Access Macedonian J Med Sci. 2019;7(24):4301.
54. Acar BT, Buttanri IB, Sevim MS, Acar S. Corneal endothelial cell loss in post-penetrating keratoplasty patients after cataract surgery: phacoemulsification versus planned extracapsular cataract extraction. J Cataract Refract Surg. 2011;37(8):1512–6, (35)
55. Leccisotti A, Islam T, McGilligan VE, Moore TCB. Phacoemulsification after deep anterior lamellar keratoplasty. Eur J Ophthalmol. 2010;20(4):680–3(39).
56. Hiratsuka Y, Sasaki S, Nakatani S, Murakami A. Traumatic wound dehiscence after penetrating keratoplasty. Jpn J Ophthalmol. 2007;51(2):146–7.
57. Musa FU, Cabrerizo J, Quilendrino R, et al. Outcomes of phacoemulsification after Descemet membrane endothelial keratoplasty. J Cataract Refract Surg. 2013;39(6):836–40.
58. Lombardo M, Terry MA, Lombardo G, et al. Investigation of corneal topography after deep lamellar endothelial keratoplasty. Eur J Ophthalmol. 2010;20(6):971–8.
59. Price MO, Price DA, Fairchild KM, Price FW Jr. Rate and risk factors for cataract formation and extraction after Descemet stripping endothelial keratoplasty. Br J Ophthalmol. 2010;94(11):1468–71.
60. Dapena I, Ham L, Moutsouris K, Melles GRJ. Incidence of recipient Descemet membrane remnants at the donor-to-stromal interface after descemetorhexis in endothelial keratoplasty. Br J Ophthalmol. 2010;94(12):1689–90.
61. Dapena I, Yeh R-Y, Quilendrino R, Melles G. Surgical step to facilitate phacoemulsification after Descemet membrane endothelial keratoplasty. J Cataract Refract Surg. 2012;38(6):1106–7.
62. Den S, Shimmura S, Shimazaki J. Cataract surgery after deep anterior lamellar keratoplasty and penetrating keratoplasty in age-and disease-matched eyes. J Cataract Refract Surg. 2018;44(4):496–503.
63. Musa FU, Cabrerizo J, Quilendrino R, Dapena I, Ham L, Melles GR. Outcomes of phacoemulsification after Descemet membrane endothelial keratoplasty. J Cataract Refract Surg. 2013;39(6):836–40.

15 Cataract Surgery in Previous Refractive Corneal Surgery Cases

Kate Xie, Li Wang, and Douglas D. Koch

Bullet Points

1. In this chapter, we offer an approach to IOL power calculations in post-PRK, post-LASIK, and post-RK eyes.
2. Key elements in the selection of candidates for toric, multifocal, and extended depth-of-focus lenses are provided.
3. A review of upcoming technology that may allow for postoperative lens adjustment is discussed.
4. Surgical pearls and intraoperative considerations are also provided.
5. Postoperative considerations and management of patient expectations are extensively discussed.

Overview

Patients who have undergone prior refractive corneal surgery, such as photorefractive keratectomy (PRK), laser in situ keratomileusis (LASIK), or radial keratotomy (RK), pose a unique challenge to the cataract surgeon. They often desire spectacle independence and expect excellent results overnight. In these patients, the majority of the surgeon's task occurs outside of the operating room – in the preoperative evaluation, planning, and management of postoperative expectations.

Preoperative Evaluation

A thorough ophthalmic examination with particular attention to the ocular surface is warranted. Tear breakup time, corneal staining with lissamine green or fluorescein, and presence of corneal haze or scarring should be noted. If a patient reports fluctuating vision throughout the day, this may reflect biomechanical instability of the cornea and swelling of prior corneal incisions.

Topography or tomography should be obtained to identify areas of steepening or flattening and assess ablation centration. Patients with post-refractive surgery ectasia can present with a progressive change in refraction and a decline in quality of vision, which may mimic symptoms of cataract progression. A hard contact lens or scleral lens evaluation can help distinguish between corneal and lenticular contributions to the patient's decline in vision. Toric IOL implantation should be avoided if it is likely that the patient will wear contact lenses in the future. Our

Supplementary Information The online version contains supplementary material available at [https://doi.org/10.1007/978-3-030-94530-5_15].

K. Xie · L. Wang · D. D. Koch (✉)
Cullen Eye Institute, Baylor College of Medicine, Houston, TX, USA
e-mail: liw@bcm.edu; dkoch@bcm.edu

J. L. Alió et al. (eds.), *Cataract Surgery*, Essentials in Ophthalmology,
https://doi.org/10.1007/978-3-030-94530-5_15

topographic criteria for toric IOL implantation are discussed later in this chapter.

Post-radial keratotomy eyes are particularly prone to irregular astigmatism. A careful evaluation of the patient's ocular surface and identification of contributing corneal scarring are warranted. Superficial keratectomy possibly combined with phototherapeutic keratectomy may be beneficial in some cases to reduce scarring and improve irregular astigmatism prior to cataract surgery.

IOL Power Calculations in Post-Refractive Eyes

Intraocular lens selection is arguably the most challenging aspect of performing cataract in eyes that have undergone corneal refractive surgery. In eyes with previous LASIK, PRK, or RK, two factors primarily contribute to challenges in IOL power calculations: (1) difficulties in determining corneal refractive power and (2) difficulties in predicting effective lens position [1].

Corneal refractive surgery changes the relationship between the front and back surfaces of the cornea and results in a large variation in central corneal curvatures. As a result, the standardized value used for the refractive index of the cornea (1.3375) is no longer accurate, and current topography/tomography methods struggle to obtain accurate measurements of central corneal power [1]. Because many current methods for predicting effective lens position (ELP) rely on corneal power values, utilizing post-refractive surgery corneal power values results in inaccurate ELP estimates. Post-myopic LASIK or PRK eyes result in flattening of the central cornea, resulting in falsely shallow ELP predictions and an underpowered IOL power estimation. This yields a postoperative hyperopic surprise. The opposite is true in post-hyperopic ablations, which may result in postoperative myopic surprises.

To improve the accuracy of IOL power calculations in post-corneal refractive surgery eyes, many approaches have been proposed. Methods utilizing solely historical data (i.e., the clinical history method [2], Feiz-Mannis IOL power adjustment method [3], and the corneal bypass

Table 15.1 Methods using a combination of historical data and current corneal power values [6–9]

	Methodology
Adjusted EyeSys EffRP	Corneal power modification based on the ΔMR from the EyeSys topographer (EyeSys Vision, Houston, TX)
Adjusted Atlas Ring Values	Corneal power modification based on the ΔMR from the Atlas 9000 topographer (Carl Zeiss Meditec AG)
Adjusted Atlas Zone Value	Corneal power modification based on the ΔMR from the Atlas 9000 topographer (Carl Zeiss Meditec AG)
Adjusted ACCP	Corneal power modification based on the ΔMR from the TMS topographer (Topographic Modeling System [TMS]; Tomey Corp., Phoenix, AZ)
Masket	Calculates the IOL power using the current corneal power value and then adjusts it by 32.6% of the ΔMR [9]
Modified Masket	Hill modification of Masket formula
Barrett true K	Unpublished methodology

Table 15.2 Formulas using anterior corneal measurement only

Formula	Methodology
Wang-Koch-Maloney	Anterior corneal power derived from atlas 4-mm zone value [6]
Shammas	Adjusts post-LASIK/PRK keratometry readings to estimate post-refractive corneal power [10, 11]
Haigis-L	Haigis formula using modified corneal radius based on historical method using regression model [12]
Potvin-Hill Pentacam	Corneal power estimated from Pentacam TNP apex zone, axial length, and ACD [13]. IOL power from Shammas-PL formula [10]
Barrett true K no history	Modified version of Barrett true K that does not require historical data. Detailed methodology unpublished

Table 15.3 Formulas using both anterior and posterior corneal measurements

	Methodology
OCT-based	Net corneal power calculated from anterior, posterior corneal powers and central corneal thickness measured on RTVue (Optovue, Inc., Fremont, CA) [14]. IOL power calculation based on vergence formula
Total keratometry	Anterior and posterior corneal curvatures determined by a combination of telecentric keratometry and swept source OCT technology on the IOLMaster 700 (Carl Zeiss Meditec AG, Jena, Germany) [15]

method [4]) should theoretically be the most accurate but are highly sensitive to errors in historically obtained data [5]. Furthermore, historical data are often unavailable.

Other methods use a combination of the change in manifest refraction (ΔMR) with current corneal power values or current corneal power values alone. They are summarized in Tables 15.1, 15.2, and 15.3.

These formulas have been consolidated in the web-based ASCRS post-refractive IOL power calculator (www.ascrs.org). The Barrett True K Formula is additionally available at apascrs.org.

In a recent review of the literature of outcomes of cataract surgery in post-LASIK, post-PRK, and post-RK eyes, we found that best outcomes in most studies did not exceed 75% accuracy within ±0.5 D in post-myopic LASIK/PRK [1]. Studies of accuracy in post-hyperopic LASIK/PRK tended to be slightly lower, ranging from 38.1% to 71.9%, with no study reaching 80% accuracy within ±0.5 D of targeted refraction. Studies of post-RK eyes reported the lowest accuracy overall, with a range from 29% to one outlier study at 87.5% [1].

Our recommendation is to obtain IOL calculations using as many approaches as possible and to select the IOL power based on the consensus of multiple methods. We place more weight on the newer IOL power calculation formulas, such as the Barrett True K No History and OCT-based IOL formulas. In general, we aim for a spherical equivalent of −0.25 D in a post-myopic or post-hyperopic LASIK/PRK patient and – 0.50 D in a post-RK patient desiring a distance goal. When choosing between two lens powers, we will err closer to plano in the patient's dominant eye.

After the patient has had surgery on the first eye, it is very helpful to review the post-refractive IOL calculator results for that eye when planning for the second eye. We will place more weight on the individual formula that was the most accurate for the first eye when planning for the second.

Intraoperative Wavefront Aberrometry

The Optiwave Refractive Analysis (ORA) (Alcon Lab, Fort Worth, TX) is an intraoperative wavefront aberrometer designed to calculate IOL power based on aphakic refraction obtained intraoperatively after the cataract has been removed [16]. It is important to note that it also utilizes preoperatively measured axial length, keratometry, and corneal diameter. Estimated ELP is calculated using a proprietary algorithm. In 246 eyes with previous myopic LASIK/PRK, Ianchulev and colleagues [16] reported that ORA achieved accuracy of ±0.5 D in 67%. Fram et al. [17] reported that the ORA produced 74–75% of eyes with refractive prediction errors within ±0.5 D. In 52 eyes of 34 post-RK patients, Curado et al. reported 48% of eyes achieving accuracy within ±0.5 D using ORA [18].

Measurements can be variable and can be influenced by intraocular pressure, the amount of viscoelastic fill, ocular surface variability, wound hydration, and pressure induced by the eyelid speculum. These factors should all be evaluated and standardized by the surgeon as much as possible.

IOL Selection

Aspheric IOL

Aspheric IOLs have been designed to compensate for the inherent positive corneal spherical aberration (SA) in normal eyes. Normal unoperated corneas have an estimated average corneal SA of +0.28 μm for a 6.0 mm pupil [19].

An increase in corneal SA is seen after myopic LASIK and PRK and RK due to central corneal flattening. To compensate for this, an IOL with negative asphericity can be selected. The greatest amount of negative SA in a commercially available IOL is −0.27 μm in the TECNIS series (Johnson and Johnson Vision, Jacksonville, FL). While this will not correct all positive ocular SA, implanting negative aspheric multifocal IOLs in these eyes may result in improved contrast sensitivity and intermediate visual acuity [20, 21]. In hyperopic LASIK/PRK eyes, central corneal steepening induces a negative shift in corneal SA [22]. Our previous study has shown that a wide range of SA results with a mean near zero SA [23].

With these considerations in mind, we recommend selecting IOLs with negative SA in eyes with prior myopic LASIK/PRK or RK and IOLs with zero SA in eyes with prior hyperopic LASIK/PRK.

Toric IOL

Due to the presence of varying amounts of irregular astigmatism, correcting corneal astigmatism in post-LASIK/PRK/RK eyes can be challenging. In a recent study of toric IOL implantation in LASIK/PRK [24], we found that ideal candidates for recommending toric IOL implantation are (1) regular bow-tie corneal astigmatism within the central 3-mm zone, (2) difference of ≤0.75D in corneal astigmatism magnitude between two ocular biometers, and (3) difference of ≤15° in the astigmatism meridians from two biometers. In the myopic LASIK/PRK and hyperopic LASIK/PRK groups that met these criteria, respectively, 80% and 84% of eyes had ≤0.50 D postoperative astigmatism. Similarly, in 72 eyes with previous RK, 69% of eyes meeting these criteria had ≤0.50 D postoperative astigmatism (unpublished data).

Multifocal and Extended Depth-of-Focus IOLs

Studies have reported that implantation of multifocal IOLs and EDOF IOLs can have successful outcomes in patients with prior corneal refractive surgery [20, 25–34]. However, their preoperative topographic inclusion criteria were not specified. In our practice, we consider EDOF IOLs primarily for post-LASIK/PRK eyes whose corneas have variation of <1 D in corneal power along meridians within the 3-mm central zone of the axial topographic map.

Figure 15.1 shows the Galilei topography of a 70-year-old male with prior hyperopic LASIK in both eyes. Preoperative manifest refraction was +1.5 + 0.75 × 135 OD and + 1.5 + 0.25 × 65

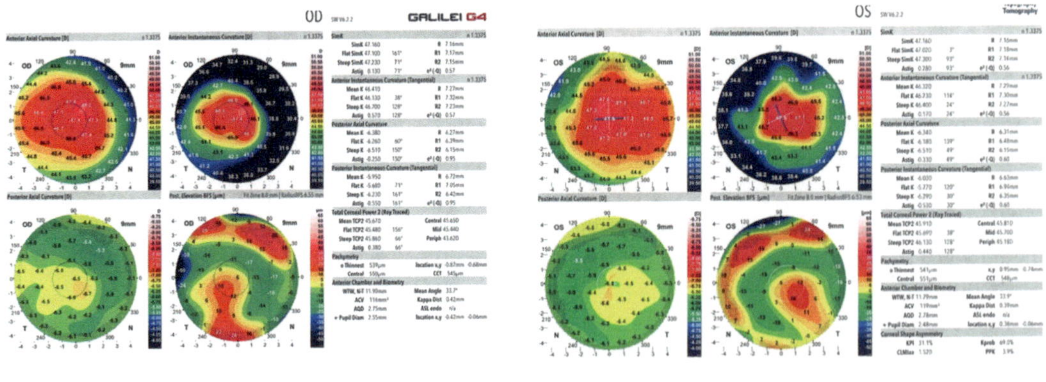

Fig. 15.1 Dual-Scheimpflug Placido topography of a patient with prior hyperopic LASIK and extended depth-of-focus intraocular lenses implant

OS. The ZXR00 EDOF IOLs were implanted in both eyes, targeting full-distance correction. Postoperatively, both eyes had UDVA of 20/20 and near vison of J1+ with complaints of minimal starburst at night.

We do not routinely recommend EDOF or multifocal IOLs in RK eyes, as these eyes are especially prone to refractive error and dysphotopsias. A study by Martin-Escuer et al. [35] of multifocal IOL implantation in 17 post-RK eyes showed that only 29% of eyes were within ±0.50 D of the target refraction and 53% had lost one line of DCVA, concluding that multifocal IOL implantation following RK did not result in good visual outcomes.

Small-Aperture IOL

Small-aperture optics offers a different approach to reduce the impact of higher-order aberrations and achieve an extended depth of focus by using the pinhole effect. Recently, Shajari et al. [36] reported a series of 17 patients with severe irregular corneal astigmatism due to penetrating keratoplasty, keratoconus, or radial keratotomy who underwent implantation of the IC-8 small-aperture IOL. All patients had improvement in uncorrected distance, intermediate, and near vision. Barnett and colleagues [37] reported a case of implantation of the IC-8 small-aperture IOL and secondary piggyback sulcus IOL in the nondominant right eye of a patient with bilateral previous RK. The dominant eye had received a monofocal lens implant for distance vision. Postoperatively, the UDVA was −0.10 logMAR in both eyes, and the patient did not require spectacles for near, intermediate, or distance vision.

Future Directions: Postoperative IOL Adjustment

The light-adjustable lens (LAL; RxSight, Inc., Pasadena, CA) allows correction of residual postoperative errors by targeted ultraviolet activation of lens macromers, which changes the shape of the IOL [38–40]. Once the target refraction is achieved, a lock-in treatment is performed. In 34 eyes of 21 cataract patients with a history of myopic LASIK or PRK, Brierley et al. [38] reported an accuracy within ±0.25 D in 74% of eyes, within ±0.50 D in 97% of eyes, and within ±1.00 D in 100% of eyes.

Perfect Lens (Perfect Lens, LLC, Irvine) utilizes a femtosecond laser to change the refractive index of defined concentric zones within a standard IOL [41]. This allows for modification of an IOL's spherical power, asphericity, toricity, and multifocality. This technology is still under development. Sahler et al. [41] performed an in vitro study using the EC-1Y IOL (Aaren Scientific, Inc., Ontario, CA). They were able to alter the power of the IOL to within ±0.1 D without compromising optical quality of the lens and were able to change the power up to 2.0 D. Similarly, Nguyen et al. [42] performed an in vitro evaluation of CT Lucia 601PY single-piece blue light filtering hydrophobic acrylic IOL and were able to produce an accuracy of ±0.1 D for attempted changes up to 2.0 D.

Surgical Considerations

A discussion of surgical pearls in the setting of radial keratotomy can be found in Video 1. It is important to avoid prior radial keratotomy incisions when making the main incision or paracentesis, as RK incisions may gape open with progressive hydration or manipulation – especially when the corneal entry of the cataract incision intersects a radial cut. The surgeon should be familiar with scleral tunnel techniques to avoid intersection with prior radial keratotomy incisions. At the close of surgery, wound hydration should be undertaken carefully, as it can also cause radial keratotomy incisions to splay open. In these cases, the surgeon should have a lower threshold for the placement of a suture.

Similar principles apply to the post-LASIK eye, where progressive manipulation and hydration can cause refractive shifts related to LASIK flap edema. Care should be taken to avoid intersection of the LASIK flap when creating incisions, which can result in epithelial ingrowth.

If intraoperative aberrometry is used, minimization of the amount of wound manipulation and hydration in the preceding steps is even more important, as this will affect aberrometry readings. Additionally, intraocular pressure, quality of the ocular surface, and external pressure from the eyelid speculum can also affect aberrometry readings.

Postoperative Considerations

Following cataract surgery, post-refractive surgery patients are more prone to ocular surface disease and refractive error. These eyes may exhibit corneal flattening due to edema, resulting in an initial outcome that is more hyperopic than intended. This may take 3 months to resolve in the setting of RK. However, we have seen early but transient postoperative flattening and astigmatic shifts in post-LASIK eyes. Prior to consideration of any further intervention, topography and manifest refractions should be repeated until stable and ocular surface disease should be addressed. Treatment of residual refractive error includes LASIK/PRK enhancement, IOL exchange, or piggyback IOL.

Discussion

Post-refractive surgery patients typically have high expectations from cataract surgery. Despite advances in IOL calculations and currently available technology, IOL power calculations remain less accurate in eyes with prior LASIK, PRK, or RK compared to previously unoperated eyes. Toric, multifocal, and EDOF lenses may be considered in select cases; however, the issue of refractive accuracy remains. A small-aperture IOL may be considered in highly aberrated corneas to improve quality of vision and depth of focus. A frank and thorough discussion with the patient should be undertaken at the preoperative visit to set appropriate expectations. Further advances are needed to improve outcomes – we may see this in the form of postoperative IOL adjustment, improved formulas, better measurements of the anterior and posterior cornea, or more accurate prediction of ELP.

Take-Home Notes

- Obtain IOL power calculations using as many approaches as possible, and select IOL power based on the consensus of preferred methods, especially Barrett True K, Avanti OCT, Haigis L, and Masket.
- Consider selection of IOLs with negative spherical aberration in eyes with prior myopic treatment and zero spherical aberration in eyes with prior hyperopic treatment.
- Ideal candidates for toric lens implantation should exhibit (1) regular bow-tie corneal astigmatism in the central 3-mm zone, (2) difference of ≤0.75D in corneal astigmatism magnitude between two ocular biometers, and (3) difference of ≤15 degrees in the astigmatism meridians from two biometers.
- Consider EDOF IOLs primarily for post-LASIK/PRK eyes whose corneas have variation of <1 D in corneal power along meridians within the 3-mm central zone of the axial topographic map. The role of trifocal IOLs is yet to be defined, but some early data are promising.
- Accuracy of IOL power prediction in the post-refractive eye is at best 80% in post-myopic LASIK/PRK and less in post-hyperopic and RK eyes. Patients' expectations should be managed accordingly.

References

1. Wang L, Koch DD. Intraocular lens power calculations in eyes with previous corneal refractive surgery: review and expert opinion. Ophthalmology. 2020;S0161–6420(20)30625–4.
2. Holladay JT. Consultations in refractive surgery (letter). Refract Corneal Surg. 1989;5:203.
3. Feiz V, Mannis MJ, Garcia-Ferrer F, Kandavel G, Darlington JK, Kim E, Caspar J, Wang JL, Wang W. Intraocular lens power calculation after laser in situ keratomileusis for myopia and hyperopia: a standardized approach. Cornea. 2001;20:792–7.
4. Walter KA, Gagnon MR, Hoopes PC Jr, Dickinson PJ. Accurate intraocular lens power calculation after myopic laser in situ keratomileusis, bypassing corneal power. J Cataract Refract Surg. 2006;32:425–9.
5. Wang L, Hill W, Koch DD. Evaluation of intraocular lens power prediction methods using the American Society of Cataract and Refractive Surgeons Post-Keratorefractive Intraocular Lens Power Calculator. J Cataract Refract Surg. 2010;36:1466–73.
6. Wang L, Booth MA, Koch DD. Comparison of intraocular lens power calculation methods in eyes that have undergone LASIK. Ophthalmology. 2004;111:1825–31.
7. Awwad ST, Dwarakanathan S, Bowman RW, Cavanagh HD, Verity SM, Mootha VV, McCulley JP. Intraocular lens power calculation after radial keratotomy: estimating the refractive corneal power. J Cataract Refract Surg. 2007;33:1045–50.
8. Awwad ST, Manasseh C, Bowman RW, Cavanagh HD, Verity S, Mootha V, McCulley JP. Intraocular lens power calculation after myopic laser in situ keratomileusis: estimating the corneal refractive power. J Cataract Refract Surg. 2008;34:1070–6.
9. Masket S, Masket SE. Simple regression formula for intraocular lens power adjustment in eyes requiring cataract surgery after excimer laser photoablation. J Cataract Refract Surg. 2006;32:430–4.
10. Shammas HJ, Shammas MC. No-history method of intraocular lens power calculation for cataract surgery after myopic laser in situ keratomileusis. J Cataract Refract Surg. 2007;33:31–6.
11. Shammas HJ, Shammas MC, Garabet A, Kim JH, Shammas A, LaBree L. Correcting the corneal power measurements for intraocular lens power calculations after myopic laser in situ keratomileusis. Am J Ophthalmol. 2003;136:426–32.
12. Haigis W. Intraocular lens calculation after refractive surgery for myopia: Haigis-L formula. J Cataract Refract Surg. 2008;34:1658–63.
13. Potvin R, Hill W. New algorithm for intraocular lens power calculations after myopic laser in situ keratomileusis based on rotating Scheimpflug camera data. J Cataract Refract Surg. 2015;41:339–47.
14. Tang M, Li Y, Huang D. An intraocular lens power calculation formula based on optical coherence tomography: a pilot study. J Refract Surg. 2010;26:430–7.
15. Wang L, Spektor T, de Souza RG, Koch DD. Evaluation of total keratometry and its accuracy for intraocular lens power calculation in eyes after corneal refractive surgery. J Cataract Refract Surg. 2019;45:1416–21.
16. Ianchulev T, Hoffer KJ, Yoo SH, Chang DF, Breen M, Padrick T, Tran DB. Intraoperative refractive biometry for predicting intraocular lens power calculation after prior myopic refractive surgery. Ophthalmology. 2014;121:56–60.
17. Fram NR, Masket S, Wang L. Comparison of intraoperative aberrometry, OCT-based IOL formula, Haigis-L, and Masket formulae for IOL power calculation after laser vision correction. Ophthalmology. 2015;122:1096–101.
18. Curado S, Hida W, Vilar X, Ordones V, Chaves M, Tzelikis P. Intraoperative aberrometry versus preoperative biometry for IOL power selection after radial keratotomy: a prospective study. J Refract Surg. 2019;35(10):656–61.
19. Wang L, Dai E, Koch DD, Nathoo A. Optical aberrations of the human anterior cornea. J Cataract Refract Surg. 2003;29:1514–21.
20. Fernández-Vega L, Madrid-Costa D, Alfonso JF, Montés-Micó R, Poo-López A. Optical and visual performance of diffractive intraocular lens implantation after myopic laser in situ keratomileusis. J Cataract Refract Surg. 2009;35:825–32.
21. Alfonso JF, Madrid-Costa D, Poo-López A, Montés-Micó R. Visual quality after diffractive intraocular lens implantation in eyes with previous myopic laser in situ keratomileusis. J Cataract Refract Surg. 2008;34:1848–54.
22. Wang L, Koch DD. Anterior corneal optical aberrations induced by laser in situ keratomileusis for hyperopia. J Cataract Refract Surg. 2003;29:1702–8.
23. Wang L, Shoukfeh O, Koch DD. Custom selection of aspheric intraocular lens in eyes with previous hyperopic corneal surgery. J Cataract Refract Surg. 2015;41:2652–63.
24. Cao D, Wang L, Koch DD. Outcome of toric intraocular lens implanted in eyes with previous corneal refractive surgery. J Cataract Refract Surg. 2020;46:534–9.
25. Gros-Otero J, Garcia-Gonzalez M, Teus M. Multifocal intraocular lens after hyperopic laser in situ keratomileusis. J Cataract Refract Surg. 2018;44:1298–9.
26. Vrijman V, van der Linden JW, van der Meulen IJE, Mourits MP, Lapid-Gortzak R. Multifocal intraocular lens implantation after previous hyperopic corneal refractive laser surgery. J Cataract Refract Surg. 2018;44:466–70.
27. Vrijman V, van der Linden JW, van der Meulen IJE, Mourits MP, Lapid-Gortzak R. Multifocal intraocular lens implantation after previous corneal refractive laser surgery for myopia. J Cataract Refract Surg. 2017;43:909–14.
28. Fisher B, Potvin R. Clinical outcomes with distance-dominant multifocal and monofocal intraocular lenses in post-LASIK cataract surgery planned using an intraoperative aberrometer. Clin Exp Ophthalmol. 2018;46:630–6.

29. Chang JS, Ng JC, Chan VK, Law AK. Visual outcomes, quality of vision, and quality of life of diffractive multifocal intraocular lens implantation after myopic laser in situ keratomileusis: a prospective, observational case series. J Ophthalmol. 2017;2017:6459504.
30. Muftuoglu O, Dao L, Mootha VV, Verity SM, Bowman RW, Cavanagh HD, McCulley JP. Apodized diffractive intraocular lens implantation after laser in situ keratomileusis with or without subsequent excimer laser enhancement. J Cataract Refract Surg. 2010;36:1815–21.
31. Alfonso JF, Fernández-Vega L, Baamonde B, Madrid-Costa D, Montés-Micó R. Refractive lens exchange with spherical diffractive intraocular lens implantation after hyperopic laser in situ keratomileusis. J Cataract Refract Surg. 2009;35:1744–50.
32. Christopher KL, Miller DC, Patnaik JL, Lynch AM, Davidson RS, Taravella MJ. Comparison of visual outcomes of extended depth of focus lenses in patients with and without previous laser refractive surgery. J Refract Surg. 2020;36:28–33.
33. Palomino-Bautista C, Carmona-González D, Sánchez-Jean R, Castillo-Gómez A, Romero-Domínguez M, Elías de Tejada M, Piñero DP. Refractive predictability and visual outcomes of an extended range of vision intraocular lens in eyes with previous myopic laser in situ keratomileusis. Eur J Ophthalmol. 2019;29:593–9.
34. Ferreira TB, Pinheiro J, Zabala L, Ribeiro FJ. Comparative analysis of clinical outcomes of a monofocal and an extended-range-of-vision intraocular lens in eyes with previous myopic laser in situ keratomileusis. J Cataract Refract Surg. 2018;44:149–55.
35. Martín-Escuer B, Alfonso JF, Fernández-Vega-Cueto L, Domíngez-Vicent A, Montés-Micó R. Refractive correction with multifocal intraocular lenses after radial keratotomy. Eye (Lond). 2019;33:1000–7.
36. Shajari M, Mackert M, Langer J, Kreutzer T, Wolf A, Kohnen T, Priglinger S, Mayer W. Safety and efficacy of a small-aperture capsular bag-fixated intraocular lens in eyes with severe corneal irregularities. J Cataract Refract Surg. 2020 Feb;46(2):188–92.
37. Barnett V, Barsam A, Than J, Srinivasan S. Small-aperture intraocular lens combined with secondary piggyback intraocular lens during cataract surgery after previous radial keratotomy. J Cataract Refract Surg. 2018;44:1042–5.
38. Brierley L. Refractive results after implantation of a light-adjustable intraocular lens in postrefractive surgery cataract patients. Ophthalmology. 2013;120:1968–72.
39. Villegas EA, Alcon E, Rubio E, Marín JM, Artal P. Refractive accuracy with light-adjustable intraocular lenses. J Cataract Refract Surg. 2014;40:1075–84.
40. Ford J, Werner L, Mamalis N. Adjustable intraocular lens power technology. J Cataract Refract Surg. 2014;40:1205–23.
41. Sahler R, Bille JF, Enright S, Chhoeung S, Chan K. Creation of a refractive lens within an existing intraocular lens using a femtosecond laser. J Cataract Refract Surg. 2016;42:1207–15.
42. Nguyen J, Werner L, Ludlow J, Aliancy J, Ha L, Masino B, Enright S, Alley RK, Sahler R. Intraocular lens power adjustment by a femtosecond laser: in vitro evaluation of power change, modulation transfer function, light transmission, and light scattering in a blue light-filtering lens. J Cataract Refract Surg. 2018;44:226–30.

Complications of Phakic Intraocular Lenses

16

Veronica Vargas, Jorge Alió del Barrio, and Jorge L. Alió

Bullet Points

- Phakic intraocular lenses are a great option for the correction of high ametropia.
- Sight-threatening complications like corneal decompensation were presented with the first phakic intraocular lenses models.
- Due to the improvement of the lens design, the presence of complications has decreased; nevertheless, they still happen.
- Intraoperative complications are usually related to the phakic intraocular lens implantation learning curve.
- Few complications can lead to the explantation of a phakic intraocular lens.

Introduction

Angle-supported (AS) and iris-fixated (IF) pIOLs were introduced in the 1950s. Both models presented with sight-threatening complications like corneal decompensation and uveitis [1]. Therefore, in the 1980s, Baikoff and Momose improved the AS pIOL design, and since then, several models were developed . Although having good visual outcomes [2], most of AS pIOLs have been phased out due to chronic endothelial cell density (ECD) loss. Iris-fixated pIOLs remain in the market with two different models available: the Verisyse or Artisan (non-foldable IOL) and the VeriFlex or Artiflex (foldable IOL) (Ophtec, Netherlands).

Posterior chamber pIOLs were introduced in the 1990s [1]. First models presented with complications such as pupillary block glaucoma, pigment dispersion, anterior subcapsular cataracts, and dislocation into the vitreous. Some models like the phakic refractive lens (PRL, Zeiss-Meditec, Jena, Germany) were phased out due to such complications. However, two PC pIOLs models are still available (and dominating pIOL market): the implantable collamer lens V4c and V5 (ICL, Staar Surgical Co, Monrovia, California) and the implantable phakic contact lens (IPCL, Care Group Sight solutions, India).

Phakic IOLs have several advantages: correction of high ametropias, higher quality of vision by the avoidance of corneal aberrations, no risk

V. Vargas
Cornea, Cataract and Refractive Surgery Department, VISSUM Alicante, Alicante, Spain

Research & Development Department, VISSUM Alicante, Alicante, Spain

J. Alió del Barrio · J. L. Alió (✉)
Cornea, Refractive and Cataract Surgery Unit, Vissum Miranza Alicante, Alicante, Spain

Division of Ophthalmology, School of Medicine, Miguel Hernandez University, Alicante, Spain
e-mail: jlalio@vissum.com

J. L. Alió et al. (eds.), *Cataract Surgery*, Essentials in Ophthalmology,
https://doi.org/10.1007/978-3-030-94530-5_16

for postoperative corneal ectasia or surface disease, and reversibility as they can be explanted at any time. Nevertheless, some complications like ECD loss and cataract development remain a concern for the refractive surgeon.

In this chapter, we will discuss the most common intraoperative and postoperative complications of phakic intraocular lenses.

Intraoperative Complications

Iris-Fixated pIOLs

Intraoperative complications are minimal and are often related to the pIOL implantation learning curve. The most frequent intraoperative complication reported by Budo et al. [3] was IOL corneal touch (2.7%), followed by wound hemorrhage (1.9%). Complications like iris prolapse and anterior chamber collapse are related to large incisions (5.5 mm in average in case of Artisan – a not foldable IOL) and high vitreous pressure. The latter is related mostly to patient anxiety and high volume of retrobulbar/peribulbar anesthetic. These two complications are very rarely observed with Artiflex (foldable IOL), as the smaller incision required (3.2 mm) allows us to work in a closed system [4–6]. Surgical iris trauma may occur if the iris is pulled too vigorously during the enclavation process or while performing iridectomy, leading to bleeding from the iris root. Generally, this complication is avoided with gentle surgery and by performing Nd:YAG iridotomy before surgery. If bleeding does occur during surgery, it can be controlled by injecting ophthalmic viscoelastic device (OVD) in the bleeding site. During learning curve, several enclavations may be necessary in order to achieve the correct lens centration or alignment (in case of toric IOLs), and multiple enclavation attempts can lead to significant iris damage or even a full thickness iris defect, mainly in light irises with low pigmentation. For novel surgeons with this technique, brown thick irises are recommended to start with in order to minimize the risk of iatrogenic lesion of the iris.

Posterior Chamber pIOLs

Intraoperative complications of PC pIOLs include the following: surgical trauma to the crystalline lens, inverted IOL implantation, broken IOL, surgical trauma to the iris, and pupillary block [7].

Surgical trauma to the crystalline lens can occur if one accidentally touches the anterior capsule with the keratome during construction of the main incision. Even though the surgical technique is relatively easy, it should be performed with extreme caution in order to avoid any injury to the crystalline lens.

The most frequent cause of an inverted IOL implantation is an incorrect loading technique. This complication was more frequent with the first ICL models, which did not have landmarks on the footplates. The current ICL models (V4c, V5) have a landmark on the footplate, which makes the implantation easier. If, however, an inverted implantation does occur, the surgeon should never try to turn the lens around inside the anterior segment, because of the high risk of damaging the crystalline lens or the corneal endothelium. The recommended solution is to enlarge the incision to 3.5–4.0 mm, remove the phakic IOL under the protection of an ocular viscoelastic device, and reload it correctly [7].

Given their reduced thickness (less than 100 μm) in the footplate and the thinnest part of the optic, ICLs are extremely delicate and should be handled with great care to avoid splits and tears [7].

Intraoperative pupillary block occurred with previous ICL models, especially if the surgeon did not perform preoperative iridotomies or if they were nonpermeable. The latest ICL version has a central hole in the lens optic which allows the flow of aqueous humor (Aquaport), so iridotomies are no longer necessary [7].

Cyclodialysis cleft and ciliochoroidal detachment provoked by a straightforward prophylactic surgical iridectomy have been reported [8], although these complications are extremely rare.

Postoperative Complications

Optical Quality: Glare/Halos

Edge effects and halos can be present in patients with anterior chamber (AC) pIOLs because they are positioned in front of the pupil. These complications are often related to poor pIOL centration (Fig. 16.1) or large pupil diameters [3]. In a series of 263 eyes, Alió et al. reported that 10% of patients implanted with an AS pIOLs (models ZB5M, ZB5MF (Chiron, Domilens, Lyon, France) and ZSAL-4 (Morcher, Stuttgart, Germany) presented halos and glare 7 years after surgery [9]. Budo et al. [3] reported in a 3-year follow-up study that 6% of the eyes presented glare and 8% halos after Artisan pIOL implantation.

Posterior chamber pIOLs can also cause glare and halos in patients with large scotopic pupil diameters. The presence of the central hole (Aquaport) in the latest ICL model does not have a detrimental effect on contrast sensitivity, although it may cause positive dysphotopsia [10]. Perez-Vives et al. [11] reported no significant differences in wave front aberrations between the ICL with the central port and the ICL without the port. Lim et al. [12] reported the incidence of night vision disturbances in patients implanted with ICL V4 model 6 months after surgery: 34% of patients reported halos, which were significantly related to the ICL optic diameter, the difference between mesopic pupil size and ICL optic diameter, and the white-to-white diameter of the cornea. 26% of patients reported glare, which was significantly related to the toricity of the ICL. Nevertheless, these symptoms were never severe. Kojima et al. [13] compared the visual disturbances at night in patients that were implanted with the V4c model in one eye and the V5 model in the other eye: the V4c model has an optical diameter of 4.9–5.8 mm, depending on the lens power, while the V5 model has a larger optical diameter (5–6.1 mm). Three months after surgery, 89% of the patients reported a change in night vision although the symptoms were not severe. They reported to see better at night and with less halos with the eye that received the V5 ICL model.

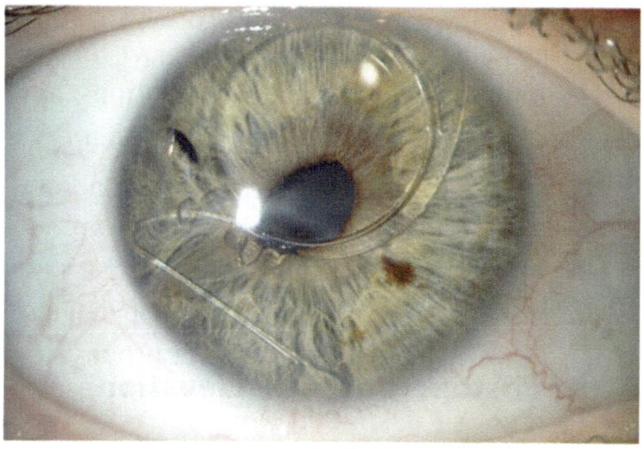

Fig. 16.1 Decentered angle-supported AC pIOL

Scotopic and photopic pupil size should be evaluated before surgery, and patients with large pupils should be warned about the presence of optic phenomena after the implantation of a pIOL (mainly at night). These optical phenomena represent less than 2% of the causes of pIOL explantation [14].

Pupil Ovalization

This complication is more specific for anterior chamber pIOLs, especially angle-supported pIOLs. Haptic compression of the iris root vessels may lead to ischemic iridopathy and inflammation, resulting in pupil ovalization (Fig. 16.2) [9]. The French multicenter study reported an overall incidence of significant pupil ovalization of 22.6% [15] after the implantation of the ZMB5M AS pIOL, while our group reported it in 5.9% of the cases (models ZB5M, ZB5MF, and ZSAL-4) [9]. Pupil ovalization is also associated with the presence of halos, glare, anterior synechia, and atrophic iris changes (Fig. 16.3) [9, 15].

Pupil ovalization may also occur after iris-fixated pIOL implantation if the haptics are fixated asymmetrically [16]. No cases of pupil ovalization have been reported with posterior chamber pIOLs [17].

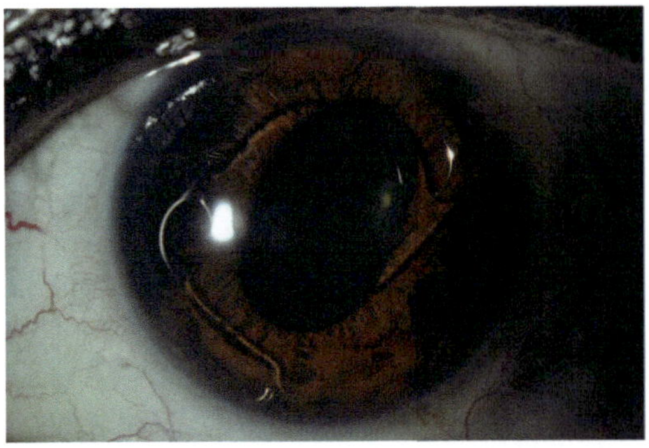

Fig. 16.2 Pupil ovalization in a patient implanted with an angle-supported AC pIOL

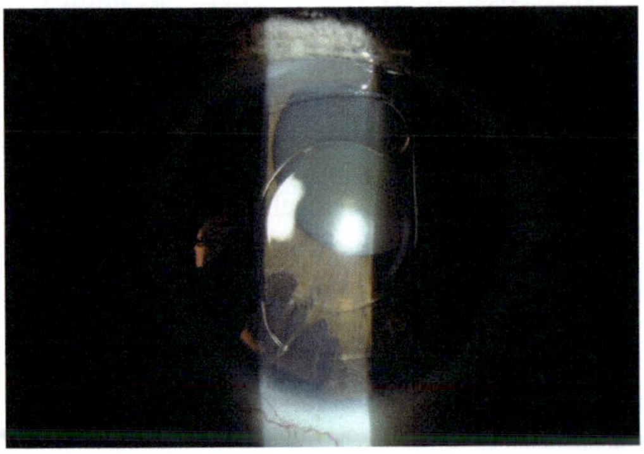

Fig. 16.3 Significant pupil ovalization and severe iris damage with iatrogenic policoria 20 years after angle-supported pIOL implantation

Pigment Dispersion

Pigment deposits may be seen with some frequency after the implantation of IF pIOLs, while they are much less frequent after the implantation of ICL. They are secondary to surgical trauma [16], patients are asymptomatic, and no treatment is required as they tend to disappear over time. Stulting et al. [18] reported an incidence of iris pigment deposits of 6.8% (45/550 eyes) during the few first days after the implantation of the Verisyse (Artisan) pIOL, but at the last follow-up visit (3 years after the pIOL implantation), no pigment deposits were reported. In a [10–]year follow-up study, Menezo et al. [19] reported an incidence of 6.57% (9/137 eyes) of pigment deposits in patients implanted with Artisan pIOL. In a 2-year follow-up study, Dick et al. reported a pigment deposit rate of 4.8% after the implantation of Artiflex pIOL [20] (Fig. 16.4).

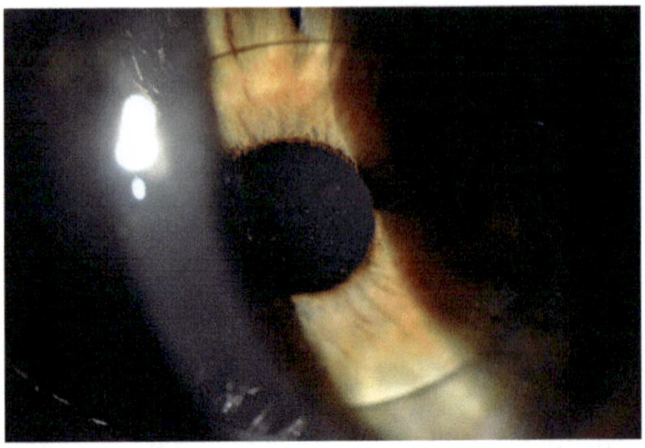

Fig. 16.4 Pigment deposits on the anterior surface of an Artiflex pIOL 6 months after surgery

Pigment dispersion syndrome is secondary to the chronic abrasion between the iris and the pIOL. Iris pigment is released into the aqueous humor, which can accumulate in the trabecular meshwork and may increase the intraocular pressure (IOP); therefore, a close observation of these patients is necessary. In very exceptional cases, the IOP cannot be controlled with medication, and the explantation of the pIOL is necessary [21].

Inflammatory Reactions

Inflammatory reactions may present as giant cell precipitates on the IOL surface, especially after the implantation of IF pIOLs. Giant cell precipitates are secondary to the foldable polysiloxane material of the Artiflex pIOL. Patients might present with a decreased visual acuity, which improves with topical steroids [22].

No long-term inflammatory reactions have been reported after the implantation of PC pIOLs [23].

Intraocular Pressure Elevation

Acute Postoperative IOP Elevation

Early postoperative IOP elevation may occur if there is incomplete removal of OVD during surgery [24]. Therefore, we recommend to measure the IOP 1 hour after the implantation of any pIOL. It is important to take into account that the presence of an Aquaport in the ICL does not prevent this complication, as the OVD may also obstruct the Aquaport, increasing the risk of pupillary block and IOP rise. If left untreated, severe IOP rise during the early postoperative period can lead to an irreversible mydriasis (Urrets-Zavalia syndrome) and/or anterior subcapsular lens opacities (glaukomflecken) [25, 26].

The presence of an excessive vault (>750um) increases the risk of pupillary block in eyes implanted with a PC pIOL without Aquaport [24]. Excessive ICL vault is usually present if there is an overestimation of the ICL size; therefore, an adequate sizing is crucial to avoid this complication. Patients implanted with ICLs models that do not have an Aquaport (V4 model or hyperopic ICL) and all IF pIOLs must have a permeable peripheral iridotomy before surgery or an intraoperative surgical iridectomy in order to avoid a pupillary block postoperatively (Fig. 16.6a, b). A rare but potential source for pupillary block might be fibrin strands from a toxic anterior segment syndrome (TASS). Actually our group recently reported a case of TASS after the implantation of an ICL V4c toric pIOL [27]. TASS-related fibrin strands blocked the Aquaport hole leading to a pupillary block (Fig. 16.7).

Chronic IOP Elevation

Synechia formation in patients with AS pIOLs can predispose to the development of chronic IOP elevation [16]. Alió et al. reported in a 7-year follow-up study that 7% of the patients implanted with an AS pIOL had an increase in IOP, all of them were successfully treated with topical medication [9].

Iris-fixated pIOL, either for myopia or for hyperopia, did not increase IOP in a 1-year follow-up study [28], although in a long-term follow-up (mean follow-up 69.3 ± 52.8 months) study, which evaluated 1037 eyes, 5 pIOLs had to be explanted because of high IOP [29].

Almaki et al. [30] reported the causes of elevated IOP after ICL V4 implantation. Elevated IOP occurred in 58 eyes (10.8%) of 534 eyes that were implanted with an ICL. Retained viscoelastic was the most common cause (39.7%) in the early postoperative period (1 day postop), followed by steroid response (37.9%) which presented 2–4 weeks after surgery. Other causes of high IOP were high ICL vault and pupillary block (10.3%) and synechial angle closure (6.9%). None of the eyes required glaucoma surgery to control the IOP.

Corneal Endothelial Cell Loss

All pIOLs can actually cause an accelerated decrease in ECD (Fig. 16.5) [16, 31, 32]. A three-year follow-up study comparing the effect of different pIOLs on the corneal ECD showed that the VeriFlex (Artiflex) pIOL induced a 25% rate of ECD loss, Verisyse (Artisan) a 15.7%, and ICL a 13.4% loss [31]. Many causes for ECD loss have been described (especially for IF pIOLs): direct contact between the pIOL and the endothelium during implantation, a close distance between the central and peripheral pIOL edges to the endothelium, a shallow anterior chamber depth (ACD), altered aqueous flow, and subclinical inflammation [16, 22].

A shallow anterior chamber depth (ACD) and a close distance between the central and peripheral pIOL edges to the endothelium have been

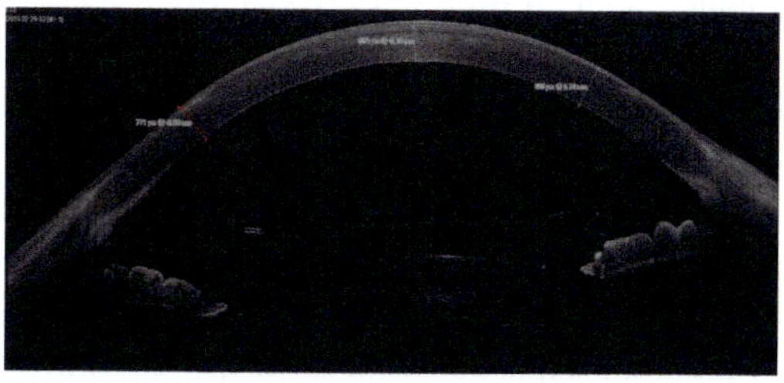

Fig. 16.5 Early corneal edema and secondary fluid within an old LASIK flap interface, on a patient with an angle-supported AC pIOL implanted years before

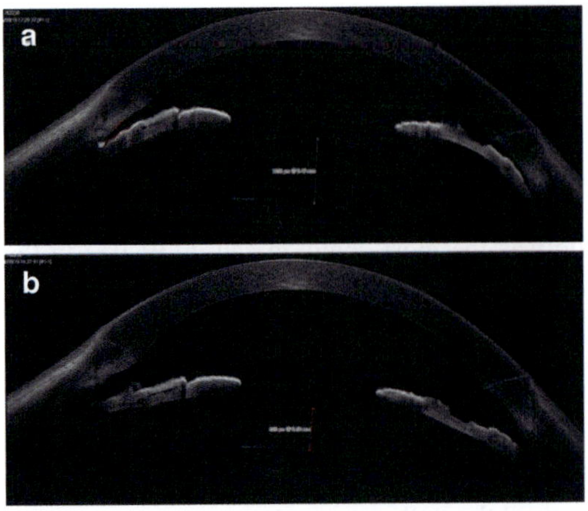

Fig. 16.6 Pupillary block after a hyperopic ICL implantation due to a non-patent peripheral iridotomy (**a**). Observe the resolution of the iris bombe and ICL hypervault after a reopening of the previous iridotomy with YAG laser (**b**)

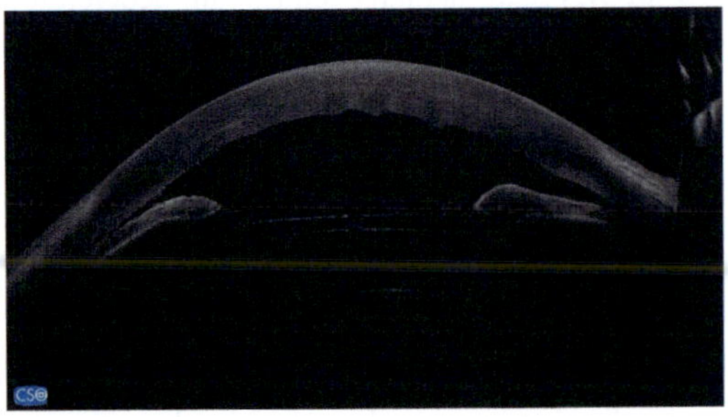

Fig. 16.7 Severe corneal edema and pupillary block with iris bombe on a patient implanted with a myopic toric ICL. This case developed a toxic anterior segment syndrome (TASS) 48 h after implantation, and the secondary anterior chamber fibrin blocked the central Aquaport of the IOL causing the acute and severe IOP rise and subsequent corneal edema

described as the main risk factors for ECD loss in patients with IF pIOLs: [32] Shajari et al. [33] reported a higher ECD loss after 4 years in patients implanted with an IF pIOL and an ACD <3.0 mm, compared to those with an ACD > 3.4 mm; Eldanasoury et al. [34] also reported in a long-term follow-up study a significant ECD loss (ECD <1500cells/mm [2]) in 86% of the eyes implanted with an IF pIOL with an ACD <3.2 mm and no loss in the eyes with an ACD >3.5 mm. Nevertheless, some discrepancies are still present among studies reporting the chronic ECD loss in eyes implanted with IF pIOLs: a 10-year follow-up study [35] reported no significant ECD loss after the implantation of IF pIOL as long as the inclusion criteria for pIOL implantation is strictly met; Budo et al. [3] reported a mean ECD loss of 7.1% during the first year after IF pIOL implantation (Artisan), which decreased to a mean physiological loss of 0.7% per year in the following 2 years. However, several studies have shown that the presence of an IF pIOL accelerates the rate of ECD loss: [36–38] one study found a linear chronic endothelial cell loss after the implantation of IF pIOL (Artisan), with a mean annual ECD loss of 48 cells/mm [2] and 61 cells/mm [2] with the myopic and toric IF pIOLs, respectively [32]. A 5-year follow-up study also reported a significant endothelial cell loss in a low percentage of eyes implanted with IF pIOLs [38].

Jonker et al. [22] reported an annual decline in ECD of 64 cells/mm [2] and 62 cells/mm [2] with the Artiflex myopia and Artiflex toric pIOL, respectively. After 5 years, an ECD decrease greater than 25% occurred in 4.4% and 4.3% of the eyes, respectively. 3.1% of the eyes implanted with the myopic model required explantation due to ECD loss, while none of the toric pIOLs had to be explanted. They did not find any correlation between ECD loss and ACD depth or pIOL distance from the corneal endothelium. Nevertheless, Jonker et al. believed that the silicone optic material might cause subclinical inflammation leading to ECD loss.

A 10-year follow-up study reported an ECD loss of 12% after Artiflex implantation [39].

Posterior chamber pIOLs seem to cause less damage to the endothelial cells because there is a wider space between the pIOL and the corneal endothelium. In a 1-year follow-up study that included 351 eyes implanted with an ICL (Aquaport model), Kamiya et al. [40] reported a mean decrease in ECD of 0.1% ± 9.7%. Shimizu et al. [41] reported an ECD loss of 0.5% ± 5.4% 5 years after the implantation of the ICL with an Aquaport, versus 1.2 ± 7.2% in eyes with a conventional ICL (no Aquaport). Lisa et al. [42] reported a decrease of 1.7% 1 year after the implantation of the ICL V4c model in 147 eyes.

Igarashi et al. [43] reported an ECD loss of 6.2 ± 8.6% 8 years after the implantation of the ICL V4 model.

The reported ECD loss after implantable phakic contact lens (IPCL) implantation was not statistically significant after a 3-year and 1-year follow-up period [44–45].

Although there are no guidelines on when to explant a pIOL due to ECD loss, some authors suggest that if the ECD decreases below 1500 cells/mm [2], the pIOL should be explanted [32]. Moreover, the distance between the center of the pIOL and the corneal endothelium should be greater than 1.5 mm and > 1.3 mm at the periphery in order to keep a healthy endothelium [16].

On this regard, annual follow-up visits to perform specular microscopy and anterior segment optical coherence tomography are always recommended after a pIOL implantation.

Cataract

Cataract development is the most frequent cause for pIOL explantation [14]. Usually patients implanted with a pIOL have high myopia, which is a risk factor for the development of posterior subcapsular and nuclear cataract [46]. Therefore, most of the cataracts developed in these patients are secondary to high myopia and aging.

Iris-Fixated pIOLs

Jonker et al. [29] reported in a 14-year follow-up study an explantation rate of IF pIOL of 12%; 59% of the causes were secondary to cataract formation. According to the authors, cataract development was not related to the pIOL due to the long time between pIOL implantation and the presence of cataract (mean time of 181.4 months).

Cataract development after Artiflex pIOL implantation is extremely rare; in a 10-year follow-up study, none of the patients developed cataract [39]. Also, in a meta-analysis by Chen et al. [47], no cataracts were reported with the Artiflex model, while the incidence of cataract after Artisan pIOL implantation was 1.11%.

Most of the cataracts developed after IF pIOL implantation are nuclear, and no direct relationship between the pIOL and cataract development has been clearly shown [29, 48].

Posterior Chamber pIOLs

Cataract development is more frequent in patients with PC pIOLs than in patients with IF pIOLs due to the proximity of the pIOL to the crystalline lens. The most common type of cataract is anterior subcapsular (ASC) (Figs. 16.8 and 16.9). Its development is secondary to insufficient aqueous humor circulation, lens trauma from preoperative Nd:YAG laser peripheral iridotomy, and inflammation [49–51]. Early cataract formation is usually secondary to surgical trauma, while late-onset cataract is related to contact between the pIOL and the crystalline lens [47] and aging.

Sanders and Vukich [52] reported an incidence of ASC of 12.6% in eyes implanted with the V3 model versus 2.9% in eyes implanted with the V4 model. Cataract development with the V3 model was secondary to insufficient vaulting which leads to crystalline lens touch. The FDA

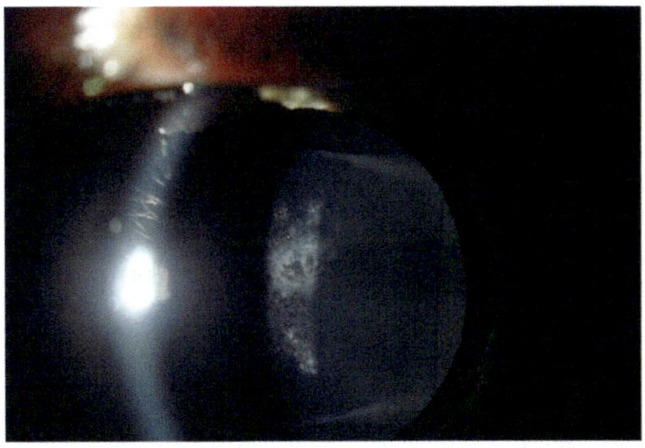

Fig. 16.8 ASC on a patient with a PRL PC pIOL. Its development is secondary to intermittent trauma of the pIOL to the lens during accommodation, iatrogenic during surgery, and insufficient vaulting

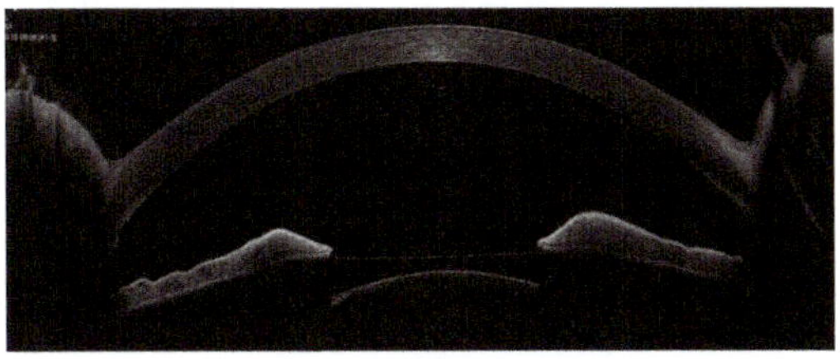

Fig. 16.9 ASC on a patient implanted with an old ICL model without Aquaport and no residual vault, with subsequent long-standing contact between the ICL and the anterior capsule of the crystalline lens

study reported an incidence of ASC of 2.7% 3 years after the implantation of the ICL V4 [53].

Due to the improvement in ICL design (V4c, V5 models), cataract development has decreased in recent years [24, 51, 54, 55]. The central port in the current ICL models allows the normal flow of aqueous humor across the anterior lens capsule [54], reducing the incidence of cataract development. Alfonso et al. [51] evaluated the prevalence of cataract after the implantation of three different ICL models (V4, V4b, and V4c). Twenty-one eyes (0.61%) implanted with the V4 model developed cataract 3–4 years after pIOL implantation. None of the eyes implanted with the V4b or V4c model developed cataract.

The reported incidence of ASC development after IPCL is very similar among the studies. Vasadava et al. reported an incidence of 3.33%, and Sachdev et al. reported an incidence of 2.9% [44–45].

Retinal Detachment

Myopic patients who receive pIOL implantation usually have long axial lengths (AL), so, they have a higher risk for developing retinal detachment (RD). High myopia is a risk factor for rhegmatogenous retinal detachment because of increased prevalence of lattice degeneration, premature vitreous liquefaction, and posterior vitreous detachment [56]. The presence of an AL >26 mm or lattice degeneration has an eightfold and tenfold excess risk of RD, respectively [57]. The percentage of retinal detachment after pIOL implantation ranges from 4.8% to 2.07%, but no correlation has been found between pIOL implantation and the development of RD. [(58–60)] In some cases, RD can be managed successfully without the need for pIOL explantation [58–60].

Endophthalmitis

The incidence of endophthalmitis secondary to pIOL implantation is extremely rare, and it has been reported after ICL implantation to be 1 in 6000 [61], which is lower than the incidence of endophthalmitis after cataract surgery [62]. Coagulase negative *Staphylococcus epidermidis*, *Aspergillus*, and *Rhizobium* (formerly *Agrobacterium*) are some of the pathogens responsible for endophthalmitis after pIOL implantation. The range of visual acuity after proper treatment ranges from 20/50 to 20/20 [63–65]. In a similar fashion as for cataract surgery, we suggest the use of intracameral antibiotics at the end of surgery in order to minimize the risk of endophthalmitis.

Take-Home Notes

- Intraoperative complications are rare and usually related to the learning curve process.
- Visual disturbances (halos and glare) are usually mild and related to large pupils and small optic size.
- Cataract development remains the main reason for pIOL explantation, although majority of the explantations are related to the high myopia and age and not less likely to the presence of the pIOL itself.
- The risk of secondary anterior subcapsular cataract after PC pIOL implantation has dramatically dropped since the optimization of such pIOLs with central openings.
- Chronic ECD loss remains the main limitation for iris-fixated AC pIOLs; if implantation criteria are strictly met (ACD over 3 mm and ideally over 3.5 mm), the risk for endothelial damage may be similar to PC pIOLs.
- Endothelial cell density loss is the most common sight-threatening complication presented in patients with pIOLs. Therefore, an annual ECD count is recommended.
- IOP monitoring is critical immediately after surgery and during the first 24 hrs, in order to avoid severe IOP spikes in relation with retained OVD or pupillary block. Consequences of such complication could be irreversible changes on the iris and/or the crystalline lens.

References

1. Lovisolo CF, Reinstein DZ. Phakic intraocular lenses. Surv Ophthalmol. 2005;50(6):549.
2. Knorz MC, Lane SS, Holland SP. Angle-supported phakic intraocular lens for correction of moderate to high myopia: three year interim results in international multicenter studies. J Cataract Refract Surg. 2011;37:469–80.
3. Budo C, Hessloehl JC, Izak M, et al. Multicenter study of the artisan phakic intraocular lens. J Cataract Refract Surg. 2000;26:1163–71.
4. Artiflex MA. A new phakic IOL. In: Garg A, Pandey S, Chang D, et al., editors. Advances in ophthalmology 2. New Delhi: Jaypee Brothers; 2005.
5. Artiflex MA. A new Phakic IOL. In: Garg A, Alio J, Marinho A, et al., editors. Lens based refractive surgery (Phakic IOLs). New Delhi: Jaypee Brothers; 2005.
6. Tehrani M, Dick H. Short term follow-up after implantation of a foldable iris-fixated intraocular lens in Phakic eyes. Ophthalmology. 2005;112(12):2189–95.
7. Lovisolo CF, Zaldivar R. Complications of posterior chamber Phakic IOLs. In: Alió JL, Azar DT, editors. Management of complications in Refractive Surgery. 2nd ed. Switzerland: Springer; 2018;289–310.
8. Arnalich-Montiel F, Ruiz-Casas D, Muñoz-Negrete F, et al. Inadvertent cyclodialysis cleft and annular ciliochoroidal detachment after hyperopic phakic intraocular lens implantation and prophylactic surgical iridectomy. J Cataract Refract Surg. 2015;41:2319–22.
9. Alió JL, De la Hoz F, Pérez-Santoja JJ, et al. Phakic anterior chamber lenses for the correction of myopia. A 7-year cumulative Analysis of Complications in 263 cases. Ophthalmology. 1999;106:458–66.
10. Eppig T, Spira C, Tsintarakis T, et al. Ghost-image analysis in phakic intraocular lenses with central hole as a potential cause of dysphotopsia. J Cataract Refract Surg. 2015;41:2552–9.
11. Perez-Vives C, Ferrer-Blasco T, Madrid-Costa D, et al. Optical quality comparison of conventional and hole-visian implantable collamer lens at different degrees of decentering. Am J Ophthalmol. 2013;156(1):69–76.
12. Lim DH, Lyu IJ, Choi S, et al. Risk factors associated with night vision disturbances after phakic intraocular lens implantation. Am J Ophthalmol. 2014;157:135–41.
13. Kojima T, Kitazawa Y, Nakamura T, et al. Prospective randomized multicenter comparison of the clinical outcomes of V4c and V5 Implantable Collamer Lenses: a contralateral eye study. J Ophthalmol. 2018;2018:7623829.
14. Alió JL, Toffaha BT, Peña-Garcia P, Sádaba LM, Barraquer RI. Phakic intraocular lens explantation: causes in 240 cases. J Refract Surg. 2015;31(1):30–5.
15. Baikoff G. ZMB5M multicenter study. Phakic lens product monograph. Claremont: Chiron Vision Corporation; 1997.
16. Kohnen T, Kook D, Morral M, Güell JL. Phakic intraocular lenses. Part 2: results and complications. J Cataract Refract Surg. 2010;36:2168–94.
17. Balakrishnan SA. Complications of Phakic intraocular lenses. Int Ophthalmol Clin. 2016;56(2):161–8.
18. Stulting RD, John ME, Maloney RK, et al. Three-year results of Artisan/Verisyse phakic intraocular lens implantation: results of the United States Food and Drug Administration Clinical Trial; the U.S. Verisyse Study Group. Ophthalmology. 2008;115:464–72.
19. Menezo JL, Peris-Martinez C, Cisneros AL, et al. Phakic intraocular lenses to correct high myopia: Adatomed, Staar, and Artisan. J Cataract Refract Surg. 2004;30:33–44.
20. Dick HB, Budo C, Malecaze F, et al. Foldable Artiflex phakic intraocular lens for the correction of myopia: two-year follow-up results of a prospective European multicenter study. Ophthalmology. 2009;116:671–7.
21. Ye C, Patel CK, Momont AC, et al. Advanced pigment dispersion glaucoma secondary to phakic intraocular collamer lens implant. Am J Ophthalmol Case Rep. 2018;10:65–7.
22. Jonker SMR, Berendschot TTJM, Ronden AE, Saelens IEY, Bauer NJC, Nuijts RMMA. Five year endothelial cell loss after implantation with Artiflex myopia and Artiflex toric phakic intraocular lenses. Am J Ophthalmol. 2018;194:110–9.
23. ICL in Treatment of Myopia (ITM) Study Group. Postoperative inflammation after implantation of the implantable contact lens. Ophthalmology 2003; 110:2335–2341. Available at: http://download.journals.elsevierhealth.com/pdfs/journals/0161-6420/PIIS0161642003008261.pdf.
24. Fernandes P, Gonzalez-Méijome JM, Madrid-Costa D, et al. Implantable collamer posterior chamber intraocular lenses: a review of potential complications. J Refract Surg. 2011;27(10):765–76.
25. Pérez-Cambrodí RJ, Piñero-Llorens DP, Ruiz-Fortes JP, et al. Fixed mydriatic pupil associated with an intraocular pressure rise as a complication of the implant of a phakic refractive lens (PRL). Semin Ophthalmol. 2014;29:205–9.
26. Al Habash A, Al Arfaj K. Al Abdulsalam. Urrets-Zavalia syndrome after implantable Collamer lens placement. Digit J Ophthalmol. 2015;21(3):1–11.
27. Mimouni M. Alió del barrio JL, Alió JL. Occlusion of AquaPORT flow in a case of toxic anterior segment syndrome following implantable collamer lens surgery causing severe pupillary block. J Refract Surg. 2020;36(12):856–9.
28. Alió JL, Mulet E, Shalaby A. Artisan phakic iris claw intraocular lens for high primary and secondary hyperopia. J Refract Surg. 2002;18(6):697–707.
29. Jonker SMR, Van Averbeke AAC, Berendschot TTJM, et al. Risk factors for explantation of iris-fixated phakic intraocular lenses. J Cataract Refract Surg. 2019;45(8):1092–8.

30. Almaki S, Abubaker A, ALsabaani NA, et al. Causes of elevated intraocular pressure following implantation of phakic intraocular lenses for myopia. Int Ophthalmol. 2016;36(2):259–65.
31. Shaaban YM, Badran TAF. Three-year effect of phakic intraocular lenses on the corneal endothelial cell density. Clin Ophthalmol. 2020;14:149–55.
32. Jonker SM, Berendschot T, Ronden AE, et al. Long-term endothelial cell loss in patients with artisan myopia and artisan toric phakic intraocular lenses 5 and 10 year results. Ophthalmology. 2017;125:486–94.
33. Shajari M, Scheffel M, Janusz Koss M, et al. Dependency of endothelial cell loss on anterior chamber depth within first 4 years after implantation of iris-supported phakic intraocular lenses to treat high myopia. J Cataract Refract Surg. 2016;42:1562–9.
34. Eldanasoury AM, Roozbahani M, Tolees S, Arana C. Long-term effect of anterior chamber depth on endothelial cell density in patients with iris-fixated phakic intraocular lenses. J Refract Surg. 2019;35(8):493–500.
35. Morral M, Güell JL, El Husseiny MA, et al. Paired-eye comparison of corneal endothelial cell counts after unilateral iris-claw phakic intraocular lens implantation. J Cataract Refract Surg. 2016;42:117–26.
36. Tahzib NG, Nuijts RM, Wu WY, Budo CJ. Long-term study of Artisan phakic intraocular lens implantation for the correction of moderate to high myopia: ten-year follow-up results. Ophthalmology. 2007;114:1133–42.
37. Saxena R, Boekhoorn SS, Mulder PG, et al. Long-term follow-up of endothelial cell change after Artisan phakic intraocular lens implantation. Ophthalmology. 2008;115:608–13.
38. Galvis V, Villamil JF, Acuña MF, et al. Long-term endothelial cell loss with the iris-claw intraocular phakic lenses (Artisan). Graefes Arch Clin Exp Ophthalmol. 2019;257(12):2775–87.
39. Castro de Luna G, Ramos-López D, Castaño Fernandez AB, et al. Artiflex foldable lens for myopia correction results of 10 years of follow up. Eye. 2019;33:1564–9.
40. Kamiya K, Shimizu K, Igarashi A. Posterior chamber phakic intraocular lens implantation: comparative, multicenter study in 351 eyes with low-to-moderate of high myopia. Br J Ophthalmol. 2018;102(2):177–81.
41. Shimizu K, Kamiya K, Igarashi A, et al. Long-term comparison of posterior chamber phakic intraocular lens with and without a central hole (Hole ICL and Conventional ICL) implantation for moderate to high myopia and myopic astigmatism; consort-compliant article. Medicine. 2016;95(14):e3270.
42. Lisa C, Naveiras M, Alfonso-Bartolozzi B, et al. Posterior chamber collagen copolymer phakic intraocular lens with a central hole to correct myopia: one-year follow-up. J Cataract Refract Surg. 2015;41(6):1153–9.
43. Igarashi A, Shimizu K, Kamiya K. Eight-year follow-up of posterior chamber phakic intraocular lens implantation for moderate to high myopia. Am J Ophthalmol. 2014;157:532–9.
44. Vasadava V, Srivastava S, Vasadava SA, et al. Safety and efficacy of a new phakic posterior chamber IOL for correction of myopia: 3 years of follow up. J Refract Surg. 2018;34(12):817–23.
45. Sachdev G, Ramamurthy D. Long-term safety of posterior chamber implantable phakic contact lens for the correction of myopia. Clin Ophthalmol. 2019;13:137–42.
46. Ikuno Y. Overview of the complications of high myopia. Retina. 2017;37:2347–51.
47. Chen LJ, Chang YJ, Kuo JC, Rajagopal R, Azar DT. Meta-analysis of cataract development after phakic intraocular lens surgery. J Cataract Refract Surg. 2008;34:1181–200.
48. Van Rijn GA, Gaurisankar ZS, Ilgenfritz AP, et al. Middle- and long-term results after iris-fixated phakic intraocular lens implantation in myopic and hyperopic patients: a meta-analysis. J Cataract Refract Surg. 2020;46:125–37.
49. Jonker SMR, Berendschot TTJM, Saelens IEY, et al. Phakic intraocular lenses: an overview. Indian J Ophthalmol. 2020;68(12):2779–69.
50. Khalifa Y, Moshirfar M, Mifflin M, et al. Cataract development associated with collagen copolymer posterior chamber phakic intraocular lenses: clinicopathological correlation. J Cataract Refract Surg. 2010;36:1768–74.
51. Alfonso JF, Lisa C, Fernández-Vega L, et al. Prevalence of cataract after collagen polymer phakic intraocular lens implantation for myopia, hyperopia and astigmatism. J Cataract Refract Surg. 2015;41:800–5.
52. Sanders DR, Vukich JA, for the ICL in Treatment of Myopia (ITM) study group. Incidence of lens opacities and clinically significant cataracts with the implantable contact lens: comparison of two lens designs. J Refract Surg. 2002;18:673–82.
53. ICL in treatment of myopia (ITM) Study group. United States Food and Drug Administration clinical trial of the Implantable Collamer Lens (ICL) for moderate to high myopia; three-year follow-up. Ophthalmology. 2004;111:1683–92.
54. Packer M. Meta-analysis and review: effectiveness, safety, and central port design of the intraocular collamer lens. Clin Ophthalmol. 2016;10:1059–77.
55. Packer M. The implantable collamer lens with a central port: review of the literature. Clin Ophthalmol. 2018;12:2427–38.
56. Martinez-Castillo BA, Verdugo A, et al. Rhegmatogenous retinal detachment in phakic eyes after posterior chamber phakic intraocular lens implantation for severe myopia. Ophthalmol. 2005;112:580–5.
57. Tielsch JM, Legro MW, Cassard SD, et al. Risk factors for retinal detachment after cataract surgery: a population-based case-control study. Ophthalmology. 1996;103:1537–45.
58. Ruiz-Moreno JM, Alió JL, Perez-Santoja JJ. Retinal detachment in phakic eyes with anterior chamber

intraocular lenses to correct severe myopia. Am J Ophthalmol. 1999;127:270–5.
59. Kim YJ, Chung JK, Lee SJ. Retinal detachment surgery in eyes with iris-fixated phakic intraocular lenses: short-term clinical results. J Cataract Refract Surg. 2014;40:2025–30.
60. Alió JL, Ruiz-Moreno JM, Artola A. Retinal detachment as a potential hazard in surgical correction of severe myopia with phakic anterior chamber lenses. Am J Ophthalmol. 1993;115:145–8.
61. Allan BD, Argeles-Sebate I, Mamalis N. Endophthalmitis rates after implantation of the intraocular Collamer lens: survey of users between 1998 and 2006. J Cataract Refract Surg. 2009;35:766–9.
62. Taban M, Behrens A, Newcomb RL, et al. Acute endophthalmitis following cataract surgery: a systematic review of the literature. Arch Ophthalmol. 2005;123:613–20.
63. Jalili M, Hashemi H, Jabarvand M, et al. Aspergillus endophthalmitis in one eye subsequent to bilateral anterior chamber phakic intraocular lens implantation. J Refract Surg. 2012 May;28(5):363–5.
64. Davis MJ, Epstein RJ, Dennis RF, et al. Culture-positive endophthalmitis after implantation of intraocular collamer lens. J Cataract Refract Surg. 2009;35:1826–2828.
65. Al-Abdullah AA, Al-Falah M, Al-Rashaed, et al. Endophthalmitis caused by Rhizobium radiobacter after posterior chamber phakic intraocular lens implantation to correct myopia. J Refract Surg. 2015;31(8):561–3.

17 Safety and Visual Outcomes Following Phakic Intraocular Lens Bilensectomy

Veronica Vargas and Jorge L. Alió

Bullet Points

In this chapter, we will discuss the following:

- Frequency of phakic intraocular lenses explantation
- Bilensectomy surgical technique
- Refractive outcomes
- Intraoperative and postoperative complications

Supplementary Information The online version contains supplementary material available at [https://doi.org/10.1007/978-3-030-94530-5_17].

V. Vargas
Cornea, Cataract and Refractive Surgery Department, VISSUM Alicante, Alicante, Spain

Research & Development Department, VISSUM Alicante, Alicante, Spain

J. L. Alió (✉)
Division of Ophthalmology, School of Medicine, Miguel Hernandez University, Alicante, Spain

Cornea, Refractive and Cataract Surgery Unit, Vissum Miranza Alicante, Alicante, Spain
e-mail: jlalio@vissum.com

Introduction

The term bilensectomy was introduced in the early 2000s by Joseph Colin; it refers to the explantation of a pIOL at the time of cataract extraction [1].

All pIOLs will be explanted at some point; therefore, it is important to know the long-term outcomes and surgical technique of bilensectomy. In this chapter, we will discuss the main causes, surgical technique, refractive outcomes, and complications of bilensectomy.

Historical Overview

Angle-Supported pIOLs

The first pIOLs were implanted in the 1950s by Baron and Strampelli in the irido-corneal angle [2, 3]. Baron's pIOL was designed to float in the anterior chamber (AC), which led to frequent corneal decompensation. Therefore, Strampelli designed a new pIOL model with three points that were fixated in the chamber angle. Because the haptics were not flexible, some complications like recurrent inflammation with anterior synechiae, sectorial iris atrophy, pupil distortion, and high intraocular pressure (IOP) were frequently seen [3]. Sight-threatening complications such as corneal decompensation and the uveitis-glaucoma-hyphema syndrome gave a bad reputation to these

J. L. Alió et al. (eds.), *Cataract Surgery*, Essentials in Ophthalmology,
https://doi.org/10.1007/978-3-030-94530-5_17

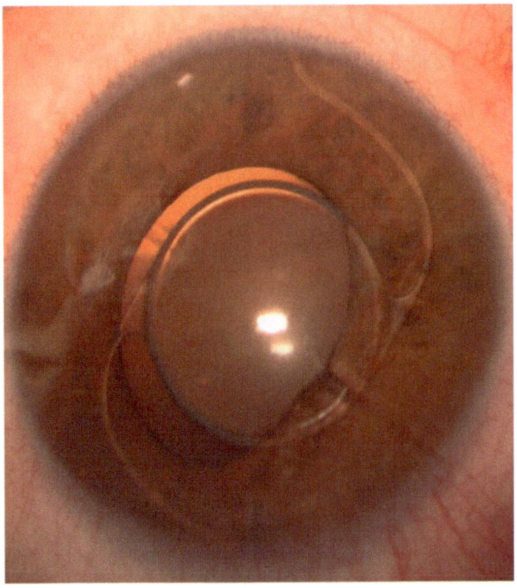

Fig. 17.1 Angle-supported pIOL, observe the pupil distortion due to posterior synechiae

pIOLs, and more than 60% of them had to be explanted [3]. In the 1980s, Baikoff and Momose decided to improve the AC pIOL models, and since then, several models of angle-supported (AS) pIOLs were developed (i.e., Baikoff ZB lens (Domilens, Lyon, France) (Fig. 17.1), NuVita MA20 (Bausch & Lomb, Salt Lake City, UT, USA), ZSAL-4/Plus lens (Morcher, Stuttgart, Germany), Kelman Duet Implant (Tekia, Irvine, CA, USA), and AcrySof Cachet (Alcon, Fort Worth, TX, USA)). Although having good visual outcomes [4], most of them have been phased out due to chronic endothelial cell density (ECD) loss.

Iris-Fixated pIOLs

In 1953, the first iris-fixated (IF) pIOLs were fixated in the iris sphincter. They had complications such as uveitis and glaucoma, so Worst designed an iris-claw pIOL that was fixated in the mid-peripheral iris stroma, which is an immobile portion of the iris [3]. It was not until 1986 that Fechner implanted an iris-claw pIOL in a myopic eye [5], the Fechner-Worst lens, which was discontinued due to progressive endothelial cell loss. The model has been improved through the years, and today, two IF pIOLs are available: Artisan and Artiflex (Ophtec, Netherlands) (see Fig. 17.2).

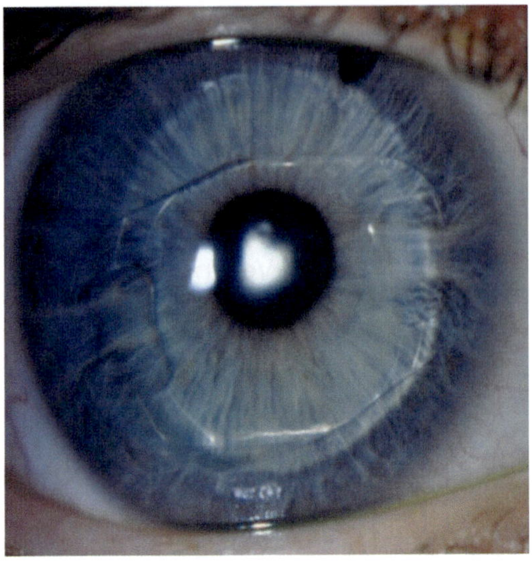

Fig. 17.2 Iris fixated phakic intraocular lens

Posterior Chamber pIOLs

These pIOLs were developed several years after the AC pIOLs. It was not until the 1990s that the first posterior chamber (PC) pIOLs were implanted [3]. Complications such as pupillary block glaucoma, pigment dispersion, anterior subcapsular cataracts, and dislocation into the vitreous were seen with early models, and even some of the PC pIOLs were phased out due to these complications like the phakic refractive lens (PRL, Zeiss-Meditec, Jena, Germany).

Two PC pIOL models are available today: the implantable collamer lens (ICL, Staar Surgical Co, Monrovia, California) (see Fig. 17.3) and the implantable phakic contact lens (IPCL, Care Group Sight solutions, India).

Phakic Intraocular Lens Explantation: Timing and Reasons

Alió et al. [6] reported the main causes of pIOL explantation in 240 eyes. Patients' mean age at explantation was 46.30 ± 11.84 years (range

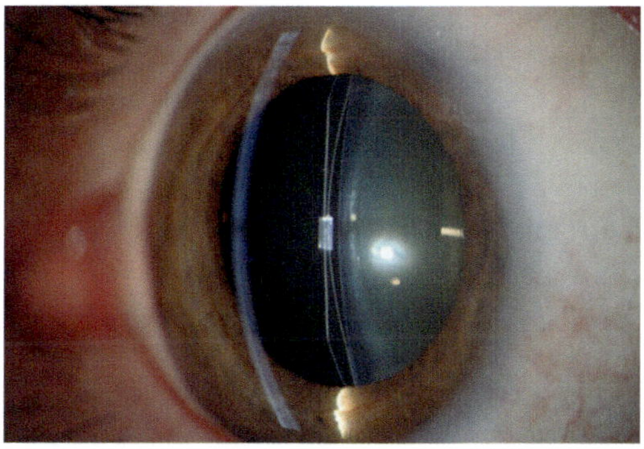

Fig. 17.3 Posterior chamber pIOL

25–80 years). The mean time between implantation and explantation was 381.14 ± 293.55 weeks. Main causes of explantation were the following: cataract formation (55%), endothelial cell loss (10.83%), corneal decompensation (9.17%), pIOL dislocation/decentration (6.67%), inadequate pIOL size or power (5%), and pupil ovalization (4.17%).

Bilensectomy Technique

Ancillary Tests

Preoperative ocular biometry is performed as usual. If the patient has an axial length (AL) greater than 28 mm, we suggest the use of the Barrett Universal II formula [7].

A corneal topography is necessary to evaluate and correct any corneal astigmatism.

All patients must have an ECD count before bilensectomy.

Surgery

Surgeries can be performed under topical anesthesia in cases with a PC pIOL. In cases with an AC pIOL the use of peribulbar anesthesia is preferred as iris manipulation may induce some pain. The surgical technique varies depending on the pIOL to be explanted.

For AC pIOL bilensectomy, the pupil should be dilated after the pIOL has been explanted; for PC pIOLs, the pupil should be dilated before pIOL explantation.

Angle-supported and the Artisan pIOLs require a 6-mm scleral frown incision to explant the pIOL; this incision must be sutured after explanting the pIOL in order to proceed with regular phacoemulsification.

The Artiflex and all PC pIOLs can be explanted through a 3-mm clear corneal incision. After explanting the pIOL, this incision is used as the main incision for phacoemulsification.

Angle-Supported pIOL Bilensectomy Technique

A 6-mm sclerocorneal incision is placed superiorly. Through a side-port incision, the AC is filled with dispersive viscoelastic to coat the endothelium. After penetrating the AC with a keratome, the haptic of the pIOL can be carefully explanted using a hook (see Video 17.1). After suturing the scleral incision with running 10-0 nylon, regular phacoemulsification can be performed.

Artisan pIOL Bilensectomy Technique

A 6-mm sclerocorneal incision is placed superiorly. Through a side-port incision, the AC is filled with dispersive viscoelastic to coat the endothelium. The optic of the pIOL is grabbed with a forceps, and the haptics are de-enclavated from the iris using the microholding forceps developed by MST (Redmond, Washington State, USA), MST Economic Touch II. The pIOL should be rotated to a vertical position for its explantation. The scleral incision is sutured with running 10-0 nylon in order to continue with phacoemulsification.

Artiflex pIOL Bilensectomy Technique

Bilensectomy of the Artiflex pIOL requires a 3-mm clear corneal incision. The de-enclavation process is the same as for the Artisan pIOL, except that the pIOL is explanted through the

3-mm corneal incision. This incision is used as the main incision for phacoemulsification (see Video 17.2). Another option is to cut the optic of the pIOL along its longer axis using the Osher-Snyder cutting device, from one enclavation to the opposite enclavation, with the haptics cut in half. By cutting the pIOL in half, it can be explanted through a 2.75-mm corneal incision.

Posterior Chamber pIOL Bilensectomy Technique

For PC pIOL bilensectomy, a broad pharmacological mydriasis is essential. After lifting the four footplates of the pIOL into the anterior chamber, the pIOL can be explanted through a 3-mm clear corneal incision, which is used as the main incision for phacoemulsification (see Video 17.3).

Clinical Outcomes

We analyzed our bilensectomy outcomes in 188 eyes. We evaluated the causes of bilensectomy, time between pIOL implantation and bilensectomy, efficacy, and visual and refractive outcomes with a follow-up of 1 year. Fifty-eight eyes underwent AS pIOL bilensectomy, 43 eyes underwent IF pIOL bilensectomy, and 87 eyes underwent PC pIOL bilensectomy.

Visual and refractive outcomes of bilensectomy are shown in Table 17.1.

PIOL Models Explanted

Angle-supported: Kelman Duet IOL (Tekia, Inc., Irvine, CA), Baikoff ZB (Domilens, Lyon, France), ZSAL-4 (Morcher, Stuttgart, Germany), and Phakic 6 IOL (Ophthalmic Innovations International, Ontario, CA)

Iris-fixated: Artisan pIOL (Ophtec BV, Groningen, Netherlands)

Posterior chamber: Visian Implantable Collamer Lens V3 and V4 models (STAAR Surgical Co., Monrovia, CA), Phakic Refractive Lens (Zeiss Meditec, Jena, Germany), and the Implantable Phakic Contact Lens (IPCL, Care Group Sight solutions, India)

Causes of Bilensectomy

The main causes of bilensectomy are depicted in Fig. 17.4.

Cataract

Cataract development is the most common cause of bilensectomy. Its development can be secondary to intermittent trauma from accommodation or during surgery, insufficient vaulting, or lens trauma from preoperative Nd:YAG laser peripheral iridotomy [8, 9]. The presence of high myopia in these patients is also a predisposing factor as it has been associated with the development of posterior subcapsular and nuclear cataract [10] (Fig. 17.5).

Endothelial Cell Loss

Endothelial cell loss is an important cause of bilensectomy especially in eyes with an IF pIOL. Intraoperative bleeding and excess iris manipulation during surgery can affect endothelial cell survival [11]. There is some controversy regarding ECD loss after the implantation of pIOLs. Some studies have reported an accelerated rate of ECD loss in the presence of a pIOL [12–14], while others have reported no significant ECD loss [15]. To maintain a healthy endothelium in patients with AC pIOLs, the minimum distance between the edge of the optic and the endothelium should be >1.5 mm [16, 17]. If the pIOL is 1.0 mm from the endothelium, it should be explanted [18].

Pupil Ovalization

Pupil ovalization is usually present in eyes with an AS pIOL. It is secondary to ischemic iridopa-

Table 17.1 Visual and refractive results of bilensectomy

	Angle-supported			Iris-fixated			Posterior chamber		
	Preop	Postop	*P* value	Preop	Postop	*P* value	Preop	Postop	*P* value
UDVA	0.91 ± 0.66	0.53 ± 0.60	.00	0.85 ± 0.49	0.45 ± 0.28	.00	0.88 ± 0.63	0.31 ± 0.28	.00
CDVA	0.48 ± 0.48	0.32 ± 0.56	.00	0.45 ± 0.42	0.23 ± 0.22	.00	0.43 ±0.44	0.15 ± 0.19	.00
Sphere	−1.6 ± 2.7	0.68 ± 1.1	.00	−1.5 ± 3.0	−0.2 ± 1.7	.00	−0.6 ± 2.6	0.6 ± 1.1	.00
Cylinder	−1.0 ± 0.78	−1.1 ± 1.0	.39	−1.2 ± 1.1	−1.5 ± 1.0	.17	−0.9 ± 1.0	−0.9 ± 0.8	.71
SE	−2.1 ± 2.6	0.11 ± 1.1	.00	−2.5 ± 3.0	−0.78 ± 1.7	.00	−1.1 ± 2.5	0.2 ± 1.2	.00
ECD	1803 ± 856	1733 ± 841	.57	1474 ± 633	1142 ± 537	.00	2212 ± 743	2169 ± 579	.67
Efficacy	0.8			0.7			0.8		
Time (m)	165.8 ± 186.7			146.6 ± 64			85.2 ± 61.5		

UDVA uncorrected distance visual acuity, *CDVA* corrected distance visual acuity, *SE* spherical equivalent, *ECD* endothelial cell density, time in months between pIOL implantation and bilensectomy

thy and inflammation secondary to the haptic compression of the iris root vessels [19]. Bilensectomy is extremely difficult in these eyes due to adhesions between the pIOL, iris, and anterior chamber [6, 19].

Complications

Intraoperative complications were the following: posterior capsule rupture and bleeding from the iris root in an eye with an IF pIOL.

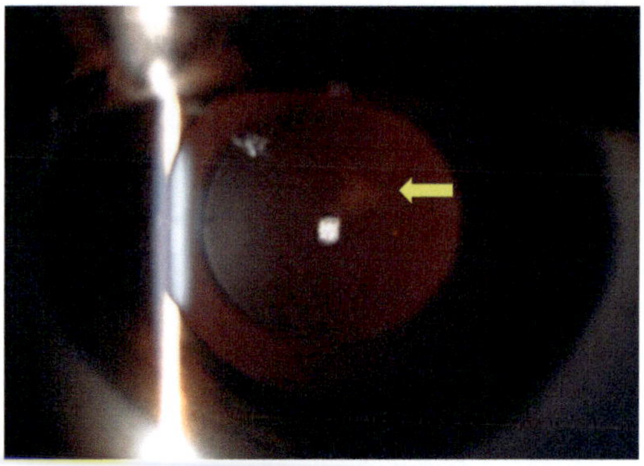

Fig. 17.5 Posterior subcapsular cataract in a patient with an ICLV4c pIOL

Postoperative complications in patients with AC pIOL were the following: severe ocular hypertension (two eyes), severe endothelial cell loss (one eye), and hyphema (two eyes). Two eyes developed a retinal detachment, one after an IF pIOL bilensectomy and the other after a PC pIOL bilensectomy.

Hyphema

It occurs especially in AS and IF pIOL bilensectomy due to iris manipulation and presence of angle synechiae. An AC washout may be necessary in some cases.

Posterior Capsule Rupture

Posterior capsule rupture (PCR) is a common intraoperative complication in cataract surgery [20]. Risk factors for capsular complications include the following: pupil size <3 mm and pseudoexfoliation; patients with high axial myopia have weaker zonules due to excessive stretch-

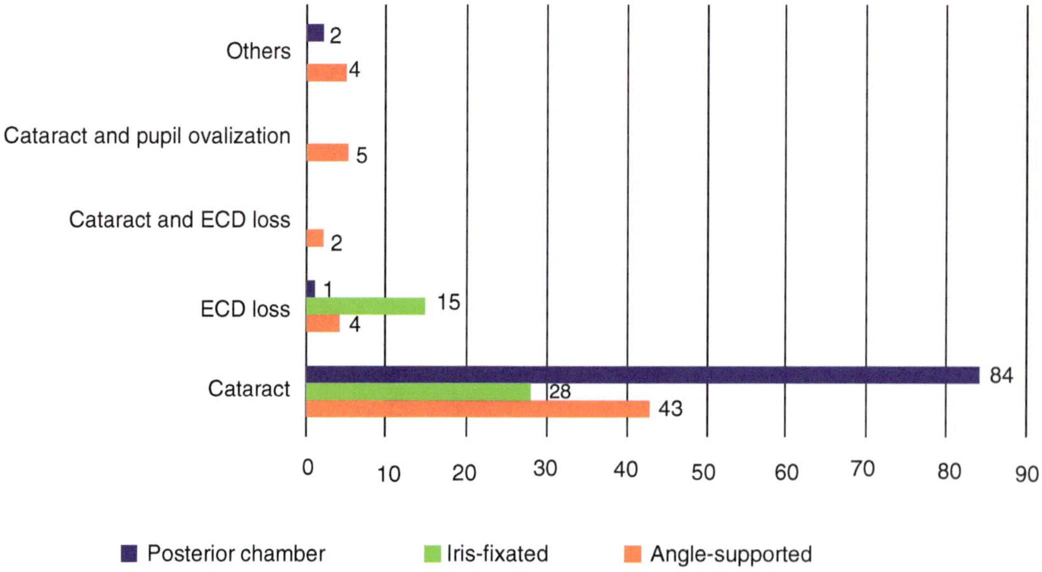

Fig. 17.4 Causes of bilensectomy in different pIOL models

ing of the zonular fibers that can predispose to PCR [20, 21]. If managed properly, the IOL can be placed into the ciliary sulcus and has good visual outcomes.

Ocular Hypertension

High intraocular pressure (IOP) can be secondary to pigment dispersion over the trabecular meshwork due to chronic chafing by the pIOL. If high IOP is presented in the early postoperative period, it might be secondary to retained viscoelastic material. In our study [22], two eyes required a combined procedure (bilensectomy and trabeculectomy), and other two had postoperative high IOP that was successfully treated with intravenous mannitol [22].

Severe Endothelial Cell Loss

Phacoemulsification and implantation of pIOLs are procedures that tend to decrease the ECD count [11–13, 23]. Early bilensectomy should be performed if the ECD is less than 1500 cells/mm^2 [24].

Retinal Detachment

Retinal detachment after cataract surgery in highly myopic eyes has an incidence of 2.2%. Axial length elongation and stretching of the posterior eye wall predispose to this vision-threatening complication [9]. In our studies [22, 25], one eye presented an RD immediately after bilensectomy, and the other eye developed it 11 months after surgery. Both eyes had a good visual outcome after pars plana vitrectomy.

Conclusions

All pIOLs will be eventually explanted; therefore, it is important to know the clinical outcomes, surgical technique, and complications of bilensectomy.

Cataract development remains the main reason of bilensectomy followed by ECD loss.

Bilensectomy is more challenging in eyes with AS pIOLs due to the presence of synechiae. Although most of the patients have a good visual and refractive outcome [26], sight-threatening complications such as retinal detachment and low ECD count may occur, so a close follow-up is necessary in all patients.

Take-Home Notes

- The main cause of bilensectomy is cataract development.
- Endothelial cell density loss is also an important cause of bilensectomy especially in AC pIOLs. Regular ECD count is necessary in all patients implanted with a pIOL. Early bilensectomy should be performed if the ECD is less than 1500 cells/mm^2.
- Retinal detachment was one of the vision-threatening complications presented after bilensectomy; this complication is related to the high myopia presented in these patients.
- Bilensectomy provides good visual and refractive outcomes.

Financial Support and Sponsorship This study has been financed in part by the Network for Cooperative Research in Health "OFTARED," Nodo Dioptrio Ocular, Biobanco Iberia (Reference: RD16/0008/0012), funded by the Instituto de Salud Carlos III, and co-funded by the European Regional Development Fund (ERDF), Project "A way to make Europe."

References

1. Colin J. Bilensectomy: the implications of removing phakic intraocular lenses at the time of cataract extraction. J Cataract Refract Surg. 2000;26(1):2–3.
2. Baron A. Prothèses cornèennes et cristalliniennes en matière plastique. Bull Mem Soc Fr Ophthalmol. 1954;67:386–90.
3. Lovisolo CF, Reinstein DZ. Phakic intraocular lenses. Surv Ophthalmol. 2005;50(6):549–87.

4. Knorz MC, Lane SS, Holland SP. Angle-supported phakic intraocular lens for correction of moderate to high myopia: three year interim results in international multicenter studies. J Cataract Refract Surg. 2011;37:469–80.
5. Fechner PU, Strobel J, Wichmann W. Correction of myopia implantation of a concave Worst-iris claw lens into phakic eyes. Refract Corneal Surg. 1991;7:286–98.
6. Alió JL, Toffaha BT, Peña-Garcia P, et al. Phakic intraocular lens explantation: causes in 240 cases. J Refract Surg. 2015;31(1):30–5.
7. Rong X, He W, Zhu Q, et al. Intraocular lens power calculation in eyes with extreme myopia: comparison of Barret Universal II, Haigis, and Olsen formulas. J Cataract Refract Surg. 2019. https://doi.org/10.1016/j.jcrs.2018.12.025.
8. Khalifa Y, Moshirfar M, Mifflin M, et al. Cataract development associated with collagen copolymer posterior chamber phakic intraocular lenses: clinicopathological correlation. J Cataract Refract Surg. 2010;36:1768–74.
9. Alfonso JF, Lisa C, Fernández-Vega L, et al. Prevalence of cataract after collagen polymer phakic intraocular lens implantation for myopia, hyperopia and astigmatism. J Cataract Refract Surg. 2015;41:800–5.
10. Ikuno Y. Overview of the complications of high myopia. Retina. 2017;37:2347–51.
11. Na KS, Jeon S, Joo CK. Effect of intraoperative manipulation during iris-claw phakic IOL implantation on endothelium. Can J Ophthalmol. 2013;48(4):259–64.
12. Tahzib NG, Nuijts RM, Wu WY, Budo CJ. Long-term study of Artisan phakic intraocular lens implantation for the correction of moderate to high myopia: ten-year follow-up results. Ophthalmology. 2007;114:1133–42.
13. Saxena R, Boekhoorn SS, Mulder PG, et al. Long-term follow-up of endothelial cell change after Artisan phakic intraocular lens implantation. Ophthalmology. 2008;115:608–613.e1.
14. Galvis V, Villamil JF, Acuña MF, et al. Long-term endothelial cell loss with the iris-claw intraocular phakic lenses (Artisan). Graefes Arch Clin Exp Ophthalmol. 2019. https://doi.org/10.1007/s00417-019-04506-9.
15. Morral M, Güell JL, El Husseiny MA, et al. Paired-eye comparison of corneal endothelial cell counts after unilateral iris-claw phakic intraocular lens implantation. J Cataract Refract Surg. 2016;42:117–26.
16. Pérez-Santonja JJ, Alió J, Jiménez-Ifaro I, Zato MA. Surgical correction of severe myopia with an angle supported phakic intraocular lens. J Cataract Refract Surg. 2000;26:1288–302.
17. Ferreira de Souza R, Allemann N, Forseto A, et al. Ultrasound biomicroscopy and Scheimpflug photography of angle-supported phakic intraocular lens for high myopia. J Cataract Refract Surg. 2003;29:1159–66.
18. Baikoff G. Anterior segment OCT and phakic intraocular lenses: a perspective. J Cataract Refract Surg. 2006;32:1827–35.
19. Alió JL, De la Hoz F, Pérez-Santoja JJ, et al. Phakic anterior chamber lenses for the correction of myopia. A 7-year cumulative analysis of complications in 263 cases. Ophthalmology. 1999;106:458–66.
20. Ergun SB, Kocamis SI, Cakmak HB, et al. The evaluation of the risk factors for capsular complications in phacoemulsification. Int Ophthalmol. 2018;38(5):1851–61.
21. Eleftheriadis H, Amoros S, Bilbao R, Teijeiro MA. Spontaneous dislocation of a phakic refractive lens into the vitreous cavity. J Cataract Refract Surg. 2004;30:2013–6.
22. Vargas V, Alió JL, Barraquer RI, et al. Safety and visual outcomes following posterior chamber phakic intraocular lens Bilensectomy. Eye Vis (Lond). 2020;7:34.
23. Reuschel A, Bogatsch H, Barth T, Wiedemann R. Comparison of endothelial changes and power settings between torsional and longitudinal phacoemulsification. J Cataract Refract Surg. 2010;36(11):1855–61.
24. Doors M, Berendschot TTJM, Webers CAB, et al. Model to predict endothelial cell loss after iris-fixated phakic intraocular lens implantation. Invest Ophthalmol Vis Sci. 2010;51:811–5.
25. Vargas V, Marinho A, El Sayyad F, Alio Del Barrio JL, Alio JL. Safety and visual outcomes following Iris-claw phakic intraocular lens bilensectomy.Eur J Ophthalmol. 2021;31(4):1795–1801. https://doi.org/10.1177/1120672120944033.
26. Vargas V, Alió JL. Refractive outcomes and complications following angle supported. Iris-fixated and posterior chamber phakic intraocular lenses bilensectomy. Curr Opin Ophthalmol. 2021;32(1):25–30.

Intraocular Lens Explantation and Exchange

18

Ali Nowrouzi, Jorge Alió del Barrio, Olena Al-Shymali, and Jorge L. Alió

Bullet Points

In this chapter, you can find the following information:

- The main causes leading to IOL explantation
- The main causes leading to IOL in-the-bag dislocation/decentration and surgical approaches to correct this dislocation/decentration and a comparison between these approaches
- The main causes of incorrect lens power calculation and how to decrease this error and the approaches to overcome this problem
- Explantation of multifocal intraocular lenses (MF-IOLs) due to neuroadaptation failure followed by the reimplantation of a different MF optical technology
- IOL explantation techniques

Introduction

Cataract surgery with intraocular lens (IOL) implantation is one of the most frequently performed surgical procedures in the world nowadays. The total number of cataract surgery has increased because of the excellent outcomes and high predictability of the technique. Such outcomes have further promoted the indication of refractive lensectomy (lens removal with IOL substitution aiming to correct a refractive error), especially in high refractive errors and presbyopia [1]. Moreover, longer lifespans have also contributed to the pseudophakic population growing very quickly. Intraocular lens explantation is infrequent today but may be potentially associated with serious complications. The reasons for explantation are diverse and related to multiple factors, including intraocular comorbidities [2, 3]. IOL explantation sometimes occurs after uneventful cataract surgery. In other cases, it may represent inadequate IOL selection, intraoperative complication, or problems

Supplementary Information The online version contains supplementary material available at [https://doi.org/10.1007/978-3-030-94530-5_18].

A. Nowrouzi
Cornea, Cataract and Refractive Surgery Unit, Department of Ophthalmology, Hospital Quironsalud Marbella, Alicante, Spain

J. Alió del Barrio · O. Al-Shymali · J. L. Alió (✉)
Cornea, Refractive and Cataract Surgery Unit, Vissum Miranza Alicante, Alicante, Spain

Division of Ophthalmology, School of Medicine, Miguel Hernandez University, Alicante, Spain
e-mail: jlalio@vissum.com

J. L. Alió et al. (eds.), *Cataract Surgery*, Essentials in Ophthalmology,
https://doi.org/10.1007/978-3-030-94530-5_18

related to the quality of IOL material or design, especially in multifocal IOLs. Further, it may be related to other intraocular comorbidities that may be affected by the presence of the IOL, with the subsequent potential for problems that may even end in the decision to explant the lens. The overall rate of explantation in different studies varies from 0.032% to 0.28% in some studies to 0.77% [4–6].

Main Causes Leading to IOL Explantation

Twenty years ago, about 70% of the IOLs explanted were anterior chamber IOLs, and the main causes of explantation were pseudophakic bullous keratopathy (PBK), uveitis-glaucoma-hyphema syndrome, and cystoid macular edema [7–10]. The IOL complication profile requiring explantation has considerably changed in recent years. In a study comparing the causes for explantation in the same clinical setting a decade later, the main reason for explantation changed from PBK to incorrect lens power and decentration/dislocation [4].

A retrospective multicenter study was published a few years ago [11]. This study aimed to analyze the demographics and reasons for pseudophakic IOL explantation in Spain, a developed country where modern cataract surgery is performed.

The main causes for explantation were dislocation/decentration in 145 cases (56.3%) and incorrect lens power in 33 cases (12.8%). The rest of the causes were IOL opacification, neuroadaptation failure, endophthalmitis, and pseudophakic bullous keratopathy.

Regarding decentration/dislocation, the authors used classifications for lens in the bag and lens out of the bag as other authors have done before [14]. Explantation surgery was only performed, as is generally recommended when the IOL was dislocated out of the visual axis causing symptoms and IOL repositioning was not possible. It is necessary to emphasize in the case of IOL decentration that repositioning would be another consideration in many cases. Dislocation of IOL especially to the vitreous cavity makes the repositioning approach not possible without vitrectomy.

Buenaga et al. [15] found that in a series of 257 eyes, 60% of the cases (145 eyes) were late in-the-bag IOL decentration. This was due to progressive zonular dehiscence in 40% of the cases and to capsule contraction syndrome in 20% of the cases. The rest of the IOLs (40%) were luxated out of the bag and were related to surgical complications. Incorrect lens power was the second cause of explantation, accounting for 12.8% of the cases. Although some authors, such as Mamalis et al., have shown in their surveys even higher rates of explantation because of incorrect lens power [12, 13], the rate found in Buenaga et al.'s study was relatively high in the context of modern cataract surgery [16]. Most of the participants in this study were treated at refractive centers; hence, the hypothesis is that probably a significant number of patients that underwent cataract surgery had a previous corneal refractive procedure which is a special group with a greater risk of calculation errors [17–19].

IOL in-the-Bag Dislocation/Decentration

Late in-the-bag dislocation of IOLs is a rare but potentially serious complication after cataract surgery. In an observational study, it was shown that the cumulative risks of IOL dislocation at 5, 10, 15, 20, and 25 years after cataract extraction were 0.1%, 0.1%, 0.2%, 0.7%, and 1.7%, respectively [20]. Nevertheless, the pseudophakic population has been growing very quickly in recent years as a result of longer lifespans, new phacorefractive procedures, and improvements in the quality and safety of phacoemulsification surgery. As a result, late in-the-bag dislocation may become a more common issue in the future.

Bag dislocation may occur due to progressive zonular dehiscence many years after uneventful surgery. The risk factors for this condition include pseudoexfoliation (PEX), connective tissue disorders, uveitis, retinitis pigmentosa, high myopia, and patients who underwent vitreoretinal surgery [21–23]. Pseudoexfoliation is probably the most recognized predisposing factor for late dislocation, as has been shown in several publications [5, 14, 23–25].

Pseudoexfoliation is likely to produce zonular insufficiency by two mechanisms. Firstly, PEX accumulations mechanically weaken the zonular lamella and impair zonular anchoring to the epithelial basement membrane at both its origin and insertion [26]. Furthermore, patients with PEX also exhibit an increase in elastinolysis that weakens the zonula. Secondly, PEX has been shown to facilitate anterior capsule contraction syndrome, which, if left untreated, usually leads to zonular failure [27, 28].

In a study published by Buenaga et al. from the IBERIA Biobank [29], it was found that high myopia was the most prevalent risk factor, followed by PEX [29]. Highly myopic eyes show some typical alterations due to thinning and degeneration of several eye layers as lacquer cracks, chorioretinal atrophy, or posterior staphyloma [32]. They hypothesized that along with the previously mentioned alterations, these eyes may also be more prone to zonular failure due to excessive elongation of the zonular fibers that have to support greater stress than in eyes with normal axial length. This theory is supported by the outcomes of a study using high-resolution magnetic resonance imaging, which demonstrated that myopic eyes are larger in all three dimensions (i.e., equatorial, anteroposterior, and vertical axes) [33, 34]. The mean time interval from cataract surgery to explantation due to late dislocation was 7.5 ± 5.2 years in this study. Some other reports have also shown a mean interval of around 8 years between both surgeries [5, 22–25].

Different surgical techniques can be used to reposition a dislocated IOL. In the Buenaga et al. series, all the patients had IOL explantation because this was one of the inclusion criteria. A new IOL was placed after explantation during the same surgery. A scleral-fixated IOL was placed in most cases (36.1%).

In conclusion, PEX is overall the most frequently reported risk factor for late in-the-bag IOL dislocation. However, some other risk factors such as high myopia are important to recognize. Furthermore, dislocation in high myopia has been reported to occur at a younger age than in PEX, hence affecting patients with greater visual demands [29].

In many cases, a dislocated IOL can be repositioned by different surgical techniques and lens explantation is not the only approach for these cases.

Although refixation of dislocated IOL is more difficult than implanting a new IOL, especially given the fact that the selection of suture position and operation technique is highly restricted, both methods share the same stability if the IOL was sutured to the sclera or iris successfully. Recently, a retrospective single-surgeon study of 118 eyes reported that scleral fixation sutures with 10-0 polypropylene provided an excellent long-term fixation of posterior chamber IOLs, resulting in suture breakage in fewer than 0.5% of cases for periods of 24 years and longer.

Several factors influence the stability of the sutured IOL, including fixation technique, suture type, and knot stability. Experienced fixation technique and knot technique may contribute to lower incidence of IOL redislocation, and 10–0 polypropylene suture and the knot technique requiring two separate sutures in one knot seem to be an ideal choice to keep knot stability [30].

Another option for IOL suturing and/or capsular bag fixation would be the Gore-Tex sutures as confirmed by other authors [31].

Some authors described other methods for fixation of the dislocated intraocular lens-capsular bag complex. This includes suturing the complex of the capsular bag and IOL to the iris at two points 180° apart using 9-0 polypropylene sutures on long needles, considered as a safe method without major complications [35].

Shangfei et al. [36] compared the repositioning approach with IOL explantation in a meta-analysis involving 1082 eyes. The average follow-up time was 13.7 months. Based on this meta-analysis, both IOL repositioning and IOL exchange were safe and effective procedures for treating IOL dislocation. Pooled analysis of ten studies showed that the two procedures had a similar effect on best-corrected visual acuity (MD −0.00; 95%CI: −0.08 to 0.08; $P = 0.99$). IOL exchange was superior to repositioning in terms of the postoperative refractory outcomes as measured by spherical equivalent, but IOL repositioning was associated with a lower incidence of anterior vitrectomy and potentially lower incidence of cystoid macular edema.

Incorrect Lens Power

Cataract surgery outcomes have greatly improved due to advancements in surgical technique, intraocular lens (IOL) technology, and preoperative testing and calculations. With the improvements have come increased expectations from patients regarding postoperative visual acuity and independence from spectacle correction. Studies on cataract surgery outcomes showed that 50–70% and 79–94% of patients will achieve postoperative refractions within 0.5 D and 1.0 D of the intended target, respectively [37–40].

Toric IOLs and limbal relaxing incisions and astigmatic keratectomy now provide the opportunity to correct astigmatism with good results. A study of patients undergoing placement of toric IOLs found that 88% had less than 1.0 D of astigmatism postoperatively [41].

If the refractive error does occur after surgery, numerous options may provide the patient with a satisfactory outcome. These are especially important in certain populations such as patients with a history of keratorefractive surgery where there is a higher rate of postoperative refractive error in general and in particular patients undergoing premium IOL implantation who are more sensitive to refractive error. Refractive error after cataract surgery may be decreasing but is still a relatively common occurrence that is critical to patient satisfaction. Therefore, cataract surgeons should take all precautions to prevent its occurrence as well as diagnose and manage the refractive error effectively.

Refractive error after cataract surgery typically manifests with blurred vision at distances where the patient was expecting to have good uncorrected visual acuity. Patients who are 20/20 uncorrected at distance with plano refraction may be unhappy if the goal was clear near vision. The amount of deviation from the target refraction at which the patient becomes symptomatic is largely dependent on the individual. The most commonly used end points for measuring refractive error in the literature are the percentage of patients achieving final refraction within 0.5 D and 1.0 D of the intended target [42].

These intervals are the highest practical levels of accuracy, as IOL powers change in 0.5 D increments. The expectation of spectacle independence at distance, near, or both in the cases of premium IOLs has led to dissatisfaction with cataract surgery that does not result in spectacle independence. Thus, even though the refractive error may be corrected with glasses or contact lenses, patients are often not happy with this result as the main goal of these surgeries is to be spectacle-free. Another issue that refractive error may create is anisometropia if the refractive error is unilateral or asymmetric. This is usually quite symptomatic and requires additional surgery.

The importance of refractive predictability has become increasingly important since the advent of premium IOLs. Bifocal, trifocal, extended depth of focus (EDOF), and pseudo-accommodative lenses require precision in postoperative refraction to maximize visual acuity. These lenses are associated with an increased rate of visual phenomena such as glare, halos, and night vision problems that are significantly worsened by any refractive error. Contrast sensitivity and subjective visual acuity are also disproportionately affected in these patients if any refractive error is present [43].

Despite new advances in cataract surgery, unsatisfactory visual outcomes because of a residual refractive error are a major cause of dissatisfaction. This may be due to different causes, such as inaccuracies in the biometric analysis [44–46].

Patients with a history of refractive surgery have a higher likelihood of refractive error after cataract surgery. This condition is frequently known as "refractive surprise." In cases of PRK, it can be impossible to determine if there was prior surgery on exam unless corneal topography is performed, and despite thorough history taking, patients may not volunteer this information. Hyperopic surprise most commonly results if the history of refractive surgery is not taken into account when calculating IOL power.

All patients should be asked about contact lens use, and if present, the specific type and date of last use must be noted. Patients must stop soft contact lens use 1 week and rigid gas-permeable (RGPs) contact lenses at least 1 month before preoperative testing. After 1 month out of RGPs, topography should be done and then should be repeated 2–4 weeks later.

Keratoconic eyes have deeper anterior chamber depths and longer axial lengths, which may lead to hyperopic surprise due to errors in the estimated lens position. One review found that the SRK II formula had the best refractive outcomes in mild keratoconus, whereas no formula performs particularly well in severe keratoconus. Some authors advocate for the use of the standard keratometry value of 43.25 D and target refraction of −2.0 D in severe keratoconus.

Sources of error unrelated to the eye may also contribute to refractive error. These include poor patient cooperation, data entry error, and placement of the wrong lens into the wrong eye. The largest study on wrong IOL implantations was a retrospective review of all reported cases in Wales from 2003 to 2010. Of the 164 reported incidents, the following etiologies were most common [47, 48]:

1. Inaccurate biometry
2. Wrong IOL selection
3. Transcription errors
4. Handwriting misinterpretation

Based on previous studies, analysing refractive data form more than 17,000 eyes after cataract surgery, it was shown that emmetropia was only achieved in 55% of eyes planned for the aim of ±0.50 D [49]. Based on recent advances in optical biometry by Swept-source OCT and utilizing the fourth-generation formulas such as Barrett II for IOL calculation as well as the incorporation of new formulas based on artificial intelligence, it was shown that emmetropia was achieved in more than 75% of eyes planned for the goal of ±0.50 D in a study of 3241 eyes of 3241 patients reported on a specific IOL type. The same study reported five of the commonly used formulas (Haigis, Hoffer Q, Holladay 1, Holladay 2, and SRK/T) and two formulas (Barrett Universal II and T2) that have never been retested in a large series across the entire AL range despite the promising results in their initial publications.

Over the entire AL range, the Barrett Universal II was the most accurate formula by a significant margin, having a lower mean absolute error and a higher percentage of eyes with prediction errors between ±0.25 D, ±0.50 D, and ± 1.00 D than the other six formulas assessed [50].

It is critical to determine the etiology of refractive error after cataract surgery. This begins with accurate refraction that is stable. The time to refractive stability may vary from 1 day to 3 months postoperatively. Patients with one-piece acrylic lenses may typically be refracted within the first week postoperatively, whereas those with premium IOLs need more time to gain their final stable refraction even up to 1 month postoperatively. Post-RK patients may take 3 months for refractive stability [51].

Auto-refraction is not enough evaluation and subjective refraction is necessary. A thorough dilated exam is critical to assess for corneal irregularity, lens malposition or distention, and/or retinal pathology. Corneal decompensation or irregularity due to surgery, eye drops, or trauma may result in pathology that was not present preoperatively. Preoperative measurements and formulas used for surgery should be double-checked. An OCT of the macula may reveal clinically inapparent macular edema or other previously undetected pathologies. If these measures do not identify a source of error, it may be assumed that there was an error in the estimated lens position and IOL formula used.

If the refractive error is decided to be treated, one option is corneal refractive surgery. This is a highly accurate means of correcting residual refractive error with 92% of pseudophakic cases achieving a result within 0.5 D of the intended target. Additionally, it is very effective in multifocal intraocular lens (MF-IOL) patients, as one large review showed that 90% of patients who underwent LASIK or PRK after MF-IOL placement were within 0.5 D and 99.5% were within 1.0 D of the intended refractive target. These patients all underwent conventional ablation, and 99.2% of the patients were 20/40 or better at the final visit, demonstrating the safety of this option [51].

It is recommended that LASIK is delayed 3 months after cataract surgery to allow for refractive and incisional stability. PRK may be pursued once manifest refraction is stable [52].

Thorough history and exam are necessary before LASIK to ensure that contraindications such as Fuchs' dystrophy, epithelial basement membrane dystrophy (EBMD), severe dry eyes, or history of herpetic eye disease are not present. PRK may be used in many cases when LASIK is contraindicated due to corneal pathology.

Pseudophakic IOL exchange may be an effective option if the source of the error and the reason behind it can be allocated. The IOL should be known, and the same IOL platform should be used for the second surgery. Exchange is technically easiest to perform in the early postoperative period (within 4 months). Exchange is more commonly used in refractive errors greater than 1 D, as other methods such as corneal refractive surgery are more precise in correcting smaller degrees of refractive error. A vergence formula is recommended to be utilized for IOL exchange calculations, which can be found via this link: https://www.doctor-hill.com/physicians/download.html.

Jin et al. [53] compared the efficacy and safety of correcting residual refractive error after cataract surgery between laser-assisted in situ keratomileusis (LASIK) and lens-based correction methods, including piggyback IOL implantation and IOL exchange in the same group. These authors found comparable results between the LASIK group and the lens-based group in the final spherical equivalent (SE) and safety. Fernández-Buenaga et al. [54] established a retrospective comparison among LASIK, piggyback IOLs, and IOL exchange as separate groups. The three different methods were compared in terms of refractive predictability and safety. All correcting methods were capable of improving refraction in myopic and hyperopic eyes. In the comparative analysis among groups, statistically, significant differences were found in SE and refractive cylinder. When compared with the IOL explantation group, the LASIK group had statistically significantly better outcomes for SE and refractive cylinders. Significant differences were also detected between the LASIK and the piggyback IOL groups in the cylinder, favoring the former. Therefore, there are no big differences in the final sphere among groups. Nevertheless, the cylinder outcome was what made the LASIK procedure more accurate than the IOL explantation or the piggyback IOL technique. In the LASIK group, the refractive cylinder was decreased after surgery, whereas in the piggyback IOL group the refractive cylinder remained stable and in the IOL explantation group the refractive cylinder was increased.

The efficacy index showed better outcomes in the LASIK group than in the IOL explantation and piggyback IOL groups. However, no statistically significant difference was found between IOL explantation and piggyback IOL implantation in this index. In the predictability analysis, the authors also detected differences among groups with the best outcome in the LASIK group followed by the piggyback group. The worst predictability was found in the IOL exchange group – remarkably that the percentage of eyes within ±0.50 dioptres of final refractive spherical equivalent in the LASIK group was 92.9%.

Regarding the safety index, no statistically significant differences were found among groups. However, the proportion of eyes that lost one or more lines of best spectacle-corrected visual acuity (BSCVA) was significantly different among groups. This percentage was four to five times higher in the IOL explantation and piggyback IOL groups in comparison with the LASIK group (7.14%). Indeed, no eye of those treated with LASIK lost more than two lines of vision, compared to one eye in the IOL explantation group and three eyes in the piggyback IOL group.

The results of this study showed that LASIK was the most accurate procedure to correct residual ametropia after cataract surgery. Lens-based procedures (IOL explantation or piggyback IOLs) are also effective methods and should be a choice in cases with extreme ametropia and corneal abnormalities or when there is no excimer laser platform available. A randomized controlled prospective study comparing the three procedures is necessary to confirm these findings.

IOL rotation or repositioning may be the best option for eyes with residual cylinder error after toric IOL placement. Rotation is indicated in cases where the IOL was placed in an improper position during surgery, as well as in cases where the IOL was initially properly placed but in the postoperative period has rotated. IOL rotation (angle correction) should be done in the early postoperative period before the healing and fibrosis that occur within a few months of surgery [51]. The postoperative refractive axis of astigmatism should be used for proper IOL repositioning, rather than the values used at the time of the initial surgery.

Specific IOL calculations for toric IOL exchange or rotation may be found at this website: https://www.astigmatismfix.com/.

If it is not possible to reduce astigmatism via IOL rotation, another option such as keratorefractive surgery will likely be necessary.

An add-on IOL may be the optimal choice for patients with a hyperopic outcome, especially if the IOL power is not known. It is also an alternative to IOL exchange when the procedure would be at high risks, such as in cases of posterior capsule tears or zonulopathy. For this procedure to be successful, the primary IOL optic capture must be fully in the capsular bag, and the anterior chamber should be deep with an open angle to allow for adequate space for the secondary IOL. Silicone IOLs are preferred, especially if the primary IOL was acrylic. Square edge and acrylic IOLs should not be used for add-on IOLs. This technique is associated with an increased risk of mechanical complications such as uveitis-glaucoma-hyphema (UGH) syndrome, iris chafing, and uveitis [55, 56].

The following rules have been used in calculating IOL power for add-on IOLs:

- Hyperopic error: 1.5 × manifest SE diopters
- Myopic error: 1.3 × manifest SE diopters

However, current vergence formulas (https://www.doctor-hill.com/physicians/download.html) provide more accurate IOL power calculations and are recommended. It is always necessary to use these formulas in cases of refractive error greater than 7 D, as the above general rules become increasingly inaccurate with larger refractive error [54].

IOL Opacification

In the middle and late 1990s, foldable IOLs became very popular and came into use worldwide due to easy implantation through smaller corneal incisions. However, some foldable hydrophilic acrylic IOLs fell into disrepute as a result of increasing reports of postoperative opacification [57–60].

Because of the widespread implantation of these IOLs before the opacification problem was noticed, IOL opacification became a common indication for IOL explantation during the past decade [11–13]. Different causes can lead to intraoperative IOL opacification or early postoperative IOL opacification/discoloration. Regarding late IOL opacification, it has been described with different materials, but as previously mentioned, most of the reports were associated with hydrophilic acrylic designs. The four major models implicated in this problem were the HydroView (Bausch & Lomb) [60, 61], MemoryLens (Ciba Vision) [62], SC60B- OUV (MDR, Inc.) [62], and AquaSense (Ophthalmic Innovations International, Inc.) [63, 64]. It was later known that in these four models, the reason for opacification was related to the manufacturing process instead of a problem associated with the lens material itself. Although these IOLs were introduced in the market more than a decade ago, IOL exchange surgery due to late opacification is still performed, as can be seen in recent reports [65, 66].

Intraocular lens opacification usually leads to decreased visual acuity and also to poor quality of vision with high levels of light scattering and decreased contrast sensitivity [67]. Hence, the decision for explantation should be based on the examination findings combined with decreased visual acuity or quality of vision.

Most of the published papers show a long interval between the original cataract surgery and the exchange surgery. In a paper published by Buenaga et al. research group [68], it was 89.1 ± 33.6 months, which is longer than what has been reported in other series [69–71]. In the majority of these reports, it was shown that the mean uncorrected visual acuity (UCVA) and best spectacle-corrected visual acuity (BSCVA) for far significantly improved after surgery [72–74]. However, some other authors did not notice a gain of vision after the IOL exchange surgery [72]. The final BSCVA achieved in Kermani et al.'s study was better than that given in most of the previous reports. A final BSCVA of 0.7 or better was achieved in 68.2% of the eyes. This difference may be explained by the existence of fewer ocular comorbidities in their cases and because most of their explanted IOLs were HydroView (63.6%) which are easier to remove than other hydrogel models, as stated by other authors [75]. In this study, the IOL exchange was uneventful in most cases. However, it was not exempt from complications. Anterior vitrectomy had to be performed in almost one-third of the eyes because of vitreous prolapse to the anterior chamber, and the new IOL had to be implanted in the ciliary sulcus in most of the patients (63.6%); it is important to emphasize the risk of retinal detachment as a potential complication although it was not reported in any of these cases.

The IOL opacification is still an important issue. There may be still patients requiring treatment now for this reason. In fact, in recent reports, it has been shown that hydrophilic IOL calcification can still occur in association with certain eye conditions like a history of air/gas fill in DMEK [65]. It has also been described in a quite recent hydrophilic IOL model with a hydrophobic surface associated with certain medical conditions like diabetes, hypertension, or glaucoma [66].

The only therapeutic option is the IOL exchange. This surgery, although associated with a high incidence of complications [75], restores and significantly improves visual acuity with no eye losing one or more lines of vision in the Kermani et al.'s series.

There are many newly designed IOLs every year in the market. However, most of the studies of the new IOL models only focus on the refractive and optical quality performance, whereas the long-term biocompatibility is not usually checked. To avoid this type of complication, it should be mandatory for every new IOL model to be tested for a prolonged period before large-scale use, as the lenses will usually remain inside the eye for decades.

Multifocal IOL Explantation

Dissatisfaction with the outcomes of multifocal IOL implantation has been reported by patients who do not achieve visual goals, with limited quality and sharpness of vision, or have new visual aberrations. A 2006 Cochrane review of multifocal IOLs found that photic phenomena are 3.5 times more likely with multifocal IOLs than with monofocal IOLs. By increasing the depth of field twofold to threefold with a multifocal IOL, contrast sensitivity can decrease up to 50% [76].

Intraocular lens explantation is the worst scenario after cataract surgery with multifocal IOL implantation because it means that the aim of the original surgery was not met and because it may be associated with new complications.

Fortunately, it is only needed in very few patients of those with complaints. Several studies show that the rate of multifocal IOL exchange among dissatisfied patients is 0.85% [77], 4% [78], and 7% [79]. If dissatisfaction continues, the main cause of this dissatisfaction should be differentiated. The main reasons for patient dissatisfaction following multifocal intraocular lens implantation are residual ametropia, posterior capsule opacification (PCO), dry eye, IOL decentration, inadequate pupil size, and wave front abnormalities [80, 81].

Residual ametropia is one of the most common reasons for patient dissatisfaction after multifocal IOL implantation as multifocal IOLs are more sensitive to residual refractive error. It may occur because of inaccuracies in the biometric analysis, inadequate selection of the IOL power, limitations of the calculation formulas, or errors in the IOL position. In situ keratomileusis or photorefractive keratectomy enhancements after cataract surgery are shown to be efficient, predictable, and safe. If excimer laser is not available, an option is the IOL exchange or "piggyback" lens implantation [80, 82].

PCO is very common and usually results in blurred vision and/or photopic phenomena in patients after long-term multifocal IOL implantation. The higher rates of PCO were found in patients with hydrogel IOLs, rounded-edged IOLs, IOLs placed in the sulcus, and large capsulorhexis when compared to other factors like another IOL material, sharp posterior optic edge, placement in the capsular bag, and small capsulorhexis, respectively [83]. The better treatment solution for it is the capsulotomy with Nd:YAG laser, which is fast and has low rates of complications. However, before the treatment with Nd:YAG laser, the surgeon should be sure that all other possible causes of patient dissatisfaction are treated or discarded as the risks of an IOL exchange is higher with a previous posterior capsulotomy [81, 82].

Dry eye is a multifactorial disease of the tear film and the ocular surface associated with discomfort, blurred vision, and photopic phenomena. Nevertheless, it is usually in the elderly population, and, in addition, cataract surgery may induce or increase it mainly by reducing corneal sensitivity through the incision although the postoperative treatment may also play a role there. The guidelines to treat dry eye include starting with eyelid hygiene and the use of artificial drops. Other options for more severe cases are the use of cyclosporine, punctual plug implantation (especially in those with aqueous deficiency and no inflammation associated), and platelet-rich plasma (PRP) drops [81, 82, 84].

Inadequate pupil size affects the visual acuity after multifocal IOL implantation because the pupil size determines the multifocal IOL zones used. Patients with very small postoperative pupils and complaining about poor near vision may be treated with the use of cyclopentolate drops or a 360° argon iridoplasty (0.5 s, 500 mW, and 500 microns). On the other hand, patients with very large postoperative pupils and complaints about increased photopic phenomena may be treated with brimonidine tartrate 0.2% drops [80, 82].

IOL decentration may affect the visual function depending on the degree of decentration, the IOL design, and the pupil size. A study comparing the performance of two diffractive and two refractive multifocal IOLs with different levels of decentration in an eye model with a 3-mm pupil found that for the total diffractive structured ZM900, both far and near modulation transfer functions (MTF) were affected at decentration of 0.75 mm. MTF is an objective metric of contrast sensitivity representing the loss of contrast produced by the optics of the eye. MTF is therefore the ability of a lens system to display the ratio of image contrast to object contrast for ocular optics as a function of the spatial frequency of a sinusoidal grating [85, 86]. For the diffractive, but with a monofocal peripheral part ReSTOR (+4) IOL, the near MTF decreases as the decentration degree increases while the far MTF tends to improve. For the refractive IOLs studied (ReZoom and SFX-MV1), the far MTF deteriorates starting at decentration of 0.75 and 1 mm, respectively, with no changes in near MTF even in 1-mm decentration [87]. The treatment with Argon laser iridoplasty avoids IOL explantation in the majority of cases [80, 81].

When necessary, the multifocal IOL explantation should be performed in the first 6 months after the surgery because of the scarring tissue that makes the surgery more difficult and comes along with higher complication risk. Another important factor to consider in the multifocal IOL explantation procedure is the presence of the capsular tension ring that makes the surgery easier [15].

Woodward et al. in a retrospective review compared 43 eyes of 32 patients dissatisfied with visual outcomes after multifocal IOL implantation, suggesting that blurred vision is the leading cause of dissatisfaction among patients with multifocal IOLs. The etiology of blurred vision was attributed to ametropia and PCO in the majority of cases. Despite overall success with less invasive interventions, 7% of eyes required IOL exchange to resolve symptoms [79].

Neuroadaptation failure may affect the visual function of multifocal IOLs. New reports proved that cortical neural areas are responsible for the long-term adaptation to such visual symptoms, suggesting that the persistence of these dysphotopsias is a neuroadaptation failure [88–91]. Eventually, the only solution in such cases would be the explantation of the MF-IOL.

The studies available in the literature report the outcomes of MF-IOL exchange to monofocal IOLs. Another acceptable approach is studied by Al-Shymali et al. [92] They conducted a study where MF-IOLs were explanted due to neuroadaptation failure followed by the reimplantation of a different MF optical technology based on the hypothesis that there may be different neuroadaptation processes for refractive and diffractive IOLs in different patients. Into neuroadaptation failure, we included all the subjective visual symptoms that did not have any clear "anatomical" cause such as photic phenomena, blurred vision, insufficient vision, and monocular diplopia. In this retrospective series of cases, MF-IOL exchange was done in 22 dissatisfied patients (38 eyes), divided into 3 groups: group 1, bilateral cases with neuroadaptation failure; group 2, unilateral cases; and group 3, dissatisfied patients due to insufficient near vision. Patients underwent an exchange of an MF-IOL with another MF-IOL of a different optical profile either in design or in power. Questionnaires including Quality of Vision (QoV), Visual Function Index (Rasch-revised version, VF-8R), and a satisfaction questionnaire were used. The mean time from explantation to implantation was 9.1 months. In group 1, the QoV scores improved significantly across all three subscales. Visual function improved with a change in VF-14 score from 60.41 ± 24.81 to 90.16 ± 10.91 ($P < 0.001$). The VF-8R score improved as well. In group 1, the uncorrected distance visual acuity improved from 20/35 to 20/26 after the exchange ($P < 0.001$), and corrected distance visual acuity improved from 20/28 to 20/22 ($P < 0.001$). Safety and efficacy indices reached 1.46 and 1.16, respectively. Patients in groups 2 and 3 had an improvement in visual outcomes, quality of vision, and visual function. For patient satisfaction, 86.4% of all the patients reported they would have the MF-IOL reimplantation procedure again. Excellent results with an increase in both far and near visual acuities and improvement of patients' quality of life and vision assessed by validated questionnaires were confirmed. This procedure showed to be feasible and able to correct the patient's dissatisfaction and keep the advantages of MF-IOLs such as spectacle independence for the benefit of the patient.

In the following videos, the surgical technique to exchange a multifocal IOL by another multifocal IOL by different optics is explained:

- Video 1. PanOptix exchange for Oculentis MF15
- Video 2. Restore exchange for Oculentis M3
- Video 3. Miniwell exchange for Oculentis M3
- Video 4. Miniwell exchange for AT Lisa Tri
- Video 5. Oculentis MF30 for Oculentis MF15
- Video 6. Oculentis MF30 for AT Lisa Tri Zeiss

IOL Explantation Techniques

There are many explantation techniques described in the scientific literature [93–100]. In recent years, interest has been focused on explanting IOLs through small incisions (2.2–2.65 mm) to avoid astigmatism induction, thus improving the predictability associated with the exchange procedure.

The explantation techniques can be divided into four different types:

1. Whole lens removal. This type is not currently used because wound enlargement is needed. It is now only used in those marginal cases of rigid polymethylmethacrylate pseudophakic IOLs. However, there is a publication about a surgical technique of explanting a single-piece acrylic hydrophobic lens through a 2.75-mm incision without cutting or folding, just pulling the lens out with toothed forceps [93].
2. Intraocular lens cutting. Intraocular lens cuts are performed inside the eye to remove the lens through a small corneal incision. This can be done in many ways: by bisecting the lens [94], partial bisections [95, 96], or, trisecting it [97].
3. Intraocular lens haptic cutting. The haptics may be cut before surgery with YAG laser [98] or at the time of the surgery with scissors [99], thus facilitating the removal of the optic. When the degree of fibrosis is so high that it is not possible to release the haptics without taking risks, it is preferable to leave the haptics in place.
4. Intraocular lens refolding. The IOL is folded in the anterior chamber and afterward explanted through a minimally enlarged incision [100]. However, this technique involves extensive manipulation and may cause more damage to clear corneal incisions and a 25% reduction in endothelial cell count.

Techniques

All explantation techniques of an in-the-bag foldable IOL begin with the same steps. Corneal incisions are made (Fig. 18.1a), after which OVD is used to dissect the IOL from the capsular bag (Fig. 18.1b). Afterward, depending on each case, the most appropriate technique is chosen. Although a lot of explantation techniques exist, we are going to list the ones mostly utilized: optic cut technique [Doctor JorgeAlióYouTube Channel. https://www.youtube.com/channel/UC9P3owJYdjwaypuvA-lcDhg].

Using a Sinskey hook and a Lester hook (Katena, USA), the IOL is loosened from the capsular bag (Fig. 18.1c) and overlapped onto the anterior capsular rim (Fig. 18.1d, e). Subsequently, a cut of the optic is performed radially to the center of the IOL (Fig. 18.1f, g), followed by its extraction through the main incision using two forceps that are alternated in grasping the IOL (Fig. 18.1h, i) while eliminating it from the anterior chamber (Fig. 18.1j).

- Haptic cut technique/"amputation": In the case of a tight adherence between the haptics and the capsular bag because of a fibrotic reaction, the haptics of the IOL are cut and left in the bag. Otherwise, the attempts to remove them may lead to zonular dehiscence. Afterward, the optic is removed.

Eguchi technique and its variation: Two radial incisions of the optic are made and are separated from a range of 35–90°. Eventually, a triangle or a quarter of the lens optic is obtained and removed from the anterior chamber through a small corneal incision followed by the rest of the IOL.

Folding technique: After elaborating the IOL from the capsular bag, it is folded onto itself in the anterior chamber and explanted through a corneal incision.

Removing the whole IOL: Mostly this technique is applied to unfoldable IOLs; however, in some cases, it may be the most comfortable technique to choose. After moving the IOL out of the capsular bag to the anterior chamber, a bigger corneal or scleral incision is performed, and the IOL is removed in one piece from the eye.

Our favorite is the cutting technique described above [Doctor JorgeAlióYouTube Channel, https://www.youtube.com/channel/UC9P3owJYdjwaypuvA-lcDhg]. In our opinion, it holds minimal risk for complications and is easier and faster than others. The folding technique has a potential risk for endothelial dam-

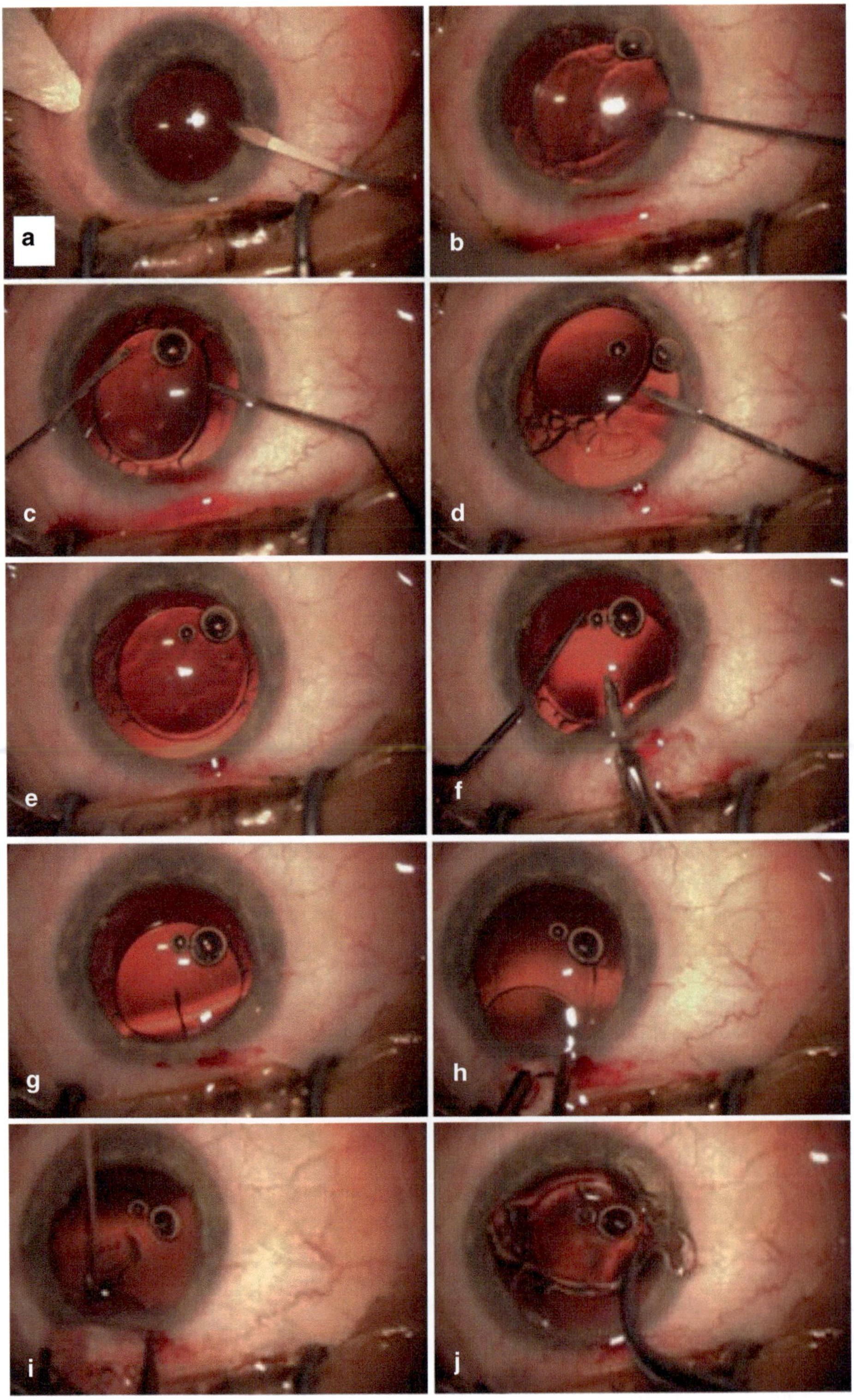

Fig. 18.1 Intraocular lens (IOL) optic cut explantation technique: (**a**) corneal incisions; (**b**) dissection of the IOL from the capsular bag using OVD; (**c**) freeing the IOL from the capsular bag; (**d**, **e**) elevation of the IOL onto the anterior capsular rim; (**f**, **g**) a radial cut of the optic is performed to the center of the IOL optic; (**h**, **i**) extraction of the IOL through the main incision using two forceps; (**j**) the IOL is completely removed from the anterior chamber

age, and removing the whole IOL needs a larger corneal incision that increases the risk of postoperative astigmatism or a scleral incision that prolongs the surgery time.

Outcomes

Explantation surgery is always challenging; however, explantation of a multifocal lens is usually easier (especially in case of capsular tension ring in place) than explantation due to other causes. First, because the decision for explantation is made only a few months after cataract surgery, the scarring process has not occurred yet. Second, because the ocular structures are undamaged, the surgery is less risky. In contrast, when performing IOL explantation due to other causes such as dislocation or IOL opacification, the surgery is potentially associated with more complications due to damage to the ocular structures in the former and the presence of fibrotic tissue in the latter, especially because in these cases IOL explantation is often performed a long time after the original cataract surgery.

The main issue regarding multifocal IOL explantation is whether the procedure is worthwhile. Is the satisfaction rate increased after explantation surgery? Is it associated with a high incidence of complications? To date, there are few publications answering these questions.

Galor et al. [73] retrospectively studied the outcomes after refractive IOL explantation in 12 eyes of 10 dissatisfied patients. The main symptoms before surgery were blurry vision, glare/halos, and contrast sensitivity loss. The CDVA and uncorrected distance visual acuity (UDVA) were 20/30 or better in all dissatisfied patients. The median time to IOL exchange after the initial cataract surgery was 13.6 months, and the median follow-up after explantation surgery was 8.9 months. The surgical outcomes were as follows: at 6 months, UDVA was 20/30 or better in 4 eyes and 20/60 or better in 8 eyes. Meanwhile, CDVA at 6 months was 20/20 or better in 8 eyes and 20/25 or better in 9 eyes. Regarding the surgical complications, one eye had corneal decompensation, one eye had IOL dislocation needing another surgery to perform IOL scleral fixation, and one eye had steroid response with elevated IOP. The aim of the surgery was achieved in eight patients who noticed an improvement of their symptoms, whereas the other two patients did not experience any change. We can draw some conclusions from this paper. First, the symptoms leading to the explantation surgery were improved in most of the patients (8 of 10). Second, there was a refractive worsening after the exchange surgery: before surgery, all the eyes had UDVA of 20/30 or better; in contrast, only four eyes achieved this result after the IOL exchange surgery. Third, in two eyes, there were severe complications such as corneal decompensation and IOL dislocation requiring scleral suturing, resulting in steroid response with elevated IOP and cystoid macular edema in the postoperative course.

Kamiya et al. [74] reported a retrospective study that included 50 eyes that required multifocal IOL explantation. Of the explanted multifocal IOLs, 84% were diffractive and 16% were refractive. Monofocal IOLs accounted for 90% of the new implanted IOLs. The most common complaints before explantation surgery were waxy vision (58%), followed by glare and halos (30%), blurred vision at far (24%), dysphotopsia (20%), blurred vision at near (18%), and blurred vision at intermediate (6%). The main objective reasons for explantation were decreased contrast sensitivity (36%), photic phenomena (34%), unknown origin including neuroadaption failure (32%), and incorrect lens power (20%). Patient satisfaction for overall quality of vision was graded on a scale of 1 (very dissatisfied) to 5 (very satisfied). After the IOL exchange surgery, patient satisfaction was significantly increased from 1.22 ± 0.55 preoperatively to 3.78 ± 0.98. The logMAR mean preoperative UDVA and CDVA were 0.23 ± 0.27 and − 0.01 ± 0.16, respectively. Before the explantation surgery, 30% and 68% of the patients had a UDVA and CDVA of 20/20 or better, respectively. The visual outcomes after the explantation surgery showed that 42% and 86% of eyes achieved UDVA and CDVA of 20/20 or better. Contrast sensitivity function also significantly improved after the IOL exchange. The authors state that CDVA is not always a good measure of patient symptoms. In this study, despite visual complaints, CDVA was 20/20 or better in almost 70% of the eyes. Therefore, more specific tests such as contrast sensitivity measurement are needed, especially in those cases with excellent CDVA. Regarding complications, anterior vitrectomy was necessary in three cases (6%). The IOL was placed in the bag in 38 eyes (76%), out of the bag in the sulcus in 11 eyes (22%), and in the sulcus with scleral suture in 1 eye (2%).

Tassignon et al. [101] reported a retrospective case series consisting of 30 eyes of 21 consecutive patients scheduled for MF-IOL exchange with complaints including diplopia, uncomfortable binocular vision, blurred vision, glare, halos (causing an inability for night driving), loss of contrast sensitivity (expressed subjectively by the need of more light during reading), and photophobia in such degree that IOL exchange was deemed to be the only solution. Of the explanted multifocal IOLs, diffractive MF-IOL was more frequently explanted (25, 83%) when compared with refractive MF-IOL (4, 13%) and progressive optic IOL (1, 4%). This depends on the MF-IOL type preferred by the surgeon. The favored technique of IOL implantation in this study was the bag in the lens, which in primary intervention allows for sizing of the anterior capsulorhexis and IOL centration by aligning the Purkinje reflections. In secondary interventions, centration with bag in the lens was not possible, albeit less problematic than when an in-the-bag IOL is implanted. In most eyes with prior Nd:YAG laser capsulotomy, an anterior vitrectomy was necessary to be performed due to vitreous loss because of rupture of the anterior vitreous hyaloid face by the YAG laser. Complications were rare, but in the one eye, a choroidal hemorrhage did occur. In 21 out of the 30 eyes (70%), a bag in the lens could be implanted. In 7 out of the 30 eyes (23%), the capsule was not considered sufficiently stable to accommodate an IOL. An iris-fixated IOL or a sulcus-fixated IOL was then implanted. In 2 out of the 30 eyes (6%), the remaining capsular bag could accommodate a traditional lens in the bag only. Eyes that underwent Nd:YAG laser capsulotomy before the MF-IOL exchange needed anterior vitrectomy (11 eyes, 37%). Visual acuity improved postoperatively in 13 out of the 30 eyes and remained stable in 17 out of the 30 eyes.

Kim et al. [102] in a retrospective case series study of 35 eyes (29 patients) confirmed multifocal IOL exchange can be performed safely with good visual outcomes using different types of IOLs. They implanted different types of IOLs after multifocal IOL explantation including in-the-bag IOLs (74%), iris-sutured IOLs (6%), sulcus-fixated IOLs with optic capture (9%), sulcus-fixated IOLs without optic capture (9%), and anterior chamber IOLs (3%). The surgical indication for exchange included blurred vision (60%), photic phenomena (57%), photophobia (9%), loss of contrast sensitivity (3%), and multiple complaints (29%). The CDVA was 20/40 or better in 94% of eyes before the exchange and 100% of eyes after the exchange. The mean refractive prediction error significantly decreased from 0.22–0.81 diopter (D) before the exchange to 0.09–0.53 D after the exchange ($P < .05$). The median absolute refractive prediction error significantly decreased from 0.43 D before the exchange to 0.23 D after the exchange ($P < .05$).

Kamiya et al. [74] in a retrospective observational study of 50 eyes of 37 patients confirmed that IOL exchange surgery appears to be a feasible surgical option for dissatisfied patients. In this study, the most common complaints about IOL explantation were waxy vision, followed by glare and halos, blurred vision at far, dysphotopsia, blurred vision at near, and blurred vision at intermediate. The most common reasons for IOL explantation were decreased contrast sensitivity, followed by photic phenomena, unknown origin including neuroadaptation failure, incorrect IOL power, preoperative excessive expectation, IOL dislocation/decentration, and anisometropia. The axial length was 25.13 ± 1.83 mm. Of the explanted multifocal IOLs, 84% were diffractive and 16% were refractive. Monofocal IOLs accounted for 90% of the exchanged IOLs. Patient satisfaction was significantly improved from 1.22 ± 0.55 preoperatively to 3.78 ± 0.97 postoperatively, which was graded on a scale of 1 (very dissatisfied) to 5 (very satisfied) (Wilcoxon signed-rank test, $P < .001$).

In conclusion, these papers show that multifocal IOL explantation in dissatisfied patients is a feasible option that significantly improved patient satisfaction. It emphasizes the importance of performing specific tests for accurate assessment of visual function, especially in patients with good visual acuity who complain of poor vision. Decreased contrast sensitivity was found in most of these cases. However, it is important to remember that IOL exchange is not free from complications. In this series, the IOL had to be placed in the ciliary sulcus in 24% of the cases, and anterior vitrectomy was performed in 6% of the eyes.

Conclusions

Intraocular lens explantation is usually a challenging surgery for the anterior segment surgeon as it might be associated with complications. However, it is important to be familiar with the causes for IOL explantation, the prognosis for each of the causes, and the explantation techniques because the number of explanted IOLs is predicted to increase in the future as a result of the growing pseudophakic population. In the vast majority of recent publications, the main cause for IOL explantation is late in-the-bag IOL dislocation years after successful cataract surgery. There are four known types of IOL explantation surgical approaches including whole lens removal, intraocular lens cutting, intraocular lens haptic cutting, and intraocular lens refolding.

The main recognizable risk factors for this condition are pseudoexfoliation and high myopia, the latter being less frequent but affecting younger patients. The IOL explantation surgery in these patients significantly improves their vision (according to data published in most reports), but it is not free of complications. The second most frequently reported cause for explantation is incorrect lens power. In these patients, IOL explantation surgery is usually easier to perform because the ocular structures are intact and because the interval between cataract surgery and explantation is usually shorter. However, it has been shown that LASIK is a safer and more accurate method to correct residual ametropia than IOL explantation; thus, IOL exchange surgery should only be performed to correct large ametropias, when the cornea is not adequate for LASIK or when the surgeon does not have a laser platform available. Intraocular lens opacification is still another important reason for explantation, not only due to old IOL models. In these cases, explantation surgery is very challenging and associated with a significant incidence of complications because the opacification usually occurs many years after cataract surgery and it is subsequently difficult to release the IOL due to the presence of fibrotic tissue.

Finally, multifocality is a known cause of IOL exchange, although, thanks to the improvement in IOL designs, multifocal IOLs are currently well tolerated by patients and the risk of explantation is low, as has been described previously. In

Take-Home Notes

- The main causes for IOL explantation after cataract surgery are dislocation/decentration, incorrect lens power, IOL opacification, neuroadaptation failure, endophthalmitis, and pseudophakic bullous keratopathy.
- There are four main methods of IOL explantation surgical approaches including whole lens removal, intraocular lens cutting, intraocular lens haptic cutting, and intraocular lens refolding.
- LASIK is the most accurate procedure to correct residual ametropia after cataract surgery. Lens-based procedures (IOL explantation or piggyback IOLs) are also effective methods and are recommended as a choice in cases with extreme ametropia and corneal abnormalities or when there is no excimer laser platform available.
- The IOL opacification issue is a relatively old problem, but there are still patients requiring IOL substitution and explantation for this reason. In recent reports, it has been shown that hydro-

philic IOLs, even with a hydrophobic surface, may develop IOL calcification. That may be associated with a history of intraocular gas use or production errors and may be associated with certain medical conditions such as diabetes, hypertension, or glaucoma.

these cases, IOL explantation is usually not very complicated, as it is performed a few months after cataract surgery. Although there are not many case series, patient satisfaction increases significantly after explantation surgery.

Although exchanging MF-IOLs to monofocal IOLs is an accepted approach for neuroadaptation failure, another acceptable approach is an explantation of MF-IOLs due to neuroadaptation failure followed by the reimplantation of a different MF optical technology based on the hypothesis that there may be different neuroadaptation processes for refractive and diffractive IOLs in different patients.

In summary, it is essential for the anterior segment surgeon to know the different reasons that may lead to explantation surgery, to recognize the risk factors, to explain the prognosis of the surgery to the patient, and to perform the best explantation technique, taking into consideration both the cause for the explantation and the IOL model to be explanted.

Financial Support This study has been supported in part by the Red Temática de Investigación Cooperativa en Salud (RETICS), reference number RD16/0008/0012, funded by the Instituto de Salud Carlos III, and co-funded by the European Regional Development Fund (ERDF), "A way to make Europe."

References

1. Alió JL, Fine IH. Minimizing incisions and maximizing outcomes in cataract surgery. Berlin: Springer; 2009. p. 1–319.
2. Stringham J, Werner L, Monson B, et al. Calcification of different designs of silicone intraocular lenses in eyes with asteroid hyalosis. Ophthalmology. 2010;117:1486–92.
3. Foot L, Werner L, Gills JP, et al. Surface calcification of silicone plate intraocular lenses in patients with asteroid hyalosis. Am J Ophthalmol. 2004;137:979–87.
4. Jin GJ, Crandall AS, Jones JJ. Changing indications for and improving outcomes of intraocular lens exchange. Am J Ophthalmol. 2005; 140:688–94.
5. Jakobsson G, Zetterberg M, Lundstrom M, et al. Late dislocation of in-the- bag and out-of-the bag intraocular lenses: ocular and surgical characteristics and time to lens repositioning. J Cataract Refract Surg. 2010;36:1637–44.
6. Clark A, Morlet N, Ng JQ, et al. Whole population trends in complications of cataract surgery over 22 years in Western Australia. Ophthalmology. 2011;118:1055–61.
7. Mamalis N, Crandall AS, Pulsipher MW, et al. Intraocular lens explantation and exchange. A review of lens styles, clinical indications, clinical results, and visual outcome. J Cataract Refract Surg. 1991;17:811–8.
8. Doren GS, Stern GA, Driebe WT. Indications for and results of intraocular lens explantation. J Cataract Refract Surg. 1992;18:79–85.
9. Leaming DV. Practice styles and preferences of ASCRS members--1998 survey. J Cataract Refract Surg. 1999;25:851–9.
10. Leaming DV. Practice styles and preferences of ASCRS members--2000 survey. American Society of Cataract and Refractive Surgery. J Cataract Refract Surg. 2001;27:948–55.
11. Fernández-Buenaga R, Alio JL, Muñoz-Negrete FJ, et al. Causes of IOL explantation in Spain. Eur J Ophthalmol. 2012;22:762–8.
12. Mamalis N, Davis B, Nilson CD, et al. Complications of foldable intraocular lenses requiring explantation or secondary intervention--2003 survey update. J Cataract Refract Surg. 2004;30:2209–22018.
13. Mamalis N, Brubaker J, Davis D, et al. Complications of foldable intraocular lenses requiring explantation or secondary intervention--2007 survey update. J Cataract Refract Surg. 2008;34:1584–91.
14. Hayashi K, Hirata A, Hayashi H. Possible predisposing factors for in- the-bag and out-of-the-bag intraocular lens dislocation and outcomes of intraocular lens exchange surgery. Ophthalmology. 2007;114:969–75.
15. Fernández-Buenaga R, Alio JL, Muñoz-Negrete FJ, Barraquer Compte RI, Alio-Del Barrio JL. Causes of IOL explantation in Spain. Eur J Ophthalmol. 2012;22(5):762–8.
16. Leysen I, Bartholomeeusen E, Coeckelbergh T, et al. Surgical outcomes of intraocular lens exchange: five-year study. J Cataract Refract Surg. 2009;35:1013–8.
17. McCarthy M, Gavanski GM, Paton KE, et al. Intraocular lens power calculations after myopic laser refractive surgery: a comparison of methods in 173 eyes. Ophthalmology. 2010;118:940–4.

18. Savini G, Hoffer KJ, Carbonelli M, et al. Intraocular lens power calculation after myopic excimer laser surgery: clinical comparison of published methods. J Cataract Refract Surg. 2010;36:1455–65.
19. Hamilton DR, Hardten DR. Cataract surgery in patients with prior refractive surgery. Curr Opin Ophthalmol. 2003;14:44–53.
20. Pueringer SL, Hodge DO, Erie JC. Risk of late intraocular lens dislocation after cataract surgery, 1980–2009: a population-based study. Am J Ophthalmol. 2011;152:618–23.
21. Gimbel HV, Condon GP, Kohnen T, et al. Late in-the-bag intraocular lens dislocation: incidence, prevention, and management. J Cataract Refract Surg. 2005;31:2193–204.
22. Jehan FS, Mamalis N, Crandall AS. Spontaneous late dislocation of intraocular lens within the capsular bag in pseudoexfoliation patients. Ophthalmology. 2001;108:1727–31.
23. Gross JG, Kokame GT, Weinberg DV. In-the-bag intraocular lens dislocation. Am J Ophthalmol. 2004;137:630–5.
24. Davis D, Brubaker J, Espandar L, et al. Late in-the-bag spontaneous intraocular lens dislocation: evaluation of 86 consecutive cases. Ophthalmology. 2009;116:664–70.
25. Lorente R, de Rojas V, de Vazquez PP, et al. Management of late spontaneous in-the-bag intraocular lens dislocation: retrospective analysis of 45 cases. J Cataract Refract Surg. 2010;36:1270–82.
26. Lorente R, de Rojas V. Luxación tardía del complejo saco capsular y lente intraocular. In: Lorente R, Mendicute J, editors. Cirugía del Cristalino. Madrid: Sociedad Española de Oftalmología; 2008. p. 1751–67.
27. Davison JA. Capsule contraction syndrome. J Cataract Refract Surg. 1993;19:582–9.
28. Auffarth GU, Tsao K, Wesendahl TA, et al. Centration and fixation of posterior chamber intraocular lenses in eyes with pseudoexfoliation syndrome. An analysis of explanted autopsy eyes. Acta Ophthalmol Scand. 1996;74:463–7.
29. Fernández-Buenaga R, Alio JL, Pérez-Ardoy AL, et al. Late in-the-bag intraocular lens dislocation requiring explantation: risk factors and outcomes. Eye (Lond). 2013;27:795–801.
30. Kokame GT, Yanagihara RT, Shantha JG. Long term outcome of pars plana vitrectomy and sutured scleral-fixated posterior chamber intraocular lens implantation or repositioning. Am J Ophthalmol. 2018;189:10–6.
31. Can E, Koçak N, Yücel ÖE, Gül A, Öztürk HE, Sayin O. Ab-interno scleral suture loop fixation with cow-hitch knot in posterior chamber intraocular lens decentration. Indian J Ophthalmol. 2016;64(2):124–6. https://doi.org/10.4103/0301-4738.179712.
32. Kanski JJ. Clinical ophthalmology. A systematic approach. 6th ed. Edinburgh: Elsevier; 2009.
33. Cheng HM, Singh OS, Kwong KK, et al. Shape of the myopic eye as seen with high-resolution magnetic resonance imaging. Optom Vis Sci. 1992;69:698–701.
34. Wilbrandt HR, Wilbrandt TH. Pathogenesis and management of the lens-iris diaphragm retropulsion syndrome during phacoemulsification. J Cataract Refract Surg. 1994;20:48–53.
35. Faramarzi A, Feizi S, Yazdani S. Trans-iris fixation of dislocated in-the-bag intraocular lenses. Eur J Ophthalmol. 2020;30(3):538–42.
36. Yang S, Nie K, Jiang H, Feng L, Fan W. Surgical management of intraocular lens dislocation: a meta-analysis. PLoS One. 2019;14(2):e0211489.
37. Lagrasta JM, Allemann N, Scapucin L, et al. Clinical results in phacoemulsification using the SRK/T formula. Arq Bras Oftalmol. 2009;72(2):189–93.
38. Cooke DL, Cooke TL. Comparison of 9 intraocular lens power calculation formulas. J Cataract Refract Surg. 2016;42(8):1157–64.
39. Kane JX, Van Heerden A, Atik A, Petsoglou C. Accuracy of 3 new methods for intraocular lens power selection. J Cataract Refract Surg. 2017;43(3):333–9.
40. Aristodemou P, Knox Cartwright NE, Sparrow JM, Johnston RL. Formula choice: Hoffer Q, Holladay 1, or SRK/T and refractive outcomes in 8108 eyes after cataract surgery with biometry by partial coherence interferometry. J Cataract Refract Surg. 2011;37(1):63–71.
41. Holland E, Lane S, Horn JD, Ernest P, Arleo R, Miller KM. The AcrySof Toric intraocular lens in subjects with cataracts and corneal astigmatism: a randomized, subject-masked, parallel-group, 1-year study. Ophthalmology. 2010;117(11):2104–11.
42. Gale RP, Saldana M, Johnston RL, Zuberbuhler B, McKibbin M. Benchmark standards for refractive outcomes after NHS cataract surgery. Eye (Lond). 2009;23(1):149–52.
43. Lee ES, Lee SY, Jeong SY, et al. Effect of postoperative refractive error on visual acuity and patient satisfaction after implantation of the Array multifocal intraocular lens. J Cataract Refract Surg. 2005;31(10):1960–5.
44. Chan CC, Crandall AS, Ahmed II. Ab externo scleral suture loop fixation for posterior chamber intraocular lens decentration: clinical results. J Cataract Refract Surg. 2006;32:121–8.
45. Hoffman RS, Fine IH, Packer M. Scleral fixation without conjunctival dissection. J Cataract Refract Surg. 2006;32:1907–12.
46. Mello MO Jr, Scott IU, Smiddy WE, et al. Surgical management and outcomes of dislocated intraocular lenses. Ophthalmology. 2000;107:62–7.
47. Kelly SP, Jalil A. Wrong intraocular lens implant; learning from reported patient safety incidents. Eye (Lond). 2011;25(6):730–4.
48. Kristianslund O, Råen M, Østern AE, et al. Late in-the-bag intraocular lens dislocation: a randomized clinical trial comparing lens repositioning and lens exchange. Ophthalmology. 2017;124:151–9.

49. Snead MP, Rubinstein MP, Lea SH, et al. Calculated versus A-scan result for axial length using different types of ultrasound probe tip. Eye (Lond). 1990;4(Pt 5):718–22.
50. Kane JX, Van Heerden A, Atik A, Petsoglou C. Intraocular lens power formula accuracy: comparison of 7 formulas. J Cataract Refract Surg. 2016;42(10):1490–500.
51. Stephenson M. Refractive surprises after cataract surgery. Rev Ophthalmol. 2014;21(1):32.
52. Schallhorn SC, Venter JA, Teenan D, et al. Outcomes of excimer laser enhancements in pseudophakic patients with multifocal intraocular lens. Clin Ophthalmol. 2016;10:765–76.
53. Jin GJ, Merkley KH, Crandall AS, et al. Laser in situ keratomileusis versus lens-based surgery for correcting residual refractive error after cataract surgery. J Cataract Refract Surg. 2008;34:562–9.
54. Fernández-Buenaga R, Alió JL, Pérez Ardoy AL, et al. Resolving refractive error after cataract surgery: IOL exchange, piggyback lens, or LASIK. J Refract Surg. 2013;29:676–83.
55. Sharma T, Chawdhary S. The opalescence of hydrogel intraocular lens. Eye (Lond). 2001;15:97–8.
56. Apple DJ, Werner L, Pandey SK. Newly recognized complications of posterior chamber intraocular lenses. Arch Ophthalmol. 2001;119: 581–2.
57. Werner L, Apple DJ, Kaskaloglu M, et al. Dense opacification of the optical component of a hydrophilic acrylic intraocular lens: a clinicopathological analysis of 9 explanted lenses. J Cataract Refract Surg. 2001;27:1485–92.
58. Werner L. Causes of intraocular lens opacification or discoloration. J Cataract Refract Surg. 2007;33:713–26.
59. Werner L, Apple DJ, Escobar-Gomez M, et al. Postoperative deposition of calcium on the surfaces of a hydrogel intraocular lens. Ophthalmology. 2000;107:2179–85.
60. Pandey SK, Werner L, Apple DJ, et al. Calcium precipitation on the optical surfaces of a foldable intraocular lens: a clinicopathological correlation. Arch Ophthalmol. 2002;120:391–3.
61. Tehrani M, Mamalis N, Wallin T, et al. Late postoperative opacification of MemoryLens hydrophilic acrylic intraocular lenses: case series and review. J Cataract Refract Surg. 2004;30:115–22.
62. Frohn A, Dick HB, Augustin AJ, et al. Late opacification of the foldable hydrophilic acrylic lens SC60B-OUV. Ophthalmology. 2001;108:1999–2004.
63. Werner L, Hunter B, Stevens S, et al. Role of silicon contamination on calcification of hydrophilic acrylic intraocular lenses. Am J Ophthalmol. 2006;141:35–43.
64. Izak AM, Werner L, Pandey SK, et al. Calcification of modern foldable hydrogel intraocular lens designs. Eye (Lond). 2003;17:393–406.
65. Dhital A, Spalton DJ, Goyal S, et al. Calcification in hydrophilic intraocular lenses associated with injection of intraocular gas. Am J Ophthalmol. 2012;153:1154–60.
66. Bompastor-Ramos P, Póvoa J, Lobo C, et al. Late postoperative opacification of hydrophilic-hydrophobic acrylic intraocular lens. J Cataract Surg. 2016;42:1324–31.
67. Michelson J, Werner L, Ollerton A, et al. Light scattering and light transmittance in intraocular lenses explanted because of optic opacification. J Cataract Refract Surg. 2012;38:1476–85.
68. Fernández-Buenaga R, Alió JL, Pinilla-Cortés L, et al. Perioperative complications and clinical outcomes of intraocular lens exchange in patients with opacified lenses. Graefes Arch Clin Exp Ophthalmol. 2013;251:2141–6.
69. Yu AK, Ng AS. Complications and clinical outcomes of intraocular lens exchange in patients with calcified hydrogel lenses. J Cataract Refract Surg. 2002;28:1217–22.
70. Gashau AG, Anand A, Chawdhary S. Hydrophilic acrylic intraocular lens exchange: five-year experience. J Cataract Refract Surg. 2006;32:1340–4.
71. Dagres E, Khan MA, Kyle GM, et al. Perioperative complications of intraocular lens exchange in patients with opacified Aqua-Sense lenses. J Cataract Refract Surg. 2004;30:2569–73.
72. Dahlmann AH, Dhingra N, Chawdhary S. Acrylic lens exchange for late opacification of the optic. J Cataract Refract Surg. 2002;28:1713–4.
73. Galor A, Gonzalez M, Goldman D, et al. Intraocular lens exchange surgery in dissatisfied patients with refractive intraocular lenses. J Cataract Refract Surg. 2009;35:1706–10.
74. Kamiya K, Hayashi K, Shimizu K, et al. Multifocal intraocular lens explantation: a case series of 50 eyes. Am J Ophthalmol. 2014;158:215–20.
75. Kermani O, Gerten G. Explantation of multifocal intraocular lenses. Klin Monatsbl Augenheilkd. 2016;233:928–32.
76. Leyland M, Pringle E. Multifocal versus monofocal intraocular lenses after cataract extraction. Cochrane Database Syst Rev. 2006;(3):CD003169. https://doi.org/10.1002/14651858. CD003169. pub2.
77. Venter JA, Pelouskova M, Collins BM, Schallhorn SC, Hannan SJ. Visual outcomes and patient satisfaction in 9366 eyes using a refractive segmented multifocal intraocular lens. J Cataract Refract Surg. 2013;39:1477–84.
78. Dissatisfaction after implantation of multifocal intraocular lenses. J Cataract Refract Surg. 2011;37:859–65.
79. Dissatisfaction after multifocal intraocular lens implantation. J Cataract Refract Surg. 2009;35:992–7.
80. Alio JL, Plaza-Puche AB, Férnandez-Buenaga R, Pikkel J, Maldonado M. Multifocal intraocular lenses: An overview. Surv Ophthalmol. 2017;62(5):611–34.

81. Rosen E, Alió JL, Dick HB, Dell S, Slade S. Efficacy and safety of multifocal intraocular lenses following cataract and refractive lens exchange: meta-analysis of peer-reviewed publications. J Cataract Refract Surg. 2016;42:310–28.
82. Alió JL, Pikkel J. Multifocal intraocular lenses: the art and the practice. Essentials in ophthalmology. Switzerland: Springer International Publishing; 2014.
83. Findl O, Buehl W, Bauer P, Sycha T. Interventions for preventing posterior capsule opacification. Cochrane Database Syst Rev. 2010:CD003738.
84. Alio JL, Colecha JR, Pastor S, Rodriguez A, Artola A. Symptomatic dry eye treatment with autologous platelet-rich plasma. Ophthalmic Res. 2007;39:124–9.
85. Kawamorita T, Uozato H. Modulation transfer function and pupil size in multifocal and monofocal intraocular lenses *in vitro*. J Cataract Refract Surg. 2005;31:2379–85.
86. Prieto PM, Vargas-Martín F, Goelz S, Artal P. Analysis of the performance of the Hartmann-Shack sensor in the human eye. J Opt Soc Am A Opt Image Sci Vis. 2000;17:1388–98.
87. Soda M, Yaguchi S. Effect of decentration on the optical performance in multifocal intraocular lenses. Ophthalmologica. 2012;227:197–204.
88. Cillino S, Casuccio A, Di Pace F, Morreale R, Pillitteri F, Cillino G, Lodato G. One-year outcomes with new-generation multifocal intraocular lenses. Ophthalmology. 2008;115:1508–151.
89. Hayashi K, Hayashi H, Nakao F, Hayashi F. Correlation between pupillary size and intraocular lens decentration and visual acuity of a zonal-progressive multifocal lens and a monofocal lens. Ophthalmology. 2001;108:2011–7.
90. Rosa A, Miranda Â, Patrício M, McAlinden C, Silva F, Murta J, et al. Functional magnetic resonance imaging to assess the neurobehavioral impact of Dysphotopsia with multifocal intraocular lenses. Ophthalmology. 2017;124(9):1280–9.
91. Rosa A, Miranda Â, Patrício M, McAlinden C, Silva F, Castelo-Branco M, et al. Functional magnetic resonance imaging to assess neuroadaptation to multifocal intraocular lenses. J Cataract Refract Surg. 2017;43(10):1287–96. 623.
92. Al-Shymali O, McAlinden C, Alio Del Barrio JL, Canto-Cerdan M, Alio JL. Patients' dissatisfaction with multifocal intraocular lenses managed by exchange with other multifocal lenses of different optical profiles. Eye Vis (Lond). 2022;1;9(1):8.
93. Henderson BA, Yang EB. Intraocular lens explantation technique for one- piece acrylic lenses. J Refract Surg. 2012;28:499–502.
94. Koo EY, Lindsey PS, Soukiasian SH. Bisecting a foldable acrylic intraocular lens for explantation. J Cataract Refract Surg. 1996;22(Suppl 2):1381–2.
95. Batlan SJ, Dodick JM. Explantation of a foldable silicone intraocular lens. Am J Ophthalmol. 1996;122:270–2.
96. Mehta JS, Wilkins MR, Gartry DS. Explantation of an acrylic Acrysof intraocular lens without wound enlargement. Acta Ophthalmol Scand. 2005;83:262–3.
97. Por YM, Chee SP. Trisection technique: a 2-snip approach to intraocular lens explantation. J Cataract Refract Surg. 2007;33:1151–4.
98. Marques FF, Marques DM, Smith CM, et al. Intraocular lens exchange assisted by preoperative neodymium:YAG laser haptic fracture. J Cataract Refract Surg. 2004;30:247–9.
99. Geggel HS. Simplified technique for acrylic intraocular lens explantation. Ophthalmic Surg Lasers. 2000;31:506–7.
100. Neuhann TH. Intraocular folding of an acrylic lens for explantation through a small incision cataract wound. J Cataract Refract Surg. 1996;22(Suppl 2):1383–6.
101. Tassignon MJ, Bartholomeeusen E, Rozema JJ, Jongenelen S, Mathysen DG. Feasibility of multifocal intra-ocular lens exchange and conversion to the bag-in-the-lens implantation. Acta Ophthalmol. 2014;92(3):265–9.
102. Kim EJ, Sajjad A, Montes de Oca I, Koch DD, Wang L, Weikert MP, Al-Mohtaseb ZN. Refractive outcomes after multifocal intraocular lens exchange. J Cataract Refract Surg. 2017;43(6):761–6.

19 Cataract Surgery in Uveitis

Bahram Bodaghi, Thierry Burtin, and Phuc LeHoang

Bullet Points

In this chapter, we will discuss the following:

- The risk factors that must be considered before cataract surgery in patients with uveitis
- Special features of cataract surgery in this group of patients
- The importance of perioperative medical treatment
- Main complications and their management
- The challenging case of cataract surgery in children with uveitis

Modern surgical management of cataract in uveitis has been dramatically improved based on recent technological advances [1, 2], but its general practice remains controversial [3]. Indeed, despite the progress in the surgical procedure, there are many medical protocols governing the perioperative period. It is also a relatively common situation that many ophthalmologists would come to deal with [4]. Cataract is a major complication of uveitis, occurring in 50–80% of cases, all etiologies combined [5]. It occurs in anterior uveitis, mainly by a direct inflammatory mechanism, and in posterior uveitis more often by an iatrogenic mechanism linked to the extensive or prolonged use of corticosteroids. The number of steroid-induced cataracts in uveitis is constantly increasing, especially with the recent use of intravitreal corticosteroid implants, which have obtained an approval for the treatment of predominantly intermediate, posterior, or total noninfectious uveitis [6, 7].

A surgical procedure such as phacoemulsification may generate a certain degree of inflammation, increasing with the difficulty of the intervention and the preexisting associated lesions. It becomes even more challenging in the context of uveitis as it is performed on an eye with a higher risk of postoperative inflammatory flare-up. There are two closely related levels of care: on the one hand, surgical, currently well-standardized and reproducible, and, on the other hand, medical, more controversial by its level of complexity but also the absence of evidence-based data. Each of these strategies must be evaluated and adapted to the different preoperative, perioperative, and postoperative steps.

Supplementary Information The online version contains supplementary material available at [https://doi.org/10.1007/978-3-030-94530-5_19].

B. Bodaghi (✉) · T. Burtin · P. LeHoang
Department of Ophthalmology, IHU FOReSIGHT, Sorbonne-APHP, Paris, France

J. L. Alió et al. (eds.), *Cataract Surgery*, Essentials in Ophthalmology,
https://doi.org/10.1007/978-3-030-94530-5_19

Preoperative Time

Surgical Evaluation

Before operating a patient with cataract and uveitis, it is necessary to ensure that the lens opacities are indeed the main cause of the visual loss, by carrying out a careful and complete examination which will determine the absence of other associated causes or complications, such as:

- Active inflammation (anterior or posterior)
- Corneal and/or vitreous opacities
- Macular involvement (edema, epiretinal membrane, hole, atrophy, ischemia, or choroidal neovascularization)
- Optic neuropathy or atrophy
- Secondary glaucoma

It is also necessary to focus on identifying the elements that may represent intraoperative difficulties, because, if anticipated, the management will be better adapted during surgery. The elements that may become challenging during the procedure are:

- Extended band keratopathy
- The presence of posterior synechiae or fibrotic cyclitic membrane in the pupillary area
- The importance and type of cataract

Combined cataract and glaucoma surgery remains controversial given the risk of failure of filtering surgery. It is rather advisable to control the pressure before proceeding with phacoemulsification.

Medical Evaluation

Even though well-standardized, the major difficulty in the surgical management of uveitic cataract lies in the medical control of ocular inflammation, as well as the choice of the most appropriate moment to schedule surgery. Sometimes ocular inflammation is triggered by lens proteins inducing lens-induced or phacogenic uveitis [8]. Surgery on an "inflammatory" eye has a high potential for severe relapse, on the anterior and posterior segments, which could threaten postoperative visual recovery. It is essential to control preoperative inflammation as best as possible; otherwise, the risk of severe inflammatory complications will increase, and the final visual prognosis will be affected. The control of inflammation is evaluated on anterior chamber flare and cells according to the SUN (Standardization of Uveitis Nomenclature) criteria [9].

A 3-month minimum period of quiescence (stable or inactive inflammation according to the SUN) is consensually required for any cataract surgery in a patient with uveitis. In addition, recent experience shows that a certain number of pejorative risk factors must be sought during the preoperative examination in order to adapt the best postoperative prevention protocol.

Risk Factor # 1: Etiology of Uveitis

Some types of uveitis are at greater risk than others (Figs. 19.1 and 19.2) (Table 19.1). Thus, birdshot retinochoroidopathy is at a lower risk of inflammatory relapse [10] than active juvenile idiopathic arthritis (JIA)-associated uveitis [11]. Fuchs uveitis does not require any special protocol and is usually considered as a nonuveitic cataract [1]. However, early inflammatory reactions are still possible with the presence of giant cells on the implant. In general, the importance of anterior synechiae is the major prognostic ele-

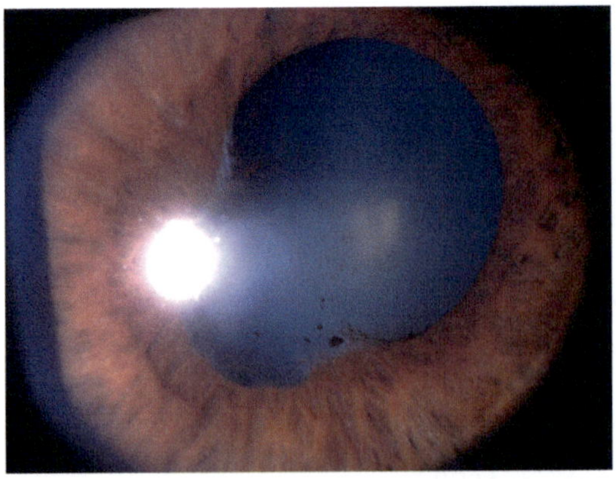

Fig. 19.1 Dense cataract in a patient with Behçet's disease

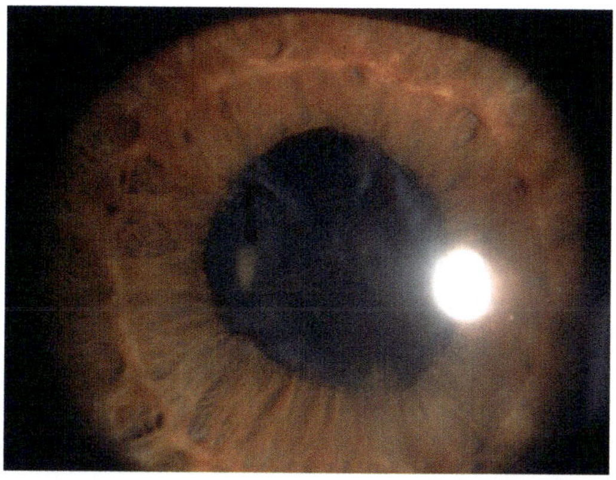

Fig. 19.2 Cataract and extensive posterior synechiae in a young child with JIA-associated uveitis

Table 19.1 Postoperative risk of complications associated with different etiologies of uveitis

High	JIA-uveitis Late-stage severe VKH disease Sarcoidosis (anterior) Tuberculosis (anterior) Syphilis (anterior) Idiopathic chronic anterior uveitis
Moderate	Behçet's disease B27-uveitis Posner-Schlossman disease HSV-VZV uveitis Acute retinal necrosis syndrome Multiple sclerosis Sympathetic ophthalmia Fuchs uveitis
Mild	Toxoplasmic retinochoroiditis Birdshot retinochoroiditis White dot syndromes

ment for further glaucomatous complications. *It is obvious that all cases with extensive posterior synechiae such as JIA-associated uveitis, sarcoidosis, tuberculosis, and late Vogt-Koyanagi-Harada disease are at high postoperative risk of relapse. They deserve a close follow-up in order to adapt the therapeutic strategy.*

Risk Factor # 2: Degree of Anterior Chamber Inflammation

The degree of inflammation of the anterior and posterior segments should be clinically assessed. Slit-lamp examination is mandatory to evaluate the number of cells in the anterior chamber. Breakdown of the blood-aqueous barrier (BAB) is important to identify cases of chronic inflammation. The aforementioned SUN criteria will be used to define whether uveitis is stable or not.

Cataract surgery causes a breakdown of the BAB promoting postoperative relapses. The barrier can be defective even before surgery, especially in cases of chronic or recurrent anterior uveitis. A defective preoperative barrier is a risk of stronger inflammatory flare-up. Signs in favor of a breakdown of the BAB associated with chronic inflammation are the presence of AC flare or cells even though uveitis is not significantly active. In case of chronic inflammation that cannot be improved, surgery is not contraindicated as long as this level of inflammation is stable for at least 3 months. Laser flare photometry is a major tool for the accurate evaluation of AC flare. It is an excellent, objective, and reproducible witness of the BAB status. Measurement is noninvasive and rapid to perform [12]. In the absence of a chronic rupture of the BAB, a value above 30 photons/milliseconds represents an increased risk of postoperative inflammatory relapse.

Risk Factor # 3: Presence or History of Macular Edema

Before any surgery performed in a patient followed for uveitis, the presence or history of macular edema (OM) should be evaluated. This indicates an active inflammation and contraindicates cataract surgery as long as ME is not fully controlled. A history of ME is a marker of the severity of uveitis and therefore a greater risk of severe relapse. Close follow-up is highly recommended in these patients [13].

The posterior segment assessment may be limited by the extent of posterior synechiae and/or cataract density. B-mode ultrasound will be mandatory in order to exclude a retinal detachment.

Risk Factor # 4: Use of a DMARD (Disease-Modifying Antirheumatic Drug)

Uveitis requiring substantial background treatment to control inflammation is considered severe, whatever the cause, and as such should benefit from a prevention protocol adapted to an increased risk of recurrence.

Risk Factor # 5: History of Inflammatory Relapse in the First Operated Eye

Caution will then be required since the same complication could occur in the second eye in patients with bilateral uveitis. A 3-month quiescence period is mandatory, although it may be reduced for some etiologies. Since cataract is not a surgical emergency (apart from lens-induced uveitis or the risk of amblyopia in children), all inflammatory parameters should be controlled as much as possible before surgery.

The eye must be quiet for a minimal period of 3 months prior to cataract surgery. Ocular inflammation is evaluated by slit-lamp examination, OCT, and laser flare photometry if available. Prevention of postoperative flare-up is achieved by the use of systemic or local corticosteroids. The strategy will be discussed on a case-to-case basis (Cf *below II-2).*

Interoperative Time

Surgical Strategy

The surgical procedure is fully standardized. Extracapsular extraction by phacoemulsification and implantation in the bag, under local anesthesia, is used as for conventional surgery in an adult patient. The incision size is reduced in order to decrease the level of BAB breakdown. Capsulorhexis should be relatively large, and the optic diameter should be at least 6 mm to maintain proper access to the fundus. Hydrophobic acrylic implants are preferred, preventing granulocyte adhesion and therefore less secondary capsular opacification, requiring early Nd:YAG laser treatment [14–16]. New generation of heparin surface-modified IOLs may improve postoperative reactions especially in patients with Fuchs uveitis. *In young patients with uveitis, multifocal or extended depth-of-focus (EDOF) IOLs are an important and tempting issue to consider. Even though progress has been made on this type of technology, caution is required. To date, evidence on long-term tolerance of multifocal or EDOF IOLs is lacking. A few papers in the literature are reporting challenging cases of displaced or dislocated lenses. Explantation is much more difficult in patients with a history of uveitis and may induce major sight-threatening complications. It is important to consider that astigmatism correcting intraocular lenses may be used in selected cases.* The posterior capsule must be polished with care in order to reduce the risk of posterior capsule opacification while preserving its integrity.

The choice of intraocular implants in uveitis remains controversial, especially in children. It depends above all on:

- The patient's age
- The type of uveitis
- Its severity
- The evolving profile
- The importance of complications of the anterior segment (synechiae, glaucoma)
- The condition of the posterior segment when accessible (vitrectomized eye, presence of silicone oil)

What will differ from classic cataract surgery depends on whether or not there are clinical elements related to chronic inflammation:

- Presence of advanced band keratopathy: An EDTA corneal treatment will then be carried out, preceding the extraction of the lens in order to obtain sufficient visibility to secure the procedure. Some prefer to perform the scraping a few weeks before or, if necessary, after phacoemulsification.
- Presence of posterior synechiae: Simple release of the synechiae using viscoelastic products with, if necessary, placement of iris hooks or more recently Malyugin ring [17, 18]. The softer and more atraumatic this gesture, the less risk there is of a postoperative inflammatory relapse [19]. Sphincterotomies are generally not recommended because in addition to the inflammatory risk, they can cause bleeding of varying intensities.
- Presence of a cyclitic membrane in the pupillary area: It is essential to identify and must be

carefully removed before the release of posterior synechiae or the installation of the hooks under penalty of tearing of the iris sphincter and major postoperative pupillary alterations.

Medical Strategy

There are different trials studying cataract surgery in uveitic patients, but only a few of them have provided an update on the intraoperative medical protocol for the prevention of inflammatory relapse. Perioperative oral corticosteroids (before and after surgery) have been prescribed frequently for over 60 years, but their dose and duration remain controversial. They are increasingly associated with or replaced by a local injection of corticosteroids at the end of the surgical period (Table 19.2).

There are two types of molecules:

- Corticosteroids with an immediate effect:
  - Dexamethasone, which can be used subconjunctival or peribulbar
- Sustained-release corticosteroids which may be offered, depending on the series, preoperatively, interoperatively, or postoperatively:
  - Subtenon or subconjunctival triamcinolone
  - Intravitreal dexamethasone implant: Ozurdex® [20]

Table 19.2 Perioperative management of ocular inflammation in a uveitic patient undergoing cataract surgery

Preoperative	Prednisone : 0.5 mg/kg/d 3d prior to surgery Or Intravitreal Ozurdex/Subtenon TM 1 month prior to surgery Valaciclovir: 3g/d 3 to 1 week prior to surgery Antibiotics for toxoplasmosis (controversial)
Intraoperative	For noninfectious uveitis Pulse of methylprednisolone (4mg/kg) Subconjunctival corticosteroid
Postoperative	Progressive tapering of topical corticosteroids adapted to immediate postoperative inflammation Tapering of systemic corticosteroids based on clinical evaluation

Studies have been carried out to compare these different protocols either with each other or against perioperative corticosteroid therapy alone. In 2010, a trial compared a group with 1 month of oral cortisone ½ mg/kg/day postoperatively versus a peribulbar injection of delayed corticosteroids at the end of surgery, in patients with chronic noninfectious uveitis. The results showed no significant difference in visual acuity, in the rate of postoperative complications (anterior uveitis or macular edema), or in secondary glaucoma.

Topical rather than oral use was considered ideal for patients with metabolic diseases such as diabetes which may be decompensated by systemic corticosteroids [21].

Before the second decade of the century, many teams have studied intravitreal triamcinolone at the end of surgery (Kenacort®: 0.1 ml/4 mg of triamcinolone). In 2007, Dada et al. compared intraoperative IVT of triamcinolone versus oral corticosteroid therapy during cataract surgery for chronic anterior and intermediate uveitis. They did not find a significant difference in the postoperative inflammatory relapse, but they deplored more ocular hypertension in the IVT group [22].

Okhravi also showed good results in 17 patients followed for chronic uveitis and treated with intraoperative IVT triamcinolone instead of oral corticosteroids. The result on postoperative inflammation was similar, but the rate of ocular hypertension was higher in the triamcinolone group even though it was controlled by topical treatment [23].

Thus, intravitreous triamcinolone compared to oral corticosteroids seems effective on the gain of visual acuity and the prevention of risk of inflammatory relapse in cataract surgery on uveitis, but it is necessary to deplore more postoperative IOP increase, controlled by local treatment. It is important to emphasize that triamcinolone does not have an approval for intravitreal use.

In another study comparing corticosteroids, Roesel et al. showed an equally effective action of the intravitreal route as the peribulbar route on postoperative inflammation, as well as a greater reduction in the rate of macular edema by the intravitreal route, with an incidence of side effects comparable in both cases [21].

The injection of triamcinolone was also studied intracameral at the end of surgery, against the protocol of intravenous methylprednisolone corticosteroid therapy, in a group of juvenile idiopathic arthritis-associated (JIA) uveitis. Li et al. showed the superiority of intracameral cortisone versus oral or intravenous corticosteroid therapy on the risk of postoperative inflammatory rebound [24].

A recent study has shown that an intraoperative injection of a sustained-release intravitreous implant of 750 µg of dexamethasone, Ozurdex®, did not prevent the postoperative formation of fibrin in the anterior chamber. But it showed that by preventively injecting the second eye 5 days before surgery, there was no postoperative inflammatory reaction. Thus, Ozurdex® could represent, in preoperative injection better than in intraoperative, an additional therapeutic tool in the arsenal of prevention of inflammatory rebound in cataract surgeries on uveitis [20]. A randomized study seems necessary to corroborate this hypothesis.

The best timing for the use of Ozurdex® and full effectiveness seems to be a month prior to lens removal.

Another more recent study showed the effectiveness of the same Ozurdex® implant placed 1 month before cataract surgery in a 6-year-old child suffering from uveitis in the context of JIA, treated with adalimumab (anti-TNF alpha). This implant was used alone as prevention of inflammatory relapse, and the follow-up at 10 months was satisfactory without side effects. However, it should be remembered that in many countries, Ozurdex® does not have approval in children.

We therefore currently have multiple therapeutic tools to control inflammation in cataract surgery on uveitis. The difficulty still lies in the choice of the protocol according to the patient and his clinical condition.

Postoperative Time

The major difference with conventional cataract surgery is the increased risk of postoperative inflammation in the uveitis population [25]. The various complications to be feared include:

Inflammatory Recurrences

This is an upsurge in inflammation of the anterior segment: increased number of cells or flare by more than 2+ compared to the preoperative state, according to the SUN criteria (Fig. 19.3). At a more severe stage, it may be associated with the formation of iridocapsular synechiae with a risk of angle closure glaucoma *(iris bombé). This complication occurs mainly in the postoperative month, but preliminary signs may be detected as early as first hours after surgery.* It is considered that if an inflammatory relapse occurs more than 3 months after surgery, it is not related to surgery but rather to the progression of the inflammatory disease. In the absence of endophthalmitis and in acute situations, intracameral injection of thrombolytics such as rt-PA (recombinant tissue-plasminogen activator) allows a very rapid cleansing of the inflammatory reaction [26].

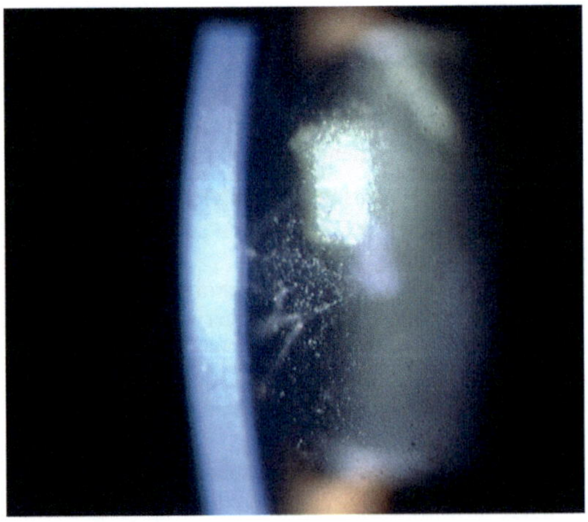

Fig. 19.3 Early postoperative flare-up in a patient with anterior uveitis

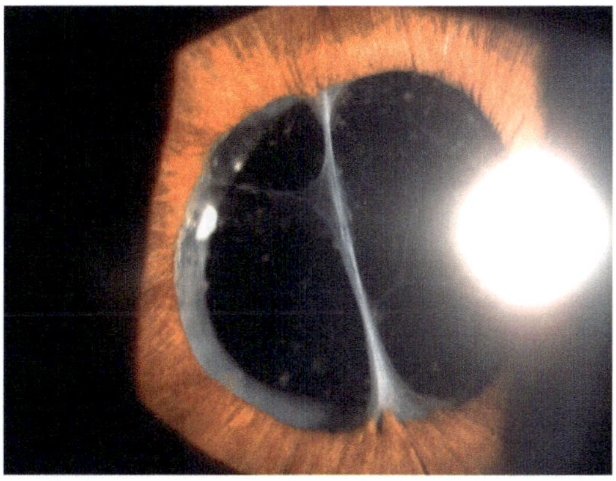

Fig. 19.4 Pupillary fibrosis complicating an acute postoperative relapse

Pupillary fibrosis may result from severe postoperative inflammation (Fig. 19.4).

Ocular Hypertension and Glaucoma

This is a mild complication if detected early enough but can be very serious if treated late. It is potentially more common in patients with uveitis, due to secondary inflammation and as they receive cortisone-based anti-inflammatory prevention protocols. Postoperative elevated IOP rates vary between 4.6% and 28.9% [25, 27]. Close follow-up allows the clinician to detect high IOP and to act rapidly. Glaucoma is more frequent in patients with Fuchs uveitis and other conditions associated with anterior synechiae.

Macular Edema

It is defined by a relative increase in retinal thickness assessed by OCT, with or without the presence of cysts and reduction or not in visual acuity (clinical or subclinical macular edema) [28]. It is the essential element of the visual functional prognosis in the postoperative period.

It occurs in 33–56% of cases in inflammatory patients after cataract surgery [29, 30].

Its risk can be reduced by careful control of preoperative inflammation with corticosteroids, as well as observing a period of inflammatory quiescence of at least 3 months [13]. The place of topical NSAIDs remains controversial.

Endophthalmitis

It is one of the most frightening complications of classic cataract surgery. Its frequency would theoretically be greater in cataract surgery in patients with uveitis, probably because many of these patients are under immunosuppressive or immunomodulatory treatments. The antiseptic rules must therefore be all the stricter, as well as systematic intraoperative antibiotic prophylaxis.

Posterior Capsule Opacification (PCO)

It remains a common complication (Fig. 19.5), occurring in nearly half of the patients after 2 years [25]. The incidence is correlated with the duration of follow-up [29]. The mean period between surgery and PCO seems to be 15 months, even though it may occur very rapidly if uveitis is not fully controlled. One-piece hydrophobic acrylic IOLs significantly reduce the rate of PCO. Fuchs uveitis, Behçet's disease, and rheumatological uveitis seem to be at a higher risk. Nd:YAG laser posterior capsulotomy should not be performed before the first semester and requires a quiet eye as relapses may occur.

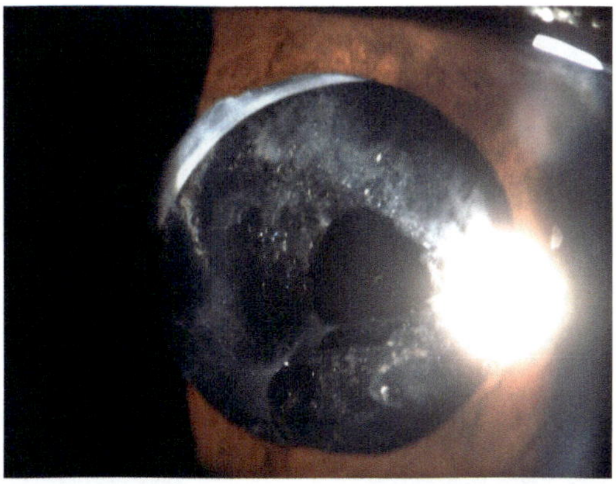

Fig. 19.5 Nd:YAG laser treatment of a posterior capsule opacification in a patient with idiopathic granulomatous anterior uveitis

Inflammatory relapses seem to be rare [31]. Late obstruction by the visual axis by freed lens cortex is a differential diagnosis (Fig. 19.6). Laser therapy is inefficient and surgical aspiration is mandatory.

Late Dislocation of in-the-Bag Intraocular Lens

Late subluxation or dislocation of an intraocular lens is a rare but serious event occurring in 2–16% of cases [32, 33]. It is mainly associated with zonular weakness associated with different types of uveitis (Fig. 19.7) or contraction of the capsular bag [32]. Surgery is not immediately required in mild cases, but repositioning by scleral suture or new IOL implantation (scleral sutured or iris-claw) may be necessary [34–36]. The decision must be made on a case-to-case basis. In some patients, explantation and aphakia remain the best alternative.

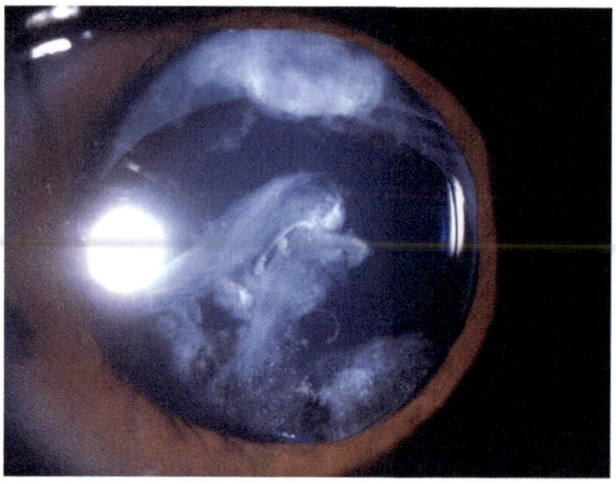

Fig. 19.6 Late obstruction of the visual axis by freed lens cortex in a patient with chronic anterior uveitis

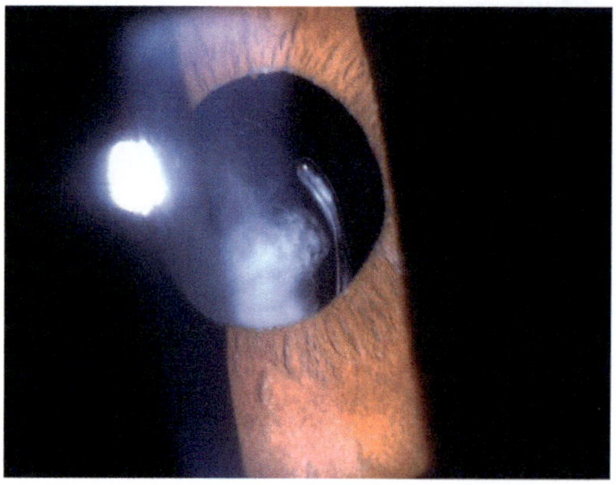

Fig. 19.7 Late dislocation of in-the-bag intraocular lens in a case of tuberculous uveitis

Postoperative follow-up consultations should be more frequent in patients followed for uveitis because of the increased risk of inflammatory relapse. To date, there are no recommendations regarding the pace of postoperative follow-up. In practice, a checkup on D1, D8, M1, M3, and M6 seems reasonable in the absence of any functional symptom giving rise to fear of an inflammatory complication. Currently, the functional results of cataract surgery on an inflammatory eye tend to be ever better in relation to strict control of inflammation before surgery, as well as continuous improvement in surgical techniques.

At each checkup, the following elements will be monitored:

- The BCVA
- The intraocular pressure
- The degree of inflammation of the aqueous humor (with, if possible, measurement of the flare)
- The correct position and stability of the implant
- The state of the vitreous and the retina (macular edema will be detected by OCT)

Prevention of postoperative inflammation is based primarily on a topical combination of corticosteroids/antibiotics for a period of 2–4 weeks, as well as topical nonsteroidal anti-inflammatory drugs for 4–6 weeks. To this can be added gradually decreasing oral corticosteroid therapy. It should be noted above all not to forget to continue the basic treatment as cataract surgery does not reduce the risk of developing postoperative uveitis, apart from the exceptional case of Fuchs uveitis. *Recent studies have shown the safety of cataract surgery when risk factors have been identified and anti-inflammatory procedures appropriately followed* [25, 37]. *However, it is interesting to highlight the importance of risk factors that may lead to postoperative complications. A recent study performed in the UK has identified patients of Asian and Afro-Caribbean ethnicity, small intraoperative pupil size, use of iris hooks or Malyugin ring, and posterior capsule rupture as challenging situations, requiring early assessment and aggressive management of postoperative relapses.*

Challenging Situations

Childhood Uveitis

These uveitis are rarely accompanied by functional complaints and are therefore potentially serious [38]. Rheumatic diseases are the most common etiologies, especially juvenile idiopathic arthritis. The prevention of ocular damage in children at risk and the increasingly early treatment including biologic agents explain the significant decrease in the incidence of ocular complications [39]. However, cataract remains a common complication of rheumatic uveitis in children [40]. These uveitis are associated with the two main types of conditions, JIA and juvenile spondyloarthropathies (JSA). JIA is arguably the most insidious etiology of uveitis in children. It occurs preferably during the oligoarticular form of the disease in young girls. It is generally of anterior topography, chronic evolution, and non-granulomatous type.

Cataract and glaucoma are the two main complications of uveitis in children. They are sometimes the consequence of an inadequate and prolonged corticosteroid therapy [41]. The surgical management of complications must take several factors into consideration [16, 42, 43]. It is preferably performed, when possible, on a quiet eye for at least 3 months. It is associated with general and local corticosteroid therapy. This will be strengthened if necessary. The surgical technique depends on the type of uveitis and the presence of chronic hypotonia by involvement of the ciliary processes. Pars plana lensectomy and vitrectomy are mainly offered when:

- Uveitis is linked to JIA.
- The child is less than 5 years old.
- There is chronic hypotonia witnessing an inflammatory membrane inducing detachment of the ciliary body.

It should be emphasized that implantation is not recommended in the case of uveitis associated with JIA and occurring in early childhood (below the age of 5), except in special cases (unilateral uveitis, social problems making lens adaptation impossible). For older children or when it is not a case of uveitis associated with JIA, conventional phacoemulsification may be performed. Iris hooks or Malyugin ring will be used when necessary. When the age of the children and the local condition allow it, an implantation is possible under good conditions [44–46]. The hydrophobic acrylic implant must be placed in the bag after posterior capsulorhexis and anterior vitrectomy in young children. Extremely rigorous postoperative monitoring is mandatory. The inflammatory flare-up can be particularly violent and result in definite blindness, if not treated early and aggressively. It is therefore essential to continue an anti-inflammatory treatment regimen and, if necessary, an immunosuppressive drug or a biologic agent. Laser flare photometry has revolutionized the monitoring of children who have had surgery and implantation. The treatment is modulated in an objective manner and avoids any overdosing or therapeutic insufficiency. The deposition of giant cells on the surface of the implant is also evidence of the BAB breakdown. Finally, Elschnig pearls readily occur several months or years after surgery and generally do not affect the quality of vision (Fig. 19.8). Laser flare photometry is a useful tool for the assessment of postoperative inflammatory flare-up and the precise tapering of corticosteroids [47].

Cataract Surgery and Viral Uveitis

Cataract surgery in patients with viral ocular inflammation has benefited from advances in microsurgery and the efficacy of the antiviral therapeutic strategies. HSV and VZV remain the two main agents responsible for ocular involve-

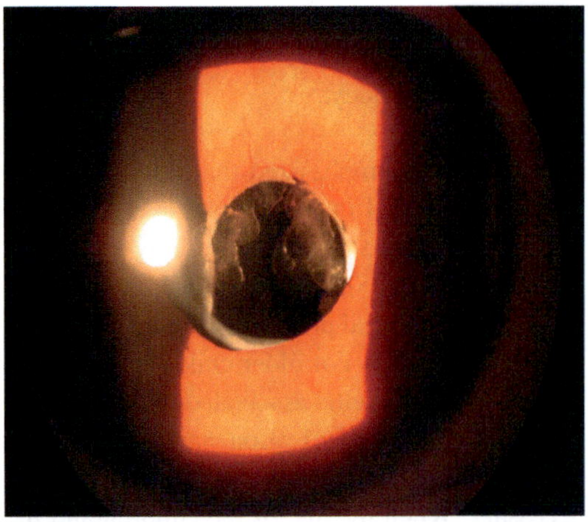

Fig. 19.8 Favorable post-surgical outcome in a 7-year-old girl with severe chronic anterior uveitis. VA is 20/20 10 years after surgery, despite extensive posterior irido-capsular synechiae and Elschnig's pearls

ment in immunocompetent patients, but CMV is also emerging recently. It is important to include Fuchs uveitis in this group as it has been associated with rubella virus infection [48]. Respecting a few fundamental rules allows a satisfactory functional result to be obtained in the long term. Unlike keratoplasty on herpetic eyes, few studies are available on the modalities and results of cataract surgery in these patients. Prophylactic antivirals are recommended in order to prevent postoperative relapses [49].

Indications

Three situations are mainly encountered:

- Cataract in patients with herpetic kerato-uveitis: The risk of viral reactivation is real even though no predictive criteria currently exist regarding this risk. Cataract surgery is rarely combined with a keratoplasty. Antiviral prophylaxis is essential.
- Cataract complicating herpetic uveitis: These are previous uveitis, granulomatous or not, often complicated with posterior synechiae and high IOP. Cataract can be related to inflammation or to corticosteroid therapy. Perioperative antiviral and anti-inflammatory prophylaxis is mandatory.
- Cataract complicating the progression of a viral retinal necrosis: Necrotizing retinitis can be accompanied by a more or less significant inflammation of the anterior segment, but this generally occurs following the surgical management of a retinal detachment associated with necrosis.

Perioperative Management

Antiviral prophylaxis: Antivirals are proposed in all these patients and started the week before surgery. Antiviral treatment is adapted to each clinical situation. In the event of keratitis, the dosage of 2 tabs to 500 mg of valaciclovir per day may be proposed and continued for the duration of corticosteroid therapy. In moderate uveitis and retinitis, the dosage is increased to 3 g/day of valaciclovir. All patients receive antibiotic prophylaxis. For patients with uveitis, corticosteroid therapy is combined with antiviral prophylaxis. The duration of treatment should be adapted on a case-by-case basis. In patients with CMV anterior uveitis, topical ganciclovir or systemic valganciclovir is used in order to prevent viral replication due to the surgical procedure.

Conclusion

Cataract surgery is a safe procedure in patients with uveitis, but it must be performed in a quiet eye. A perioperative anti-inflammatory or anti-infectious protocol is necessary in order to reduce the risk of further relapses. Close monitoring of these patients is a key element for long-term successful outcome. The final visual prognosis depends on the type of uveitis and its previous complications especially at the level of the posterior segment. Pediatric cataract surgery remains a challenging issue even though early diagnosis and biologic agents have dramatically delayed the onset of cataract.

Take-Home Notes

- Corticosteroids remain the first risk factor for the development of cataract in patients with uveitis.
- A 3-month period of quiescence is mandatory before lens removal.
- Development of surgical procedures and tools makes surgery safe and efficient in most of the cases.
- Hydrophobic intraocular lenses should be the only type of material used in this indication.
- The medical control of intraocular inflammation remains one of the last challenges facing the surgeon.
- Complications may occur years after surgery, requiring rigorous and prolonged follow-up.

References

1. Mehta S, Linton MM, Kempen JH. Outcomes of cataract surgery in patients with uveitis: a systematic review and meta-analysis. Am J Ophthalmol. 2014;158(4):676–692 e677.
2. Moshirfar M, Somani AN, Motlagh MN, Ronquillo YC. Management of cataract in the setting of uveitis: a review of the current literature. Curr Opin Ophthalmol. 2020;31(1):3–9.
3. Pistilli M, Gangaputra SS, Pujari SS, Jabs DA, Levy-Clarke GA, Nussenblatt RB, Rosenbaum JT, Sen HN, Suhler EB, Thorne JE, et al. Contemporaneous risk factors for visual acuity in non-infectious uveitis. Ocul Immunol Inflamm. 2021:1–8.
4. Chu CJ, Dick AD, Johnston RL, Yang YC, Denniston AK, Group UKPMES. Cataract surgery in uveitis: a multicentre database study. Br J Ophthalmol. 2017;101(8):1132–7.
5. Jancevski M, Foster CS. Cataracts and uveitis. Curr Opin Ophthalmol. 2010;21(1):10–4.
6. Lowder C, Belfort R Jr, Lightman S, Foster CS, Robinson MR, Schiffman RM, Li XY, Cui H, Whitcup SM, Ozurdex HSG. Dexamethasone intravitreal implant for noninfectious intermediate or posterior uveitis. Arch Ophthalmol. 2011;129(5):545–53.
7. Callanan DG, Jaffe GJ, Martin DF, Pearson PA, Comstock TL. Treatment of posterior uveitis with a fluocinolone acetonide implant: three-year clinical trial results. Arch Ophthalmol. 2008;126(9):1191–201.
8. Nche EN, Amer R. Lens-induced uveitis: an update. Graefes Arch Clin Exp Ophthalmol. 2020;258(7):1359–65.
9. Jabs DA, Nussenblatt RB, Rosenbaum JT, Standardization of Uveitis Nomenclature Working G. Standardization of uveitis nomenclature for reporting clinical data. Results of the First International Workshop. Am J Ophthalmol. 2005;140(3):509–16.
10. Nghiem-Buffet MH, Gatinel D, Fajnkuchen F, Chaine G. Cataract in uveitis patients: extracapsular and intraocular posterior implantation results. A retrospective study of 14 eyes. J Fr Ophtalmol. 2001;24(7):704–9.
11. Gueudry J, Touhami S, Quartier P, Bodaghi B. Therapeutic advances in juvenile idiopathic arthritis – associated uveitis. Curr Opin Ophthalmol. 2019;30(3):179–86.
12. Ladas JG, Wheeler NC, Morhun PJ, Rimmer SO, Holland GN. Laser flare-cell photometry: methodology and clinical applications. Surv Ophthalmol. 2005;50(1):27–47.
13. Belair ML, Kim SJ, Thorne JE, Dunn JP, Kedhar SR, Brown DM, Jabs DA. Incidence of cystoid macular edema after cataract surgery in patients with and without uveitis using optical coherence tomography. Am J Ophthalmol. 2009;148(1):128–135 e122.
14. Alio JL, Chipont E, BenEzra D, Fakhry MA, International Ocular Inflammation Society SGoUCS. Comparative performance of intraocular lenses in eyes with cataract and uveitis. J Cataract Refract Surg. 2002;28(12):2096–108.
15. Tomlins PJ, Sivaraj RR, Rauz S, Denniston AK, Murray PI. Long-term biocompatibility and visual outcomes of a hydrophilic acrylic intraocular lens in patients with uveitis. J Cataract Refract Surg. 2014;40(4):618–25.
16. Terrada C, Julian K, Cassoux N, Prieur AM, Debre M, Quartier P, LeHoang P, Bodaghi B. Cataract surgery with primary intraocular lens implantation in children with uveitis: long-term outcomes. J Cataract Refract Surg. 2011;37(11):1977–83.
17. Balal S, Jbari AS, Nitiapapand R, Cook E, Akhtar W, Din N, Sharma A. Management and outcomes of the small pupil in cataract surgery: iris hooks, Malyugin ring or phenylephrine? Eye (Lond). 2021;35(10):2714–8.
18. Nderitu P, Ursell P. Iris hooks versus a pupil expansion ring: operating times, complications, and visual acuity outcomes in small pupil cases. J Cataract Refract Surg. 2019;45(2):167–73.
19. Shingleton BJ, Campbell CA, O'Donoghue MW. Effects of pupil stretch technique during phacoemulsification on postoperative vision, intraocular pressure, and inflammation. J Cataract Refract Surg. 2006;32(7):1142–5.
20. Li YT, Cui XX, Yang XT, Li B, Ren XJ, Li XR, Zhang XM. Utilizing dexamethasone intravitreal implant to control postoperative inflammation in refractory uveitis undergoing cataract surgery. Int J Ophthalmol. 2021;14(2):317–22.

21. Roesel M, Heinz C, Koch JM, Heiligenhaus A. Comparison of orbital floor triamcinolone acetonide and oral prednisolone for cataract surgery management in patients with non-infectious uveitis. Graefes Arch Clin Exp Ophthalmol. 2010;248(5):715–20.
22. Dada T, Dhawan M, Garg S, Nair S, Mandal S. Safety and efficacy of intraoperative intravitreal injection of triamcinolone acetonide injection after phacoemulsification in cases of uveitic cataract. J Cataract Refract Surg. 2007;33(9):1613–8.
23. Okhravi N, Morris A, Kok HS, Menezo V, Dowler JG, Hykin PG, Lightman S. Intraoperative use of intravitreal triamcinolone in uveitic eyes having cataract surgery: pilot study. J Cataract Refract Surg. 2007;33(7):1278–83.
24. Li J, Heinz C, Zurek-Imhoff B, Heiligenhaus A. Intraoperative intraocular triamcinolone injection prophylaxis for post-cataract surgery fibrin formation in uveitis associated with juvenile idiopathic arthritis. J Cataract Refract Surg. 2006;32(9):1535–9.
25. Ozates S, Berker N, Cakar Ozdal P, Ozdamar Erol Y. Phacoemulsification in patients with uveitis: long-term outcomes. BMC Ophthalmol. 2020;20(1):109.
26. Osaadon P, Belfair N, Lavy I, Walter E, Levy J, Tuuminen R, Achiron A, Knyazer B. Intracameral r-tPA for the management of severe fibrinous reactions in TASS after cataract surgery. Eur J Ophthalmol. 2021:1120672121 1002064.
27. Ram J, Gupta A, Kumar S, Kaushik S, Gupta N, Severia S. Phacoemulsification with intraocular lens implantation in patients with uveitis. J Cataract Refract Surg. 2010;36(8):1283–8.
28. Kim SJ, Belair ML, Bressler NM, Dunn JP, Thorne JE, Kedhar SR, Jabs DA. A method of reporting macular edema after cataract surgery using optical coherence tomography. Retina. 2008;28(6):870–6.
29. Estafanous MF, Lowder CY, Meisler DM, Chauhan R. Phacoemulsification cataract extraction and posterior chamber lens implantation in patients with uveitis. Am J Ophthalmol. 2001;131(5):620–5.
30. Krishna R, Meisler DM, Lowder CY, Estafanous M, Foster RE. Long-term follow-up of extracapsular cataract extraction and posterior chamber intraocular lens implantation in patients with uveitis. Ophthalmology. 1998;105(9):1765–9.
31. Kolli H, Evers C, Murray PI. Nd:YAG laser posterior capsulotomy in adult patients with uveitis. Ocul Immunol Inflamm. 2020:1–3.
32. Gross JG, Kokame GT, Weinberg DV, Dislocated In-The-Bag Intraocular Lens Study G. In-the-bag intraocular lens dislocation. Am J Ophthalmol. 2004;137(4):630–5.
33. Gimbel HV, Condon GP, Kohnen T, Olson RJ, Halkiadakis I. Late in-the-bag intraocular lens dislocation: incidence, prevention, and management. J Cataract Refract Surg. 2005;31(11):2193–204.
34. Jones NP, Jalil A, Steeples LR. Management of subluxed and dislocated intraocular lenses in patients with uveitis: a practical approach. Ocul Immunol Inflamm. 2020:1–6.
35. Ohta K, Sato A, Fukui E. Late dislocation of in-the-bag intraocular lens in three patients with multiple chorioretinal atrophy associated with sarcoidosis. Int Med Case Rep J. 2021;14:95–100.
36. Negretti GS, Chan WO, Pavesio C, Muqit MMK. Artisan-style iris-claw intraocular lens implantation in patients with uveitis. J Cataract Refract Surg. 2019;45(11):1645–9.
37. Takai N, Kobayashi T, Kida T, Ikeda T. Clinical features of Japanese patients with ocular inflammation and their surgical procedures over the course of 20 years. Clin Ophthalmol. 2020;14:2799–806.
38. de Boer J, Wulffraat N, Rothova A. Visual loss in uveitis of childhood. Br J Ophthalmol. 2003;87(7):879–84.
39. Tappeiner C, Schenck S, Niewerth M, Heiligenhaus A, Minden K, Klotsche J. Impact of antiinflammatory treatment on the onset of uveitis in juvenile idiopathic arthritis: longitudinal analysis from a nationwide pediatric rheumatology database. Arthritis Care Res (Hoboken). 2016;68(1):46–54.
40. Blum-Hareuveni T, Seguin-Greenstein S, Kramer M, Hareuveni G, Sharon Y, Friling R, Sharief L, Lightman S, Tomkins-Netzer O. Risk factors for the development of cataract in children with uveitis. Am J Ophthalmol. 2017;177:139–43.
41. Thorne JE, Woreta FA, Dunn JP, Jabs DA. Risk of cataract development among children with juvenile idiopathic arthritis-related uveitis treated with topical corticosteroids. Ophthalmology. 2010;117(7):1436–41.
42. BenEzra D, Cohen E. Cataract surgery in children with chronic uveitis. Ophthalmology. 2000;107(7):1255–60.
43. Quinones K, Cervantes-Castaneda RA, Hynes AY, Daoud YJ, Foster CS. Outcomes of cataract surgery in children with chronic uveitis. J Cataract Refract Surg. 2009;35(4):725–31.
44. Grajewski RS, Zurek-Imhoff B, Roesel M, Heinz C, Heiligenhaus A. Favourable outcome after cataract surgery with IOL implantation in uveitis associated with juvenile idiopathic arthritis. Acta Ophthalmol. 2012;90(7):657–62.
45. Guindolet D, Dureau P, Terrada C, Edelson C, Barjol A, Caputo G, LeHoang P, Bodaghi B. Cataract surgery with primary lens implantation in children with chronic uveitis. Ocul Immunol Inflamm. 2018;26(2):298–304.
46. Leinonen S, Kotaniemi KM, Kivela TT, Krootila K. Results 5 to 10 years after cataract surgery with primary IOL implantation in juvenile idiopathic arthritis-related uveitis. J Cataract Refract Surg. 2020;46(8):1114–8.

47. Ores R, Terrada C, Errera MH, Thorne JE, Doukhan R, Cassoux N, Penaud B, LeHoang P, Quartier PM, Bodaghi B. Laser flare photometry: a useful tool for monitoring patients with juvenile idiopathic arthritis-associated uveitis. Ocul Immunol Inflamm. 2020:1–11.
48. Wang H, Tao Y. Relationship between the higher inflammatory cytokines level in the aqueous humor of Fuchs uveitis syndrome and the presence of cataract. BMC Ophthalmol. 2021;21(1):108.
49. Lu LM, McGhee CNJ, Sims JL, Niederer RL. High rate of recurrence of herpes zoster-related ocular disease after phacoemulsification cataract surgery. J Cataract Refract Surg. 2019;45(6):810–5.

20 Prevention and Treatment of Negative and Positive Dysphotopsia

Samuel Masket, Zsofia Rupnik, Nicole R. Fram, Ananya Jalsingh, Andrew Cho, and Jessie McLachlan

What the Reader Should Find Interesting

- Categories of Dysphotopsia
- Various Causes for Dysphotopsia
- Management Strategies for Positive Dysphotopsia
- Management Strategies for Negative Dysphotopsia
- Preventing Dysphotopsia

Introduction

Dysphotopsias (positive and negative) represent undesirable subjective optical phenomena that may occur after uncomplicated, seemingly "perfect" cataract surgery. As such, dysphotopsia can be quite frustrating for surgeon and patient alike. They are, in part, related to IOL design and IOL position. Positive dysphotopsia (PD) is described by patients as light streaks, light arcs, flashes, and starbursts that are all induced by an external light source, whereas negative dysphotopsia (ND) is manifest as a temporal arc-shaped or linear dark shadow that is typically stimulated by temporally oriented light sources (Figs. 20.1, 20.2, and 20.3) [1]. The etiology and symptomatology of PD and ND are different; however, they can coexist in the same patient [1]. While an "ND scotoma" may be plotted by Goldmann kinetic perimetry, there are no specific objective tests to diagnose PD; the clinician relies primarily on patient-reported outcomes [2–4]. Moreover, there are some atypical cases in symptoms, causes, and course of both conditions that make diagnosis and treatment potentially more difficult. It has been suggested that dysphotopsia is a leading cause of patient dissatisfaction following cataract surgery as reported by Tester et al. [5] Indeed, they indicated that 49% of their cases had some form of dysphotopsia following surgery and Bournas et al. reported that 19.5% of patients complained of dysphotopsia on the first postoperative day [5, 6]. As the dysphotopsias seemingly have different causes, patients may experience both types. However, for discussion and understanding, they can be considered as separate conditions.

Supplementary Information The online version contains supplementary material available at [https://doi.org/10.1007/978-3-030-94530-5_20].

S. Masket (✉)
Stein Eye Institute, Geffen School of Medicine UCLA, Los Angeles, CA, USA

Advanced Vision Care, Los Angeles, CA, USA

Z. Rupnik · N. R. Fram · A. Jalsingh · A. Cho
J. McLachlan
Advanced Vision Care, Los Angeles, CA, USA

J. L. Alió et al. (eds.), *Cataract Surgery*, Essentials in Ophthalmology,
https://doi.org/10.1007/978-3-030-94530-5_20

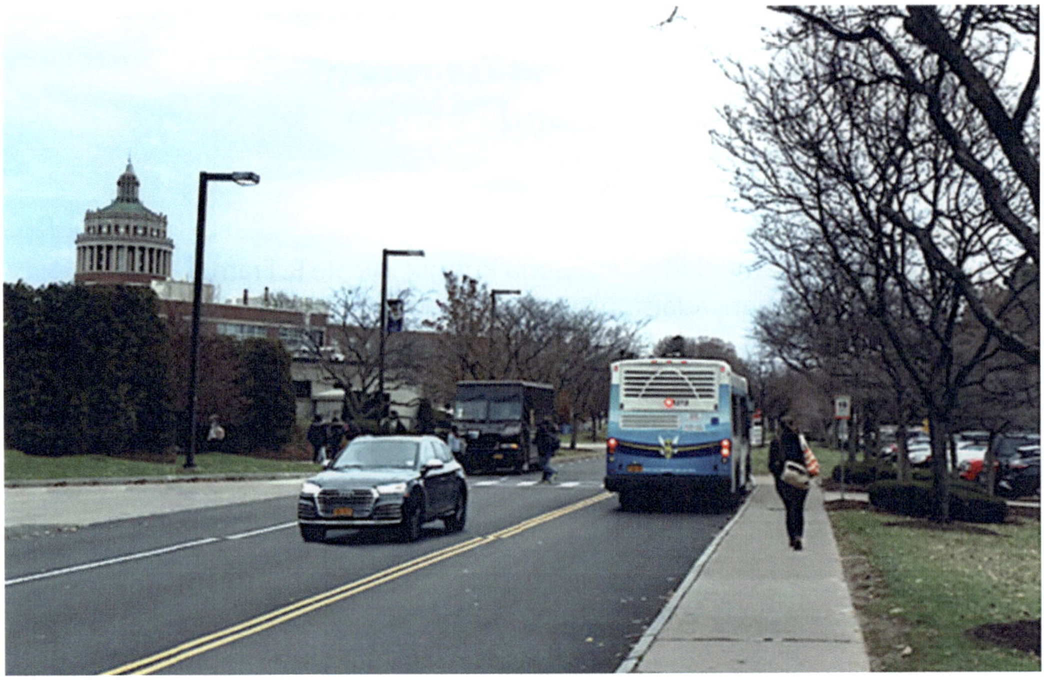

Fig. 20.1 Reference image for street scene on a cloudy day without direct sunlight. (Courtesy Drs. Geunyoung Yoon and Scott MacRae, University of Rochester)

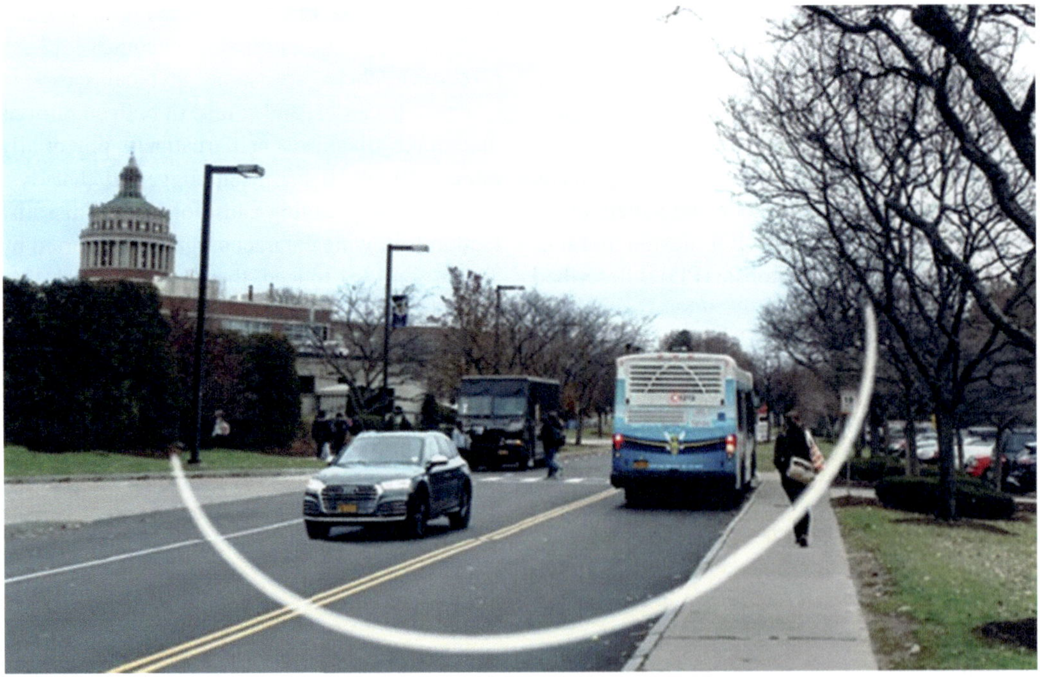

Fig. 20.2 Reference photo with superimposed white arc simulating positive dysphotopsia. (Courtesy Drs. Geunyoung Yoon and Scott MacRae, University of Rochester)

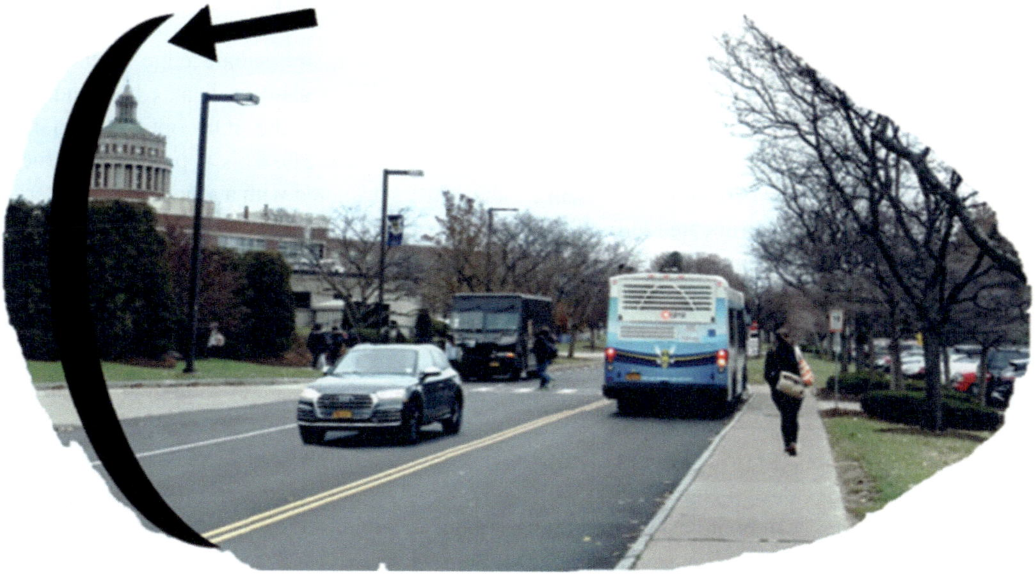

Fig. 20.3 Reference photo with superimposed temporal dark arc simulating negative dysphotopsia. (Courtesy Drs. Geunyoung Yoon and Scott MacRae, University of Rochester)

Positive Dysphotopsia

Positive dysphotopsia (PD) is described by patients as light streaks, light arcs, central flashes, and starbursts that are induced by an external light source (Fig. 20.2). PD must be distinguished from entoptic light flashes caused by vitreoretinal traction, noted under dark conditions, whereas PD requires an external light source as a stimulus in order to be realized by the patient. Also, PD must be distinguished from a Maddox rod effect that is caused by posterior capsule striae and generated by a point source of light; this condition may be managed by Nd:YAG laser posteriorly capsulotomy as indicated by patient symptoms (Fig. 20.4).

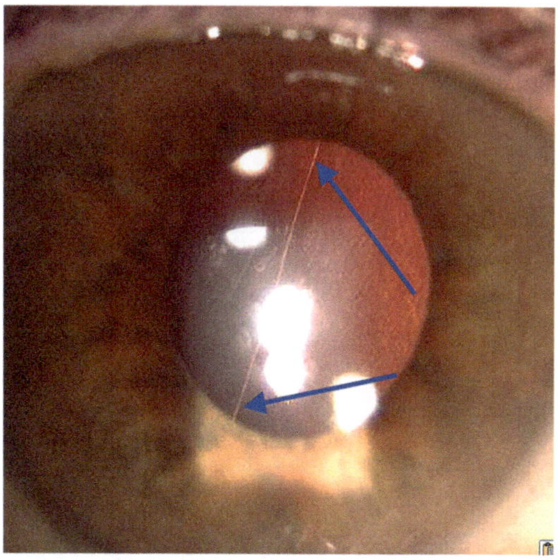

Fig. 20.4 Stria in posterior capsule (delineated by arrows) that induce a Maddox rod effect with point sources of light

The etiology of PD is reasonably well understood, given good correlation between the optical laboratory and the clinical findings. IOL edge design, index of refraction of the optic material, and overall optic design have all been implicated as causative factors. Truncated or square edge design of ovoid intraocular lenses (IOL) was first reported as a source of undesired optical images by Masket et al. [7] They used ray tracing and reflectometry to demonstrate that light of oblique incidence (between 40° and 70°) may strike the truncated square edge of the IOL and reflect onto the retinal surface, inducing PD symptoms [7]. In the era prior to foldable IOLs, rigid PMMA (poly methyl-methacrylate) was essentially the only

IOL optic material available, and oval PMMA IOLs were manufactured by truncating parallel edges of a round optic, reducing the diameter in one meridian (from 6.0 to 5.0 mm) so that the IOL could be implanted through a smaller incision. The Masket et al. investigation found a nearly fourfold greater likelihood for PD symptoms with oval versus round-shaped IOLs, owing to the squared edge of the truncated side of the optic [7]. Supporting this finding, the work of Holladay revealed that square-edged IOLs concentrate stray light into an arc that is projected onto the retina opposite the image of the light source, while round-edged IOLs disperse stray light over a larger portion of the retina, thus reducing PD symptoms [8]. Franchini et al. also found that square edge design is associated with halos, rings, and arcs of light and suggested that rounding the anterior edge of a square-edged IOL could be beneficial [9]. All of that stated, the square edge of an IOL can have a significant impact on the retardation and/or reduction of PCO as the posterior square edge of the optic inhibits lens epithelial cell migration from the equator of the capsule bag onto the posterior capsule (Fig. 20.5) [10]. As such, it is unlikely that square edge design will be removed from the marketplace, despite its causal relationship to PD.

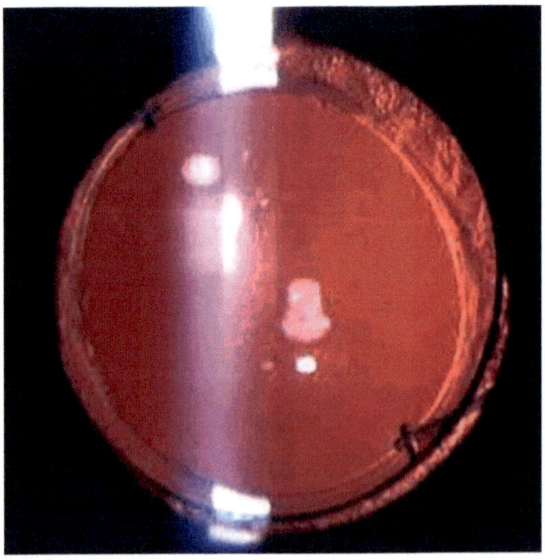

Fig. 20.5 Square-edged IOL (AcrySof, Alcon Labs, Ft. Worth Texas) with extensive posterior capsule opacification peripheral to the IOL, but minimal opacity behind the optic, indicating that optic edge retards lens epithelial cell migration onto the posterior capsule

In addition to the square edge of the optic, existing evidence also implicates high index of refraction (I/R) of the IOL optic material as another cause for PD. This is particularly true if the optic is designed with a relatively flat anterior radius of curvature as has been reported by Erie et al. [11] Their work revealed that high *I/R* when combined with a flat anterior radius of curvature was a key cause of patient-reported central light flashes from reflection off the back of the flat anterior surface of the optic. Other authors found that PMMA IOLs and round-edged silicone IOLs were associated with a decreased incidence of PD. These studies also suggest that square edge design is associated with a higher incidence of PD irrespective of IOL material [12, 13]. *I/R* also plays a major role in the reflectivity of the optic material, impacting both patient symptoms and the "cats eye" phenomenon of an accentuated 3rd Purkinje image from the anterior surface of the IOL. Table 20.1 indicates index of refraction and other characteristics of IOLs in common use in the United States. Table 20.1 lists the material, *I/R*, and design of several IOLs in use in the United States that are associated with PD.

Given a good overall understanding of the causes, the ophthalmic IOL industry has addressed PD by rounding the anterior portion of the optic's edge, reducing square-edged IOL thickness, leaving the IOL edge unpolished, and moving the IOL optical power more to the anterior rather than the posterior optic [14]. Although these logical improvements have helped, the incidence of PD is still significant in large part due to the square edge of the optic. Unless and until better means for preventing or retarding PCO are developed, PD will persist as an undesired subjective postsurgical phenomenon.

Nonsurgical Management of PD

Although not well studied, unlike ND (see below), it appears that there is no meaningful neuro-adaptation to PD, and highly symptomatic

Table 20.1 Positive dysphotopsia inciting IOLs: index of refraction and edge design

PCIOL	IOL material	Manufacturer	Refractive index	Edge design
ZCBOO	Hydrophobic acrylic	Johnson & Johnson	1.47	Frosted, posterior square edge
ZCTXXX	Hydrophobic acrylic	Johnson & Johnson	1.47	Frosted, posterior square edge
ZMBOO	Hydrophobic acrylic	Johnson & Johnson	1.47	Frosted, posterior square edge
ZKBOO	Hydrophobic acrylic	Johnson & Johnson	1.47	Frosted, posterior square edge
ZXTXXX	Hydrophobic acrylic	Johnson & Johnson	1.47	Frosted, posterior square edge
ZXROO	Hydrophobic acrylic	Johnson & Johnson	1.47	Frosted, posterior square edge
SN60WF	Hydrophobic acrylic	Alcon	1.55	Square edge
SN6ATX	Hydrophobic acrylic	Alcon	1.55	Square edge
SN6AD1	Hydrophobic acrylic	Alcon	1.55	Square edge
Softec HDO	Hydrophilic acrylic	Lenstec	1.43	Square edge, oval optic
Akreos AO60	Hydrophilic acrylic	Bausch & Lomb	1.6	Square edge
CZ70BD	PMMA	Alcon	1.49	Round thin
AQ2010V	Silicone	Staar surgical	1.41	Round edge
L161AO	Silicone	Bausch & Lomb	1.41	Square edge
ZA9002	Silicone	Johnson & Johnson	1.46	Rounded anteriorly, square posteriorly
Crystalens	Silicone	Bausch & Lomb	1.43	Square edge
CC4204A	Collamer/Co-polymer	Staar surgical	1.44	Plate haptic
CQ2015A	Hydrophilic acrylic/ Co-polymer	Staar surgical	1.45	Rounded anteriorly, square posteriorly

cases require treatment in some fashion. Conservative management methods for PD include correction of any refractive error, treatment of any coexisting ocular surface disease, treatment of posterior capsule opacification (PCO), and pharmacologic miosis. The latter may be accomplished with pilocarpine HCL 0.5% or brimonidine 0.15%. Regarding PCO and laser capsulotomy, the clinician must be certain that the posterior capsule is the offending agent; otherwise its opening could complicate future attempts at IOL exchange, should it be necessary. As a rule of thumb, if the patient was asymptomatic early after surgery (perhaps other than the Maddox rod effect) and developed symptoms later as PCO evolved, capsulotomy may be helpful. On the other hand, if the patient was symptomatic with PD immediately after surgery when the capsule was clear, it is unlikely that capsulotomy will improve PD symptoms. Moreover, posterior capsule openings, once made, should be generous in size, as the edges of a small capsulotomy can be the source of additional light-induced symptoms, particularly at night.

Should conservative measures fail and patients remain significantly symptomatic, IOL exchange can be considered as the most definitive step (see below).

Negative Dysphotopsia

Negative dysphotopsia (ND) is reported by patients as an arc-shaped dark shadow or line in the temporal periphery after otherwise uncomplicated cataract surgery (Fig. 20.3) [1]. One of the most frustrating aspects of ND for both patient and surgeon is that it occurs after what surgeons believe to be anatomically "perfect" surgery as it tends not to accompany complicated surgery that may result in malpositioned IOLs, etc. ND can be very disturbing to some patients, and the incidence is reported as high as 15–20% early after surgery when patients are specifically queried about presence of the condition [15, 16]. However, presumably due to neuro-adaptation, the incidence reduces to approximately 3% at 1-year post-op [15]. Curiously, and as yet unexplained, the incidence is higher in women and in left eyes. While there are no specific objective testing devices for ND, recent reports demonstrate far peripheral visual field changes on Goldmann kinetic VF testing that are missed with standard 30 degree static Humphrey visual field (HVF) testing [2–4]. Interestingly, patient symptoms may appear to exceed what would be expected from the Goldmann visual field changes reported by Makhotkina et al. under monocular testing [2]. More recent *binocular* Goldmann VF testing suggests that the ND "scotoma" is significantly greater with both eyes open and reduces with contralateral eye occlusion or use of a peripherally opaque contact lens on the contralateral eye, affording an understanding of the depth of some patients' symptoms and suggesting a central nervous system (CNS) component to ND (Figs. 20.6 and 20.7) [4]. In general, the clinician relies primarily on patient-reported outcomes to determine the presence and course of symptomatic ND. Moreover, there are occasional atypical cases regarding symptoms and course that make diagnosis and understanding even more difficult. Indeed, Olsen and others have suggested that a temporal "shimmering" effect, reported by some patients, is a manifestation of ND, simulating positive dysphotopsia in some manner (2014, "personal communication").

ND appears to be more enigmatic than PD. However, there seems to be general agreement about certain conditions: In the susceptible patient, ND is stimulated by light from the temporal side and improves if the temporal light source is blocked; ND symptoms are reduced with pupil dilation and worsened with pupil constriction; despite seemingly similar anatomy, ND may not occur bilaterally, having a greater incidence in the LE; ND has not been reported with ciliary sulcus, anterior chamber, or scleral suture fixated IOLs; ND has only been reported with "in the bag" IOLs after what is considered to be anatomically perfect surgery [17]. Unlike PD, the etiology seems to be less well-understood as there appears to be a gap between optical laboratory findings and clinical assessment. As an example, initial ray tracing studies from Holladay et al. implicated square edged, high I/R IOLs as likely causal of ND [18]. However, in a clinical analysis of patients requiring secondary surgery for chronic ND (persisting beyond 6 months), it was reported that 13% of cases had low I/R silicone IOLs with round edges [19]. Indeed, in that report virtually all types of IOLs on the US market were noted to be associated with ND. Additionally, a report from Burke and Benjamin indicated that high I/R, square-edged IOLs would "cure" ND if the lenses were placed in the ciliary sulcus, rather than the capsule bag [20]. That report, in combination with others, suggests that the final common clinical pathway for ND is an "in-the-bag" IOL with an overlapping anterior capsulotomy and that material or design of the IOL is less relevant [17, 19, 20–22]. Indeed, the Masket and Fram et al. study revealed that 42 of 43 eyes were improved, cured, or prevented from ND by placing the optic anterior to the anterior capsulotomy in reverse optic capture fashion, with the haptic supports remaining in the capsule bag (Fig. 20.8) [19]. Therefore, in clinical terms, ND may occur if the anterior capsule overlies the optic, but if the optic overlies the capsule, ND will be avoided. This phenomenon has not been well investigated in the optical laboratory setting. This tenet is furthered by the observation that by removing the nasal capsule edge with the Nd:YAG laser, ND will be improved in the majority of cases [23, 24]. Additionally, in one case, the nasal portion of the optic was truncated surgically, successfully eliminating ND and furthering the concept that for ND to occur, the capsule must overlap the optic, in particular on the nasal side [25]. These reports also firmly suggest that alteration of posterior chamber depth is not a likely causal factor, given that no movement of the IOL occurs with capsulectomy or optic truncation [23–25]. Further suggesting that varying posterior chamber depth does not contribute

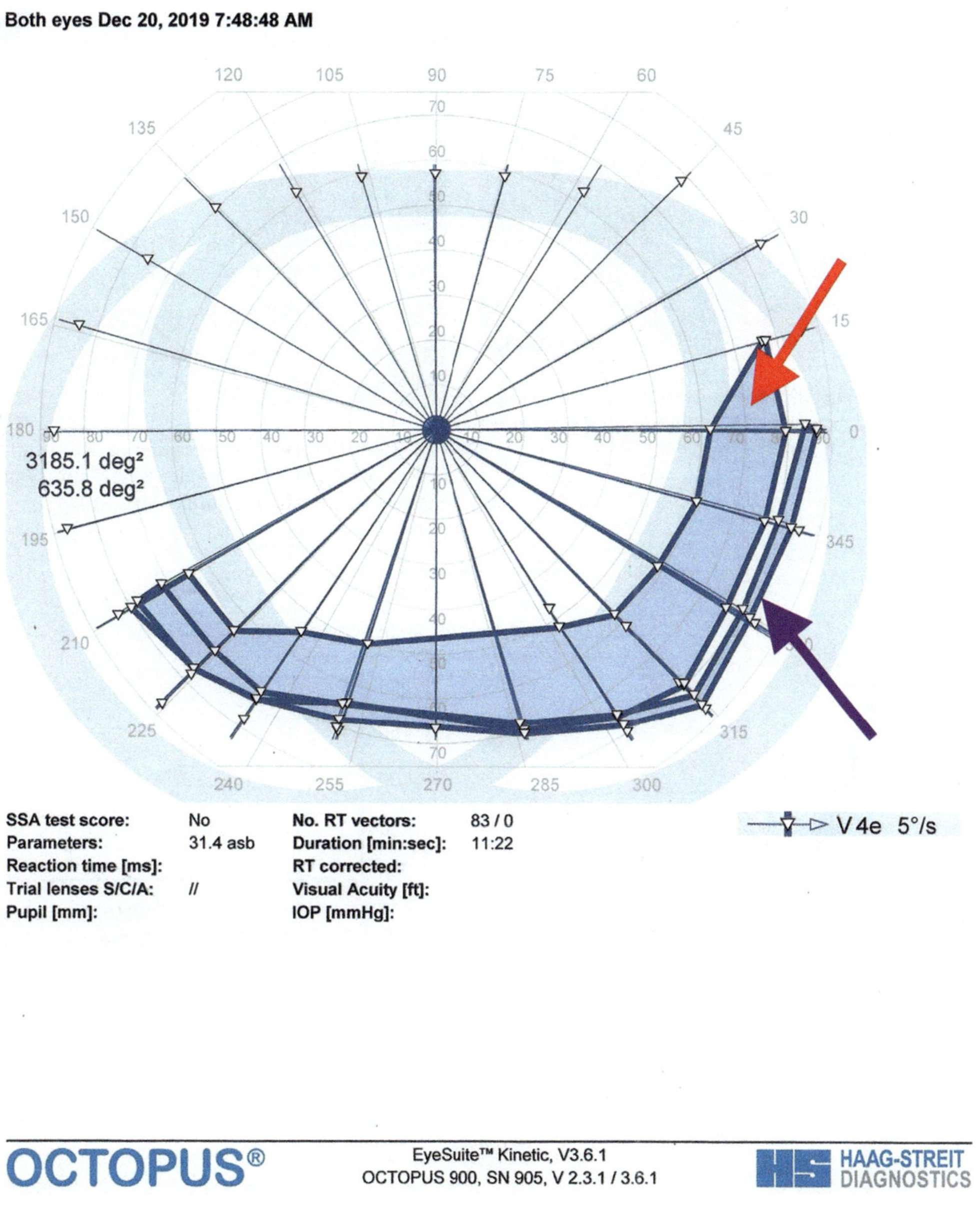

Fig. 20.6 Binocular Goldmann kinetic visual field for patient with negative dysphotopsia right eye. Note the large inferotemporal scotoma (red arrow) with both eyes fully open. However, note the markedly reduced size of the scotoma after application of a peripherally opaque contact lens on the fellow left eye (purple arrow)

to ND is the 2010 report from Vamosi et al. in which they found no difference in posterior chamber depth between a group of cases with ND and an asymptomatic control group [22]. Similarly, Masket and Fram found that reducing posterior chamber depth alone did not reduce ND symptoms [17]. However, working non-clinically with ray tracing analysis in the optical laboratory, Holladay et al. reported that increased depth and volume of the posterior chamber of the pseudophakic eye contributes to ND [18].

While there is an apparent disconnect between the clinical findings of ND and what has been garnered from the optical lab, more recent ray

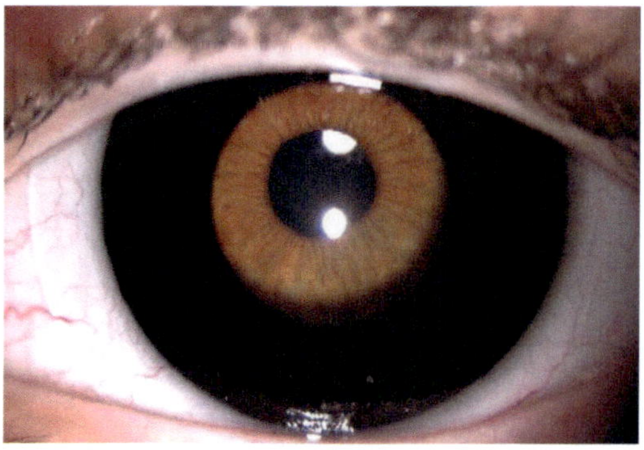

Fig. 20.7 Peripherally opaque contact lens applied to LE caused marked reduction of ND scotoma for RE of patient in Fig. 20.6

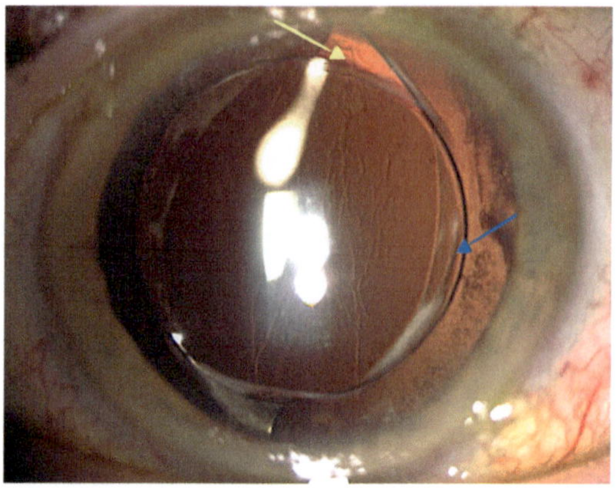

Fig. 20.8 Reverse optic capture in RE with haptics underneath the anterior capsule (yellow arrow) and optic edge above the anterior capsule (blue arrow)

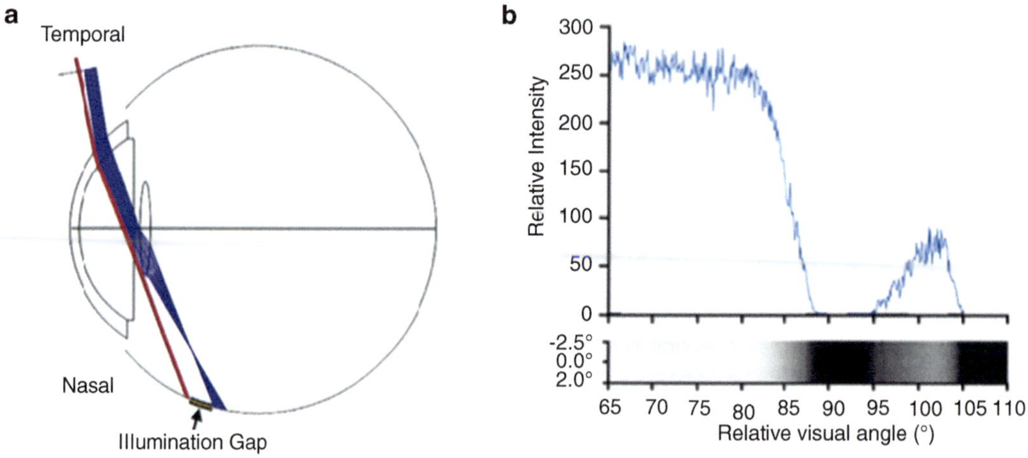

Fig. 20.9 Schematic ray trace demonstrating the proposed "illumination gap" between the light rays that are incident anterior to the optic and those that are refracted by it (**a**) and the resultant reduced relative light intensity near 90 degrees temporal (**b**). (From: Erie et al. [27]. Reproduced with permission)

tracing analyses describe an "illumination gap" between temporally incident light rays that pass anterior to the IOL optic and those that are refracted by the lens (Fig. 20.9) [26–28]. These theoretical reports are widely accepted, seem quite plausible, and possibly offer an understanding of the focal optical mechanism for ND. However, there are clinical findings that cannot be explained by the illumination gap theory: Why should ND occur more frequently in women and in the left eye; why does ND occur in only one of two eyes in many cases; why wouldn't ND occur more frequently with thick, low I/R IOLs as the illumination gap would be wider? Moreover, recent binocular far peripheral kinetic Goldmann VF testing (see above) suggests the possibility that ND has CNS manifestations, confirming that ND is a complex clinical issue that cannot be explained solely by a focal "illumination gap" [4].

Nonsurgical Management of ND

Given all of the above, how can we best manage patients with existing ND and how can we prevent it? ND is an exclusionary diagnosis in which no observable ocular pathology exists. Therefore, a dilated fundus examination and standard VF testing are necessary to rule out a disease condition that could mimic ND, such as retinal detachment or optic neuropathy. Most importantly, patients with ND early after surgery should have a thorough explanation of the condition (as best we understand it), be encouraged that it will likely improve over time, and given support. Also, there are some nonsurgical approaches that may aid: Given that temporally incident oblique light appears to be the chief inciting source for ND, use of spectacles with a thick temple piece has been beneficial to some patients, and, based on findings from recent investigations, occlusion of the fellow eye with part-time patching or use of peripherally opaque contact lenses on one or both eyes can reduce symptoms and might help patients achieve neuro-adaptation, although the latter is speculative (Fig. 20.7) [4]. However, patients with chronic ND, persisting more than 6 months, are unlikely to benefit from nonsurgical approaches, and surgery offers the best opportunity to alleviate symptoms of ND (see below). Our surgical experience indicates that nearly 100% of cases will have ND prevented or improved with primary or secondary reverse optic capture [19].

IOLS Designed to Prevent Dysphotopsia

Unfortunately, in the United States, there are no foldable IOLs available with round edges, and there are no IOLs that are specifically designed to prevent *PD*. However, as noted above, modifications to IOL edge design and optic configuration have been made over time in attempt to reduce the incidence of *PD*. In our practice we have had success with PD by exchanging for IOLs with a lower index of refraction, hence reduced surface reflectivity. Our surgical experience with 46 eyes requiring IOL exchange for chronic PD suggests an overall success rate between 85% and 90% with both silicone and co-polymer IOLs when exchanged for hydrophobic acrylic IOLs as the inciting device (Fig. 20.10) [29]. Unfortunately, at this time, round edge IOLs are only available as PMMA material, and they require large (7.0 mm) incisions.

On the other hand, with regard to specific IOLs and *ND*, Masket designed an optic (90S IOL, Morcher, Stuttgart, Germany) to mimic reverse optic capture by placing a groove on the optic edge that captures the anterior capsulotomy; in that fashion, there is a portion of the optic over capsule, rather than capsule over optic (Figs. 20.11 and 20.12) [30]. In European limited clinical trials, none of the 175 cases with that IOL experienced ND. At present, there are two other IOLs in use in Europe that provide anterior capsulotomy fixation of the IOL, and no cases of ND have been reported with these either, confirming the concept that optic over capsule prevents ND. One device, the Femtis IOL, has also been studied for other facets of anterior capsule fixation, including positional stability and more predictable effective lens positioning (ELP) (Fig. 20.13) [31]. Another is the "Bag-in-the-Lens" IOL designed by Tassignon (Fig. 20.14); it is a non-haptic IOL that requires anterior *and* posterior capsulotomies that are captured in the equatorial groove of the IOL [32]. Although not published to date, reportedly none of thousands of cases with that lens have experienced ND, giving further testimony that anterior capsulotomy optic fixation precludes ND. The design strategy of capsulotomy fixated IOLs has theoretical advantages, other than elimination of ND, that are under investigation. They include absence of rotation of toric IOLs, reduced tilt and decentration of the optic, reduced higher-order aberrations with diffractive optic IOLs, absence of capsule contraction, and more predictable and stable ELP.

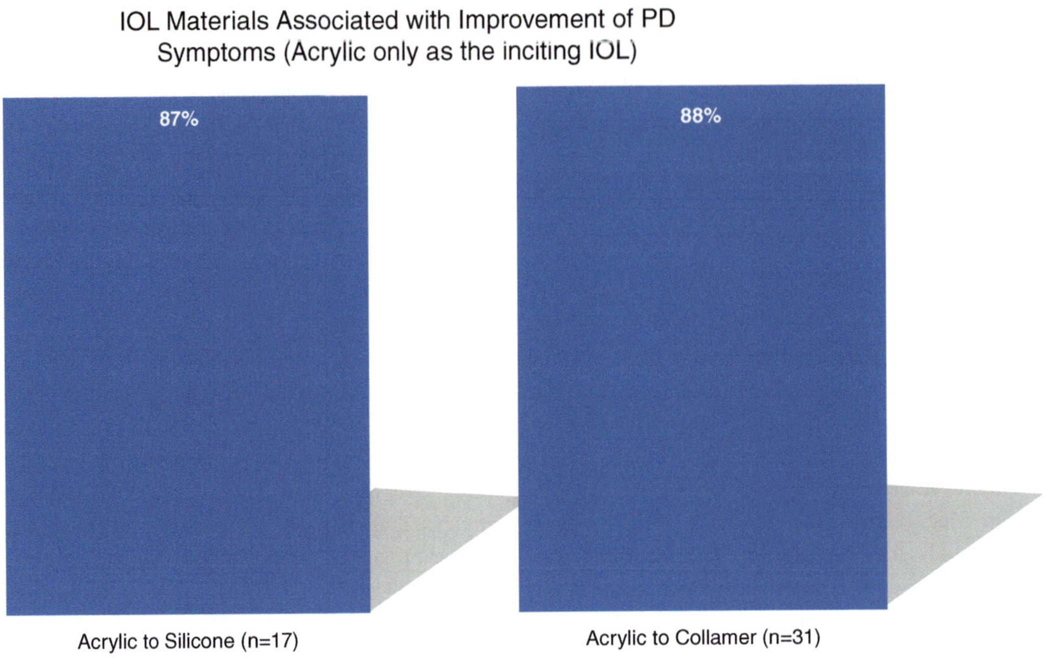

Fig. 20.10 Success rates for improving PD symptoms associated with acrylic IOLs achieved with silicone (left) and copolymer IOLs as the exchanged material. (From: Masket et al. [29]. Reproduced with permission)

Surgical Strategies for Management of Dysphotopsia

Surgery is indicated if the dysphotopsia is chronic, if nonsurgical means (see above) have failed, and if the patient is intolerant of the condition. Given that ND, PD, and DD have varied causal mechanisms, their surgical management differs. That said, patients may exhibit more than one type of dysphotopsia, and surgery should address all related problems. Surgical planning is based on a combination of patient symptoms and ocular findings and that no single form of treatment will be appropriate for all cases. To our understanding, PD appears purely related to the IOL whether in the capsule bag or ciliary sulcus; position seems to be non-contributory. Moreover, it appears that the square optic edge is the chief causal factor, but high index of refraction with high surface reflectivity is also contributory. The latter can be addressed by IOL exchange for one of lower I/R, whereas as virtually all foldable IOLs have square edges, only large diameter PMMA rigid IOLs are available with round or knife edge design for exchange. Positioning of the new or exchanged IOL depends on the condition of the anterior capsulotomy, the status of the posterior capsule, and the integrity of the zonule. Typically, PD has been associated with high *I/R* hydrophobic acrylic IOLs, and our experience dictates that exchange for either silicone or copolymer (Collamer, Staar Surgical, Monrovia CA) optic IOLs will bring success in 85–90% of cases under that circumstance (Fig. 20.9) [29]. Unfortunately, the 3-piece copolymer IOL model is no longer manufactured.

On the other hand, clinically, ND appears to be associated with any IOL, irrespective of design, that is within the confines of the capsule bag, generally underlying an intact circular anterior capsulotomy. In this situation, change in IOL position relative to the anterior capsule is more significant for reducing symptoms than

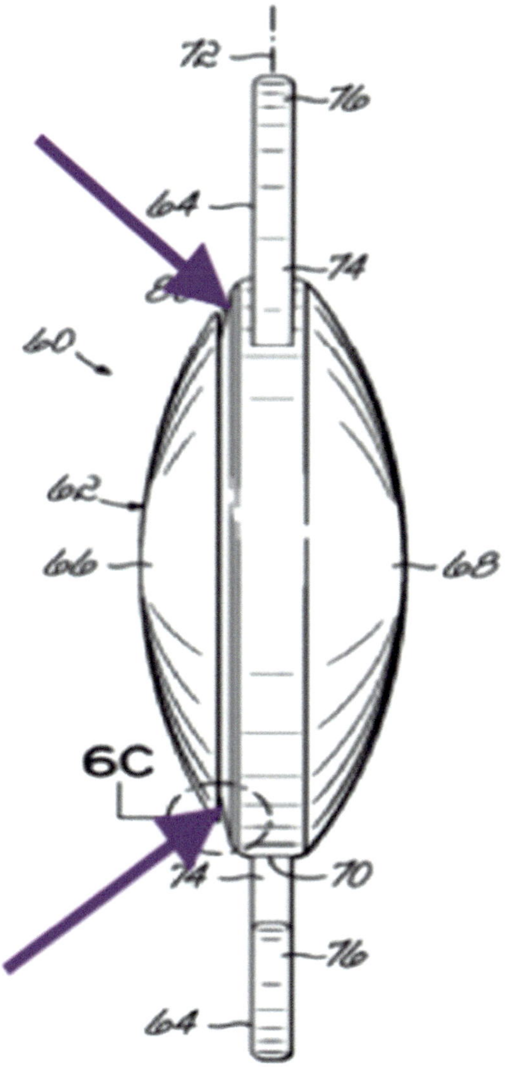

Fig. 20.11 Anti-dysphotopic IOL design from US patent drawings (Masket) with groove (noted by arrows) to accept anterior capsulotomy, simulating reverse (anterior) optic capture. (Masket [34])

is IOL design or material. Surgical strategies generally require that the optic of the IOL is brought anterior to the anterior capsulotomy either by reverse (anterior) optic capture or sulcus placement. Though we prefer the former options, there is good evidence that add-on or "piggy-back" IOLs also reduce ND, but carry added risks of decentration and late iris chafe [17, 27, 33].

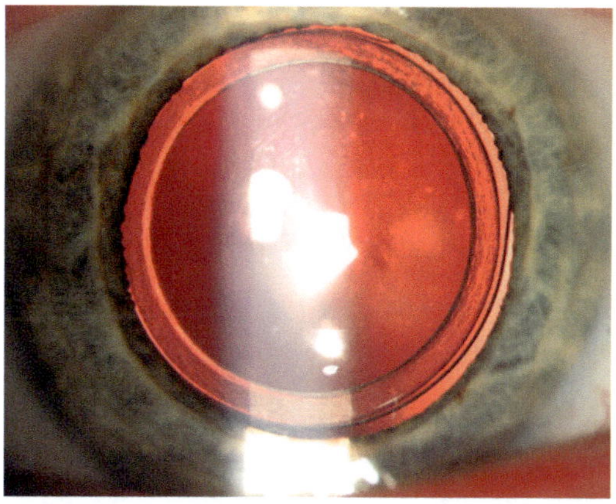

Fig. 20.12 Postoperative clinical photograph of early generation 90S IOL (Morcher) demonstrating excellent centering. Note peripheral groove that accepts the anterior capsulotomy. (Courtesy Burkhard Dick MD and Tim Schultz MD)

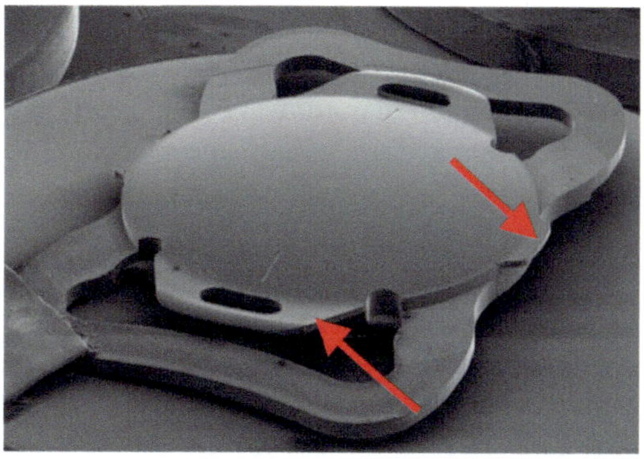

Fig. 20.13 Scanning electron photomicrograph (SEM) of the Femtis (Oculentis) IOL. Note that the optic has four tabs (two are illustrated by arrows) that keep optic edge anterior to the anterior capsulotomy

Patients who experience more than one type of dysphotopsia must have all conditions addressed by surgery. Position of the optic for the new IOL will be determined by the condition of the capsule remnant. Surgical strategies, listed below, are applied as appropriate for the existing dysphotopic condition(s), the status of the posterior capsule, and the size and centration of the anterior capsulotomy. Incision size may vary 2.2–7.0 mm depending on the technique required to remove the existing IOL or the IOL to be implanted. For a clear corneal approach, the inci-

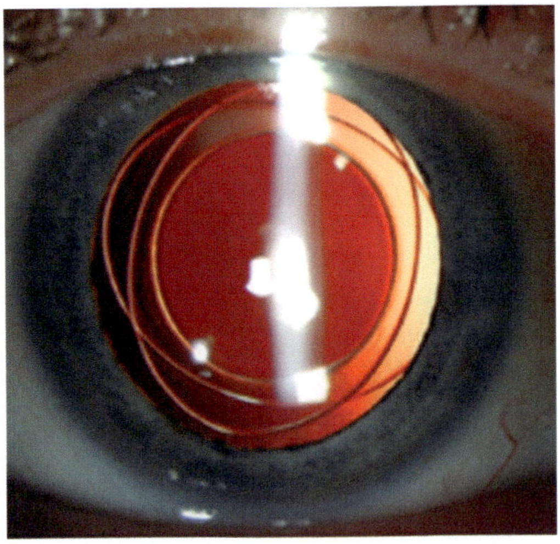

Fig. 20.14 Bag-in-the-lens (BIL) (Morcher) design of Tassignon. This non-haptic IOL design has opposing ovals with a groove that accepts both anterior and posterior capsulotomies

sion size should range from 2.2 to 3.5 mm. For eyes requiring a scleral tunnel, incisions may be 7 mm or greater. Sutures or wound sealants are used when appropriate.

Bag-to-bag PCIOL exchange *This technique involves the removal of the original IOL and the replacement of a different IOL in the capsular bag.* ***This method is appropriate for patients with isolated PD symptoms; this strategy is NOT to be applied for patients with ND*** (Video 20.1).

Primary reverse (anterior) optic capture *Either a 3-piece or single piece IOL is placed in the capsule bag after which the optic is prolapsed anteriorly to sit above the capsule, leaving the haptics in the bag. It is key that the nasal portion of the optic overly the anterior capsule edge.* ***This technique is used for the fellow eye of patients who are highly symptomatic with ND in their previously operated eye*** (Video 20.2).

Secondary reverse (anterior) optic capture *The anterior capsule edge is freed from the anterior surface of the previously placed IOL by blunt dissection, aided by an ophthalmic viscosurgical device (OVD). The optic edge is elevated above the anterior capsule nasally and temporally with a spatula. This requires that the haptics are oriented near 6 o'clock and 12 o'clock. Non-toric IOLs with horizontal or oblique haptic orientation can be rotated into vertical orientation prior to optic capture.* ***This technique is applicable to patients with persistent ND associated with an in-the-bag IOL*** (Video 20.3).

IOL exchange with reverse (anterior) optic capture (ROC) *This technique requires removal of the originally placed IOL from the capsular bag and replacement with a different IOL (for the PD symptoms) in a reverse optic capture position (for the ND symptoms).* ***This method is applied to patients with both PD and ND symptoms.*** *PD symptoms are addressed by changing the material or design of the IOL, and the ND symptoms are addressed by placing the IOL in the ROC position above the (nasal and temporal) anterior capsule* (Video 20.4).

Ciliary sulcus PCIOL placement with iris suture fixation (ISF) *An existing bag fixated IOL is removed from the capsular bag and replaced (for* ***PD****) with a 3-piece IOL in the ciliary sulcus. This strategy is employed if the posterior capsule is open and not suitable for in-the-bag placement or if the patient also has* ***ND*** *and the capsule cannot accommodate ROC positioning. We opt to use ISF with 10-0 polypropylene for long-term fixation stability. We believe that secondary IOLs should not be placed passively in the sulcus due to the concern of movement or dislocation over time.* ***This technique is used in cases with either PD or combined PD/ND when the condition of the capsule bag so dictates*** (Video 20.5).

Ciliary sulcus PCIOL placement with posterior (traditional) optic capture *An existing capsule bag placed PCIOL with a previously opened posterior capsule is removed from the capsule bag and replaced with a different 3-piece IOL positioned in the ciliary sulcus and the optic prolapsed behind the anterior capsulotomy, typically following limited vitrectomy.* ***This strategy is applied for PD but not ND.*** *This strategy requires that the anterior capsulotomy be well centered and of appropriate size and the zonule has normal integrity* (Video 20.6).

Take-Home Messages for the Reader

- The patient with dysphotopsia needs assurance that nothing is wrong with the surgery or with them.
- Negative dysphotopsia and positive dysphotopsia are separate conditions with different causes and management strategies.
- Negative dysphotopsia appears to have central nervous system manifestations; positive dysphotopsia does not.
- Positive dysphotopsia can be addressed by using an IOL with a lower index of refraction or one with a round edge, although almost all IOLs have square edges.
- Negative dysphotopsia can be addressed or prevented by elevating the optic above the anterior capsule (reverse optic capture).

References

1. Davison JA. Positive and negative dysphotopsia in patients with acrylic intraocular lenses. J Cataract Refract Surg. 2000;26(9):1346–55.
2. Makhotkina NY, Berendschot TT, Nuijts RM. Objective evaluation of negative dysphotopsia with Goldmann kinetic perimetry. J Cataract Refract Surg. 2016;42(11):1626–33.
3. Masket S, Rupnik Z, Fram NR. Neuroadaptive changes in negative dysphotopsia during contralateral eye occlusion. J Cataract Refract Surg. 2019;45(2):242–3.
4. Masket S, Rupnik Z, Fram NR, Vikesland RJ. Binocular Goldmann visual field testing of negative dysphotopsia. J Cataract Refract Surg. 2020;46(1):147–8.
5. Tester R, Pace NL, Samore M, Olson RJ. Dysphotopsia in phakic and pseudophakic patients: incidence and relation to intraocular lens type. J Cataract Refract Surg. 2000;26(6):810–6.
6. Bournas P, Drazinos S, Kanellas D, Arvanitis M, Vaikoussis E. Dysphotopsia after cataract surgery: comparison of four different intraocular lenses. Ophthalmologica. 2007;221(6):378–83.
7. Masket S, Geraghty E, Crandall AS, Davison JA, Johnson SH, Koch DD, Lane SS. Undesired light images associated with ovoid intraocular lenses. J Cataract Refract Surg. 1993;19(11):690–4.
8. Holladay JT, Lang A, Portney V. Analysis of edge glare phenomena in intraocular lens edge designs. J Cataract Refract Surg. 1999;25(6):748–52.
9. Franchini A, Gallarati BZ, Vaccari E. Computerized analysis of the effects of intraocular lens edge design on the quality of vision in pseudophakic patients. J Cataract Refract Surg. 2003;29(2):342–7.
10. Nishi O, Nishi K, Wickstrom K. Preventing lens epithelial cell migration using intraocular lenses with sharp rectangular edges. J Cataract Refract Surg. 2000;26(10):1543–9.
11. Erie JC, Bandhauer MH, McLaren JW. Analysis of postoperative glare and intraocular lens design. J Cataract Refract Surg. 2001;27(4):614–21.
12. Farbowitz MA, Zabriskie NA, Crandall AS, Olson RJ, Miller KM. Visual complaints associated with the AcrySof acrylic intraocular lens. J Cataract Refract Surg. 2000;26(9):1339–45.
13. Ellis MF. Sharp-edged intraocular lens design as a cause of permanent glare. J Cataract Refract Surg. 2001;27(7):1061–4.
14. Meacock WR, Spalton DJ, Khan S. The effect of texturing the intraocular lens edge on postoperative glare symptoms: a randomized, prospective, double-masked study. Arch Ophthalmol. 2002;120:1294–8.
15. Osher RH. Negative dysphotopsia: long-term study and possible explanation for transient symptoms. J Cataract Refract Surg. 2008;34(10):1699–707.
16. Makhotkina NY, Nijkamp MD, Berendschot T, van den Borne B, Nuijts R. Effect of active evaluation on the detection of negative dysphotopsia after sequential cataract surgery: discrepancy between incidences of unsolicited and solicited complaints. Acta Ophthalmol. 2018;96(1):81–7.
17. Masket S, Fram N. Pseudophakic negative dysphotopsia: surgical management and new theory of etiology. J Cataract Refract Surg. 2011;37(7):1199–207.
18. Holladay JT, Zhao H, Reisin CR. Negative dysphotopsias: the enigmatic penumbra. J Cataract Refract Surg. 2012;38(7):1251–65.
19. Masket S, Fram NR, Cho A, Park I, Pham D. Surgical management of negative dysphotopsia. J Cataract Refract Surg. 2018;44(1):6–16.
20. Burke TR, Benjamin L. Sulcus-fixated intraocular lens implantation for the management of negative dysphotopsia. J Cataract Refract Surg. 2014;40(9):1469–72.
21. Trattler WB, Whitsett JC, Simone PA. Negative dysphotopsia after intraocular lens implantation irrespective of design and material. J Cataract Refract Surg. 2005;31(4):841–5.
22. Vámosi P, Csákány B, Németh J. Intraocular lens exchange in patients with negative dysphotopsia symptoms. J Cataract Refract Surg. 2010;36(3):418–24.
23. Folden DV. Neodymium: YAG laser anterior capsulectomy: surgical option in the management of negative dysphotopsia. J Cataract Refract Surg. 2013;39(7):1110–5.
24. Cooke DL, Kasko S, Platt LO. Resolution of negative dysphotopsia after laser anterior capsulotomy. J Cataract Refract Surg. 2013;39(7):1107–9.
25. Alapati NM, Harocopos GJ, Sheybani A. In-the-bag nasal intraocular lens optic truncation for treatment of negative dysphotopsia. J Cataract Refract Surg. 2016;42(12):1702–6.

26. Holladay JT, Simpson MJ. Negative dysphotopsia: causes and rationale for prevention and treatment. J Cataract Refract Surg. 2017;43:263–75.
27. Erie JC, Simpson MJ, Bandhauer MH. Effect of a sulcus-fixated piggyback intraocular lens on negative dysphotopsia: ray-tracing analysis. J Cataract Refract Surg. 2019;45:443–50.
28. Simpson MJ. Mini-review: far peripheral vision. Vis Res. 2017;140:96–105.
29. Masket S, Rupnick Z, Fram NR, Kwong S, McLachlan J. Surgical management of positive dysphotopsia: US perspective [published online ahead of print, 2020 Jul 13]. J Cataract Refract Surg. 2020. https://doi.org/10.1097/j.jcrs.0000000000000307.
30. Masket S. Development of an anti-dysphotopic IOL. Expert Rev Ophthalmol. https://doi.org/10.1080/17469899.2018.1560263.
31. Darian-Smith E, Versace P. Visual performance and positional stability of a capsulorhexis-fixated extended depth-of-focus intraocular lens. J Cataract Refract Surg. 2020;46(2):179–87.
32. Tassignon MJ, Dhubhghaill S, Van Os L. Innovative implantation technique. In: Bag-in-the lens cataract surgery. Basel: Springer; 2019.
33. Makhotkina NY, Dugrain V, Purchase D, Berendschot TTJM, Nuijts RMMA. Effect of supplementary implantation of a sulcus-fixated intraocular lens in patients with negative dysphotopsia. J Cataract Refract Surg. 2018;44:209–18.
34. Masket S, inventor. Anti-dysphotopsia intraocular lens and method. US patent 8652206. April 11, 2011.

Cataract Surgery in the Vitrectomized Eye

21

E. Di Carlo and A. J. Augustin

5 Top Issues
- Phacoemulsification technique
- Intraoperative complications
- Posterior capsule instability
- Zonular weakness
- Silicone oil

Epidemiology

The indications of pars plana vitrectomy are numerous, including non-clearing vitreous haemorrhage, retinal detachment, macular pucker and hole, vitreo-macular traction and endophthalmitis. Despite its high efficacy and safety in the treatment of the aforementioned retinal diseases, vitrectomy may induce the formation and facilitate the progression of cataract in phakic patients, thereby compromising visual acuity [1].

Various studies report an incidence of cataract formation after 20-gauge PPV varying from 12.5% to 80% [2, 3]. The use of small gauge (23/25 gauge) systems has proven to be less risky to promote the onset of cataract as compared to 20-gauge PPV systems [4]. It seems to depend on the reduced amount of balanced salt solution used during the surgery, lower fluid flow in the vitreous cavity, shorter surgical time and diminished ocular manipulation [5].

Recently, Feng et al. [6] evaluated the incidence and prevalence of cataract formation and progression in patients that underwent vitreoretinal procedures in order to determine factors that can potentially predispose patients to postoperative cataracts. The study asserts that eyes that underwent the combination between PPV and scleral buckle (SB) showed the most lenticular changes, followed by 20-gauge PPV and small-gauge procedures. In contrast, eyes that underwent either SB or pneumatic retinopexy exhibited only mild postoperative lens opacification.

Pathogenesis of Cataract Formation After Pars Plana Vitrectomy

Cataract formation after vitreoretinal surgery shows two main pathophysiological mechanisms. The first is based on time of presentation of lens opacities distinguishing early and late subcapsular cataracts. The other mechanism, based on modality of onset, is typical of cases where an accidental contact with the lens is caused by the intraocular surgical instrumentation. Regarding

Supplementary Information The online version contains supplementary material available at [https://doi.org/10.1007/978-3-030-94530-5_21].

E. Di Carlo (✉) · A. J. Augustin
Department of Ophthalmology, Staedtisches Klinikum Karlsruhe, Karlsruhe, Germany

J. L. Alió et al. (eds.), *Cataract Surgery*, Essentials in Ophthalmology,
https://doi.org/10.1007/978-3-030-94530-5_21

the latter mechanism, the formation of nuclear sclerosis after PPV is not well understood [7].

An early subcapsular opacity has been shown to be caused by an alteration of the water and electrolyte balance of the lens fibres [8]. Specifically, some authors assume that gas or silicone oil, often used as intraocular tamponade in the vitreoretinal procedures, disrupt the function of the Na+-K+-ATPase. As a consequence of this process, sodium is not transported out of the cells, Cl- and water come out and thus swell the lens fibres [3].

Late subcapsular opacities occur mainly after silicone oil tamponade [9]. However, not only occur a proliferation and migration of the epithelial cells along the posterior capsule but also a fibrous metaplasia of these epithelial cells [10]. The reason for the proliferation, migration and pseudometaplasia of epithelial cells with silicone oil is unclear. Mechanical, toxic and metabolic causes are still under discussion, but a clear mechanism has not yet been discovered.

Cataract formation following contact between the lens and surgical instrumentation is also due to water influx inside the lens fibres. In this case the water influx is irreversible and leads to a change in the refractive index and thus to light scattering [11].

The nuclear sclerosis after PPV is probably based on a different pathophysiological mechanism as compared to subcapsular opacities. The interaction between the vitreous body and oxygen metabolism plays a fundamental role in the development of postvitrectomy nuclear cataract. The vitreous body acts as a barrier preventing the diffusion of free oxygen radicals from the surface of the retina to the posterior lens. For this reason, after the vitreous removal, this barrier function is lost, leading to an accumulation of oxygen free radicals in the lens and thus promoting the development of a nuclear sclerosis [12].

Clinical Presentation

The most common cataract that forms after vitreoretinal surgery is nuclear sclerotic and posterior subcapsular. A nuclear sclerotic opacity represents the typical cataract appearance after pars plana vitrectomy mostly in older patients. This particular type may occur independently from the type of retinal procedure and even without the use of air, gas or silicone oil, as described by Panozzo et al. [13]. On the other hand, younger patients and those affected by diabetes are more likely to develop a posterior subcapsular cataract [6].

The typical clinical sign of eyes that previously underwent vitrectomy is represented by a decreased visual acuity, independently from the anatomical and functional success of the vitreoretinal procedure. Postvitrectomy eyes may also show a reduced visual acuity or other visual disturbances compared to the preoperative situation. For this reason it may be possible that patients who develop a postvitrectomy cataract exhibit a poorer vision than patients with typical age-related cataracts.

As with other forms of cataracts, the diagnosis is made with slit-lamp biomicroscopy, which allows to differentiate a nuclear sclerosis from a subcapsular cataract. In addition, the use of optical coherence tomography (OCT) may help the physician to detect the absence of vitreous gel.

Preoperative Assessment and IOL Power Calculation

Before performing cataract surgery in a previously vitrectomized eye, it is essential to obtain as much information as possible regarding the patient's medical history and to conduct a thorough ophthalmic examination. The most difficult aspect to deal with is certainly to determine how much the visual acuity reduction depends on the cataract formation. In this regard additional tests, such as the potential acuity pinhole test, the potential acuity meter, the retinal acuity meter, the illuminated near card and laser interferometer and also the Amsler grid, have been demonstrated as valuable tools to predict postsurgical visual acuity and may help the surgeon in deciding to perform cataract surgery [14].

The preoperative evaluation has also the aim to recognize any possible complications of the previous surgery, such as zonular weakness, the presence of silicon oil in the anterior chamber, small pupil difficult to dilate or iatrogenic injury to the posterior lens capsule. All these factors may represent an additional risk for the planned cataract surgery, and therefore the accurate identification of those conditions allows the surgeon to prepare for a safer surgery avoiding unwanted complications [15].

Some additional testing may be necessary preoperatively, such as B-scan ultrasonography, fluorescein angiography and optical coherence tomography, in order to assess any ocular disease that should be addressed before, in combination with or after cataract surgery.

Special attention must be paid to the intraocular lens power (IOL) calculation that can be more challenging than in nonvitrectomized eyes due to the alteration of ocular morphology or the vitreoretinal disease itself, as in case of tractional macular oedema. The utilization of ocular biometry has recently improved the accuracy and repeatability of IOL measurements. Some authors demonstrated, using optical biometry and Haigis formula, no statistically significant differences in terms of refractive outcomes between patients who underwent combined phacovitrectomy and those who underwent phacoemulsification after PPV [16, 17]. Nevertheless, they also reported a better postoperative result in the patients not previously vitrectomized. In addition to these results, further studies [17, 18] asserted that no myopic shift was found using ultrasound biometry in patients undergoing cataract surgery after PPV, as previously reported in the scientific literature. Thus, optical biometry enables more precise measurements than ultrasound in previously vitrectomized eyes, although still not as accurate as in the nonvitrectomized eye.

The use of optical biometry instead of ultrasound offers several advantages in the vitrectomized eye. For example, in case of high myopia or myopic staphyloma, conditions frequently associated with vitreoretinal surgery, it could be challenging to obtain the correct axial length measurement through the visual axis with the ultrasound biometry. The optical biometry has proven to be superior in terms of accuracy and repeatability when compared to ultrasound biometry for calculating the axial lenght [19]. Recently, an interesting paper has been published by Tan et al. [20], comparing the prediction accuracy of new IOL calculation formulas (Barrett Universal II [BUII], Emmetropia Verifying Optical [EVO], Kane and Ladas Super formula) and traditional formulas (Haigis, Hoffer Q, Holladay 1, and SRK/T) with Wang-Koch (WK) axial length (AL) adjustment in vitrectomized eyes. The authors concluded that the BUII, EVO, Kane and Haigis show good and comparable performance in vitrectomized eyes with optimized constants. Moreover, in vitrectomized highly myopic eyes, the new formulas and traditional formulas with WK adjustment exhibited satisfactory prediction accuracy.

The use of ultrasound biometry in silicone oil-filled eyes does not permit accurate measurements. The presence of silicone oil in the posterior chamber of the eye does not allow the transmission of sound waves to the retina, and this may lead to an overestimation of axial length measurements. For this reason, ocular biometry should be performed in those eyes with silicon oil tamponade [16, 21]. Such authors reported that silicone oil-filled eyes that underwent combined silicone oil removal and phacoemulsification showed no statistically significant difference in predictive refractive errors between preoperative optical biometry and intraoperative ultrasound biometry executed after silicone oil removal.

Surgery: Surgical Technique, Intraoperative Risks and Complications

A recent Cochrane database review [22] indicates that cataract surgery, typically performed using phacoemulsification and intraocular lens implantation, is commonly recommended for individuals with significant visual acuity impairment due to lens opacities after PPV.

Surgeons share the common idea that cataract surgery in previously vitrectomized eyes may have a higher complication rate as compared to standard phacoemulsification. Conditions, such as deep fluctuating anterior chamber, intraoperative miosis, an enormously instable posterior capsule, rigidity of the anterior capsule, the presence of plaques at the posterior capsule level, weakened zonules and loss of vitreous support, have proven to be associated with an increased risks of intraoperative complications during cataract surgery [23–25]. Nevertheless, evidence from comparative studies regarding efficacy and safety of phacoemulsification in nonvitrectomized and vitrectomized eyes is lacking [26, 27].

When considering the surgical technique, phacoemulsification in vitrectomized eyes has shown to be superior as compared to extracapsular cataract extraction with better outcomes in terms of both superior visual acuity improvement and fewer intra- and postoperative complications [27]. Extracapsular extraction with large incision and nuclear expression are more challenging in vitrectomized eyes with an increased complication rate due to zonular and capsular fragility [28, 29].

Recently, Fenberg et al. [30] retrospectively examined all cases (98 eyes) of complicated cataract surgery over a period of 15 years to assess the risk of complicated phacoemulsification and/or delayed IOL dislocation in patients with a previous vitrectomy. They hypothesized that vitrectomy surgery alters the zonular strength and capsular bag stability, which may increase both the risk of intraoperative complications in subsequent cataract surgery and IOL dislocation in eyes with previous phacoemulsification. The study reported that 9.2% of patients with complicated cataract surgery have undergone PPV, confirming that vitrectomy surgery represents a risk factor for complicated cataract surgery and IOL dislocation. Therefore different techniques have been suggested in order to minimize zonular stress and ultrasound power during the phacoemulsification. Nevertheless, as previously mentioned, the scientific literature lacks prospective, randomized clinical trials comparing the safety and efficacy of various surgical techniques to manage cataract surgery in vitrectomized eyes. However, we try to give some important recommendations to follow in order to achieve the better functional outcome.

The mechanisms that lead to complications during phacoemulsification in previously vitrectomized eyes are still unknown. As mentioned above, vitrectomized eyes show a deeper anterior chamber and a less stable lens. In nonvitrectomized eyes the vitreous body acts as a "damper" to stabilize the capsule and thus reducing the anteroposterior movements during the surgery.

Zonular stability plays a fundamental role to avoid complications during phacoemulsification and also to prevent postoperative IOL dislocation. In this regard, despite the presence of zonular adherence to the lens that is well documented, the role of peripheral zonular adhesions is not still well understood. Rohen et al. [31] described in great detail that the zonules were anchored between the ciliary processes at a common point, whereas the group of Fansworth [32] demonstrated that some of the zonules pass through the ciliary processes to attach more posteriorly on the pars plana near the ora serrata. According to the Fansworth's model, in which the zonular adhesions are located posteriorly, it is very likely that vitrectomy surgery may induce zonular disruption. In case of zonular instability, the surgeon has to perform a complete, possibly cortical cleaving hydrodissection in order to minimize zonular and capsular stress during the phases of nuclear rotation, emulsification with the phacotip and the cortical removal [33] (Supplementary Video 21.1). Additionally, weakened lens zonules after PPV could be the cause of late in-the-bag spontaneous IOL dislocation, described in the study by Davis [34]. The authors reported a rate of 19% IOL dislocation, occurring about 8 years after the cataract surgery. The long time elapsed between IOL implantation and episode of dislocation may suggest the dynamicity of the zonular instability that could also continue over the years. The study focuses the attention on the possibility for the surgeon to choose a different IOL implantation instead of standard in-the-bag approach, in the event of intraoperatively recognizable phacodonesis. In this case the use of capsular tension ring or implanting a 3-piece IOL in the ciliary sulcus may be good alternative options to minimize the risk of postoperative IOL dislocation. Furthermore, in extreme situations, as in case of complete absence of capsular support, the surgeon necessitates alternative surgical approaches, which include scleral fixation, iris fixation or IOL placement in the anterior chamber angle [35].

Zonular weakness and absence of vitreous support are the main causes of the presence of a deep anterior chamber, as frequently observed during phacoemulsification in vitrectomized eyes. The positive infusion pressure induced by the phaco-tip combined to the lack of vitreous support augments considerably the anterior chamber depth and the zonular stress, thus leading to additional unwanted zonular tractions. To counteract these forces, it is essential to lower the irrigating fluid bottle height, before introducing the phaco-tip into the anterior chamber [24] (Supplementary Video 21.2). Another possibility to reduce the zonular stress is to remove some viscoelastic substance out of the anterior chamber prior to the introduction of the phaco-tip. As general recommendation, care should be taken to avoid pushing on the nucleus with the instruments.

The surgeon may also deal with a particular condition associated with zonular elongation in vitrectomized eyes, called iris diaphragm retropulsion syndrome (LIDRS) and characterized by a reverse pupillary block that causes an excessively deep anterior chamber and extreme pupil widening during phacoemulsification [36]. Differently from a classical pupillary block, LIDRS occurs when the pressure in the anterior chamber is greater than that of the posterior and vitreous chamber, leading to a posterior movement of both iris and lens. The surgical goal consists in the separation of the iris from the anterior capsular rim and is achieved by depressing the anterior capsule or lifting the iris, thus allowing fluid to reach the 360° of space behind the iris.

An additional challenging scenario is the management of posterior capsule instability (Supplementary Video 21.3). In this case cortex removal may be challenging sometimes leading to an unexpected capsule rupture. If there is a high suspicion of a tear in the posterior capsule, it could be much safer to utilize the infusion line via pars plana continuing the phacoemulsification [37].

The presence of posterior synechiae with an undilatable pupil represents a further challenge for the surgeon who has to face a cataract surgery in vitrectomized eyes. The combined use of iris spatula and viscoelastic break the posterior adhesions between lens and iris, whereas the utilization of intracameral mydriatics, iris hooks or pupil expansors (i.e. Malyugin ring [38]) result to be optimal to deal with this problem.

Another possible complication that may occur after PPV and that the surgeon has to deal with is represented by the presence of a posterior capsular plaque. This can be peeled off performing a posterior capsulorhexis or, as alternative, dissected off the capsule with the aim of delicate intraocular forceps. Another option is to polish off the plaque using a vitrectomy cutter [39]. Instead, a rigid anterior capsule, as in cases of long time exposure to silicone oil, may be managed with the use of cutter or retinal microscissors [40]. Finally, in particular circumstances, for example, when the plaque does not have huge dimensions, it can be left in place and managed afterward with a posterior YAG laser capsulotomy.

Cataract removal through phacoemulsification in eyes filled with silicone oil is a challenging procedure. In this regard, a recent study evaluated the complications of cataract surgery in silicone oil-filled eyes [41]. The authors reported a 10.1% rate of posterior capsule rupture and a 5.6% rate of silicone oil migration into the anterior chamber. The buoyancy of silicone oil could explain the increased rate of complications because it may determine posterior capsule elevation and additional capsular instability. Regarding the migration of silicone oil into the anterior chamber, some authors demonstrated that breaking the integrity of the posterior chamber and anterior hyaloid membrane, caused by countless changes in intraocular pressure during phacoemulsification, may lead to anterior silicone oil migration despite the integrity of zonular structures [42, 43]. For this reason, due to the high rate of complications associated with cataract surgery in eyes filled with silicone oil, other authors recommend its removal through pars plana prior to performing phacoemulsification surgery [44].

Functional Outcomes and Complication Rate

Cataract surgery in the vitrectomized eye is generally a safe surgery with reported good results of postoperative visual acuity, which may be limited only by the concomitant retinal disease [45].

Nevertheless, peer-review data on postoperative visual acuity outcomes after surgery for postvitrectomy cataract are scarce [21]. Prior studies demonstrated that the percentage of eyes able to achieve postoperative visual acuity of 20/40 range from 20% to 77% [45–47]. Due to this wide variability of results, it is arduous to reach certain conclusions on visual outcomes in eyes previously vitrectomized.

Another important element to take into account is the conflicting results reporting in the literature regarding the safety of phacoemulsification after PPV. For example, some authors assessed an overall intraoperative complication rate of 12.5% and posterior capsule rupture rate of 13.3%, respectively [26, 46]. On the contrary, other authors reported a good safety profile for the phacoemulsification similar to eyes not previously vitrectomized [45, 47].

Recently, Soliman et al. retrospectively analysed and summarized the visual outcomes and rate of intraoperative complications of phacoemulsification surgery after prior pars plana vitrectomy in 2221 eyes [48]. This multicentre study reported that at all postoperative time points measured up to 24 weeks, mean vision was poorer in the prior PPV group (0.41 ± 0.47 vs. 0.17 ± 0.29 at 4 and 12 weeks, $P < 0.0001$) and a smaller proportion of eyes achieved postoperative visual acuity of 0.30 logMAR (Snellen 20/40) (60.8% vs. 86.5% at 4 and 12 weeks, $P < 0.0001$). The rate of posterior capsular rupture was not different between the prior PPV (1.5%) and the nonvitrectomized (1.7%) groups, but the incidences of zonular dialysis (1.3% vs. 0.6%) and dropped nuclear fragments (0.6% vs. 0.2%) were significantly higher in the prior PPV group ($P < 0.0001$).

The safety of phacoemulsification procedure in vitrectomized eyes has been also assessed by the study of Rey et al. [49], which retrospectively reported no cases of intraoperative capsule rupture and only one anterior capsule rhexis tear as complication in a cohort of 87 patients.

The latest researches show a significant and progressive improvement in postoperative outcomes, suggesting how a challenging procedure, like the phacoemulsfication in vitrectomized eyes, may be successfully managed by surgeons with huge benefits for the patients.

Conclusion

In conclusion, cataract surgery in previously vitrectomized eyes is a challenging procedure with a higher complication rate as compared to nonvitrectomized eyes. Visual acuity outcome measures have to be interpreted with caution because of the retinal disease potentially reducing visual acuity as well. Cataract surgery in previously vitrectomized eyes should be done by experienced surgeons to optimize the outcomes in those patients.

Take-Home Notes

- The most common cataract types are nuclear sclerosis and posterior subcapsular.
- Phacoemulsification with in the bag intraocular lens implantation is the standard procedure to perform in eyes previously vitrectomized.
- Zonular weakness, instable posterior capsule and deep fluctuating anterior chamber due to loss of vitreous support are the main intraoperative challenging conditions the surgeon has to deal with.
- Phacoemulsification in silicone oil-filled eyes is associated with a higher complication rate, such as posterior capsule rupture and silicone oil migration into the anterior chamber.
- Cataract surgery in previously vitrectomized eyes is a challenging procedure and should be done by experienced surgeons.

References

1. Benson WE. Vitrectomy in clinical ophthalmology. In: Duane TD, editor. Duane's clinical ophthalmology, vol. 5. Philadelphia: Lippincott; 1988. p. 15–7.
2. Cherfan GM, Michels RG, de Bustros S, Enger C, Glaser BM. Nuclear sclerotic cataract after vitrectomy for idiopathic epiretinal membranes causing macular pucker. Am J Ophthalmol. 1991;111(4):434–8.
3. Hsuan JD, Brown NA, Bron AJ, Patel CK, Rosen PH. Posterior subcapsular and nuclear cataract after vitrectomy. J Cataract Refract Surg. 2001;27(3):437–44.
4. Fujii GY, De Juan E Jr, Humayun MS, et al. Initial experience using the transconjunctival sutureless vitrectomy system for vitreoretinal surgery. Ophthalmology. 2002;109(10):1814–20.
5. Rizzo S, Genovesi-Ebert F, Murri S, et al. 25-gauge, sutureless vitrectomy and standard 20-gauge pars plana vitrectomy in idiopathic epiretinal membrane surgery: a comparative pilot study. Graefes Arch Clin Exp Ophthalmol. 2006;244(4):472–9.
6. Feng H, Adelman RA. Cataract formation following vitreoretinal procedures. Clin Ophthalmol. 2014;23(8):1957–65.
7. Petermeier K, Szurman P, Bartz-Schmidt UK, Gekeler F. Pathophysiology of cataract formation after vitrectomy. Klin Monatsbl Augenheilkd. 2010;227(3):175–80.
8. Ryan SJ, Hinton DR, Schachat AP, et al. Retina. 4th Edition (Hrsg) ed. Philadelphia: Elsevier Inc; 2008.
9. Federman JL, Schubert HD. Complications associated with the use of silicone oil in 150 eyes after retina-vitreous surgery. Ophthalmology. 1988;95:870–6.
10. Spraul CW, Jakobczyk-Zmija MJ, Aigner T, et al. Posterior fibrous pseudometaplasia of lens epithelial cells in phacic eyes filled with silicone oil. Graefes Arch Clin Exp Ophthalmol. 2002;240:829–34.
11. Pau H. Cortical and subcapsular cataracts: significance of physical forces. Ophthalmologica. 2006;220:1–5.
12. Holenkamp NM, Shui YB, Beebe DC. Vitrectomy surgery increases oxygen exposure to the lens: a possible mechanism for nuclear cataract formation. Am J Ophthalmol. 2005;139:302–31.
13. Panozzo G, Parolini B. Cataracts associated with posterior segment surgery. Ophthalmol Clin N Am. 2004;17(4):557–68.
14. Chang MA, Airiani S, Miele D, Braunstein RE. A comparison of the potential acuity meter (PAM) and the illuminated near card (INC) in patients undergoing phacoemulsification. Eye. 2006;20:1345–51.
15. Shousha MA, Yoo SH. Cataract surgery after pars plana vitrectomy. Curr Opin Ophthalmol. 2010;21(1):45–9.
16. Manvikar SR, Allen D, Steel DH. Optical biometry in combined phacovitrectomy. J Cataract Refract Surg. 2009;35:64–9.
17. Bilinska E, Nawrocki J, Suprunowicz I, Omulecki W. Refraction changes after cataract extraction with IOL implantation in the eyes with previous performed vitrectomy. Klin Ocz. 2002;104:344–6.
18. Patel D, Rahman R, Kumarasamy M. Accuracy of intraocular lens power estimation in eyes having phacovitrectomy for macular holes. J Cataract Refract Surg. 2007;33:1760–2.
19. Findl O, Drexler W, Menapace R, et al. Improved prediction of intraocular lens power using partial coherence interferometry. J Cataract Refract Surg. 2001;27:861–7.
20. Tan X, Zhang J, Zhu Y, Xu J, Qiu X, Yang G, Liu Z, Luo L, Liu Y. Accuracy of new generation intraocular lens calculation formulas in vitrectomized eyes. Am J Ophthalmol. 2020;217:81–90.
21. El-Baha SM, Hemeida TS. Comparison of refractive outcome using intraoperative biometry and partial coherence interferometry in silicone oil-filled eyes. Retina. 2009;29:64–8.
22. Do DV, Gichuhi S, Vedula SS, Hawkins BS. Surgery for postvitrectomy cataract. Cochrane Database Syst Rev. 2018;1(1):CD006366.
23. Pinter SM, Sugar A. Phacoemulsification in eyes with past pars plana vitrectomy: case–control study. J Cataract Refract Surg. 1999;25:556–61.
24. Akinci A, Batman C, Zilelioglu O. Cataract surgery in previously vitrectomized eyes. Int J Clin Pract. 2008;62:770–5.
25. Smiddy WE, Stark WJ, Michels RG, et al. Cataract extraction after vitrectomy. Ophthalmology. 1987;94:483–7.
26. Ahfat FG, Yuen CH, Groenewald CP. Phacoemulsification and intraocular lens implantation following pars plana vitrectomy: a prospective study. Eye. 2003;17(1):16–20.
27. Biro Z, Kovacs B. Results of cataract surgery in previously vitrectomized eyes. J Cataract Refract Surg. 2002;28(6):1003–6.
28. Saika S, Kin K, Ohmi S, Ohnishi Y. Posterior capsule rupture by blunt ocular trauma. J Cataract Refract Surg. 1997;23(1):139–40.
29. Angra SK, Vajpayee RB, Titiyal JS, Sharma YR, Sandramouli S, Kishore K. Types of posterior capsular breaks and their surgical implications. Ophthalmic Surg. 1991;22(7):388–91.
30. Fenberg MJ, Hainsworth KJ, Rieger FG, Hainsworth DP. Vitrectomy as a risk factor for complicated cataract surgery. Mo Med. 2016;113(1):44–7.
31. Rohen JW. Scanning electron microscopic studies of the zonular apparatus in human and monkey eyes. Invest Ophthalmol Vis Sci. 1979;18(2):133–44.
32. Farnsworth PN, Mauriello JA, Burke-Gadomski P, Kulyk T, Cinotti AA. Surface ultrastructure of the human lens capsule and zonular attachments. Investig Ophthalmol. 1976;15(1):36–40.
33. Fine IH. Cortical cleaving hydrodissection. J Cataract Refract Surg. 1992;18(5):508–12.
34. Davis D, Brubaker J, Espandar L, et al. Late in-the-bag spontaneous intraocular lens dislocation: evaluation of 86 consecutive cases. Ophthalmology. 2009;116:664–70.

35. Kim EJ, Brunin GM, Al-Mohtaseb ZN. Lens placement in the absence of capsular support: scleral-fixated versus iris-fixated IOL versus ACIOL. Int Ophthalmol Clin. 2016;56(3):93–106.
36. Cionni RJ, Barros MG, Osher RH. Management of lens-iris diaphragm retropulsion syndrome during phacoemulsification. J Cataract Refract Surg. 2004;30(5):953–6.
37. Mohammadpour M. Self-repositioned IOL in a vitrectomized eye. J Cataract Refract Surg. 2008;34:347–8.
38. Malyugin B. Small pupil phaco surgery: a new technique. Ann Ophthalmol (Skokie). 2007;39(3):185–93.
39. Grusha YO, Masket S, Miller KM. Phacoemulsification and lens implantation after pars plana vitrectomy. Ophthalmology. 1998;105:287–94.
40. Yung CW, Oliver A, Bonnin JM, Gao H. Modified anterior capsulotomy technique and histopathology of the anterior capsule in cataracts after prolonged exposure to intravitreal silicone oil. J Cataract Refract Surg. 2008;34:2020–3.
41. Kanclerz P, Grzybowski A, Schwartz SG, Lipowski P. Complications of cataract surgery in eyes filled with silicone oil. Eur J Ophthalmol. 2018;28(4):465–8.
42. Kawasaki S, Suzuki T, Yamaguchi M, et al. Disruption of the posterior chamber-anterior hyaloid membrane barrier during phacoemulsification and aspiration as revealed by contrast-enhanced magnetic resonance imaging. Arch Ophthalmol. 2009;127(4):465–70.
43. Kawasaki S, Tasaka Y, Suzuki T, et al. Influence of elevated intraocular pressure on the posterior chamber-anterior hyaloid membrane barrier during cataract operations. Arch Ophthalmol. 2011;129(6):751–7.
44. Braunstein RE, Airiani S. Cataract surgery results after pars plana vitrectomy. Curr Opin Ophthalmol. 2003;14(3):150–4.
45. Chang MA, Parides MK, Chang S, Braunstein RE. Outcome of phacoemulsification after pars plana vitrectomy. Ophthalmology. 2002;109:948–54.
46. Cole C, Charteris D. Cataract extraction after retinal detachment repair by vitrectomy: visual outcome and complications. Eye. 2009;23:1377.
47. Chung T-Y, Chung H, Lee JH. Combined surgery and sequential surgery comprising phacoemulsification, pars plana vitrectomy, and intraocular lens implantation: comparison of clinical outcomes. J Cataract Refract Surg. 2002;28:2001–5.
48. Soliman MK, Hardin JS, Jawed F, Uwaydat SH, Faramawi MF, et al. A database study of visual outcomes and intraoperative complications of postvitrectomy cataract surgery. Ophthalmology. 2018;125(11):1683–91.
49. Rey A, Jürgens I, Maseras X, Dyrda A, Pera P, Morilla A. Visual outcome and complications of cataract extraction after pars plana vitrectomy. Clin Ophthalmol. 2018;25(12):989–94.

22 Combined Cataract Surgery with Pars Plana Vitrectomy

James M. Osher, Christopher D. Riemann, Samantha L. Schockman, and Michael E. Snyder

Bullet Points

- Combined phaco/vitrectomy is almost always preferred over staged procedures.
- Surgical technique can markedly reduce the complication risk during phaco/vitrectomy.
- Intraocular lens selection may be different if posterior segment surgery is performed with phaco.
- Silicone intraocular lenses should be avoided in patients with current or potential surgical posterior segment disease.
- Certain lens and intraocular lens complications are managed better with an approach that combines pars plana vitrectomy with anterior segment surgery.

Supplementary Information The online version contains supplementary material available at [https://doi.org/10.1007/978-3-030-94530-5_22].

J. M. Osher (✉) · C. D. Riemann · M. E. Snyder
Cincinnati Eye Institute, University of Cincinnati, Cincinnati, OH, USA
e-mail: josher@cvphealth.com; criemann@cvphealth.com; msnyder@cvphealth.com

S. L. Schockman
Cincinnati Eye Institute, Cincinnati, OH, USA
e-mail: sschockman@cvphealth.com

When we encounter a patient with both cataract and surgical posterior segment pathology, there is a dilemma regarding the best approach. Is it best to remove the cataract first and then address the posterior pathology at a later date? Would it be best to manage vitreoretinal problems prior to cataract surgery in order to get optimal IOL calculations and do the cataract later? Or is combined phaco/vitrectomy the most favorable course? Of these three options, the authors strongly advocate for combined surgery, which offers many advantages when executed correctly and very few drawbacks in most scenarios.

As both phaco and vitrectomy have evolved over the past few decades to result in quicker, safer procedures, combined phaco/vitrectomy has become more common worldwide. Unfortunately, staged cataract surgery before or after vitrectomy remains common in the United States. There are several possible explanations for this departure from the worldwide standard of care. These include lacking phaco-competence among US vitreoretinal surgeons (many US retina fellowship programs do not incorporate cataract surgery as part of the training curriculum), the segmentation of many retinal surgeons into separate practices from their anterior segment colleagues, many operating rooms not being equipped with appropriate instrumentation to accomplish both surgeries, and difficulty scheduling two surgeons to be in the same place at the same time. These realities, turf battles between

J. L. Alió et al. (eds.), *Cataract Surgery*, Essentials in Ophthalmology,
https://doi.org/10.1007/978-3-030-94530-5_22

subspecialists and medical practices, and resulting referral patterns result in staged surgeries. Regrettably, it is the patient in this situation who suffers most.

In this chapter, we will discuss why phaco/vitrectomy is almost always the best option. We will review the advantages and disadvantages of our preferred phaco/vitrectomy technique, as well as management pearls to achieve a successful outcome. Finally, we will review selected complex situations for which phaco/vitrectomy remains the option of choice.

Advantages to Combined Phaco/Vitrectomy

We feel strongly that a combined approach, rather than staged, provides several benefits. The literature has long been very clear that combined phaco-vitrectomy can be performed with excellent results. Lahey et al. reported 89 eyes undergoing phaco/vitrectomy for macular hole, and results were similar to historic controls without phaco [1]. In addition, these authors reviewed 223 patients undergoing combined phaco/vitrectomy for diabetic eye disease (including 153 eyes with vitreous hemorrhage, 58 traction retinal detachments, and 12 eyes with posterior hyaloidal traction) with 10 months follow-up and excellent anatomical and visual results [2]. Demetriades et al. reported 122 eyes that underwent phaco/vitrectomy for varied indications also with excellent results and low complication rates [3]. Ling et al. reported 90 patients undergoing combined phaco/vitrectomy for retinal detachment (21), recurrent retinal detachment (7), macular hole (MH) (44), epiretinal membrane (ERM) (11), proliferative diabetic retinopathy (PDR) (3), and vitreous hemorrhage (4) with excellent anatomical and visual results [4]. Jun et al. reported 113 eyes that underwent phaco/vitrectomy for PDR, proliferative vitreoretinopathy, ERM/MH, trauma, and retinal vein occlusion with excellent results and no combined surgery-related complications [5]. Amino and Tanihara reported 42 eyes operated with phaco/vitrectomy/membrane peel for diabetic macular edema. At 18 month follow-up, there was reduced edema and improved visual acuity [6]. Several case series comparing staged and combined surgical approaches also uniformly demonstrated non-inferiority of combined phaco/vitrectomy [7–9].

In eyes with a routine cataract, the surgeon's role is to exclude other disease and causally link the patient's symptoms to the cataract. In the absence of comorbid ocular pathology, it is then the patient who determines whether alleviating the cataract symptoms is worth the downside risks of proceeding with surgical intervention. The surgical decision lies mainly with the patient.

In patients with both cataract and posterior pathology, decision-making is more complex, and the surgeon plays a more central role in the surgical decision-making process. Is the cataract visually significant? Is it likely to become so after posterior segment surgery? Will the cataract preclude adequate visualization for retinal surgery and post-op visits? Is the posterior segment pathology a *must operate* scenario (examples include fovea threatening tractional retinal detachment, intraocular foreign body, post-injection endophthalmitis with light perception vision), a *should operate* scenario (examples include 20/60 ERM, macular hole, non-clearing vitreous hemorrhage with retinal tear and sub-clinical retinal detachment), or a *may operate* scenario (examples include 20/30 ERM, visually significant floaters)? Will adding cataract surgery to the posterior surgery possibly complicate the posterior outcome (see below section on retinal detachment)? Is the symptomatology and visual loss due to cataract, the posterior pathology, or both? In the case of combined pathology, the required surgical decision-making bends more toward the surgeon than the patient for both the posterior disease and the cataract.

Posterior disease states and vitrectomy surgery are known to cause cataract or advance pre-existing cataract. Chung et al. described cataract progression in 33 eyes after vitrectomy for diabetic and hypertensive retinopathy. Thirty-one (94%) had worsened nuclear sclerosis at an average of 9.1 months post-op, 15 (47%) had worsened cortical sclerosis by an average of 8 months, and 24 (78%) had worsened posterior subcapsular changes by an average of 13.3 months after vitrectomy [10]. Thompson et al. reported a 76% of eyes underwent cataract surgery within 2 years following macular hole repair [11]. Melberg and Thomas reported 7% of patients under 50 years old vs 79% of patients over 50 years old developed significant cataract progression compared to the non-operated eye after vitrectomy with gas at 27 months post-op [12]. Cherfan et al. reported an 80% progression to visually significant cataract 29 months after vitrectomy for ERM. Patients less than 50 years old were much less likely to need cataract surgery within the follow-up period [13]. Thompson found a 700% greater chance of cataract progression in patients greater than 50 years old vs under 50 years old and a 60% greater chance of cataract progression in patients with vs without a bubble in eyes undergoing vitrectomy for various indications [14].

Given that most patients who require vitrectomy already have some degree of cataract formation and the overwhelming evidence that vitrectomy surgery almost always leads to progression to visually significant cataract – especially in patients age 50 or above – it makes sense to remove the cataract simultaneously with combined phaco/vitrectomy to allow for unidirectional visual improvement postoperatively. By performing phaco/vitrectomy together, the patients are exposed to one set of surgical risks, postoperative visits, postoperative medications, insurance co-payments, and psychological stressors associated with surgery. In addition, patients have a faster time to visual rehabilitation and require less time off from work, which can also help reduce the financial burden of multiple surgeries. It should be noted, however, that vitrectomy does not always cause cataracts, and caution should be exercised when cataract surgery is being considered in younger patients without presbyopia who do not yet have a cataract.

The above advantages are mostly from the patient perspective. What about the surgeon? There are benefits of combined surgery, both practical and technical, for the surgeon. From a practical perspective, physicians and medical practices also benefit from fewer postoperative visits, with fewer patients allowing for improved patient flow and increased productivity. Significant resource expenditure from ancillary and operating room staff is needed to schedule and prepare surgery for patients. Combined surgery reduces overall overhead and improves overall efficiency [15].

From a technical standpoint, most of the advantage to combined surgery is in the vitrectomy. A well-executed phaco affords a pristine view for posterior segment surgery. To perform meticulous, safe macular surgery, the view to the posterior segment is critical. It is preferable to operate through a clear implant lens, rather than an opaque crystalline lens. In addition, the anterior retina and vitreous base are far more easily accessed surgically in pseudophakic vs phakic eyes. Reaching across the midline of the vitreous cavity in a phakic eye risks hitting and damaging the posterior capsule of the crystalline lens, which can reduce surgical visualization and can also risk complications during future cataract surgery. Since crossing midline is unwise in phakic eyes, shaving the vitreous base requires ambidextrous surgical techniques, a skilled surgical assistant, and/or special equipment to perform scleral depression, none of which are always available. These limitations are not present in pseudophakic eyes where reaching across the midline to reach the entirety of the posterior segment is straightforward and uncomplicated.

The cataract surgeon also benefits from combined phaco/vitrectomy surgeries as it allows for surgery in a non-vitrectomized eye. If done as a staged procedure, the cataract surgeon is faced with a previously vitrectomized eye which can present its own surgical challenges. Eyes which have undergone previous vitrectomy oftentimes develop dense lenses, and the fluidics in a vitrectomized eye cause more anterior chamber instability and posterior capsule mobility. There is a higher risk of posterior capsule rupture during cataract surgery in an eye with previous vitrectomy [16].

Disadvantages of Combined Phaco/Vitrectomy

The disadvantages to combined phaco/vitrectomy are mitigated, if not eliminated, by proper procedure technique. However, we will review the drawbacks in this section and include those that may be encountered even when the technique is poor.

It is difficult to separate the disadvantages into practical and technical, as was done in the advantages section, since there are so few practical disadvantages. The main disadvantage from this perspective is when the cataract is dense enough to handicap the posterior segment examination. Missing exam findings result in the inability to properly educate the patient about the upcoming procedure and possibly postoperative recovery. For example, if exam or imaging through a dense cataract reveals an ERM, yet the co-existing inferior retinal detachment is not able to be visualized, the patient may require unexpected strict face down postoperative positioning and an extensive explanation that this was present prior to surgery but not seen. However, even in this circumstance, combined surgery was the right decision as phaco alone may have allowed the retinal detachment to progress. So when the cataract is significant enough to impair the posterior exam, the patient needs to be counseled that there may be findings intraoperatively that may need to be addressed at that time. The frequency of cataract precluding diagnosis of posterior pathology so severe that if known would have obviated the need for retinal surgery altogether (optic atrophy or end-stage glaucoma in a patient with a large ERM for example) is exceedingly rare. In addition, the patient must be counseled that a combined phaco/vitrectomy may result in less predictable refractive outcomes when the retinal pathology does not allow for accurate preoperative testing and optical measurements.

The technique for combined phaco/vitrectomy is detailed later in this chapter so it will not be discussed at length here. However, it is worth mentioning that suboptimal technique from both the anterior and posterior segment surgeries can pose significant challenges. Poor phaco wound construction can cause an unstable anterior chamber, intraocular lens (IOL) and iris movement, and prolapse during vitrectomy. This is typically seen when placing vitrectomy trocars and during scleral depression, which we perform at the end of every vitrectomy surgery. Suboptimal wound construction can also cause significant problems when different forms of tamponade are used, which can cause anterior displacement of the IOL and even IOL-corneal touch. This same scenario could also affect rotational stability of a toric IOL. Poor trocar insertion, especially if the eye was left at a low intraocular pressure after cataract surgery, can also cause these same problems with IOL stability. Poor phaco technique or excessive energy for a dense lens can cause corneal clouding making visualization for subsequent vitreoretinal surgery very difficult. Pupillary constriction can occur during cataract surgery and, if not managed appropriately, can make posterior visualization challenging. In the anterior chamber, residual air bubbles or even some residual ophthalmic viscosurgical devices (OVD) can affect the view posteriorly.

On the one hand, the phaco itself can be challenging in the setting of common posterior segment problems, like a dense vitreous hemorrhage, which often affords little to no red reflex during cataract surgery, or positive posterior pressure on the posterior capsule from the buoyancy of indwelling oil fill of the vitreous cavity from prior retinal detachment repair. On the other hand, a planned combined approach offers opportunities to use advanced anterior and posterior surgical techniques and skillsets to mitigate problems.

There are reports that postoperative inflammation is worse after combined phaco/vitrectomy but that has not been our experience in a vast majority of cases. In addition, there are published outcomes which suggest combined phaco/vitrectomy is not associated with increased risk of adverse events versus staged procedures in patients with vitreomacular diseases [17]. In their series of 122 eyes undergoing combined surgery, Demetriades et.al described complications including PCO, IOP spike, corneal epithelial defects, vitreous hemorrhage, retinal detachment, and iris capture of IOL. To mitigate these risks, the authors recommend meticulous continuous curvilinear capsulorhexis (CCC), in-the-bag IOL placement, large IOL optics at least 6 mm in diameter, secured cataract wounds, use of miotics, and the avoidance of atropine after gas exchange [3]. Iris posterior synechiae formation after phaco/vitrectomy was seen at higher rates with concurrent proliferative diabetic retinopathy, use of gas tamponade, fibrin deposition, and the amount of laser photocoagulation used to treat PDR [18]. In patients with uveitis, sequential surgery resulted in less fibrin formation compared to combined surgery, though the number of eyes in this review was very small [8].

Less predictable refractive outcomes with a myopic shift were seen in eyes undergoing combination surgery when gas tamponade was used, possibly resulting from an anterior IOL displacement [19].

One special situation when we believe that combined phaco vitrectomy is not the preferred way forward is in the setting of primary rhegmatogenous retinal detachment (RRD) repair. Proliferative vitreoretinopathy (PVR) remains a persistent and frustrating complication occurring 1–2 months after RRD repair in 5–10% of cases, resulting in permanent loss of foveal vision, even after timely reoperation, in over half of cases. Postoperative inflammation levels correlate to PVR rates, and any extra surgical manipulation beyond what is required to achieve retinal reattachment is unwise – especially when this may result in liberation of inflammation-inducing lens material into the eye. For this reason, we believe that as long as visualization is adequate for precise surgical maneuvers, phakic eyes with retinal detachment should undergo RRD repair without combined cataract surgery. Staged cataract surgery (perhaps in the setting of a combined silicone oil removal) should be performed once the eye has stabilized, usually 3–4 months after RRD repair.

As mentioned above, most of these potential disadvantages are rarely encountered if the surgical technique is sound. When these problems are faced, they typically are not difficult to manage, and rarely is the ultimate outcome adversely affected.

Preoperative Considerations

Patient Selection

Unless there is premature cataract formation, patients under the age of 50 rarely need simultaneous cataract surgery when posterior segment pathology requires vitrectomy. The threshold for combined surgery declines as the patient age increases, which often goes hand-in-hand with increasing lens opacity. Regardless of patient age, if there is not a cataract present, combined phaco/PPV should not be performed under most circumstances, with rare exceptions to include patients who require general anesthesia or a hematologic disorder mandating coagulopathy correction prior to any surgery.

As a general rule, if it is anticipated that a patient will require cataract surgery within a few years of posterior segment surgery, it is appropriate and preferred to perform a combined procedure. The use of an air, gas, or oil bubble also increases the rate of cataract progression, lowering the threshold to recommend combined surgery. A commonly encountered scenario that must also be considered is for patients who will become significantly anisometropic following cataract surgery who don't have much cataract formation in the fellow eye. The threshold to perform combined surgery in this patient population is certainly higher, and a detailed preoperative discussion with the patient is extremely important in this decision-making process. In most cases, contact lens wear in the non-operated eye alleviates this problem.

IOL Selection

A cataract surgeon needs to give careful thought and consideration when deciding on the type and power of IOL for a combined phaco/vitrectomy case. Silicone IOLs are contraindicated in patients with or at risk for surgical retinal pathology due to the fogging of the optic that occurs under air and marring of silicone IOL optics by silicone oil. The oil-related marring may be very severe precluding adequate visualization for vitreoretinal diagnosis and surgery and is extremely challenging to remove often resulting in IOL exchange. A large IOL optic (at least 6 mm) is also favored if possible, especially in situations requiring clear peripheral retinal visualization both during and after surgery. Toric IOLs are perfectly acceptable in combination with vitrectomy when using the techniques described above in appropriate patients. Toussaint et al. reported 55 eyes of 51 patients operated with combined phaco/vitrectomy and toric IOL implantation with uncorrected visual acuity outcomes comparable to cataract surgery and toric IOL implantation alone [20].

Decision-making regarding multifocal intraocular (MFIOL) placement in the setting of combined phaco/vitrectomy is more complex and nuanced. While small pilot series of phaco/vitrectomy with MFIOL for visually significant opacities and ERM revealed excellent near and distance uncorrected visual results, we urge great caution and thoughtfulness when considering a MFIOL in patients with concurrent vitreoretinal disease [21, 22]. Posterior segment disease often manifests with reduced contrast sensitivity. Contrast sensitivity reduction is the most important optical compromise that patients sacrifice to achieve multifocality, and the combined contrast sensitivity reductions of a multifocal lens and retinal pathology can be insurmountable, even after extensive periods of neuroadaptation, resulting in unhappy MFIOL patients. Preoperative optical coherence tomography (OCT) testing to carefully evaluate the integrity of all retinal layers is essential in these scenarios.

Determining the necessary IOL power can sometimes be tricky in this patient population. Various pathologies such as vitreous hemorrhage, macular edema/fibrosis, macula-involving RD, dense cataract, and others can result in inaccurate preoperative biometric testing. When this occurs, IOL calculations are directly affected, and the surgeon must be acutely aware of this when determining which IOL power should be used. In addition, substitute media in the vitreous cavity, such as silicone oil, must be taken into account when performing IOL calculations to avoid a refractive surprise.

Highly myopic eyes typically have longer than normal axial lengths and are associated with more retinal pathology than eyes of normal axial length. In such cases with unilateral pathology, significant anisometropia may result postoperatively, and a plan for postoperative vision must be determined beforehand. If the fellow eye has a cataract, a plan for eventual phaco/IOL in that eye may be the answer. If the fellow eye does not have lens opacity, post-op anisometropia may be ameliorated by (1) making the surgical eye myopic postoperatively, (2) using a contact lens in the non-surgical eye, or (3) having refractive surgery.

In cases in which retinal detachment repair is planned by both vitrectomy and scleral buckle, both surgeons should openly communicate and attempt to incorporate the myopic effect of a buckle on the IOL power selection, recognizing that refractive target accuracy will be less than in vitrectomy-only cases.

Regardless of which IOL is chosen, it is imperative to have a thorough discussion with the patient to review realistic expectations for visual acuity and refractive needs after surgery. It is always important to under promise while emphasizing the likelihood of needing glasses after surgery.

Surgical Planning

As discussed previously, there is some logistical planning required for a phaco/vitrectomy procedure. In particular, a surgery center with both a cataract and retina surgeon having overlapping surgical times is required. In addition, there needs to be clear communication between the two surgeons, particularly if one or both surgeons will need to deviate from the routine. The surgeons must plan for possible challenges that may ensue for each unique patient. For example, if a patient has a substantial amount of fibrosis on the posterior capsule that is not amenable to polishing, should the cataract surgeon perform a posterior continuous capsulorhexis to improve the retina surgeon's view, or would the retina surgeon prefer to use the vitrector on the posterior capsule? If there is a small pupil, will an expanding device be needed and which surgeon will place and remove it? To address these challenges, good communication between the surgeons is required to determine the best way to address each dilemma.

Intraoperative Technique and Considerations

The principles of combined phaco/vitrectomy are quite straightforward, and there are many iterations that result in good outcomes. The main goals of phaco are to put the IOL in the desired position, keep the IOL in position by creating a stable anterior chamber, provide a clear view through which to perform retina surgery, and establish water-tight, secured wounds. The goals for the posterior portion share some similarities: keep the IOL in good position; leave the eye with appropriate, stable intraocular pressure; and position the patient appropriately postoperatively if necessary.

Surgical Management Pearls

In combined phaco/vitrectomy surgery, routine cataract surgery should be performed with attention to a few important details. If a peribulbar or retrobulbar block is given, excess volume should be avoided to minimize posterior pressure and chemosis, which can cause fluid pooling and frustrate visualization for the cataract surgeon. Chemosis may also block scleral landmarks for toric IOL alignment. If needed, additional block can be given in the posterior subtenon space after the cataract surgery.

The phaco wound construction is extremely important, even if the plan is to suture the incision. The most common time for the main cataract incision to leak is when trocars are being inserted. Therefore, some surgeons advocate trocar placement prior to the cataract surgery incisions, which is a completely acceptable approach. With the advent of valved cannulas, it is quite simple to leave the cannulas in place during phaco. Pre-placement of the cannulas may make an inferonasal approach for the infusion cannula more desirable for a temporal approach cataract surgeon to avoid having two cannulas in the temporal pars plana. Cannula placement is less influenced by a superior main cataract incision, though this has established implications for induced astigmatism. The authors have found that attentive corneal wound construction, with or without a postoperative corneal suture or wound sealant, in combination with careful trocar placement, obviates the need to pre-place the cannulas.

If the red reflex is poor due to posterior segment media opacity, trypan blue can be used to facilitate capsulorhexis. We are very attentive to making our anterior capsulorhexis between 4.5 and 5.0 mm to ensure uniform coverage of the IOL edge for 360 degrees and to facilitate optic capture in the rare event of a compromised posterior capsule. We find a small gauge coaxial capsulorhexis forceps with millimeter markings (Seibel Forceps, MicroSurgical Technologies, Redmond, Washington) to make the capsulotomy creation and size reproducibly facile. Others prefer using the femtosecond laser as an automated technology to achieve the same goal.

Iris manipulation should be minimized to prevent the pupil from becoming too small during the cataract surgery. A small pupil can make visualization more difficult for the retina surgeon. Intracameral epinephrine or a combination drug like Omidria (phenylephrine and ketorolac) can be utilized during cataract surgery in attempt to maximize the pupillary size before the retina portion of the procedure. If an iris expander device is needed for cataract surgery, it can be removed either at the end of cataract surgery with the subsequent removal of the anterior chamber OVD, or it can be left in place during the retinal procedure to optimize visualization. If it is kept in place during the retinal procedure, it will need to be removed at the end of the case by the cataract surgeon, unless the retinal surgeon feels comfortable doing so.

Phaco and cortical removal can proceed in the usual fashion with attention to make the posterior capsule as clear as possible for the subsequent retina surgery. In some cases, the cataract can be quite dense and result in corneal edema from prolonged phacoemulsification. Use of additional OVD throughout phaco may reduce this edema. In addition, optimizing the settings on the phaco machine for a dense cataract may help to minimize corneal edema [23]. If corneal edema does become significant enough to reduce the retina surgeon's view, the surgeon can perform corneal scraping for a better view or potentially use a hyperosmolar corneal lubricant [24].

In eyes with indwelling silicone oil in which are undergoing combined cataract surgery and silicone oil removal, the cataract surgery may be a bit more challenging. In these cases, the silicone oil will continuously push the posterior capsule anteriorly. To combat this, it is important to keep the anterior chamber filled with OVD and to instill extra OVD when removing either the phaco or irrigation/aspiration (I/A) handpiece. A second instrument can be placed between the phaco tip and the posterior capsule to avoid inadvertent contact with an expectedly convex posterior capsule.

In the rare event of a posterior capsular tear, we would manage this similarly to a cataract surgery without a combined retina procedure. Specifically, we would either convert the tear into a posterior capsulorhexis or plan an in-the-bag IOL placement of the original planned implant, or, if a posterior capsulorhexis were not viable, we would select a three-piece IOL and place this implant in the sulcus with optic capture through the anterior capsulorhexis. It is important to recognize that in a combined phaco/PPV case, a full 3-port vitrectomy is planned so after a posterior capsular tear, it is perfectly acceptable to fill the anterior chamber with OVD and then perform a pars plana vitrectomy and lensectomy (if needed). Managing the vitreous by thorough removal through the pars plana will often back anterior chamber cleanup and IOL placement much more straightforward.

As we have suggested previously, maintaining a "pro combined surgery" ethos presents opportunities for more efficient, better care for patients. The combined cataract surgery-silicone oil (SO) removal scenario is a particularly good example. Oftentimes, SO placement for retinal detachment repair occurs in patients with more complex pathology, including proliferative vitreoretinopathy, and there is a higher risk for recurrent RD and poor visual outcome. In these cases, a microincisional approach with minimal uveal manipulation is preferred. Removing silicone oil through the pars plana valved cannula with a viscous fluid cannula works very well but can take considerable time, especially if removing 5000cs oil. We suggest the following surgical plan: phaco and I/A of the lens is followed by polishing of the capsule and placement of viscoelastic as usual. A small (approximately 2–3 mm) primary posterior capsulorhexis is then performed. A single 27 gauge pars plana trocar is placed and charged with a vitreoretinal infusion cannula. Silicone oil is removed by placing an appropriate cannula (we prefer a trimmed 18 or 20 gauge AngioCath™ for 5000cs oil and 1000cs oil, respectively) through the phaco wound, through the anterior capsulorhexis, and through the posterior capsulorhexis into the vitreous cavity. After oil removal, the capsular bag is re-inflated with OVD, an appropriate lens implant is placed into the capsular bag, OVD is removed, and self-sealing wounds are confirmed to be watertight. A pearl for this technique is to make sure the eye is positioned absolutely vertically under the microscope to allow the oil bubble to move centrally for complete removal, avoiding retention of an oil droplet hidden under the peripheral iris. Another pearl is to be mindful of pressure gradients between the anterior and posterior chambers. It is important to keep the posterior infusion high enough to keep the eye fully formed. A partially collapsed globe will immediately re-inflate when the I/A probe is inserted to remove OVD after IOL placement, with a gush of fluid from anterior to posterior risking luxation of the IOL onto the macula. An over-pressurized posterior segment, on the other hand, will lead to a flat anterior chamber and iris prolapse as soon as the main incision is opened to insert the I/A probe. Accomplishing combined approach surgery in this fashion is enormously gratifying because we avoid the sclerotomy which is a second large incision into the eye, through the uvea to remove the silicone oil.

During surgery on axially myopic eyes, especially those that have undergone prior vitrectomy for retinal detachment repair, the anterior chamber may become hyper-deep and/or hyperdynamic in the so-called lens-iris-diaphragm retropulsion syndrome (LIDRS) [25, 26]. This is not an uncommon setting to need a combined surgery in a post-RD repair eye that may now have cataract and ERM. With no vitreous to ballot the lens, when infusion is initiated, the chamber becomes rapidly very deep, dilating the pupil widely and putting the zonules on stretch. The attentive surgeon can immediately eliminate this problem by depressing the anterior capsule or by gently lifting the iris margin with the second instrument, allowing infusate to pass under the iris, through the zonules, and thereby equalizing the pressure in the anterior and posterior segments. If this occurs at the start of phaco, it will certainly recur in the same eye when I/A is initiated. It can be pre-empted by lifting the iris margin with the I/A tip before infusion is started or by infusing balanced salt solution under the iris margin in the OVD filled anterior chamber to pressurize the posterior segment before the I/A device is placed into the eye. Lowered parameters (slow motion phaco) reduce the tendency for LIDRS to occur.

When performing combined cataract and vitrectomy "combo" surgery in axial myopes, it may be prudent to consider placing a capsular tension ring (CTR) prophylactically, as these eyes are prone to subsequent progressive zonulopathy and with a CTR in place, subsequent repositioning of a subluxed IOL/bag complex will be much easier. This is especially useful in eyes with peculiarly low IOL powers, since such implant powers are not readily available in models suitable for scleral fixation.

Adequate closure of the corneal incision is critical, either with wound hydration, a wound sealant, or a nylon suture. At the conclusion of the cataract surgery portion, the wounds must be sealed enough to tolerate trocar placement and potential scleral depression. Care should be taken not to overly hydrate the incision to avoid corneal edema which could impair the view to the peripheral retina.

The intraocular pressure should be left above normal at the conclusion of cataract surgery. Having a firm eye makes it much easier to place the trocars without indenting the sclera. A gentle rotation of the trocar between the fingers will also allow smooth trocar placement. The position of the trocar should be at least 15 degrees away from the main corneal incision to reduce the likelihood of wound gape during insertion.

Complex Case Example

In the introduction, we mentioned that the combined approach make the retinal surgeon's job more facile. There is one kind of case in which the retinal surgeon's expertise is crucial for the cataract surgeon's execution of the case – the dangling crystalline lens! Occasionally, zonulopathy will be so profound that the lens is hanging by just a few sparse zonules into the vitreous cavity and entangled in vitreous gel. While some would advocate a vitrectomy/lensectomy, we suggest a capsule sparing approach for selected cases. In such a case, the retina surgeon will remove the vitreous gel around the lens, and then using the vitrector and the light pipe under the lens as "crossed-swords," the lens can be lifted into the iris plane, and the cataract surgeon can initiate the capsulorhexis and then place flexible stabilization retractors to the capsule margin and/or the equator of the bag. Once phacoemulsification is complete, a fixatable (Cionni) CTR can be placed and fixated to the scleral wall. Not only does this preserve the option for toric and/or multifocal IOLs but also eliminates the risk of reverse pupillary capture of an IOL margin from a sclerally fixated implant lens, which would be required were a pars plana lensectomy performed (Videos 22.1, 22.2, and 22.3).

Postoperative Considerations

Once the combo phaco/vitrectomy procedure is completed, attention is directed toward the patient's postoperative care. The immediate postoperative instructions will largely be dependent on the retinal procedure undertaken. Per the retina surgeon, the patient may require strict precautions and positioning requirements. Intraocular pressure should be monitored and controlled. The postoperative appointments should be determined before surgery by the cataract and retina surgeon team to minimize patient appointments and avoid unnecessary duplicate appointments. A longer taper of post-op steroid and NSAID eye drops, compared to phaco alone, is often needed in patients with retinal pathology. Clear communication between the two surgeons should continue throughout the postoperative course.

Summary

Combined phaco/vitrectomy carries many benefits for both the patient and surgeons. Unfortunately, it is still underutilized in the United States, and a staged procedure is often done. Admittedly, there are some logistical and technical challenges when attempting a combo phaco/vitrectomy; however with careful planning, these can certainly be overcome, and a successful outcome can be achieved. We strongly believe a combined approach is superior to a staged procedure when there is appropriate patient selection, preoperative planning, intraoperative technique, and postoperative care.

Take-Home Notes

- Combined phaco/vitrectomy is almost always preferred over staged procedures.
- Excellent communication between the cataract and vitreoretinal surgeons is essential.
- Preoperative identification of posterior segment disease with subsequent management can help avoid an unhappy patient after cataract surgery alone.
- Proper surgical technique using the pearls discussed in this chapter will greatly reduce surgical complications and challenges encountered during phaco/vitrectomy.
- With appropriate patient selection, multifocal, accommodating, and toric IOLs are appropriate for phaco/vitrectomy.

References

1. Lahey JM, Francis RR, Fong DS, Kearney JJ, Tanaka S. Combining phacoemulsification with vitrectomy for treatment of macular holes. Br J Ophthalmol. 2002;86(8):876–8.
2. Lahey JM, Francis RR, Kearney JJ. Combining phacoemulsification with pars plana vitrectomy in patients with proliferative diabetic retinopathy: a series of 223 cases. Ophthalmology. 2003;110(7):1335–9.
3. Demetriades AM, Gottsch JD, Thomsen R, et al. Combined phacoemulsification, intraocular lens implantation, and vitrectomy for eyes with coexisting cataract and vitreoretinal pathology. Am J Ophthalmol. 2003;135(3):291–6.
4. Ling R, Simcock P, McCoombes J, Shaw S. Presbyopic phacovitrectomy. Br J Ophthalmol. 2003;87(11):1333–5.
5. Jun Z, Pavlovic S, Jacobi KW. Results of combined vitreoretinal surgery and phacoemulsification with intraocular lens implantation. Clin Exp Ophthalmol. 2001;29(5):307–11.
6. Amino K, Tanihara H. Vitrectomy combined with phacoemulsification and intraocular lens implantation for diabetic macular edema. Jpn J Ophthalmol. 2002;46(4):455–9.
7. Krepler K, Mozaffarieh M, Biowski R, Nepp J, Wedrich A. Cataract surgery and silicone oil removal: visual outcome and complications in a combined vs. two step surgical approach. Retina. 2003;23(5):647–53.
8. Senn P, Schipper I, Perren B. Combined pars plana vitrectomy, phacoemulsification, and intraocular lens implantation in the capsular bag: a comparison to vitrectomy and subsequent cataract surgery as a two-step procedure. Ophthalmic Surg Lasers. 1995;26(5):420–8.
9. Chung TY, Chung H, Lee JH. Combined surgery and sequential surgery comprising phacoemulsification, pars plana vitrectomy, and intraocular lens implantation: comparison of clinical outcomes. J Cataract Refract Surg. 2002;28(11):2001–5.
10. Chung CP, Hsu SY, Wu WC. Cataract formation after pars plana vitrectomy. Kaohsiung J Med Sci. 2001;17(2):84–9.
11. Thompson JT, Glaser BM, Sjaarda RN, Murphy RP. Progression of nuclear sclerosis and long-term visual results of vitrectomy with transforming growth factor beta-2 for macular holes. Am J Ophthalmol. 1995 Jan;119(1):48–54.
12. Melberg NS, Thomas MA. Nuclear sclerotic cataract after vitrectomy in patients younger than 50 years of age. Ophthalmology. 1995;102(10):1466–71.
13. Cherfan GM, Michels RG, de Bustros S, Enger C, Glaser BM. Nuclear sclerotic cataract after vitrectomy for idiopathic epiretinal membranes causing macular pucker. Am J Ophthalmol. 1991;111(4):434–8.
14. Thompson JT. The role of patient age and intraocular gas use in cataract progression after vitrectomy

for macular holes and epiretinal membranes. Am J Ophthalmol. 2004;137(2):250–7.
15. Seider MI, Michael Lahey J, Fellenbaum PS. Cost of phacovitrectomy versus vitrectomy and sequential phacoemulsification. Retina. 2014;34(6):1112–5.
16. Erçalık NY, Yenerel NM, Sanisoğlu HA, Kumral ET, İmamoğlu S. Comparison of intra- and postoperative complications of phaco between sequential and combined procedures of 23-gauge vitrectomy and phaco. Saudi J Ophthalmol. 2017;31(4):238–42.
17. Savastano A, Savastano MC, Barca F, Petrarchini F, Mariotti C, Rizzo S. Combining cataract surgery with 25-gauge high-speed pars plana vitrectomy: results from a retrospective study. Ophthalmology. 2014;121(1):299–304.
18. Shinoda K, O'hira A, Ishida S, et al. Posterior synechia of the iris after combined pars plana vitrectomy, phacoemulsification, and intraocular lens implantation. Jpn J Ophthalmol. 2001;45(3):276–80.
19. Suzuki Y, Sakuraba T, Mizutani H, Matsuhashi H, Nakazawa M. Postoperative complications after simultaneous vitrectomy and cataract surgery. Ophthalmic Surg Lasers. 2001;32(5):391–6.
20. Toussaint BW, Appenzeller MF, Miller DM, et al. Stability of the acrysof toric intraocular lens in combined cataract surgery and transconjunctival sutureless vitrectomy. Retina. 2015;35(6):1065–71.
21. Patel SB, Snyder ME, Riemann CD, Osher JM, Mi CW, Sisk RA. Combined phacoemulsification surgery with multifocal intraocular lens implantation and pars plana vitrectomy for symptomatic vitreous opacities. Retin Cases Br Rep. 2021;15(6):724–9.
22. Patel SB, Snyder ME, Riemann CD, Foster RE, Sisk RA. Short-term outcomes of combined pars plana vitrectomy for epiretinal membrane and phacoemulsification surgery with multifocal intraocular lens implantation. Clin Ophthalmol. 2019;13:723–30.
23. Osher RH. Slow motion phacoemulsification approach. J Cataract Refract Surg. Published online. 1993. https://doi.org/10.1016/S0886-3350(13)80025-9.
24. McCannel CA. Improved intraoperative fundus visualization in corneal edema: the Viscoat trick. Retina. 2012;32(1):189–90.
25. Wilbrandt HR, Wilbrandt TH. Pathogenesis and management of the lens-iris diaphragm retropulsion syndrome during phacoemulsification. J Cataract Refract Surg. 1994;20(1):48–53.
26. Osher RH, Osher JM, Cionni RJ. Multifocal iris sphincter ruptures: new sign of the lens-iris diaphragm retropulsion syndrome. J Cataract Refract Surg. 2010;36(1):170–2.

23 Cataract Surgery in High and Extreme Myopia

Michael J. daSilva and Uday Devgan

Preoperative Discussion, Examination, and Planning

High myopia has profound effects on ocular health and on outcomes after cataract surgery. It is therefore important for the surgeon to have a frank discussion with the patient about the general and individual risks of surgery. Of particular importance is the risk of rhegmatogenous retinal detachment (RRD.) At the initial evaluation, the patient should be counseled about the association of high axial length and retinal detachment [1, 2]. Younger age, male sex, and vitreous loss during surgery are also reported risk factors for RRD after cataract extraction [1], and the confluence of these variables can make RRD significantly more likely in certain axial myopes. The patient should be taught the symptoms of retinal tear or detachment, including new floaters, flashing lights, and curtain-like visual field deficit. The patient should seek immediate care if any of these symptoms develop.

Extremely myopic eyes with cataract are at high risk for comorbidities of the retina and optic nerve. Conditions associated with myopia include amblyopia, RRD, open angle glaucoma, and myopic macular degeneration with or without choroidal neovascularization [3, 4]. The cataract surgeon should perform a complete preoperative examination with attention to the macula, optic nerve, and retinal periphery. If significant myopic morphology is apparent, such as peripapillary atrophy, oval-shaped tilted disc, or degenerative changes of the macula, further testing is warranted. This testing should be based on the individual characteristics of the eye being evaluated. Testing may include optical coherence tomography (OCT) of the macula and nerve, visual field testing, and fluorescein angiography if choroidal neovascularization is suspected. B-scan ocular ultrasound should be obtained to assess the shape of the eye if posterior staphylomatous changes are present, as they may affect foveation and the optically measured axial length. The cataract surgeon should not hesitate to refer to a retina specialist colleague for a scleral depressed examination of the periphery. Prophylactic laser retinopexy may be necessary if any symptomatic holes, tufts, or tears are present.

Lens calculations in the axial myope are affected primarily by corneal contour and the axial length. Because a low-power lens will be implanted, changes in effective lens position (ELP) have less refractive consequence. In a simple example, a lens with zero diopters of power has no vergence and will not change with

Supplementary Information The online version contains supplementary material available at [https://doi.org/10.1007/978-3-030-94530-5_23].

M. J. daSilva (✉) · U. Devgan
Stein Eye Institute, University of California Los Angeles (UCLA) School of Medicine, Los Angeles, CA, USA
e-mail: mdasilva@bhrei.com

J. L. Alió et al. (eds.), *Cataract Surgery*, Essentials in Ophthalmology,
https://doi.org/10.1007/978-3-030-94530-5_23

ELP. Similarly, low-power positive or negative lenses are minimally affected by changes in ELP; however, very deep anterior chambers greater than 4 mm may impact the IOL calculation. It is important to have accurate measurements of the corneal curvature (K values), but the greatest challenge in high axial myopia is often to obtain an accurate axial length (AL.) Optical means of measuring AL are preferred. Here the patient is instructed to fixate on a target, which aligns the biometer measurement beam with the fovea. Care should be taken with directly applying the AL value produced by an optical biometer, as biometers generally assume a constant refractive index of the eye. This assumption does not remain accurate in extremely long eyes, in which the vitreous cavity may represent a higher proportion of the measurement beam path. With older-generation two-variable formulae, it was advisable for the surgeon to adjust AL measurements greater than 25 mm using the formula proposed by Wang and Koch [5]. Newer-generation formulae such as the Barrett Universal II, Hill-RBF, Olsen, and others automatically account for measurement characteristics in long eyes.

Highly myopic eyes will need a low-power or even negative-power lens. The geometry of the lens implant changes at very low or negative powers. The most popular US lens platforms begin at +5 to +6 diopters. Lenses below this power, or negative power lenses, are likely to employ a meniscus design. These lenses are commonly produced in one-diopter increments. Meniscus geometry shifts the optical principal plane relative to standard biconvex design and thereby alters the effective lens position. Meniscus lens geometry is compared to biconvex designs in Fig. 23.1.

Various means of adjusting lens calculation equations for high axial myopia have been employed. One strategy is to adjust the lens A-constant with each step in dioptric power of a meniscus lens platform [6, 7]. These optimized A-constants can be accessed at the User Group for Laser Interference Biometry (ULIB) online and can be applied to standard formulae. If this approach is taken, it is important to use the A-constant of the exact power lens that is expected to be implanted. A second proposed strategy is to adjust the axial length, using a formula that accounts for the effect of a longer biometry measurement beam path through the

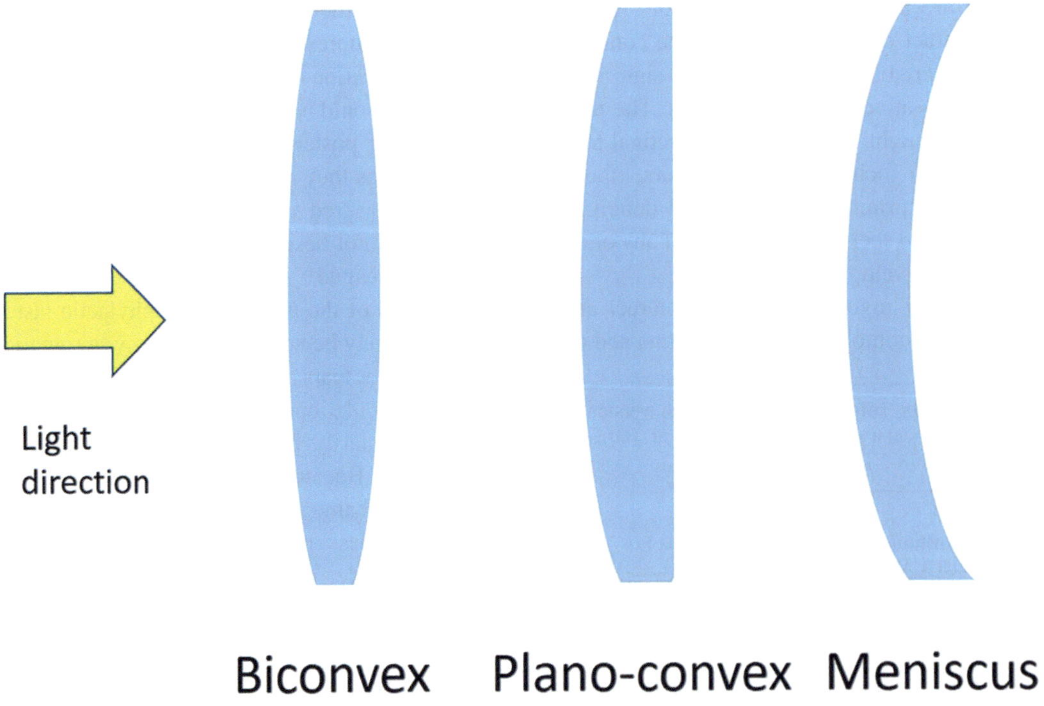

Fig. 23.1 Lens geometry of common IOL designs

vitreous cavity [5, 8]. Studies of axial myopes note that third-generation formula, after axial length adjustment, have similar lens power calculation accuracy to fourth-generation formulae [9, 10]. One study noted that the incidence of small hyperopic outcomes was reduced by using the Wang-Koch AL adjustment when compared to fourth-generation formulae [11]. It is generally accepted that the Wang-Koch AL adjustment shifts outcomes from slightly hyperopic to slightly myopic in high myopes.

Fourth-generation formulae use additional variables, such as anterior chamber depth or lens thickness, to increase accuracy in all eyes. The accuracy of these modern formulae have been analyzed repeatedly in the setting of high axial myopia. Excellent results have been achieved using the Barrett Universal II [10–14], Hill-RBF [11, 14], and Olsen [12] formulae among others. One study of Chinese patients with extreme axial myopia found the Haigis less accurate in the subgroup with AL >30 mm [12]. For practical purposes, the authors recommend the surgeon become familiar with one or two modern formulae and apply it as intended by its creator(s), as not all formulae require measurement data adjustment of any kind. High-quality outcomes can be achieved with several formulae, but all the above-referenced studies indicate high performance of the Barrett Universal II in extreme myopia. A final possibility is to use intraoperative aberrometry, which was reported to result in outcomes similar to those of fourth-generation formulae among moderate axial myopes [15]. Of note, the eyes in this study of aberrometry had an average AL of 25.9 mm, which may normalize data when compared to more extreme degrees of myopia [15].

Consider targeting residual myopia in patients with high axial length. Despite the advancement of biometry and lens calculation, it is still possible to end up with an unintentional hyperopic outcome if measurement error is introduced to any variables. The patient is habituated to myopia and may appreciate the finer near vision afforded by low degrees of myopia. The surgeon should freely discuss the option of targeting near vision. In the past, it has been common practice to target one to two diopters of residual myopia. Given the advancement of lens calculation and formulae which use anterior chamber depth as a variable, the authors recommend targeting only 0.5 to one diopter of residual myopia if an emmetropic result is desired.

The approach to astigmatism management in extreme axial myopes differs from the general population. Toric intraocular lenses are only available down to +5 or + 6 diopters depending on the manufacturer. Astigmatism management patients may therefore require cornea-based treatment. The surgeon can perform intra- or postoperative astigmatic keratotomy or limbal relaxing incisions. Another option is to plan postoperative laser vision correction, termed bioptics by the refractive surgery community. If bioptics are planned, it is beneficial to leave the astigmatic patient with pure myopic astigmatism, and not with mixed astigmatism. Outcomes from excimer laser ablation are more predictable and durable for myopic treatment, so a spherical equivalent in excess of one half the corneal astigmatism power should be targeted. This gives the laser a simple ablation pattern, as outlined in Fig. 23.2. If a spherical equivalent of plano is targeted, resulting in mixed astigmatism, the laser would attempt to steepen one axis while flattening the other; this situation should be avoided if possible. If mixed astigmatism is present postoperatively, limbal relaxing incisions are an effective means of management. A final consideration is the Light Adjustable Lens (LAL), which has been reported to be efficacious in astigmatism management in axial myopes [16]. This platform is currently limited by its dioptric range, which extends from +10.0 to +30.0 diopters, and may therefore not be suitable for extreme axial myopes. The LAL is able to correct up to two diopters of cylinder.

Intraoperative Considerations

Elongated eyes are likely to be larger in several dimensions and may have a white-to-white corneal measurement of 13 mm or more. Myopic eyes may also dilate excessively. If the surgeon proceeds to create a continuous curvilinear capsulorhexis (CCC) gauged by the pupil size, it may become larger than the IOL optic. The

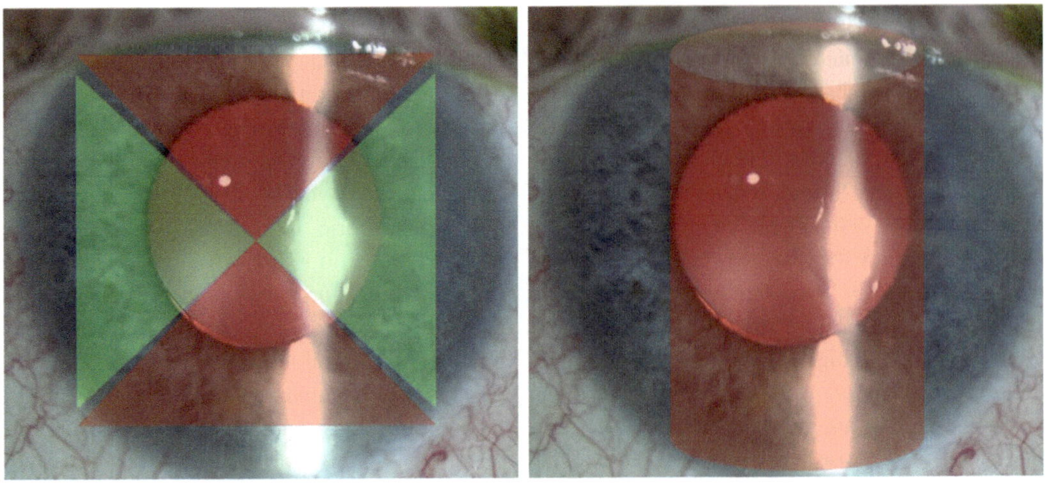

Fig. 23.2 The left image depicts an eye with postoperative refraction +1.00–2.00 × 090. The excimer laser would steepen the horizontal axis and flatten the vertical axis. The surgeon should avoid this situation or consider postoperative limbal relaxing incisions. The right image depicts an eye with postoperative refraction plano −2.00 × 090, simplifying the ablation pattern

authors recommend one of two means of ensuring a consistent capsulorhexis size. One common method is to use a ring guide to indent and thereby lightly mark the cornea; the ring guide takes into account the 20 percent magnification of the anterior lens capsule that is produced by the cornea itself [17]. The rhexis can then simply trace the mark. Another method is to mark the 2.5 and 5 mm distances from the tip of the capsulorhexis forceps, to visualize the intended capsulorhexis size prior to its creation. Before CCC, the surgeon should be aware that a larger amount of ophthalmic viscosurgical device (OVD) may be needed to adequately form the chamber and flatten the anterior lens capsule. Further alternatives include the use of a nanopulse vacuum capsulotomy device (Zepto) or femtosecond laser-assisted capsulorhexis.

The lens capsule in highly myopic eyes is prone to large anteroposterior movements, which may heighten the risk of capsular rupture. Supracapsular lens disassembly can mitigate this risk. Some surgeons favor prolapsing the lens nucleus into the anterior chamber (AC). Due to typically larger AC, safe distance can be maintained from the corneal endothelium, while the nucleus is then chopped and emulsified in the AC. In addition to capsular movement, many surgeons have noted qualitatively that zonular laxity is common in extreme axial myopia. Decades of research into the genetics of myopia have indeed found polymorphisms in proteoglycan synthesis and cell signaling pathways, which would be expected to interact with zonular strength; some of these include PAX6, WNT, and Decorin mutations [18]. It is therefore wise to avoid stressing the zonules. Some surgeons prefer chop techniques for nucleus disassembly. Most agree that thorough hydrodissection can reduce zonular trauma. It is also wise to have assistive devices such as capsular tension rings, capsular tension segments, and capsular hooks readily available in the operating room.

Lens-iris diaphragm retropulsion syndrome (LIDRS) refers to posterior movement of the iris and lens capsule complex. This typically occurs in myopic eyes during cataract surgery. It is caused by a reverse pupillary block, when fluid can no longer travel out of the posterior chamber. In addition to being painful for the patient, it may stress the zonules. The reverse pupillary block can be broken either by gently lifting the underside of the iris or by depressing the anterior capsule to re-establish fluid flow into the retro-irideal space. For persistent reverse pupillary block, an alternative that is rarely necessary is to place a single nasal iris hook.

Care should be taken throughout lens removal, and especially between steps which require removal of the handpiece, to prevent collapse of the anterior chamber. The first important step is to create an adequately long corneal incision, the architecture of which limits fluid egress. The surgeon should next lower the infusion pressure. High infusion pressure can deepen the anterior chamber excessively in myopic eyes, which causes more anteroposterior movement upon depressurization. The surgeon can also use his or her second hand to inject viscoelastic, while the handpiece is still in the eye on position one, prior to removal of the handpiece at the end of cortical cleanup. Likewise, after implantation of the intraocular lens and removal of the viscoelastic, balanced saline can be injected in the paracentesis during removal of the handpiece. These extra steps aimed at preventing chamber collapse can reduce anterior movement of the vitreous base, which may theoretically reduce the risk of vitreous traction and subsequent retinal tears.

Postoperative Follow-Up

In the postoperative period, the cataract surgeon should again carefully counsel the patient regarding the symptoms of retinal tears and of retinal detachment (RD.) The patient should resume care with their habitual retina specialist, ideally one who examined their eyes prior to surgery. Retrospective studies have found variable rates of retinal detachment in myopic eyes after cataract surgery. A large retrospective review of eyes with axial length greater than 27 mm found no increased risk of RD after cataract surgery through 2 years, when compared to reported idiopathic incidence [19]. A smaller retrospective study sorted their study population into subgroups and found a high rate of retinal detachment in eyes with lattice degeneration who first developed posterior vitreous detachment (PVD) in the postoperative period; among this smaller group, the rate of RD was reported to be 21% at 5 years [20]. This same study noted a low rate of RD (0.70%) in patients who had neither lattice nor preoperative PVD. Though the exact incidence of retinal tear or detachment is unclear and certainly varies depending on what group is selected, evidence distinctly recommends close follow-up.

Myopic patients may require prompt sequential surgery, within 2 weeks, due to intolerable degrees of aniseikonia. Patients should be alerted preoperatively, so they may plan on sequential surgery. The visual disturbance of aniseikonia is likely to be mitigated by the high residual myopia in the partner eye; if left uncorrected, this eye would be fogged and likely ignored by the patient. An alternative to prompt sequential surgery, if the patient can tolerate their degree of aniseikonia, is contact lens use.

Take-Home Points for Clinical Practice

- The cataract surgeon or a designated retina colleague should conduct a thorough preoperative survey of the highly myopic eye, to include OCT of the retina and nerve, peripheral exam, and possibly B-scan ultrasound to assess morphology.
- The authors recommend using optical biometry methods to acquire an axial length measurement; it is also recommended to use a fourth-generation formula such as the Barrett II, Ladas, or Hill-RBF for IOL calculations, as these formulae automatically account both for increased vitreous cavity depth and for changes in IOL geometry.
- Target residual myopia in the range of −0.5 to −1.0 diopters. More residual myopia may be necessary if the patient desires astigmatism management, if bioptics are planned.
- Highly myopic eyes have deeper anterior chambers and are prone to flux intraoperatively. To perform a gentle surgery, lower bottle height, be aware of

lens-iris diaphragm retropulsion syndrome, replace fluids during probe withdrawal to prevent AC collapse, and consider supracapsular nucleus disassembly.

- Patients with extreme myopia are at higher risk for postoperative retinal detachment and should be counseled thoroughly about symptoms. Follow-up visits should be more frequent for those with lattice degeneration.

References

1. Qureshi MH, Steel DHW. Retinal detachment following cataract phacoemulsification-a review of the literature. Eye (Lond). 2020;34(4):616–31. https://doi.org/10.1038/s41433-019-0575-z. Epub 2019 Oct 1. Erratum in: Eye (Lond). 2019 Oct 28;: PMID: 31576027; PMCID: PMC7093479.
2. Sheu SJ, Ger LP, Chen JF. Axial myopia is an extremely significant risk factor for young-aged pseudophakic retinal detachment in Taiwan. Retina. 2006;26(3):322–7. https://doi.org/10.1097/00006982-200603000-00011. PMID: 16508433.
3. Haarman AEG, Enthoven CA, Tideman JWL, Tedja MS, Verhoeven VJM, Klaver CCW. The complications of myopia: a review and meta-analysis. Invest Ophthalmol Vis Sci. 2020;61(4):49. https://doi.org/10.1167/iovs.61.4.49. PMID: 32347918; PMCID: PMC7401976.
4. Marcus MW, de Vries MM, Junoy Montolio FG, Jansonius NM. Myopia as a risk factor for open-angle glaucoma: a systematic review and meta-analysis. Ophthalmology. 2011;118(10):1989–1994.e2. https://doi.org/10.1016/j.ophtha.2011.03.012. PMID: 21684603.
5. Wang L, Shirayama M, Ma XJ, Kohnen T, Koch DD. Optimizing intraocular lens power calculations in eyes with axial lengths above 25.0 mm. J Cataract Refract Surg. 2011;37(11):2018–27. https://doi.org/10.1016/j.jcrs.2011.05.042. PMID: 22018365.
6. Haigis W. Biometry and intraocular lens calculation in extreme myopia. Acta Clin Croat. 2012;51(Suppl 1):65–9. PMID: 23431727.
7. Petermeier K, Gekeler F, Messias A, Spitzer MS, Haigis W, Szurman P. Intraocular lens power calculation and optimized constants for highly myopic eyes. J Cataract Refract Surg. 2009;35:1575–81.
8. Preussner P-R. Intraocular lens calculation in extreme myopia. [Letter]. J Cataract Refract Surg. 2010;36:531–2, reply by W Haigis, 532–534.
9. Zhang J, Tan X, Wang W, Yang G, Xu J, Ruan X, Gu X, Luo L. Effect of axial length adjustment methods on intraocular lens power calculation in highly myopic eyes. Am J Ophthalmol. 2020;214:110–8. https://doi.org/10.1016/j.ajo.2020.02.023. Epub 2020 Mar 12. PMID: 32171766.
10. Abulafia A, Barrett GD, Rotenberg M, Kleinmann G, Levy A, Reitblat O, Koch DD, Wang L, Assia EI. Intraocular lens power calculation for eyes with an axial length greater than 26.0 mm: comparison of formulas and methods. J Cataract Refract Surg. 2015;41(3):548–56. https://doi.org/10.1016/j.jcrs.2014.06.033. Epub 2015 Feb 21. PMID: 25708208.
11. Liu J, Wang L, Chai F, Han Y, Qian S, Koch DD, Weikert MP. Comparison of intraocular lens power calculation formulas in Chinese eyes with axial myopia. J Cataract Refract Surg. 2019;45(6):725–31. https://doi.org/10.1016/j.jcrs.2019.01.018. PMID: 31146930.
12. Rong X, He W, Zhu Q, Qian D, Lu Y, Zhu X. Intraocular lens power calculation in eyes with extreme myopia: comparison of Barrett Universal II, Haigis, and Olsen formulas. J Cataract Refract Surg. 2019;45(6):732–7. https://doi.org/10.1016/j.jcrs.2018.12.025. Epub 2019 Mar 12. PMID: 30876784.
13. Zhou D, Sun Z, Deng G. Accuracy of the refractive prediction determined by intraocular lens power calculation formulas in high myopia. Indian J Ophthalmol. 2019;67(4):484–9. https://doi.org/10.4103/ijo.IJO_937_18. PMID: 30900579; PMCID: PMC6446621.
14. Wan KH, Lam TCH, Yu MCY, Chan TCY. Accuracy and precision of intraocular lens calculations using the new Hill-RBF version 2.0 in eyes with high axial myopia. Am J Ophthalmol. 2019;205:66–73. https://doi.org/10.1016/j.ajo.2019.04.019. Epub 2019 May 10. PMID: 31078534.
15. Hill DC, Sudhakar S, Hill CS, King TS, Scott IU, Ernst BB, Pantanelli SM. Intraoperative aberrometry versus preoperative biometry for intraocular lens power selection in axial myopia. J Cataract Refract Surg. 2017;43(4):505–10. https://doi.org/10.1016/j.jcrs.2017.01.014. PMID: 28532936.
16. Hengerer FH, Hütz WW, Dick HB, Conrad-Hengerer I. Combined correction of sphere and astigmatism using the light-adjustable intraocular lens in eyes with axial myopia. J Cataract Refract Surg. 2011;37(2):317–23. https://doi.org/10.1016/j.jcrs.2010.08.037. PMID: 21241915.
17. Marques FF, Marques DMV, Osher RH. New technique to demonstrate corneal magnification using trypan blue in cataract surgery. Rev Bras Oftalmol. [online]. 2011;70(4):235–7. https://doi.org/10.1590/S0034-72802011000400006. Cited 17 May 2021. Available from: http://www.scielo.br/scielo.php?script=sci_arttext&pid=S0034-72802011000400006&lng=en&nrm=iso. ISSN 0034-7280.

18. Cai XB, Shen SR, Chen DF, Zhang Q, Jin ZB. An overview of myopia genetics. Exp Eye Res. 2019;188:107778. https://doi.org/10.1016/j.exer.2019.107778. Epub 2019 Aug 28. PMID: 31472110.
19. Neuhann IM, Neuhann TF, Heimann H, Schmickler S, Gerl RH, Foerster MH. Retinal detachment after phacoemulsification in high myopia: analysis of 2356 cases. J Cataract Refract Surg. 2008;34(10):1644–57. https://doi.org/10.1016/j.jcrs.2008.06.022. PMID: 18812113.
20. Ripandelli G, Coppé AM, Parisi V, Olzi D, Scassa C, Chiaravalloti A, Stirpe M. Posterior vitreous detachment and retinal detachment after cataract surgery. Ophthalmology. 2007;114(4):692–7. https://doi.org/10.1016/j.ophtha.2006.08.045. Epub 2007 Jan 17. PMID: 17208303.

24 Relative Anterior Microphthalmos, High Hyperopia, Nanophthalmos

Gerd U. Auffarth, Maximilian Hammer, and Tadas Naujokaitis

The Top 5 Issues Addressed in This Chapter

- How to preoperatively identify patients with relative anterior microphthalmos, high hyperopia, and nanophthalmos.
- How to handle the challenge of a small pupil diameter and a shallow anterior chamber.
- How to manage the high comorbidity load in this patient population.
- How to adequately adjust the IOL calculation.
- How to manage patient expectations after cataract surgery in small eyes.

Supplementary Information The online version contains supplementary material available at [https://doi.org/10.1007/978-3-030-94530-5_24].

G. U. Auffarth (✉) · T. Naujokaitis
Department of Ophthalmology, University of Heidelberg, Heidelberg, Germany

The David J. Apple International Laboratory for Ocular Pathology, Heidelberg, Germany
e-mail: Gerd.Auffarth@med.uni-heidelberg.de

M. Hammer
The David J. Apple International Laboratory for Ocular Pathology, Heidelberg, Germany

Introduction

In this chapter, we focus on three different conditions, relative anterior microphthalmos (RAM), high hyperopia, and nanophthalmos, that are associated with either a small anterior chamber, or a short axial length, or a combination of both. Recognizing these conditions preoperatively and preparing for surgery accordingly is the key to success when performing cataract surgery in patients with these morphological conditions.

Definitions

The three conditions belong to the clinical spectrum of simple microphthalmos. Other than being small in size, these eyes are anatomically intact [1].

The term *relative anterior microphthalmos* refers to the eyes with normal axial length but disproportionally small anterior segment [1, 2]. In terms of morphometric variables, the eyes with an axial length of >20 mm, horizontal corneal diameter of <11 mm, and an anterior chamber depth of around 2 mm are diagnosed as relative anterior microphthalmos [1, 2].

In contrast, the eyes with short axial length but normal anterior segment dimensions are described by the term *(axial) high hyperopia* [3]. The term

J. L. Alió et al. (eds.), *Cataract Surgery*, Essentials in Ophthalmology,
https://doi.org/10.1007/978-3-030-94530-5_24

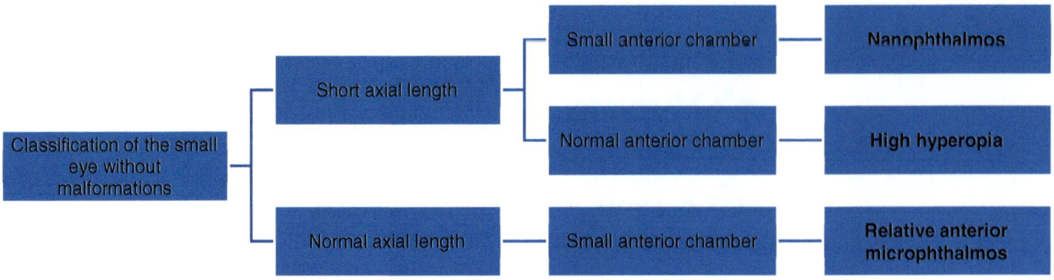

Fig. 24.1 Classification of the small eye without malformations for clinical decision making

Table 24.1 Relation between anterior segment depth and axial length modified by Holladay et al. [9] and Auffarth et al. [2]

Anterior Segment ↓ / Axial Length →	Short	Medium	Long
Small	True/Complex Microphthalmos	Relative Anterior Microphthalmos	Complex Dysgenesis
Medium	Hyperopia	Normal	Myopia
Large	Complex Dysgenesis	Megalocornea	Buphthalmus

posterior microphthalmos is also used to describe eyes with a short posterior segment [4].

Nanophthalmos (also called simple or pure microphthalmos) is instead characterized by a proportionally small eye [3]. Most recent studies consider the eyes with an axial length of <20.0 mm or <20.5 mm as nanophthalmic [3, 5–8].

Figure 24.1 and Table 24.1 present this classification in an easy manner.

Relative Anterior Microphthalmos (RAM)

Caution *RAM patients are often underrecognized and make up a substantial amount of cataract surgical patients. The prevalence of RAM is approximately 6% in the general population* [1]. *The condition is not only underrecognized but at the same time much more common than high hyperopia or nanophthalmos. We suggest a preoperative screening of the anterior chamber depth in order to identify patients at risk. Once RAM is identified, the surgeon can appropriately plan surgery and consult the patient regarding the nature and possible intra- and postoperative complications.*

Preoperative Assessment of Patients with RAM, Prevalence of Comorbidities Prevalence of glaucoma is high in patients with RAM (up to 77% in clinical studies), and most RAM patients have undergone glaucoma procedures at time of cataract surgery (approx. 62%). Additionally, corneal guttae can be observed in 45% of patients with RAM. Finally, the prevalence of synechiae and pseudoexfoliation syndromes is high compared to eyes with normal anterior chambers (approx. 12%) [1, 2]. Why is all of this important? In studies with RAM patients, a high incidence of postoperative complications can occur if the condition is not diagnosed.

Preparation and Indication for Cataract Surgery in RAM Patients

Successful cataract surgery is possible in patients with a shallow anterior chamber morphology and small pupil diameter. However, some precautions are necessary to deal with the conditions mentioned above. Additionally, cataract surgery in patients with nanophthalmos or RAM might be an approach to decrease the crowding of the anterior chamber in this patient population, therefore preventing the progression of glaucoma and unnecessary glaucoma surgery [10].

IOL Calculation

Modified formulas are recommended for IOL calculation in patients with relative anterior microphthalmos such as the modified Haigis formula [11]. Customized high-power IOLs can be used. Only in very rare cases or countries with no access to customized IOLs "piggyback" IOL implantation of two posterior chamber lenses to achieve emmetropia or the desired refraction target is needed. In some studies, none of these approaches were necessary at all [2].

Intraoperative Challenges and Surgical Approaches

Intraoperative challenges and therefore possible postoperative complications of cataract surgery in patients with a complex anterior chamber morphology can be divided in complications deriving from a *shallow anterior chamber depth/small corneal diameter*, a *small pupil diameter*, as well as *pre-existing comorbidities* such as *glaucoma*. In the following paragraphs, we share our solutions to these intraoperative problems.

Shallow Anterior Chamber Morphology/Small Corneal Diameter

Greater Intraoperative Endothelial Cell Loss and Postoperative Corneal Edema

Patients with RAM with additional corneal guttae and low endothelial cell counts showed a higher incidence of postoperative corneal edema when compared to a control group with normal anterior chamber morphology. Most likely, this is caused by lens fragments being located close to the endothelium during removal. In multiple studies, the cell count decreased somewhere between 11% and 13%. It is therefore crucial to protect the endothelium with viscoelastics, e.g., applying techniques like the soft-shell technique first presented by Arshinoff [12]. He presented a technique that uses both high-viscosity cohesive and low-viscosity dispersive viscoelastic agents in the anterior chamber at the same time. During capsulorhexis and phacoemulsification, the endothelial cells of the cornea are protected by a smoothed-out layer of low-viscosity dispersive viscoelastic material, while at the same time the anterior chamber is well pressured by the high-viscosity cohesive viscoelastic material. We most strongly suggest this technique to be used in all RAM and nanophthalmic eyes [12]. There is other options which allow the creation of space in the anterior chamber. One of them is the three-step approach first introduced by Osher et al. [13] 20 minutes before incision, mannitol is administered. The second step includes the depression of the globe against the bony orbit using a muscle hook. After several minutes, the eye softens. As the last step, Healon 5 is injected in order to deepen the anterior chamber [14, 15]. In extreme cases, a pars plana vitreous aspiration could be used to create space [16]. This should be used with caution as often the location of the pars plana cannot be adequately predicted.

Another risk of the shallow anterior chamber is, surprisingly, posterior capsule rupture: In order to protect the endothelium of the cornea a surgeon might consume parts of the lens very posteriorly in cases with this morphology. This is why we recommend the posterior plane emulsification technique by creating space with sculpting as introduced by Vasavada et al. [17] Exposing the posterior capsule early during the surgery often inherently leads to the surgeon to positioning the phaco probe anteriorly; thus the energy is dissipated closer to the endothelium than normally with the risk of hard cataract pieces causing damage. The continuous lowering of vacuum, preset energy, and the flow of the aspiration performed when using this technique also prevents posterior capsule complications [17].

Small Pupil Diameter/Pseudoexfoliation Syndrome

Phacoemulsification through a small pupil opening, mostly defined as a diameter of less than 4 mm, remains a challenge for cataract surgeons. Recently, the intake of alpha 1A- adrenergic blockers for benign prostatic hypertrophy added another cause of intraoperatively constricted pupils: the so-called intraoperative floppy iris syndrome (IRIS). While 5% of cataract surgeries are already complicated by a constricted iris, this challenge is magnified by the shallow anterior chamber in patients with RAM. The surgeon needs to work precisely in a very low range of appropriate angles. Next to preoperative pharmacological mydriasis, intraoperative medications should be the next step of escalation. There are various options such as intracameral injection of unpreserved suprarenine, which stimulates the dilator muscle through the sympathetic pathway. This sympathetic pathway can be combined with impairment of prostaglandin-induced miosis (e.g., the combination of phenylephrine and ketorolac, available in the United States as Omidria, Omeros Corporation, Seattle, Washington, USA). In some cases, pharmacological pupil dilation may not be sufficient. In these cases, mechanical pupil dilation should be considered.

There are many tools that can be used to achieve mechanical iris dilation during surgery if pharmacological mydriasis is not sufficient: mechanical stretching, sphincterotomies, iris hooks, and intraocular rings. These rings, also referred to as pupil expanders, are one of the currently most popular options due to an important advantage over the previously preferred iris hooks: Nearly all iris rings are inserted through the main corneal incision with no additional openings required when compared to iris hooks. Additionally, the placement of the iris expander is more time efficient than the previously used iris hooks [18]. While some complications of cataract surgery like endothelial cell loss are less prevalent after using pupil expanders [19], many of the previous complications are still present, especially in RAM or nanophthalmic patients with comorbidities like glaucoma, uveitis, or macular disease. Thus, there is many different types of pupil expanders that try to minimize intraocular manipulation during mechanical dilation.

Please note that all acts of mechanical pupil dilation mentioned above are most likely not necessary in RAM patients and should be saved for extraordinary cases. We suggest a stepwise escalation of pupil dilation, starting with pre- and intraoperative pharmacological mydriasis and with mechanical manipulation as the last line [20]. *Cases in which pupil expanders were used should be checked for postoperative anterior uveitis.*

The step-by-step chop technique introduced by Nagahara (later amended by a lateral separating movement by Vasavada et al. in 1998 [21]) allows the surgeon to consume most of the cataract in the middle of the iris plane often preventing the need to use mechanical dilation.

Vasavada et al. later showed that in 30 consecutive eyes with a small pupil, only synechiolysis and occasional pupil retraction with a chopper had to be used in all of them during cataract surgery [22]. This was confirmed by Nihalani et al. in solely eyes with RAM [1]. Instead of the occasional pupil retraction with the chopper, we suggest the use of the abovementioned pupil expander rings.

Comorbidities: Glaucoma

Many patients with RAM or nanophthalmos suffer from glaucoma. In some cases, cataract surgery in order to make room in a very crowded anterior chamber is at the same time a causal treatment option for some forms of underlying glaucoma. In cases with previous glaucoma surgery, a temporal approach rather than the usual superior approach might be necessary. This might have advantages such as a smaller loss of corneal endothelial cells [2]. Additionally, a near clear corneal approach allows the option for a subsequent filtering procedure if necessary, by preserving the conjunctiva.

Comorbidities: Synechiae of the Iris and Low Iris Stability

In case of low iris stability, the least possible manipulation of the iris is of great importance. Latest reports of RAM patients therefore renounce any use of retractors or other iris manipulations [1]. In case of posterior synechiae of the iris, the use of a spatula or viscodissection are possible options [1].

Nanophthalmos

Early attempts of cataract surgery in nanophthalmic eyes were associated with a high risk of complications and poor outcomes [10]. Although modern surgical techniques allow a safer procedure with better outcomes, cataract surgery in nanophthalmic eyes remains challenging [8]. Apart from the difficulties arising when working in a small anterior chamber, which have already been described above, there are several additional issues to consider. Table 24.2 summarizes the challenges of cataract surgery and proposed solutions to them in nanophthalmic eyes.

IOL Power Calculation

The prediction of postoperative refraction in nanophthalmic eyes is considerably less accurate than in normal eyes. Jung et al. compared the refractive outcomes in nanophthalmic eyes to the outcomes in a normal control group. While 90–98% of normal eyes achieved a refraction within ±1.00 D, this was the case in only 46–66% of nanophthalmic eyes [7]. The prediction error increases with decreasing axial length, and this is in part due to the high optical power of IOLs implanted in such eyes, giving more weight to errors in the prediction of IOL position [23, 24].

In studies of short eyes, Haigis, Hoffer Q, Holladay 1, and Holladay 2 formulas were reported to be more accurate than SRK/T formula [23, 25, 26]. A study by Eom et al. compared Hoffer Q and Haigis formulas in short eyes and found Haigis formula to perform better in eyes with shallow anterior chamber (<2.40 mm) [27].

Table 24.2 Challenges of performing cataract surgery in nanophthalmic eyes

Challenges	Possible approach
IOL power calculation	
Low accuracy of IOL power prediction	Informing the patient and managing expectations
High postoperative refractive error likely	Correction with spectacles postoperatively
Lack of studies on IOL power calculation in extremely short eyes	Caution when interpreting the results of the studies of short eyes
High discrepancy between formulas	Comparing the results of different formulas
High-power IOL manufacturing and availability	
Tolerance of ±1.0 D for IOL power labeling	Being aware of this source of postoperative refractive error
Increased spherical aberration	Use of aspheric IOLs
Limited availability	Researching the options available in the country of practice; considering piggyback IOL option
Intraoperative and postoperative considerations	
Suboptimal access	Performing the surgery from temporal position
High complication rate	Adequate preparation; informing the patient
Risk of uveal effusion	Use of topical or general anesthesia
Risk of postoperative corneal edema	The soft-shell technique to protect the endothelium (described in the RAM part)
Risk of posterior capsule rupture	Applying the posterior plane emulsification technique (described in the RAM part)
Higher incidence of raised intraocular pressure postoperatively	Monitoring the intraocular pressure
Worse visual outcomes; possible lack of improvement in visual acuity	Informing the patient and managing expectations

The studies that included Barrett Universal II formula found no differences in accuracy of predicting the IOL power when comparing it with other formulas in short eyes.

It should be noted that the mean axial length in studies evaluating different IOL power calculation formulas in short eyes ranges from 19.53 to 21.69 mm [7, 23, 25, 27–33]. However, there is limited data available regarding the IOL power calculation in extremely short eyes. In a study of 11 eyes with the mean axial length of 16.4 mm (simple microphthalmos group), the only formula used was Hoffer Q, and the mean absolute postoperative refractive error was 5.6 D. However, as this is an absolute value, it is not clear if there was a tendency toward myopia or hyperopia [3]. Another study of nanophthalmic eyes used a proprietary IOL calculation algorithm by Carl Zeiss Meditec AG which in most cases resulted in hyperopic outcomes [5].

Our past experience indicates high discrepancy between different formulas in extremely short eyes, an example of which is presented in the case report (see below) [34]. In some cases of very small eyes, Barrett Universal II formula cannot be used as the biometry values are out of the acceptable range for this formula. Haigis formula usually delivers relatively accurate calculation even in extremely short eyes. However, it may be useful to perform the IOL power calculation using several different formulas and compare the results [34]. A newer approach that is solely based on artificial intelligence is the RBF formula. It is available for free online and also shows good results.

High-Power IOL Manufacturing and Availability

Nanophthalmic eyes often require high-power IOLs, and there are several issues related to such IOLs. First of all, the International Organization for Standardization allows the tolerance of ±1.0 D for the IOLs of >30.0 D, while the tolerance for lower-powered IOLs is ±0.5 D or even less [24, 32]. This is a concern when trying to achieve a good refractive outcome, especially as the IOL calculation is already less accurate in very short eye [7, 27]. Another issue is the increase of spherical aberration with increasing IOL power [4]. Some manufacturers now offer aspheric aberration-free IOLs, which may be advantageous in these cases. The third issue is the rarity of cases when high-power IOLs are needed, which makes the production of such IOLs less attractive from a manufacturer's perspective. This results in limited availability of high-power IOLs. In a lot of countries, only IOLs with powers up to +30.0 to 35.0 D are available [34]. However, customized IOLs are available from a variety of companies in a growing number of countries (e.g., the Zeiss Xtreme Series).

Piggyback IOL Option

In cases when high-power IOLs are not available, piggyback IOLs are an option to minimize the postoperative refractive error in nanophthalmic eyes [34, 35]. As the primary implantation of two IOLs in the capsular bag can result in interlenticular membranes and opacifications, late hyperopic shift, and reduction of visual acuity, it is recommended to implant one IOL in the capsular bag and the other IOL in the ciliary sulcus [4]. In order to avoid the sulcus IOL scraping the posterior surface of the iris with the resulting pigment dispersion, the selection of a sulcus IOL with angulated haptics and a rounded edge has been suggested [4]. A potential benefit of piggyback IOLs is that the lower-powered sulcus IOL can be implanted later as a secondary procedure. The postoperative refraction, once stable, can be used to calculate the power of the sulcus IOL and potentially improve the refractive outcome [4]. However, the risks of an additional surgery also need to be considered [34]. Also, it has to be considered that nanophthalmic eyes with very little space inherently limit the use of piggyback IOLs. In some cases, with extremely small capsular bags, the amputation of the haptics of the IOL may be an alternate approach to account for space problems.

Intraoperative Complications

In 1982, Singh et al. reported "an extremely high complication rate with disastrous results" of intraocular surgery in nanophthalmic eyes [10]. Although the modern cataract surgery technique is safer, complications still occur often in nanophthalmic surgery and include posterior capsule rupture, vitreous loss, suprachoroidal hemorrhage, iris prolapse, iritis, persistent corneal edema, cystoid macular edema, and phthisis [3, 7, 36, 37].

Uveal effusion is another well-known complication in nanophthalmic eyes, which can lead to secondary retinal detachment, vitreous hemorrhage, malignant glaucoma, and loss of the eye [3, 38–40]. This latter complication should be considered when choosing the type of anesthesia because retrobulbar and peribulbar anesthesia increase posterior pressure that may lead to vortex vein congestion. Instead, topical or general anesthesia is preferred [4, 41]. Small ocular dimensions and suboptimal access are other aspects to be considered. It may be advantageous to perform the surgery from temporal position to facilitate access. Postoperatively, the intraocular pressure needs to be closely monitored, as the incidence of glaucoma following a cataract surgery in nanophthalmic eyes is high [4, 30].

Postoperative Outcomes

Visual outcomes after cataract surgery in nanophthalmic eyes are considerably worse than in normal eyes. Studies report the mean postoperative corrected distance visual acuity to range from +0.55 logMAR (20/80) to +0.41 logMAR (20/50) [3, 7, 8, 23]. In cases when the preoperative hyperopic refractive error is corrected with spectacles, the postoperative improvement in corrected distance visual acuity may be less than expected due to preoperative relative spectacle magnification. Ametropic amblyopia due to large preoperative hyperopic refractive error may also limit the postoperative visual acuity. The residual refractive error is also often high because of the limited accuracy of IOL power calculations [34].

Management of Patient Expectations

The increased risk of complications and worse visual prognosis should be discussed with patients before the surgery. They should also understand the limitations of the IOL power prediction accuracy and be ready to wear spectacles to correct residual refractive error. Even though an improvement in visual acuity is not always achieved, cataract surgery in nanophthalmic eyes still has the potential to significantly improve the quality of life. By reducing the preoperative refractive error, it enables patients to be less dependent on spectacles and contact lenses [34]. Cataract surgery also reduces the risk of synechiogenesis and angle closure glaucoma.

Case Report: Cataract Surgery in Extreme Nanophthalmos [34]

The 60-year-old male patient with bilateral nanophthalmos presented to our clinic for cataract surgery. He was complaining of increased glare sensitivity. The patient had been wearing rigid contact lenses since the age of 14 because of high hyperopia. Before that, spectacles had been used since the age of 5. According to the patient, the vision had never been good. Corrected distance visual acuity with rigid contact lenses of +17.5 D was +0.46 logMAR (20/63) in the right eye and +0.58 logMAR (20/80) in the left eye. No improvement could be achieved with additional lenses. IOP was 12 mm Hg in both eyes. Slit lamp examination of the anterior segment revealed progression of cataracts (Fig. 24.2). Fundoscopy and optical coherence tomography findings were unremarkable.

After performing biometry measurements with IOLMaster 700 (Carl Zeiss Meditec, Jena, Germany), the IOL power for emmetropia for the foldable acrylic Aspira-aAY IOL (HumanOptics AG, Erlangen, Germany) was calculated with different formulas. The suggested power to achieve emmetropia ranged from +55.28 to +70.09 D. Based on our past experience of selecting high-power IOLs, we had a certain preference for the Haigis formula in achieving a reliable result, but we tended to choose the average value taken from four formulas (Haigis, Holladay 1, Holladay 2, SRK/T). The IOL power of +56.0 D was selected for the right eye and one of +58.0 D for the left eye. The biometry values and IOL power calculation results are presented in Table 24.3.

With the patient under general anesthesia, both surgeries were performed by an experienced surgeon (GUA). LenSx® femtosecond laser

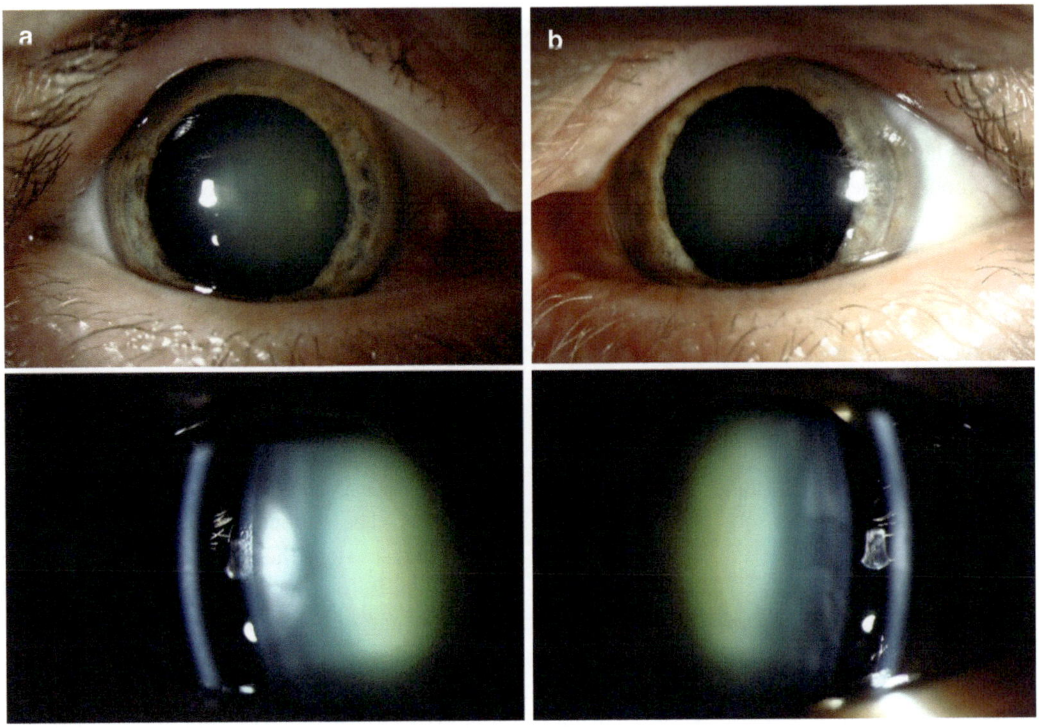

Fig. 24.2 Preoperative images of the right (**a**) and the left (**b**) eye

(Alcon Laboratories, Inc., Fort Worth, TX, USA) was used for capsulotomy and lens fragmentation. The docking of the patient interface was more complicated, due to the nanophthalmos, but was completed successfully. Considerable artifacts were visible in the LenSx® optical coherence tomography images, so the automatic detection of structures had to be manually overridden (Fig. 24.3). The femtosecond laser was in this case capable of creating only a partial capsulotomy, and it was safely completed with a manual technique. However, it should be noted that incomplete capsulotomy, if unrecognized, could have resulted in a radial tear of the capsule, potentially jeopardizing the implantation of the IOL in the capsular bag. The nucleus fragmentation was also only partial. We applied the "pizza cut" pattern, but only a few lines could be seen intraoperatively. Despite these technical difficulties, a round capsulotomy could be achieved, which we think is advantageous when implanting a high-power IOL (+56.0 and +58.0 D) into the capsular bag. A temporal position for the main incision was chosen in order to facilitate access. Due to the thickness of the IOL, the incision size of slightly more than 3.0 mm was used (Figs. 24.4 and 24.5). Despite small dimensions of the eyes, both surgeries were uneventful (Videos 24.1 and 24.2).

On the first day postoperatively, corrected distance visual acuity in the right eye was +0.38 logMAR (20/50) with the manifest refraction of +0.50–1.00 × 80°. Corrected distance visual acuity in the left eye was +0.64 logMAR (20/80) with the manifest refraction of −0.50 −0.50 × 65°. The early postoperative period was complication-free. Two months after the surgery, corrected distance visual acuity was +0.40 logMAR (20/50) and +0.60 logMAR (20/80) with the manifest refraction of +1.00–0.75 × 135° and +0.50–1.75 × 45° in the right and the left eye, respectively. Spherical equivalent refractions were +0.625 D and −0.375 D in the right and the left eye, respectively. The IOP was 12 mmHg in the right eye and 14 mmHg in the left eye. The slit lamp examination revealed slight posterior

Table 24.3 Biometry data, IOL power calculation results, and prediction error using Hoffer Q, Haigis, SRK/T, Holladay 1, and Holladay 2 formulas

Biometry data		
Parameter	Right eye	Left eye
AL	14.94 mm	15.05 mm
R	6.70 mm	7.04 mm
R1	6.75 mm @ 132°	7.10 mm @ 64°
R2	6.65 mm @ 42°	6.97 mm @ 154°
WTW	11.5 mm	11.3 mm
ACD	2.24 mm	2.33 mm
LT	5.96 mm	5.90 mm
Calculated IOL power for emmetropia (Aspira-aAY)		
Formula	Right eye	Left eye
Hoffer Q	+70.09 D	+69.96 D
Haigis	+55.28 D	+57.47 D
SRK/T	+56.04 D	+57.09 D
Holladay 1	+57.07 D	+59.20 D
Holladay 2	+57.43 D	+59.05 D
Prediction error (postoperative spherical equivalent – target refraction)		
Formula	Right eye	Left eye
Hoffer Q	−7.57 D	−7.75 D
Haigis	+1.21 D	+0.06 D
SRK/T	+0.60 D	+0.34 D
Holladay 1	−0.19 D	−1.29 D
Holladay 2	−0.45 D	−1.18 D

ACD anterior chamber depth, *AL* axial length, *IOL* intraocular lens, *LT* lens thickness, *R* corneal radius, *WTW* white-to-white distance

capsule opacification in both eyes, currently not requiring treatment.

When comparing the accuracy of different IOL calculation formulas in our case, we found the smallest difference from target refraction with Holladay 1 formula for the right eye (−0.19 D) and Haigis formula for the left eye (+0.06 D). Haigis, Holladay 1, Holladay 2, and SRK/T formulas delivered similar results, with the prediction error ranging from −1.29 D to +1.21 D. In contrast, Hoffer Q formula returned highly myopic results (−7.57 D and −7.75 D for the right and the left eye, respectively). Barrett Universal II formula could not be used in this case of extreme nanophthalmos since the biometry values were out of the acceptable range for the formula and therefore an error message was displayed in the official calculator.

This case report shows that cataract surgery in nanophthalmic eyes is challenging but can be successfully performed after adequate preparation. High-power customized IOLs allow complete correction of hyperopia, but caution is required with the results from different IOL power calculation formulas, which can be misleading. In this case, even though the axial length was extremely short, no complications occurred, and the prediction of postoperative refraction was relatively accurate.

High Hyperopia

Although the normal dimensions of the anterior segment in patients with high hyperopia make cataract surgery itself easier to perform, the issues related with IOL power calculation and high-power IOL manufacturing remain. An important aspect to consider is the IOL power calculation in highly disproportionate eyes. Due to a short axial length but normal anterior segment, it may be useful to perform the IOL power calculation using newer formulas, which require not only axial length and keratometry values, but also additional biometric parameters such as anterior chamber depth.

Intraoperative and postoperative complications depend on the exact morphology and are similar of those in nanophthalmos, with the exception of the complications related to the anterior segment dimensions. In eyes with a very short posterior segment, uveal effusion syndrome may occur. To be pointed out is the importance of carrying the tunnel incision beyond the peripheral iris. This avoids iris damage or prolapse. It might be favorable to fill the anterior chamber with OVD before performing the stab incision. In high hyperopia, clear lensectomy is also an available option with good results [42].

Video 24.3 presents a cataract surgery of a right eye of a patient with high hyperopia. The 82-year-old patient had an axial length of 19.27 mm and an anterior chamber depth of 2.84 mm. A 37.0 D IOL was used to achieve optimal refraction results.

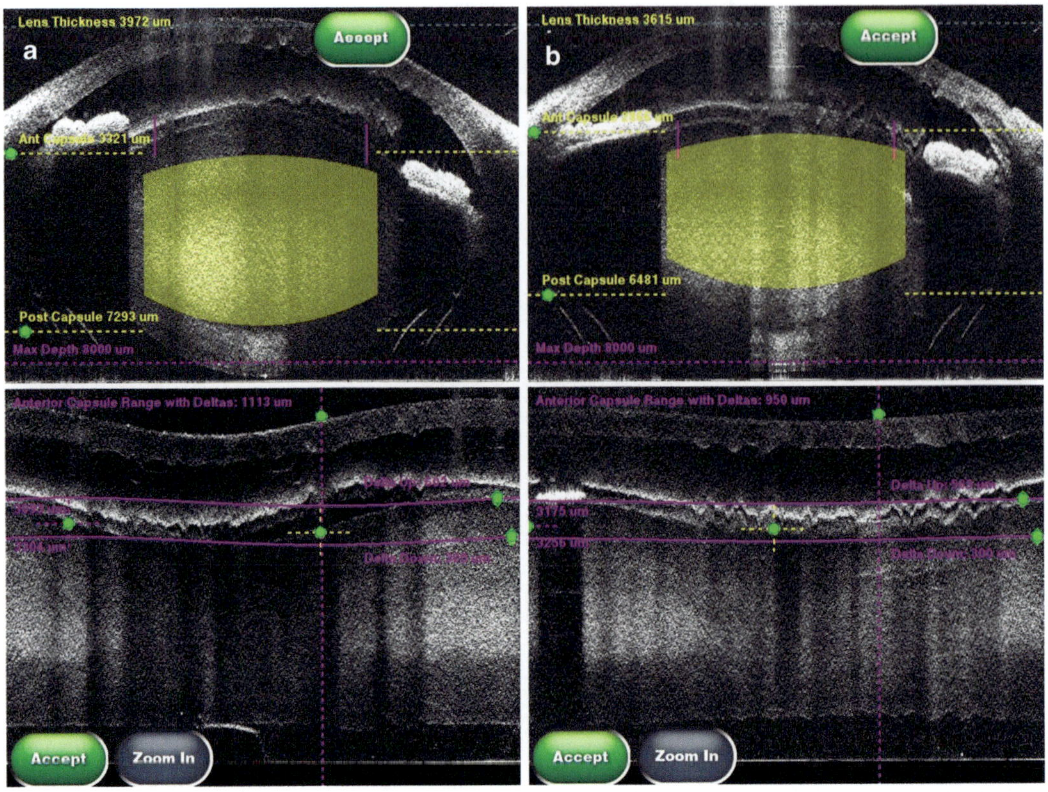

Fig. 24.3 Optical coherence tomography images of the right (**a**) and the left (**b**) eye from the LenSx® femtosecond laser

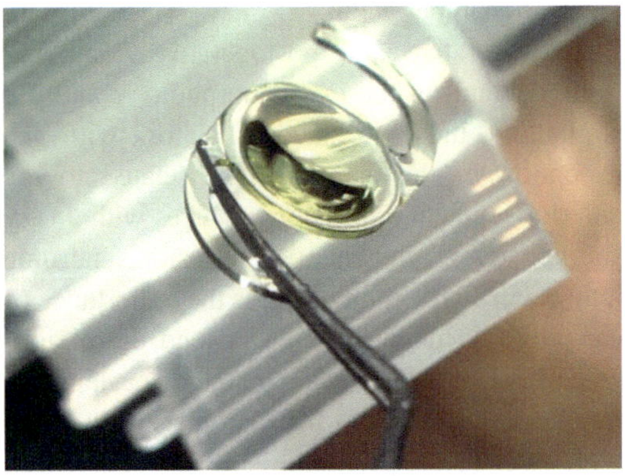

Fig. 24.4 Aspira-aAY intraocular lens (IOL) of +56.0 D before loading it into the cartridge

Take-Home Notes

- A preoperative screening of the anterior chamber depth and axis length allows to identify patients with small eye conditions.
- The soft-shell technique, posterior plane emulsification, and the step-by-step chop routine should be used to deal with the anatomical challenge of the small eye.
- Glaucoma is very frequent in this patient population: A temporal approach and the possible causal treatment of glaucoma by cataract surgery should be considered.
- Multiple formulas that integrate anatomical parameters should be compared to allow a good postoperative refractive result in small eyes.

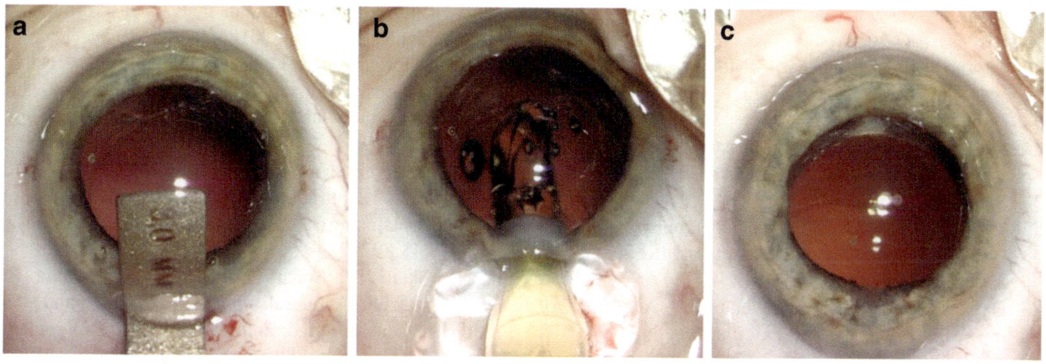

Fig. 24.5 Intraoperative images of the left eye: incision size measurement before IOL implantation (**a**), injection of +58.0 D Aspira-aAY IOL (**b**), and the eye after the IOL implantation (**c**)

- Especially patients with nanophthalmos should understand limitations of IOL power prediction accuracy. They need to be ready to wear spectacles to correct residual refractive errors.

References

1. Nihalani BR, Jani UD, Vasavada AR, Auffarth GU. Cataract surgery in relative anterior microphthalmos. Ophthalmology. 2005;112:1360–7.
2. Auffarth GU, Blum M, Faller U, Tetz MR, Völcker HE. Relative anterior microphthalmos: morphometric analysis and its implications for cataract surgery. Ophthalmology. 2000;107:1555–60.
3. Zheng T, Chen Z, Xu J, Tang Y, Fan Q, Lu Y. Outcomes and prognostic factors of cataract surgery in adult extreme microphthalmos with axial length <18 mm or corneal diameter <8 mm. Am J Ophthalmol. 2017;184:84–96.
4. Hoffman RS, Vasavada AR, Allen QB, Snyder ME, Devgan U, Braga-Mele R, ASCRS Cataract Clinical Committee, Challenging/Complicated Cataract Surgery Subcommittee. Cataract surgery in the small eye. J Cataract Refract Surg. 2015;41:2565–75.
5. Singh H, Wang JC-C, Desjardins DC, Baig K, Gagné S, Ahmed IIK. Refractive outcomes in nanophthalmic eyes after phacoemulsification and implantation of a high-refractive-power foldable intraocular lens. J Cataract Refract Surg. 2015;41:2394–402.
6. Day AC, MacLaren RE, Bunce C, Stevens JD, Foster PJ. Outcomes of phacoemulsification and intraocular lens implantation in microphthalmos and nanophthalmos. J Cataract Refract Surg. 2013;39:87–96.
7. Jung KI, Yang JW, Lee YC, Kim S-Y. Cataract surgery in eyes with nanophthalmos and relative anterior microphthalmos. Am J Ophthalmol. 2012;153:1161–1168.e1.
8. Lemos JA, Rodrigues P, Resende RA, Menezes C, Gonçalves RS, Coelho P. Cataract surgery in patients with nanophthalmos: results and complications. Eur J Ophthalmol. 2016;26:103–6.
9. Holladay JT, Gills JP, Leidlein J, Cherchio M. Achieving emmetropia in extremely short eyes with two piggyback posterior chamber intraocular lenses. Ophthalmology. 1996;103:1118–23.
10. Singh OS, Simmons RJ, Brockhurst RJ, Trempe CL. Nanophthalmos: a perspective on identification and therapy. Ophthalmology. 1982;89:1006–12.
11. Haigis W. Biometrie bei komplizierten Ausgangssituationen. In: Rochels R, Duncker G, Hartmann C, editors. 9. Kongreß der Deutschsprachigen Gesellschaft für Intraokularlinsen Implantation. Berlin, Heidelberg: Springer Berlin Heidelberg; 1995. p. 17–26.
12. Arshinoff SA. Dispersive-cohesive viscoelastic soft shell technique. J Cataract Refract Surg. 1999;25:167–73.
13. Osher RH. Extremes. Video Journal of Cataract and Refractive Surgery. 2007;23(4).
14. Osher RH. Nanophthalmos. Video Journal of Cataract and Refractive Surgery. 2006;22(1).
15. Osher RH. Slow motion phacoemulsification. 6/1998;1(2):42–6. Operative techniques in cataract and refractive surgery.
16. Chang DF. Pars plana vitreous tap for phacoemulsification in the crowded eye. J Cataract Refract Surg. 2001;27:1911–4.
17. Vasavada AR, Raj S. Step-down technique. J Cataract Refract Surg. 2003;29:1077–9.
18. Nderitu P, Ursell P. Iris hooks versus a pupil expansion ring: operating times, complications, and visual acuity outcomes in small pupil cases. J Cataract Refract Surg. 2019;45:167–73.
19. Wilczynski M, Wierzchowski T, Synder A, Omulecki W. Results of phacoemulsification with Malyugin Ring in comparison with manual iris stretching with

hooks in eyes with narrow pupil. Eur J Ophthalmol. 2013;23:196 201.
20. Grzybowski A, Kanclerz P. Methods for achieving adequate pupil size in cataract surgery. Curr Opin Ophthalmol. 2020;31:33–42.
21. Vasavada A, Singh R. Step-by-step chop in situ and separation of very dense cataracts. J Cataract Refract Surg. 1998;24:156–9.
22. Vasavada A, Singh R. Phacoemulsification in eyes with a small pupil. J Cataract Refract Surg. 2000;26:1210–8.
23. Day AC, Foster PJ, Stevens JD. Accuracy of intraocular lens power calculations in eyes with axial length <22.00 mm. Clin Exp Ophthalmol. 2012;40:855–62.
24. Hoffer KJ, Savini G. IOL power calculation in short and long eyes. Asia Pac J Ophthalmol (Phila). 2017;6:330–1.
25. Gavin EA, Hammond CJ. Intraocular lens power calculation in short eyes. Eye (Lond). 2008;22:935–8.
26. Carifi G, Aiello F, Zygoura V, Kopsachilis N, Maurino V. Accuracy of the refractive prediction determined by multiple currently available intraocular lens power calculation formulas in small eyes. Am J Ophthalmol. 2015;159:577–83.
27. Eom Y, Kang S-Y, Song JS, Kim YY, Kim HM. Comparison of Hoffer Q and Haigis formulae for intraocular lens power calculation according to the anterior chamber depth in short eyes. Am J Ophthalmol. 2014;157:818–824.e2.
28. Wang AY, Wong MS, Humbyrd CJ. Eligibility criteria for lower extremity joint replacement may worsen racial and socioeconomic disparities. Clin Orthop Relat Res. 2018;476:2301–8.
29. Roh YR, Lee SM, Han YK, Kim MK, Wee WR, Lee JH. Intraocular lens power calculation using IOLMaster and various formulas in short eyes. Korean J Ophthalmol. 2011;25:151–5.
30. Terzi E, Wang L, Kohnen T. Accuracy of modern intraocular lens power calculation formulas in refractive lens exchange for high myopia and high hyperopia. J Cataract Refract Surg. 2009;35:1181–9.
31. Shrivastava AK, Behera P, Kumar B, Nanda S. Precision of intraocular lens power prediction in eyes shorter than 22 mm: an analysis of 6 formulas. J Cataract Refract Surg. 2018;44:1317–20.
32. Hoffer KJ, Calogero D, Faaland RW, Ilev IK. Testing the dioptric power accuracy of exact-power-labeled intraocular lenses. J Cataract Refract Surg. 2009;35:1995–9.
33. Gökce SE, Zeiter JH, Weikert MP, Koch DD, Hill W, Wang L. Intraocular lens power calculations in short eyes using 7 formulas. J Cataract Refract Surg. 2017;43:892–7.
34. Naujokaitis T, Scharf D, Baur I, Khoramnia R, Auffarth GU. Bilateral implantation of +56 and +58 diopter custom-made intraocular lenses in patient with extreme nanophthalmos. Am J Ophthalmol Case Rep. 2020;20:100963.
35. Gayton JL, Sanders VN. Implanting two posterior chamber intraocular lenses in a case of microphthalmos. J Cataract Refract Surg. 1993;19:776–7.
36. Yuzbasioglu E, Artunay O, Agachan A, Bilen H. Phacoemulsification in patients with nanophthalmos. Can J Ophthalmol. 2009;44:534–9.
37. Wu W, Dawson DG, Sugar A, Elner SG, Meyer KA, McKey JB, Moroi SE. Cataract surgery in patients with nanophthalmos: results and complications. J Cataract Refract Surg. 2004;30:584–90.
38. Steijns D, Bijlsma WR, Van der Lelij A. Cataract surgery in patients with nanophthalmos. Ophthalmology. 2013;120:266–70.
39. Faucher A, Hasanee K, Rootman DS. Phacoemulsification and intraocular lens implantation in nanophthalmic eyes: report of a medium-size series. J Cataract Refract Surg. 2002;28:837–42.
40. Rajendrababu S, Babu N, Sinha S, Balakrishnan V, Vardhan A, Puthuran GV, Ramulu PY. A randomized controlled trial comparing outcomes of cataract surgery in nanophthalmos with and without prophylactic sclerostomy. Am J Ophthalmol. 2017;183:125–33.
41. Auffarth null. Cataract surgical problem: response #6. J Cataract Refract Surg. 2000;26:1709.
42. Osher RH. Clear lensectomy. In: Fine IH, editor. Clear corneal lens surgery. Thorofare (NJ): SLACK Incorporated; 1999. 281–5.

Cataract Surgery in the Diabetic Eye

25

Ronald D. Gerste and H. Burkhard Dick

Bullet Points

- Diabetics have a higher prevalence of cataract and it occurs at an earlier age than in non-diabetics.
- One rationale for timely cataract surgery is to gain a clear view of the retina which allows to schedule necessary treatment like panretinal laser coagulation or anti-VEGF injection at an appropriate time.
- There is a higher risk of diabetic macular edema (DME) in diabetic patients who tend to profit from a prophylactic treatment.
- The capsular opening should be performed larger than usual, and phacoemulsification energy should be reduced as far as possible. Operating time should be as short as possible.
- When it comes to choosing the right IOL, it seems that diabetic patients might benefit from monofocal lenses with a rather large optic zone of, for instance, 6.5 mm versus 5.5 mm.

R. D. Gerste (✉)
North Potomac, MD, USA

H. B. Dick
Ruhr University Eye Clinic, Bochum, Germany

Epidemiology and Pathology

Cataract and diabetes mellitus have something in common: in wide parts of the world with an aging population, they will both become more frequent in the future – even more frequent than they currently are. According to the International Diabetes Federation, the disease will affect close to 600 million people by the year 2035. Diabetic retinopathy currently is a leading cause of vision loss in the industrialized world [1]. This is not going to change anytime soon – some estimates predict a prevalence of diabetes mellitus as high as 33% of the US population by 2050 [2].

Diabetes mellitus has an influence on most, probably on all, structures of the eye, not the least on the lens. Some large epidemiological studies like the Beaver Dam Study in the USA and the Blue Mountains Study in Australia demonstrated a significantly increased incidence of cataract among diabetic individuals, up to a factor of 5 [3–5]. It is postulated that hyperglycemia results in production of advanced glycation end products, increased oxidative stress, and activation of the polyol pathway; each of these processes is believed to play a role in cataract formation [6]. Ocular manifestations of diabetes mellitus such as retinopathy and macular edema are in turn a risk indicator for ischemic heart disease in diabetic patients [7].

Not only is cataract more common among a diabetic population, it also generally occurs at an

J. L. Alió et al. (eds.), *Cataract Surgery*, Essentials in Ophthalmology,
https://doi.org/10.1007/978-3-030-94530-5_25

earlier age than in non-diabetics. In an analysis of 56,510 individuals with diabetes mellitus from a British database, an incidence rate of cataract of 20.4 per 1000 person-years was assessed, almost twice as much as in the general population with 10.8 per 1000 person-years. The incidence rate ratio (the ratio of incidence rates between diabetics and non-diabetics) was highest in the age group of 45–54 years. In the age group of 50–59 years, the relative risk (RR) of cataract was significantly higher than in the general population (RR 12.6). While cataract was diagnosed in patients with retinopathy to only a slightly higher degree, a diagnosis of cataract in patients with diabetic macular edema was considerably higher than in the general population. The likelihood of a cataract diagnosis increased with the duration of diabetes mellitus; for patients with a history of the disease of more than 10 years, the odds ratio (OR) of developing cataract was 5.14. Not surprisingly, the odds of cataract diagnosis were increased in patients under long-term steroid therapy (OR 1.87) [8]. Besides the duration of the diabetes, poor metabolic control is a risk factor for the development of cataract. While in older diabetics the cataract formation is irreversible, good blood sugar control might reverse some cataracts in young patients [9]. Another risk factor for cataract development demonstrated in a study from the USA was the use of insulin versus non-insulin (OR 2.11) [10].

Cataract does not only occur with a higher incidence, and frequently at a comparatively young age in adults, it is also an ocular complication in young adults and children with diabetes mellitus type 1. In some, probably in most pediatric patients with diabetes, the occurrence of cataract is the first sign of the disease. Estimates of the prevalence of cataract in diabetic children and adolescents are as high as 3.3%. High HbA_{1c} levels increase the likelihood of cataract in these young individuals. Posterior subcapsular cataract seems to be the most frequent type of cataract in diabetic children. It almost goes without saying for any cataract surgeon with experience in treating pediatric cataract that these children invariably develop posterior capsule opacification (PCO) due to the more active inflammatory response in younger age; the PCO rate after pediatric cataract surgery of diabetic eyes can be estimated at a solid 100% [11].

Timing of Cataract Surgery

Currently, up to 20% of cataract surgeries is performed in diabetic eyes [12]. There was an old paradigm according to which surgery had to wait until no other choice was left. It was not unusual to operate on eyes of diabetic patients with a visual acuity of less than 20/200 [13]. This is widely considered an outdated approach by now. Today, there is general consensus that early treatment benefits diabetics and leads to better visual outcome [14]. In addition, by not waiting for further opacification and rather operating early, the examination of the fundus is unimpaired, and the clear view of the retina allows to schedule necessary treatment like panretinal laser coagulation or anti-VEGF injection at an appropriate time. If an earlier operation also means intervening at an earlier, milder stage of retinopathy, this might also influence the risk of postoperative macular edema positively [15]. Cataract extraction before the opacification becomes too advanced also makes sense since removing the cataract and implanting an IOL enables the ophthalmologist routinely taking care of the patient to visualize the retina and the macula much better and possibly detect abnormalities earlier than with a cataract still in place.

Pre- and Intraoperative Considerations

Preoperative diagnostics should always include a thorough assessment of the posterior part of the eye, if available including SD-OCT and fluorescein angiography. If active retinal manifestations are detected, these should be treated first – usually with focal laser coagulation or by panretinal coagulation – and the date of cataract surgery be postponed until stability has been achieved. Eyes with proliferative retinopathy should undergo treatment first although there might be situations depending on the patient's circumstances where a combined approach (see below) is preferred.

Patients with diabetes mellitus but without (yet) any diabetic ocular manifestation will undergo routine cataract surgery just as anybody else. It has to be kept in mind, though, that there is a higher risk of diabetic macular edema (DME) in these patients. In the PREMED study, it was convincingly demonstrated that diabetics profit from a prophylactic treatment; it has been the only truly evidence-based study to give proof about such a treatment, while in healthy patients such pretreatment does not make sense [16].

The intravitreal application of drugs – VEGF inhibitors like bevacizumab, ranibizumab, and aflibercept or steroids like dexamethasone and triamcinolone – is now an established method to treat ocular manifestations of diabetes mellitus. This has led to the question whether these applications which in particular in the case of anti-VEGF medications have to be administered on a regular basis should be done before cataract surgery – or rather simultaneously.

The dexamethasone implant (Ozurdex®) was implanted by one surgeon during cataract surgery in a prospective randomized controlled study to treat pre-existing diabetic macular edema (DME), not as a prophylaxis. These patients had a decline of central macular thickness (CMT) during the 24-week follow-up, while eyes in the control group (without steroid injection during phacoemulsification) had an increase of CMT at every visit. The authors argued that intraoperative dexamethasone might act as an anti-inflammatory agent during the postoperative period by inhibiting mediators such as prostaglandins and VEGF. The size of that intervention group was, however, rather small ($n = 9$ eyes) [17].

In our clinical experience, it is quite legitimate, and sometimes outright necessary, to combine both procedures: the scheduled injection of, for instance, a VEGF inhibitor and cataract surgery (Fig. 25.1). In cases where the patient needs his or her next injection anyway, this reduces the number of appointments and thus eases the burden at least a bit. Scheduling the injection of a VEGF inhibitor before cataract surgery is indicated to reduce a pre-existing

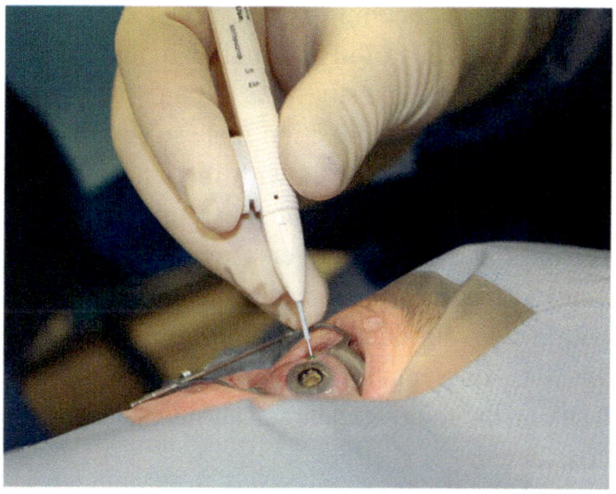

Fig. 25.1 Intravitreal Ozurdex injection at the same time as the cataract surgery in a diabetic eye suffering from diabetic macular edema

DME as much as possible. If there is any evidence in the preoperative OCT for an already existing DME, the intravitreal application of a VEGF inhibitor during cataract surgery is highly indicated [18, 19]. The initiation or progression of pre-existing DME following cataract surgery has been reported to be about 29% in eyes with non-proliferative diabetic retinopathy within 6 months [20], underlining the necessity of treating DME as effectively and timely as possible with the effect of the injection holding the increase of visual acuity in eyes with the pre-existing condition up to 6 months [21]. The other way round, in patients with DME who required cataract surgery while being participants in clinical studies on anti-VEGF therapy, continuous anti-VEGF injections secured the improved visual acuity despite a slight increase in retinal central thickness [22]. Anti-VEGF medications like Lucentis° or Eylea° (as well as bevacizumab, the drug used in earlier studies on cataract surgery and anti-VEGF therapy [23]) are, in our view, preferable to the injection of steroids or the positioning of a steroid implant. Diabetic patients tend to develop IOP increases [24] under such a therapeutic approach that often turn out to be extremely difficult to treat. A massive steroid supplementation always means an attack on the patient's immune system which increases the threat of postoperative endophthalmitis in individuals which often are already immunocompromised. A periocular steroid injection is a valid alternative; in these cases, however, topical anesthesia is not an option.

A simultaneous injection makes sense to prevent a DME also in eyes with the macula so far unaffected. Depending on the retinal situation, performing cataract surgery together with pars plana vitrectomy (ppV) is also an option. In eyes with a severely damaged retina, refraining from an IOL implantation (certainly a rather rare decision in today's cataract surgery) has to be considered.

Diabetic patients with retinal manifestations in general have a significantly increased risk of postoperative inflammation; their vitreous is already charged with inflammatory mediators. Expecting a deterioration of the retinal situation in many cases justifies a simultaneous approach with the vitreoretinal surgeon joining the cataract surgeon on these occasions (Figs. 25.2 and 25.3). Individual factors might also warrant a combined intervention. The patient might not be compliant or might not stand a second operation within a short time. Here again, doing cataract surgery and ppV in one session should be considered.

In our clinic, we have employed the femtosecond laser in thousands of interventions and have widely published our data and experience with LCS (laser cataract surgery) – an experience which overall is very positive and which has opened up new opportunities particularly in challenging cases [25, 26]. With that background, we can clearly state that LCS benefits many diabetic patients just as it benefits non-diabetics. One aspect, however, has to be kept in mind in LCS as well as in phacoemulsification: the diabetic eye's tendency to react with a strong inflammation. Therefore, pretreatment is essential [27]. This concerns particularly the pupil size: in many cases already quite small, an uninhibited inflammatory reaction will lead to an even more pronounced intraoperative miosis.

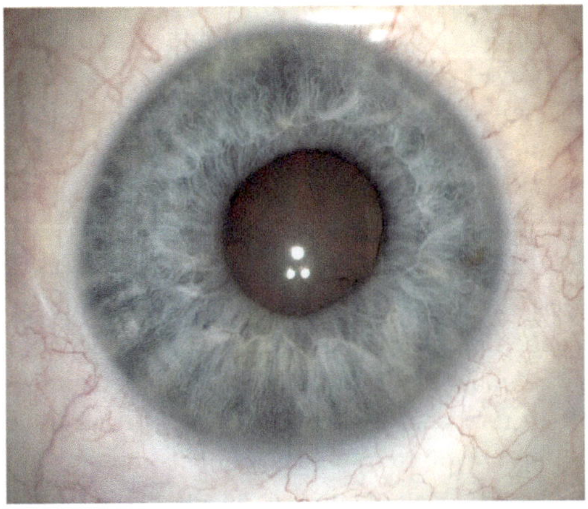

Fig. 25.2 Atrophic iris with nondilating pupil of a diabetic eye before cataract surgery

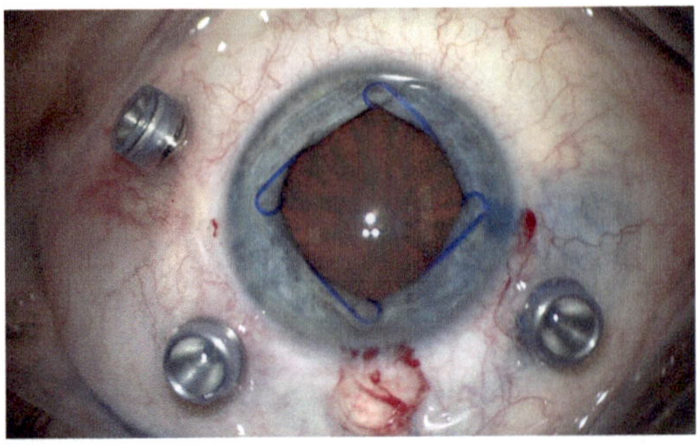

Fig. 25.3 Cataract surgery combined with pars plana 23 G vitrectomy after pupil dilation using a Malyugin ring (the same eye as in Fig. 25.2)

We tend to operate diabetic patients first during our daily program, reducing the anxiety of wait times and giving them ample opportunity to relax afterward under rather intensive care and observation. During surgery, we try to minimize any undue stress that might evoke some unfavorable reactions in these sensitive eyes like a further increase of inflammation mediators. The surface is meticulously being kept moist, usually by applying HPMC in generous portions. The capsular opening should be performed larger than usual, and phacoemulsification energy should be reduced as far as possible. To expose the eye to as little irritation as possible, the amount of fluid used should be limited; the same applies to the light exposure by the operating microscope. Operating time should be as short as possible. If the pupil does not widen as expected, the handling of the iris has to be very gentle; any stretching that might lead to bleeding has to be avoided. All these requirements point to the fact that the more experience the surgeon has, the better for the patient.

In contrast to the sometimes regular but sometimes almost explosive inflammatory reaction, there is also a slight advantage in performing cataract surgery in diabetic patients. In general, they are significantly younger than the usual cataract population which in turn means that we hardly ever have to deal with truly hard cataracts that can prove excessively difficult to fragment or emulsify.

When it comes to choosing the right IOL, it seems that diabetic patients might benefit from monofocal lenses with a rather large optic zone of, for instance, 6.5 mm versus 5.5 mm. We prefer hydrophobic acrylate IOL with sharp edges and are reluctant to implant hydrophilic IOLs which come with an even higher probability of PCO. We are equally reluctant to implant multifocal IOLs which can cause more problems and dissatisfaction in diabetics than in the general public. In eyes with significant pre-existing astigmatism, implanting a toric IOL is preferable to relaxing limbal incisions – diabetics tend to have problems of the ocular surface which is not a good condition for any kind of corneal intervention.

Complications of Cataract Surgery in Diabetic Eyes and Their Prevention

Diabetics have a higher rate of PCO and develop this postoperative complication usually faster than other patients. With this in mind, we are rather reluctant to implant silicone IOLs in patients with an active retinopathy. Removing the entire lens – i.e. removing even the capsule – as recommended now and then by some surgeons appears to be too radical in our view and is most likely unnecessary.

Cataract surgery may have implications on the ocular surface – as does diabetes itself. Diabetes is regarded as one of the risk factors for dry eye syndrome with 54% of diabetic patients suffering from this condition in one study [28]. Cataract surgery can induce dry eye syndrome or increase the existing symptoms [29]. Often, however, these symptoms are transient, and the situation gets better though recovery in the postoperative phase tends to be slower than in non-diabetic eyes. In a study by Liu et al., 17.1% of diabetic eyes and 8.1% of non-diabetic eyes developed dry eye syndrome within 7 days after cataract surgery. While in both groups the problem resolved over time, diabetic eyes took longer to return to normal [30]. Phacoemulsification exerts stress and trauma on structures that are in diabetic eyes more susceptible to these factors than in the eyes of otherwise healthy patients. This is particularly true for diabetic corneas which suffer a greater loss of endothelial cells than non-diabetic eyes over the first 3 postoperative months [31].

Diabetic corneas have a greater tendency than those of non-diabetic individuals to suffer epithelial defects, erosions, superficial punctate keratopathy, and corneal wounds and often show a slower wound healing. Thus corneal wounds as a result of cataract surgery take some time to heal and turn frequently into recurrent corneal erosions [32, 33]. What is true for the corneal epithelium seems to be true for the endothelium as well. In general, diabetics have a lower endothelial cell density than non-diabetics [34]. Their endothelium is more susceptible to surgical trauma, and further endothelial cell loss can be expected following cataract surgery [35]. In this respect, employing as little ultrasound energy as possible during lens removal is to be recommended.

Another concern with diabetic patients is their increased risk of infection. They have an increased prevalence of blepharitis and conjunctivitis which has to be taken into account when performing antiseptic measures preoperatively. The rate of conjunctival colonization in diabetics seems to be correlated to the severity of their diabetic retinopathy [36, 37]. Similarly, diabetics are at higher risk of endophthalmitis and the more so the less controlled their blood sugar is – achieving good metabolic control contributes to reducing this risk which is estimated to be almost three times as high as in non-diabetics [38]. If diabetics have to undergo vitrectomy to treat endophthalmitis, their visual outcomes are worse than in other patients: while 55% of non-diabetics achieved 20/40 vision after endophthalmitis-related vitrectomy, only 39% of diabetics did [39].

Cataract Surgery and Diabetic Retinopathy

As is well-known, risk factors for diabetic retinopathy are the duration of diabetes, an earlier age at the onset of the disease, the presence of neuropathy, and elevated HbA1c, cholesterol, and systolic blood pressure [40] – these all are factors of which the cataract surgeon has to be aware of to assess the potential benefit of the intervention for the individual diabetic patients and its limits.

The potential influence of cataract surgery on the prevalence and/or the severity of diabetic retinopathy has been debated for many years, the different views supported by studies which did or did not demonstrate such an effect. Rather typical might the analysis of a health insurance database from Taiwan which showed limited influence of the intervention. Jeng et al. found, for instance, a higher risk of diabetic patients to develop nonproliferative diabetic retinopathy after cataract surgery with an adjusted hazard ratio (HR) of 1.48. There was no significant difference, however, to develop proliferative diabetic retinopathy or diabetic macular edema between diabetics undergoing cataract surgery and a control group who did not. An increased risk to develop nonproliferative retinopathy was found for women (HR 1.68), patient's age 65 or older (HR 1.54), and patients with comorbidities such as hypertension, dyslipidemia, heart disease, or other diabetic complications (HR 1.48), statin users (2.02), angiotensin-converting enzyme inhibitor users (HR 1.57), and non-insulin users (HR 1.74). The authors stated their strong belief that the use of statins and dyslipidemia are strongly associated with cataract formation in diabetic patients that requires surgery. They also argued that the impact of cataract surgery on the risk of developing non-proliferative diabetic retinopathy persists for about 5 years [40].

To assess whether cataract surgery exacerbates the development and progression of diabetic retinopathy, 278 eyes undergoing cataract surgery and IOL implantation were compared with 60 phakic eyes in a clinic-based cohort study from Sydney, Australia. After 1 year, diabetic retinopathy developed in 28.2% of pseudophakic and 13.8% of unoperated eyes; the adjusted OR for the manifestation of diabetic retinopathy was 2.65. Nevertheless, this progression rate was lower than comparable data from earlier times when older techniques were used before the advent of phacoemulsification. The authors could not rule out the possibility that eyes which are undergoing cataract surgery are at greater risk for developing retinopathy than nonsurgical fellow eyes since the development of cataract in diabetic patients is related to poor glycemic control, rendering these eyes susceptible to retinal complications due to an impaired blood-aqueous barrier [41].

In a number of studies, though, the difference in retinopathy progression between eyes that had undergone cataract surgery and in eyes that had not were rather unimpressive. In a group of 42 patients, 12% of operated eyes showed progression during a 12-month follow-up compared to 10.8% in non-operated eyes [42]. In 50 diabetic patients undergoing unilateral cataract surgery, 20% of the operated eyes versus 16% of the non-operated eyes progressed [43].

Cataract Surgery and Diabetic Macular Edema

In diabetic patients – in those with retinopathy and often in those without – the blood-aqueous barrier is impaired which is the cause of the high risk of postoperative inflammation and specifically of sight-threatening DME following cataract surgery. Other consequences are the progression of diabetic retinopathy, other macular changes, and the induction of rubeosis iridis [44]. Macular edema can be considered the main cause of unsatisfactory visual results or even vision loss in diabetics after cataract surgery. In a large study from the UK analyzing more than 81,000 eyes undergoing cataract surgery, a risk ratio of 1.80 for developing macular edema was found for eyes of diabetics who did not have diabetic retinopathy. For those with retinopathy, the risk factor increased – depending of the severity of the retinopathy – up to a maximum of 10.34 [45].

DME is a frequent condition in patients undergoing cataract surgery. In a recent study from Italy, about one fifth of 3657 patients undergoing cataract surgery were diabetics. Among these diabetic patients, 27.5% had diabetic macular edema of any kind; a clinically significant DME was found in 6.6%. These relative high numbers suggest that a strict preoperative assessment is necessary and adequate treatment of the DME is warranted before performing cataract surgery to keep the risk of exacerbation of a pre-existing macular edema as low as possible [46].

A Finnish study has shown that eyes of diabetic patients benefit significantly more from either a steroid monotherapy to prevent postoperative macular edema or from a combination therapy of steroid and NSAID (nonsteroidal anti-inflammatory drugs) than non-diabetic patients. Under steroid monotherapy, for instance, central retinal thickness (CRT) increased on average by 38.1 μm in non-diabetic eyes compared to 7.8 μm in diabetic eyes [47]. It seems, however, that these drugs lack a protective effect in eyes with advanced vascular damage like in those with non-proliferative diabetic retinopathy [48].

Treating a pre-existing DME is strongly recommended; before the advent of anti-VEGF medications, focal or grid laser photocoagulation was the treatment of choice. Today, the effect of bevacizumab, ranibizumab, and aflibercept on central retinal thickness and visual acuity has been well proven. Preoperative stabilization and postoperative management of DME with anti-VEGF agents is crucial in establishing a positive visual outcome of cataract surgery; helpful adjunctive measures are the injections of steroids and sometimes the traditional way of treating CME, focal laser coagulation [6].

Diabetic patients may not only develop DME; they are also at a higher risk of cystoid macular edema, one of the major sight-reducing complications following cataract surgery. Pharmacological prophylaxis helps at least in patients without prior macular changes. In a large study from California with more than 89,000 patients, those who postoperatively received a topical NSAID developed CME in 1.3% compared to 1.7% in those patients without this prophylaxis. Patients with diabetic retinopathy did not profit from this topical prophylactic treatment [49].

Visual Outcomes

In the past, patients with diabetic ocular manifestations like retinopathy tended to have only a limited visual outcome or even ended up worse than before surgery. A publication from 1994 estimated that these patients are twice as likely to fail to improve after surgery than patients without ocular comorbidities [50]. With modern surgical techniques, however, the majority of diabetic patients benefits from cataract surgery (depending in their retinal situation), and many of them enjoy visual gains comparable to those of the general public. Fong et al. showed that in a cohort of 1192 surgical patients of whom 27.2% had diabetes, the average visual acuity gain 12 months after surgery was 10.8 letters among 868 patients without diabetes, 10.6 letters among 188 patients with diabetes, but no diabetic retinopathy and 10.0 letters among 95 patients with diabetic retinopathy. Only the 41 patients with diabetic retinopathy who had undergone laser treatment before did not have an improvement of their visual acuity after cataract surgery [51].

Nevertheless, patients with advanced diabetic manifestations like proliferative retinopathy can functionally benefit from cataract surgery when it is performed as a combined operation with anti-VEGF or steroid injections into the vitreous or as a phacovitrectomy. In a group of 161 eyes with 4-year follow-up available, eyes undergoing the combination technique of phacoemulsification and ppV gained on average 11 letters of visual acuity [52].

Besides the potential visual gain, cataract surgery in diabetics offers another advantage. The variations in refraction that are associated with changes of blood glucose levels and which are caused by glucose migrating into the lens and inducing swelling particularly in the lens periphery will be eliminated by lens removal and IOL implantation [19].

Conclusion

Patients with diabetes mellitus face a number of issues when undergoing cataract surgery from comorbidities to a higher risk of complications like DME and a deterioration of retinopathy. Cataract surgery should be performed in a timely manner; there is no sense in delaying what has to be done anyway. Diabetic patients require an individual approach that is based on factors like the quality of their blood sugar control, their social situation, and their compliance. They are not a homogenous group; diabetics who are successfully treated with dietetics, those who can be helped with glucose-reducing drugs, those who require insulin – they pose very different (and, in that order, increasing) challenges. Fortunately, modern cataract surgery is able to provide them with satisfying and often outright good functional results after all [47].

Take-Home Notes

- In contrast to traditional treatment patterns, early cataract surgery in diabetic eyes benefits the patients and leads to better visual outcome.
- If active retinal manifestations are detected, these should be treated and the date of cataract surgery be postponed until stability has been achieved.
- In diabetic children and adolescents, posterior capsule opacification (PCO) following cataract surgery is highly likely, indeed almost guaranteed.
- Combining a scheduled injection of a VEGF inhibitor with cataract surgery can make sense and reduces the number of appointments and thus the burden of treatment for the patient at least a bit.
- In patients with a pre-existing macular edema, it makes particularly sense to combine cataract surgery with anti-VEGF injection. A preoperative OCT seems always to be a reasonable diagnostic tool to verify (or exclude) the existence of DME.
- There is some evidence that cataract surgery might increase the risk of progression of diabetic retinopathy though this is still a matter of debate.

References

1. Haddad NM, Sun JK, Abujaber S, et al. Cataract surgery and its complications in diabetic patients. Semin Ophthalmol. 2014;29:329–37.
2. Boyle JP, Thompson TJ, Gregg EW, et al. Projection of the year 2050 burden of diabetes in the US adult population: dynamic modeling of incidence, mortality, and prediabetes prevalence. Popul Health Metrics. 2010;8:29. https://doi.org/10.1186/1478-7954-8-29.
3. Klein KR, Lee KE. Diabetes, cardiovascular disease, selected cardiovascular disease risk factors, and the 5-year incidence of age-related cataract and progression of lens opacities: the Beaver Dam Eye Study. Am J Ophthalmol. 1998;126:782–90.
4. Kanthan GL, Mitchell P, Burlutsky G, et al. Fasting blood glucose levels and the long-term incidence and progression of cataract: the Blue Mountains Eye Study. Acta Ophthalmol. 2011;89:e434–8.
5. West SK, Valmadrid CT. Epidemiology of risk factors for age-related cataract. Surv Ophthalmol. 1995;39:323–34.
6. Peterson SR, Silva PA, Murtha TJ, et al. Cataract surgery in patients with diabetes: management strategies. Semin Ophthalmol. 2018;33:75–82.
7. Klein R, Klein BE, Moss SE, et al. Association of ocular disease and mortality in a diabetic population. Arch Ophthalmol. 1999;117:1487–95.
8. Becker C, Schneider C, Aballéa S, et al. Cataract in patients with diabetes mellitus – incidence rates in the UK and risk factors. Eye. 2018;32:1028–35.
9. Kiziltoprak H, Tekin K, Inanc M, et al. Cataract in diabetes mellitus. World J Diabetes. 2019;10:140–53.
10. Klein BE, Klein R, Moss SE. Incidence of cataract surgery in the Wisconsin epidemiologic study of diabetic retinopathy. Am J Ophthalmol. 1995;119:295–300.
11. Simunovic M, Paradzik M, Skrabic R, et al. Cataract as an early ocular complication in children and adolescents with type 1 diabetes mellitus. Int J Endocrinol. 2018;2018:6763586. https://doi.org/10.1155/2018/6763586.
12. Wild S, Roglic G, Green A, et al. Global prevalence of diabetes: estimates for the year 2000 and projections for 2030. Diabetes Care. 2004;27:1047–53.
13. Pollack A, Leiba H, Bukelman A, et al. Cystoid macular oedema following cataract extraction in patients with diabetes. Br J Ophthalmol. 1992;76:221–4.
14. Chew EY, Benson WE, Remaley NA. Results after lens extraction in patients with diabetic retinopathy:

early treatment diabetic retinopathy study report number 25. Arch Ophthalmol. 1999;117:1600–6.
15. Dowler JG, Sehmi KS, Hykin PG, et al. The natural history of macular edema after cataract surgery in diabetes. Ophthalmology. 1999;106:663–8.
16. Wielders LHP, Schoutens J, Winkens B, et al. Randomized controlled European multicenter trial on the prevention of cystoid macular edema after cataract surgery in diabetics: ESCRS PREMED study report 2. J Cataract Refract Surg. 2018;44:836–47.
17. Agarwal A, Gupta V, Ram J, et al. Dexamethasone intravitreal implant during phacoemulsification. Ophthalmology. 2013;120:211–211.e5.
18. Amoaku WM, Ghanchi F, Bailey C. Diabetic retinopathy and diabetic macular oedema pathways and management: UK Consensus Working Group. Eye (Lond). 2020;34(Suppl 1):1–51.
19. Grzybowski A, Kanclerz P, Huerva V, et al. Diabetes and phacoemulsification cataract surgery: difficulties, risks and potential complications. J Clin Med. 2019;8:716. https://doi.org/10.3390/jcm8050716.
20. Funatsu H, Yamashita H, Ikeda T, et al. Angiotensin II and vascular endothelial growth factor in the vitreous fluid of patients with diabetic macular edema and other retinal disorders. Am J Ophthalmol. 2002;133:537–43.
21. Zhao LQ, Cheng JW. A systematic review and meta-analysis of clinical outcomes of intravitreal anti-VEGF agent treatment immediately after cataract surgery for patients with diabetic retinopathy. J Ophthalmol. 2019;2019:2648267. https://doi.org/10.1155/2019/2648267.
22. Moshfegi AA, Thompson D, Berliner AJ, et al. Outcomes in patients with diabetic macular edema requiring cataract surgery in VISTA and VIVID studies. J Ophthalmol Retina. 2020;4:481–5.
23. Cheema RA, Al-Mubarak MM, Amin YM, et al. Role of combined cataract surgery and intravitreal bevacizumab injection in preventing progression of diabetic retinopathy: prospective randomized study. J Cataract Refract Surg. 2009;35:18–25.
24. Chew E, Glassman AR, Beck RW, et al. Ocular side effects associated with peribulbar injections of triamcinolone acetonide for diabetic macular edema. Retina. 2011;32:284–9.
25. Grewal DS, Schultz T, Basti S, Dick HB. Femtosecond laser-assisted cataract surgery--current status and future directions. Surv Ophthalmol. 2016;61:103–31.
26. Dick HB, Schultz T. A review of laser-assisted versus traditional phacoemulsification cataract surgery. Ophthalmol Ther. 2017;6:7–18.
27. Schultz T, Joachim SC, Szuler M, et al. NSAID pretreatment inhibits prostaglandin release in femtosecond laser-assisted cataract surgery. J Refract Surg. 2015;31:791–4.
28. Manaviat MR, Rashidi M, Afkhami-Ardekani M, et al. Prevalence of dry eye syndrome and diabetic retinopathy in type 2 diabetic patients. BMC Ophthalmol. 2008;8:10. https://doi.org/10.1186/1471-2415-8-10.
29. Cetinkaya S, Mestan E, Acir NO, et al. The course of dry eye after phacoemulsification surgery. BMC Ophthalmol. 2015;15:68. https://doi.org/10.1186/s12886-015-0058-3.
30. Liu X, Gu YS, Xu YS, et al. Changes of tear film and tear secretion after phacoemulsification in diabetic patients. J Zhejiang Univ Sci. 2008;9:324–8.
31. Tang Y, Chen X, Zhang X, et al. Clinical evaluation of corneal changes after phacoemulsification in diabetic and non-diabetic cataract patients, a systemic review and meta-analysis. Sci Rep. 2017;7:14128. https://doi.org/10.1038/s41598-017-14656-7.
32. Moshirfar M, Simpson RG, Christiansen S, et al. Laser in-situ keratomileusis in patients with diabetes mellitus: a review of the literature. Clin Ophthalmol. 2012;6:1827–37.
33. Javadi MA, Zarei-Ghanavati S. Cataracts in diabetic patients: a review article. J Ophthalmic Vis Res. 2008;3:52–65.
34. Sudhir RR, Raman R, Sharma T. Changes in the corneal endothelial cell density and morphology in patients with type 2 diabetes mellitus: a population-based study. Cornea. 2012;31:1119–22.
35. Dhasmana R, Singh IP, Nagpal RC. Corneal changes in diabetic patients after small manual incision cataract surgery. J Clin Diagn Res. 2014;8:VC03–6.
36. Karimsab D, Razak SK. Study of aerobic bacterial conjunctival flora in patients with diabetes mellitus. Nepal J Ophthalmol. 2013;5:28–32.
37. Kruse A, Thomsen RW, Hundborg HH, et al. Diabetes and risk of acute infectious conjunctivitis: a population-based case-control study. Diabet Med. 2006;23:393–7.
38. Jabbarvand M, Hashemian H, Khodaparast M, et al. Endophthalmitis occurring after cataract surgery: outcomes of more than 480 000 cataract surgeries, epidemiologic features and risk factors. Ophthalmology. 2016;123:295–301.
39. Doft BH, Wisniewski SR, Kelsey SF, Endophthalmitis Vitrectomy Study Group, et al. Diabetes and postcataract extraction endophthalmitis. Curr Opin Ophthalmol. 2002;13:147–51.
40. Jeng CJ, Hsieh YT, Yang CM, et al. Development of diabetic retinopathy after cataract surgery. PLoS One. 2018;13:e0202347. https://doi.org/10.1371/journal.pone.0202347.
41. Hong T, Mitchell P, de Loryn T, et al. Development and progression of diabetic retinopathy 12 months after phacoemulsification cataract surgery. Ophthalmology. 2009;116:1510–4.
42. Krepler K, Biowski R, Schrey S, et al. Cataract surgery in patients with diabetic retinopathy: visual outcome, progression of diabetic retinopathy, and incidence of diabetic macular edema. Graefes Arch Clin Exp Ophthalmol. 2002;240:735–8.
43. Squirrell D, Bhola J, Bush S, et al. A prospective, case-controlled study of the natural history of diabetic retinopathy and maculopathy after uncomplicated phacoemulsification cataract surgery in patients with type 2 diabetes. Br J Ophthalmol. 2002;86:565–71.

44. Pollreisz A, Schmidt-Erfurth U. Diabetic cataract – pathogenesis, epidemiology and treatment. J Ophthalmol. 2010;2010:608751. https://doi.org/10.1155/2010/608751.
45. Chu CJ, Johnston RL, Buscombe C, et al. Risk factors and incidence of macular edema after cataract surgery: a data-base study of 81984 eyes. Ophthalmology. 2016;123:316–23.
46. Panozzo G, Staurenghi G, Dalla Mura G, et al. Prevalence of diabetes and diabetic macular edema in patients undergoing senile cataract surgery in Italy: the DIabetes and CATaract study. Eur J Ophthalmol. 2020;30:315–20.
47. Danni R, Taipale C, Ilveskoski L, et al. Diabetes alone does not impair recovery from uneventful cataract surgery. Am J Ophthalmol. 2019;198:37–44.
48. Grzybowski A. Diabetes alone does not impair recovery from uneventful cataract surgery. Am J Ophthalmol. 2019;200:224–5.
49. Modjtahedi BS, Paschal JF, Batech M, et al. Perioperative topical nonsteroidal anti-inflammatory drugs for macular edema prophylaxis following cataract surgery. Am J Ophthalmol. 2017;176:174–82.
50. Schein OD, Steinberg EP, Cassard SD, et al. Predictors of outcome in patients who underwent cataract surgery. Ophthalmology. 1994;102:817–23.
51. Fong CS, Mitchell P, Rochtchina E, et al. Visual outcomes 12 months after phacoemulsification cataract surgery in patients with diabetes. Acta Ophthalmol. 2012;90:173–8.
52. Silva PS, Diala PA, Hamam RN, et al. Visual outcomes from pars plana vitrectomy versus combined pars plana vitrectomy, phacoemulsification, and intraocular lens implantation in patients with diabetes. Retina. 2014;34:1960–8.

Cataract Surgery in Aniridia

26

Karl Thomas Boden and Peter Szurman

Bullet Points

- Congenital aniridia is a relatively rare condition with a reported prevalence of approximately 1:40000 to 1:100000.
- Congenital aniridia is usually a panocular disease with macular hypoplasia and also optic disc hypoplasia.
- Pronounced congenital aniridia associated with a defect of the PAX6 gene usually includes profound developmental disorders of the eye that require different ophthalmologic expertise.
- Secondary glaucoma can be a significant problem in the management of patients with aniridia. The more pronounced the aniridia, the earlier and more severe the courses.
- In 20–30% of patients with congenital aniridia, keratopathy occurs, which can vary significantly in severity depending on the mutation of the PAX6 gene.

K. T. Boden (✉) · P. Szurman
Eye Clinic Sulzbach, Knappschaft Hospital Saar, Sulzbach/Saar, Germany
e-mail: Karl.Boden@kksaar.de

Introduction

The absence of an iris has a significant influence on the function of the eye. In addition to the individual cosmetic aspect, aniridia primarily causes a glare effect with different levels of severity. Likewise, the pupil plays an essential role in accommodation, which leads to reduced-depth visual acuity in pronounced defects. Without the iris, the full functionality of the eye cannot be achieved.

Congenital aniridia is a relatively rare condition with a reported prevalence of approximately 1:40000 to 1:100000. There is no increased prevalence in relation to gender. The PAX6 gene, which is located on chromosome 11p13, plays a crucial role in the defective development.

Congenital aniridia is usually a panocular disease with macular hypoplasia and also optic disc hypoplasia. With increasing age, secondary glaucoma and limbal stem cell deficiency are often added. This makes the treatment, and especially a surgical procedure, more difficult. Pronounced congenital aniridia associated with a defect of the PAX6 gene usually includes profound developmental disorders of the eye that require different ophthalmologic expertise.

The forms of congenital aniridia with alterations in the PAX6 gene are much more frequent and not uncommonly associated with other systemic diseases. This is also called “aniridia syndrome” or “PAX6 syndrome.”

J. L. Alió et al. (eds.), *Cataract Surgery*, Essentials in Ophthalmology,
https://doi.org/10.1007/978-3-030-94530-5_26

These concomitant systemic diseases may include potentially life-threatening conditions (e.g., Wilms tumor, WAGR syndrome, Gillespie syndrome, genito-urethral abnormalities, and mental retardation) that require interdisciplinary treatment.

Aniridia as a Complex Disorder of the Eye

Congenital aniridia may be associated with a variety of ocular changes. In particular, in association with the PAX6 gene defect, microphthalmos, foveal hypoplasia, and micropapillary dysfunction occur frequently during embryonic development [1, 2]. Reduced visual acuity from 20/200 to 20/63 and nystagmus are typical. These complex developmental disorders can extend to the photoreceptor cell level and often also result in red/green weakness [3].

Aniridia and Secondary Glaucoma

Secondary glaucoma can be a significant problem in the management of these patients. The more pronounced the aniridia, the earlier and more severe the courses. Diagnosis in young patients may be complicated by reduced compliance. Measuring intraocular pressure is also difficult due to the frequently thickened cornea (either as an anomaly or due to increasing corneal decompensation) [4, 5].

The cause of secondary glaucoma is either pre-trabecular (as a result of peripheral iris remnants) or intra-trabecular (the malposition or total absence of a Schlemm's canal) with impairment of outflow facility [6]. A surgical approach is also crucial when (preservative-free) local therapeutics are no longer sufficient. If the initial corneal situation is good, trabeculotomy is the surgery of choice, especially if gonioscopic pretrabecular membranes/synechiae are detectable. Major fistulating glaucoma surgery should be avoided because of the pronounced profibrotic response, especially in children with aniridia. In childhood, non-penetrating surgery (e.g., deep sclerectomy or suprachoroidal drainage) or the use of glaucoma implants should be preferred [7, 8].

Aniridia and Corneas

In 20–30% of patients with congenital aniridia, keratopathy occurs, which can vary significantly in severity depending on the mutation of the PAX6 gene [9]. In the majority of cases, keratopathy is a limbal stem cell deficiency characterized by a corneal wound healing disorder with abnormal cell adhesion or metabolism [10, 11]. As a result, a chronic surface disorder including dryness, corneal neovascularization, pannus formation, and Salzmann keratopathy develop.

The surface disorder should be treated with hyaluronic acid-containing eye drops in the initial stage of keratopathy. In the case of incipient epithelialization disorders, autologous serum eye drops or amniotic membrane transplantation is useful.

For mild neovascularizations, local therapy with bevacizumab eye drops may be helpful [12]. More severe and deeper neovascularizations can be obliterated with fine-needle diathermy. Salzmann nodules can be ablated with excimer smoothing using phototherapeutic keratectomy.

Penetrating keratoplasty should be avoided if possible because the procedure is high risk due to impaired wound healing and surface issues, and corneal transplantation does not solve the stem cell problem. In the most severe cases, limbo keratoplasty or Boston keratoprosthesis have been described [13, 14].

Differentiation from Acquired Aniridia

Acquired aniridia is traumatic in most cases. It could also be the result of iatrogenic causes such as secondary sphincter atrophy due to postoperative pressure spikes or other complicating intraocular surgeries. Less common syndromal conditions such as iridocorneal endothelial (ICE) syndromes may also cause aniridia.

A traumatic cataract with total or subtotal aniridia usually requires extensive reconstruction, which is rarely accomplished in a singular cataract surgery. Therefore, the surgeon should have ample surgical experience in corneal surgery and vitreoretinal surgery. The surgical techniques for reconstruction of the iris in traumatic aniridia are described in detail in the "Iris Repair" chapter.

Aniridia and Cataract

In addition to the ocular comorbidities associated with aniridia, cataract surgery itself is a surgical challenge.

In the following section, the preoperative risk factors that indicate possible intraoperative difficulties during cataract surgery are described. In addition, specific details and practical tips for such special cases are discussed.

Preoperative Specificities in Patients with Cataract and Aniridia

Preoperatively, a detailed examination of the eye is necessary to determine the initial situation, which is unique for each patient. In particular, the extent of corneal opacities must be recorded, as this decisively shapes the surgical strategy.

Very often a concomitant limbal stem cell deficiency due to the PAX6 gene defect is present, which can vary in its severity [15]. If only a peripheral pannus with mild vascularization is present, cataract surgery can be performed with omission of the affected quadrants. Pannus ablation with fine-needle diathermy can be performed simultaneously. Deep vessels, on the other hand, should be obliterated with fine-needle diathermy prior to cataract surgery. This is helpful to improve the intraoperative view and to avoid postoperative corneal decompensation. In pronounced cases of aniridia-associated keratopathy (Figs. 26.1 and 26.2), limbal stem cell transplantation with or without amniotic membrane transplantation should be performed before cataract surgery. Consideration should also be given to the common ocular surface disorder associated with meibomian gland dysfunction, which should also be treated preoperatively with intensive tear-substitute therapy [16].

However, if penetrating keratoplasty is unavoidable in rare cases, it should not be combined with cataract surgery (triple procedure).

Choice of IOL for Implantation

Aniridia is often associated with high myopia. With the appropriate choice of IOL in the low diopter range, even extreme myopia can be compensated for. In individual cases, special myopic lenses in the minus diopter range are necessary.

In contrast, the use of iris diaphragm IOLs (Morcher, Stuttgart, Germany) is critical. Due to

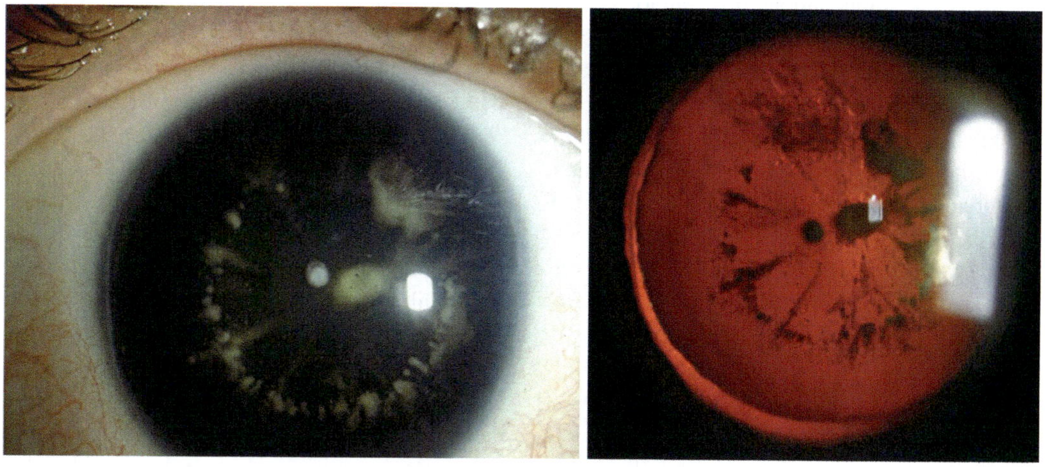

Fig. 26.1 A patient with congenital aniridia and cataract without keratopathy

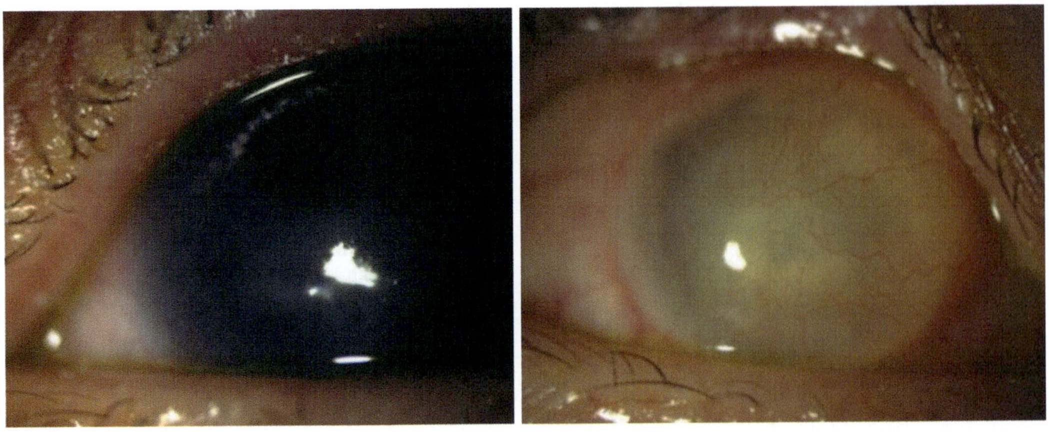

Fig. 26.2 Two eyes with different stages of keratopathy of one patient. Left: isolated pannus with vascularization. Right: severe keratopathy without red-light reflex

the nature of the commonly used PMMA material, a large limbal or corneoscleral access is necessary, which should be avoided due to the existing limbal stem cell problem [17, 18]. In addition, iris diaphragm IOLs are designed to be implanted in the sulcus, which may worsen preexisting glaucoma. Therefore, acrylate iris diaphragm IOLs have been manufactured as alternatives for several years (e.g., Ophtec, Groningen, Netherlands). These implants are foldable and can be implanted via small, clear corneal incisions. However, larger case studies on acrylate IOLs are not available.

It should be noted that the overall diameter must not be underestimated in order to avoid glare phenomena in the peripheral area. With capsular bag implantation, this cannot be prevented and can cause serious glare problems and double images. Therefore, some surgeons generally advise against the use of iris IOLs [19].

Whether the implantation of a blue-light filter lens brings about a subjective improvement of photophobia can only be assumed because no published data on this subject are available.

Anatomical Specialties in Aniridia

The intraocular anatomy of eyes with congenital aniridia is altered, and often the zonular apparatus of the lens is also compromised. Therefore, safe and stable implantation of the IOL into the capsular bag is not always possible. The surgeon should be prepared for simultaneous scleral fixation of the IOL, if necessary, to avoid a second procedure.

Zonular insufficiency may also be limited to single quadrants or caused by lens colobomas (pseudocolobomas). These findings should already have been identified during preoperative examination.

If dysregulated intraocular pressure is also present, it should be adjusted preoperatively. Combined cataract and glaucoma surgery should be avoided.

Even in the case of successful cataract surgery, the visual prognosis is limited. This is not only due to the lacking iris function but may also be a consequence of hypoplasia of the fovea.

Iris Reconstruction: Useful or Not?

Prior to any cataract surgery, it must be decided if a simultaneous reconstruction of the iris is useful. Aniridia can be partial, subtotal, or total. Both the extent of aniridia and discomfort level of the patient ultimately guide the strategy of a possible reconstruction.

While iris reconstruction in traumatic aniridia can be performed well in combination with cataract surgery, iris reconstructive procedures in congenital aniridia should only be considered in selected cases.

Not every iris defect needs to be closed. Patients with congenital aniridia are often accustomed to glare and benefit little from extensive iris reconstruction. Foveal hypoplasia and nystagmus also limit the positive effect of iris reconstruction. In addition, iris reconstruction is usually associated with a higher intra- and postoperative stimulus, which significantly increases the risk of postoperative healing disorders. In unclear cases, a wearing trial with an iris print contact lens is useful.

The strategy of reconstruction of the iris depends on the extent of the defect. In asymptomatic defects that are covered by the upper lid, the defect can be left in place. Segmental defects can be closed with a McCannel suture [22] or with the "sliding knot" technique introduced by Siepser [23]. Such minimally invasive suture techniques are often sufficient for achieving good results.

For covering large, subtotal, or total iris defects, foldable, flexible implants are preferred (Customflex Artificial Iris; HumanOptics, Erlangen, Germany). These implants are custom-made and offer a natural and cosmetically appealing result. They require smaller incisions and can be implanted in a minimally invasive manner without a capsular bag—even in complicated cases—and fixed in the sulcus without knots [20, 21].

Capsular tension rings with segmental orifices should be avoided. These require significantly larger incisions, frequently dislocate, and can often only be used intracapsularly, leaving a peripheral, uncovered ring.

Intraoperative Specificities in Patients with Cataract and Aniridia

Generally, in the case of nystagmus, surgery should be performed under general anesthesia.

In daily surgical practice, the greatest challenge in cataract surgery with congenital aniridia is reduced vision due to stromal corneal opacities. If only epithelial edema is present, glycerin-containing eye drops (5%) can be applied to deswell the cornea.

In severe cases, a corneal abrasion with postoperative insertion of a bandage contact lens is necessary. However, postoperative wound healing disturbances have to be considered. In cases of severely reduced vision, retrolental illumination is helpful, according to Oshima [24]. For this purpose, a 27 g chandelier light is introduced over the pars plana, which can replace the missing red reflex.

In capsulorhexis, it should be noted that the lens capsule is significantly thinner and more fragile in congenital aniridia [25]. This complicates capsulorhexis considerably. In most cases, visualization of the capsule by vital dyes is helpful [26]. If corneal transparency permits, the use of a femtosecond laser is recommended, especially in younger patients [27, 28].

The lens nucleus itself is usually soft in the majority of young patients and can be easily removed during phacoemulsification. However, the surgeon's focus should be on the zonular apparatus. In many cases, either a general zonular insufficiency or a lens pseudocoloboma is present. Capsular bag instability can be improved with a capsular tension ring. It is usually sufficient to implant this after lens removal. In individual cases, the capsular tension ring can be implanted earlier—after hydrodissection and before phacoemulsification—so that zonular stress is reduced by manipulation during phacoemulsification.

As an intraoperative support, iris hooks can be inserted into the capsulorhexis to temporarily fix the capsular bag [29]. However, this requires further corneal incisions, which should be considered in relation to limbal stem cell deficiency.

In the case of dislocated lens capsule, especially in the presence of a lens pseudocoloboma, special capsular tension rings can be used, which are fixed transsclerally and thus allow re-centering of the capsular bag and the IOL (Cionni ring; FCI Ophthalmics, Paris, France) [30]. The same effect is achieved with ring segments that are also fixed transsclerally with a suture (e.g., AssiAnchor, Hanita Lenses; Kibbutz Hanita, Israel). In this way, the repositioning of the dislocated capsular bag is often achieved more precisely [31].

Not infrequently, intracapsular IOL implantation is impossible. An implantation of a transscleral fixed IOL should be performed during the same procedure, if possible.

If a pronounced nystagmus is present, a primary posterior capsulorhexis should also be performed, since a subsequent YAG capsulotomy is often difficult without re-anesthetizing the patient.

Postoperative Specialties in Patients with Cataract and Aniridia

Patients with congenital aniridia require closer monitoring and more intensive postoperative care than regular cataract patients. In addition to the higher risk of postoperative corneal and pressure decompensation, increased fibrosis tendency is among the most difficult postoperative complications. "Anterior segment fibrosis syndrome," first described by Tsai and colleagues [32], is typical of patients with congenital aniridia and can occur in any intraocular surgery [33, 34]. The pathogenesis appears to be the disturbed barrier of blood vessels in the remaining iris roots. Intraocular manipulation allows profibrotic mediators to enter the anterior chamber and trigger the growth of these hypocellular fibrous membranes.

This develops into a noninflammatory fibrotic membrane in the pupillary plane, which can lead to lens dislocation and corneal decompensation. In some cases, further growth of the fibrotic membrane onto the ciliary body has been described, which may lead to hypotony or tractional retinal detachment.

Excessive capsular fibrosis up to phimosis and IOL dislocation are also possible. On the other hand, opaque capsular fibrosis can also act as a diaphragm and thus positively influence glare sensitivity.

Corneal decompensation should initially be treated with intensive local steroid therapy and osmotically active eye drops. The typical surface problems in limbal stem cell deficiency require intensive tear-substitute therapy.

In cases of persistent endothelial failure, Descemet membrane endothelial keratoplasty may be required. This procedure is preferable to penetrating keratoplasty.

Decompensated intraocular pressure is common in the postoperative course. In addition to topical therapy, systemic therapy with carbonic anhydrase inhibitors may be necessary temporarily. Glaucoma surgery should be delayed, if possible. If pressure control cannot be achieved without surgery in the longer term, the choice of procedure depends on the existing architecture of the anterior segment of the eye or the chamber angle [35].

Trabeculotomy is the operation of choice for pretrabecular faculties. This can be verified gonioscopically. Alternatively, nonpenetrating procedures (e.g., canaloplasty with suprachoroidal drainage) are reasonable [36]. However, the Schlemm's canal is often dysgenetic and thus cannot be probed; in these cases, the procedure can be converted to a deep sclerectomy with a suprachoroidal collagen implant in the short term [7]. Classic fistulizing surgery should be avoided due to the strong scarring tendency of the often young aniridia patients. Glaucoma drainage systems are preferable in the most severe courses.

Summary

In all patients with coexisting congenital aniridia and cataracts, a precise preoperative evaluation of the individual pathology is mandatory. This assessment should be carried out personally by the surgeon, who can expertly assess the possible intraoperative peculiarities preoperatively and plan the surgical procedure and possible next steps.

Due to the altered anatomical conditions, all steps of complication management in lens surgery, especially scleral fixation of IOLs, should be mastered.

Although iris reconstruction in traumatic aniridia can be well-combined with cataract surgery, reconstructing the iris in congenital aniridia should be avoided, except under special circumstances.

Cataract surgery for congenital aniridia is associated with a variety of postoperative complications and requires close monitoring. In particular, anterior fibrosis syndrome, corneal decompensation, and the frequent incidence of secondary glaucoma are postoperative challenges.

Take-Home Notes

- Preoperatively, a detailed examination of the eye is necessary to determine the initial situation, which is unique for each patient.
- While iris reconstruction in traumatic aniridia can be performed well in combination with cataract surgery, iris reconstructive procedures in congenital aniridia should only be considered in selected cases.
- The greatest challenge in cataract surgery with congenital aniridia is reduced vision due to stromal corneal opacities.
- The lens capsule is significantly thinner and more fragile in congenital aniridia.
- Patients with congenital aniridia require due to the "anterior segment fibrosis syndrome" closer monitoring and more intensive postoperative care than regular cataract patients.

References

1. Brémond-Gignac D, Bitoun P, Reis LM, Copin H, Murray JC, Semina EV. Identification of dominant FOXE3 and PAX6 mutations in patients with congenital cataract and aniridia. Mol Vis. 2010;16:1705–11.
2. Deml B, Reis LM, Lemyre E, Clark RD, Kariminejad A, Semina EV. Novel mutations in PAX6, OTX2 and NDP in anophthalmia, microphthalmia and coloboma. Eur J Hum Genet. 2016. https://doi.org/10.1038/ejhg.2015.155.
3. Pedersen HR, et al. Color vision in aniridia. Investig Ophthalmol Vis Sci. 2018. https://doi.org/10.1167/iovs.17-23047.
4. Brandt JD, Casuso LA, Budenz DL. Markedly increased central corneal thickness: an unrecognized finding in congenital aniridia. Am J Ophthalmol. 2004. https://doi.org/10.1016/j.ajo.2003.09.038.
5. Whitson JT, et al. Central corneal thickness in patients with congenital aniridia. Eye Contact Lens. 2005. https://doi.org/10.1097/01.ICL.0000152487.16012.40.
6. Bajwa A, Burstein E, Grainger RM, Netland PA. Anterior chamber angle in aniridia with and without glaucoma. Clin Ophthalmol. 2019. https://doi.org/10.2147/OPTH.S217930.
7. Szurman P, Januschowski K, Boden KT, Seuthe AM. Suprachoroidal drainage with collagen sheet implant- a novel technique for non-penetrating glaucoma surgery. Graefes Arch Clin Exp Ophthalmol. 2018. https://doi.org/10.1007/s00417-017-3873-9.
8. Brauner SC, Walton DS, Chen TC. Aniridia. Int Ophthalmol Clin. 2008. https://doi.org/10.1097/IIO.0b013e318169314b.
9. Lagali N, et al. PAX6 mutational status determines aniridia-associated keratopathy phenotype. Ophthalmology. 2020. https://doi.org/10.1016/j.ophtha.2019.09.034.
10. Latta L, et al. Human aniridia limbal epithelial cells lack expression of keratins K3 and K12. Exp Eye Res. 2018. https://doi.org/10.1016/j.exer.2017.11.005.
11. Ramaesh K, Ramaesh T, Dutton GN, Dhillon B. Evolving concepts on the pathogenic mechanisms of aniridia related keratopathy. Int J Biochem Cell Biol. 2005. https://doi.org/10.1016/j.biocel.2004.09.002.
12. Lapid-Gortzak R, Santana NTY, Nieuwendaal CP, Mourits MP, van der Meulen IJE. Topical bevacizumab treatment in aniridia. Int Ophthalmol. 2018. https://doi.org/10.1007/s10792-017-0605-4.
13. Tiller AM, Odenthal MTP, Verbraak FD, Gortzak-Moorstein N. The influence of keratoplasty on visual prognosis in aniridia: a historical review of one large family. Cornea. 2003. https://doi.org/10.1097/00003226-200303000-00004.
14. Rafaella Nascimento E Silva, et al. Glaucoma management in patients with aniridia and Boston type 1 keratoprosthesis. Am J Ophthalmol. 2019. https://doi.org/10.1016/j.ajo.2019.06.018.
15. Lee HK, Kim MK, Oh JY. Corneal abnormalities in congenital aniridia: congenital central corneal opacity versus aniridia-associated keratopathy. Am J Ophthalmol. 2018. https://doi.org/10.1016/j.ajo.2017.10.017.
16. Landsend ECS, et al. Meibomian gland dysfunction and keratopathy are associated with dry eye disease in aniridia. Br J Ophthalmol. 2019. https://doi.org/10.1136/bjophthalmol-2017-310927.
17. Wong VWY, Lam PTH, Lai TYY, Lam DSC. Black diaphragm aniridia intraocular lens for aniridia and albinism. Graefes Arch Clin Exp Ophthalmol. 2005. https://doi.org/10.1007/s00417-004-1058-9.
18. Qiu X, Ji Y, Zheng T, Lu Y. The efficacy and complications of black diaphragm intra-ocular lens implantation in patients with congenital aniridia. Acta Ophthalmol. 2016. https://doi.org/10.1111/aos.12923.
19. Seitz B, Käsmann-Kellner B, Viestenz A. Stage-related therapy of congenital aniridia. Ophthalmologe. 2014. https://doi.org/10.1007/s00347-014-3061-9.

20. Wolf A, Shajari M. Slip-and-slide technique for combined small-incision artificial iris and IOL implantation. J Cataract Refract Surg. 2020. https://doi.org/10.1097/j.jcrs.0000000000000254.
21. Yoeruek E, Bartz-Schmidt KU. A new knotless technique for combined transscleral fixation of artificial iris, posterior chamber intraocular lens, and penetrating keratoplasty. Eye. 2019. https://doi.org/10.1038/s41433-018-0202-4.
22. McCannel MA. A retrievable suture idea for anterior uveal problems. Ophthalmic Surg. 1976. https://doi.org/10.3928/1542-8877-19861101-10.
23. Siepser SB. The closed chamber slipping suture technique for iris repair. Ann Ophthalmol. 1994;26(3):71–2.
24. Oshima Y, Shima C, Maeda N, Tano Y. Chandelier retroillumination-assisted torsional oscillation for cataract surgery in patients with severe corneal opacity. J Cataract Refract Surg. 2007. https://doi.org/10.1016/j.jcrs.2007.07.055.
25. Schneider S, Osher RH, Burk SE, Lutz TB, Montione R. Thinning of the anterior capsule associated with congenital aniridia. J Cataract Refract Surg. 2003. https://doi.org/10.1016/S0886-3350(02)01602-4.
26. Melles GRJ, De Waard PWT, Pameyer JH, Beekhuis WH, Van Vroonhoven CCJ. Trypan blue capsule staining to visualize the capsulorhexis in cataract surgery. J Cataract Refract Surg. 1999. https://doi.org/10.1016/S0886 3350(99)80004-2.
27. Gazzola LN, Ghem MRD, Serpe C, Santhiago MR, Mello GR. The role of a femtosecond laser in congenital cataract associated with aniridia. Arq Bras Oftalmol. 2018. https://doi.org/10.5935/0004-2749.20180083.
28. Dick HB, Schultz T. Femtosecond laser-assisted cataract surgery in infants. J Cataract Refract Surg. 2013. https://doi.org/10.1016/j.jcrs.2013.02.032.
29. Merriam JC, Zheng L. Iris hooks for phacoemulsification of the subluxated lens. J Cataract Refract Surg. 1997. https://doi.org/10.1016/S0886-3350(97)80105-8.
30. Moreno-Montañés J, Sainz C, Maldonado MJ. Intraoperative and postoperative complications of Cionni endocapsular ring implantation. J Cataract Refract Surg. 2003. https://doi.org/10.1016/S0886-3350(02)01604-8.
31. Ton Y, Naftali M, Gortzak RL, Assia EI. Management of subluxated capsular bag–fixated intraocular lenses using a capsular anchor. J Cataract Refract Surg. 2016. https://doi.org/10.1016/j.jcrs.2016.04.002.
32. Tsai JH, et al. A progressive anterior fibrosis syndrome in patients with postsurgical congenital aniridia. Am J Ophthalmol. 2005. https://doi.org/10.1016/j.ajo.2005.07.035.
33. Kothari M, Rao K, Moolani S. Recurrent progressive anterior segment fibrosis syndrome following a descemet-stripping endothelial keratoplasty in an infant with congenital aniridia. Indian J Ophthalmol. 2014. https://doi.org/10.4103/0301-4738.128635.
34. Lee H, Khan R, O'keefe M. Aniridia: current pathology and management. Acta Ophthalmol. 2008. https://doi.org/10.1111/j.1755-3768.2008.01427.x.
35. Viestenz A, et al. Clinical anatomy of the anterior chamber angle in congenital aniridia and consequences for trabeculotomy/cyclophotocoagulation. Clin Anat. 2018. https://doi.org/10.1002/ca.22935.
36. Szurman P, Januschowski K, Boden KT, Szurman GB. A modified scleral dissection technique with suprachoroidal drainage for canaloplasty. Graefes Arch Clin Exp Ophthalmol. 2016. https://doi.org/10.1007/s00417-015-3234-5.

Floppy Iris Syndrome

27

Argyrios Tzamalis and Boris Malyugin

Bullet Points

- Pathophysiology of IFIS: What causes iris floppiness?
- Risk factors for the appearance of IFIS: What are the chances our cataract patients will develop IFIS?
- Medication and IFIS: Which medication could lead to floppy iris? Should they be discontinued prior to surgery?
- Prophylaxis: Is there any way to prevent the appearance of floppy iris?
- Intraoperative management: How to avoid complication when IFIS occurs?

Introduction

Since its original description by Chang and Campbell, intraoperative floppy iris syndrome (IFIS) has been widely established as one of the most challenging conditions for cataract surgeons [1]. Although most of the syndrome signs had long ago been identified during phacoemulsification, IFIS was systematically described in 2005. It was defined as the presence of one or more intraoperative features of a typical triad occurring during phacoemulsification surgery (Fig. 27.1a, b). These features were:

A. Floppy iris stroma that ripples and billows in response to phaco fluidics
B. Tendency of the iris stroma to prolapse through incisions
C. Progressive intraoperative miosis despite the use of mydriatic agents

Based on the characteristics mentioned above, the following classification of IFIS in grades of severity has been proposed.

- *Grade 0:* none
- *Grade 1:* mild IFIS (A only)
- *Grade 2*: moderate IFIS (A&B or A&C)
- *Grade 3*: severe IFIS (A&B&C) [2]

The reported prevalence of IFIS at its first description was almost 2% (10/511 patients) and was entirely associated with the use of tamsulosin in males with benign prostate hyperplasia [1]. More contemporary studies have estimated the incidence of IFIS in cataract surgery to vary between 1.1% and 12.6% [1, 3, 4]. Beyond the

Supplementary Information The online version contains supplementary material available at [https://doi.org/10.1007/978-3-030-94530-5_27].

A. Tzamalis
2nd Department of Ophthalmology, Aristotle University of Thessaloniki, Papageorgiou General Hospital, Thessaloniki, Greece

B. Malyugin (✉)
S. Fyodorov Eye Microsurgery Federal State Institution, Moscow, Russian Federation

J. L. Alió et al. (eds.), *Cataract Surgery*, Essentials in Ophthalmology,
https://doi.org/10.1007/978-3-030-94530-5_27

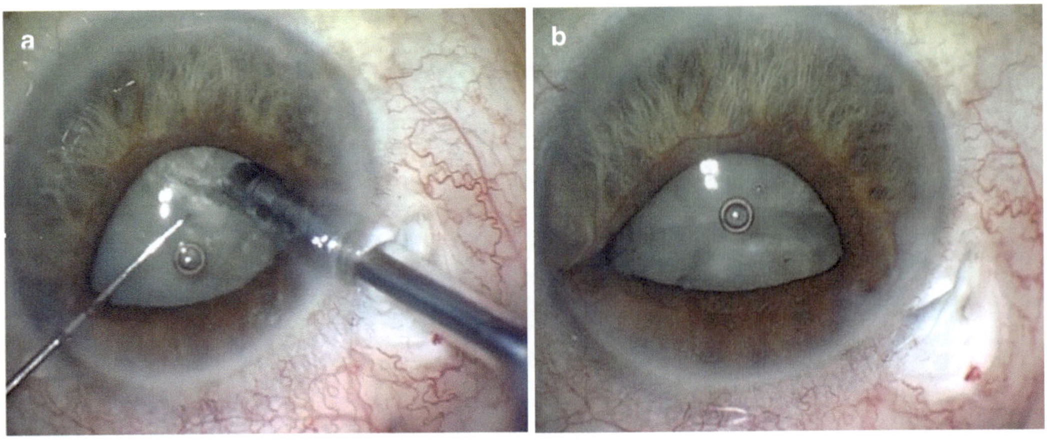

Fig. 27.1 (**a**) Intraoperative floppy iris syndrome in patient with white cataract. Note the iris starting to prolapse through the side port incision (**b**) After withdrawing the phaco tip, the iris prolapses through the main incision in addition to the paracentesis

initial correlation with tamsulosin intake [1], IFIS has been associated with numerous risk factors which among others comprise male gender, older age, arterial hypertension and related medication, poor preoperative pupillary dilation, antipsychotics, benzodiazepines, finasteride, and other α1- adrenergic receptor antagonists (α1-blockers) [5–10].

The careful preoperative assessment of these predisposing factors is essential in the stratification of the preoperative risk. As a matter of fact, several studies have been published in the last 15 years proving that the appearance of IFIS significantly increases the risk of intraoperative complications, especially when not anticipated [1, 9, 11, 12]. Subsequently, it is of outmost importance for cataract surgeons to be aware of factors predisposing to the appearance of IFIS and be able to employ possible preventive measures and surgical technique modifications that will address the needs of IFIS management and minimize complications.

Pathophysiology of IFIS

Many factors and medical conditions have been proposed so far to be associated with the appearance of floppy iris during cataract surgery [5–10]. However, the intake of α1-blockers and specifically tamsulosin, which was the initially described risk factor, represents by far the strongest correlation. This association became much more apparent after the establishment of α1-blockers as first-line treatment for benign prostatic hyperplasia (BPH) instead of surgical intervention [13]. Subtype A of α1 adrenergic receptors represents the main regulator of smooth muscle tone in the human urinary system, and, therefore, α1-blockers are widely used for BPH and other urinary disorders. However, such receptors also exist on the iris dominating the tone of musculus dilatator pupillae [14]. Subsequently, α1-blockers antagonize these receptors too preventing the iris from fully dilating.

Based on the above explanation, one could hypothesize that the discontinuation of α1-blockers could significantly increase the tone of the pupil dilator muscle providing thus better mydriasis and minimizing the risk of IFIS appearance. Although this may happen in some cases, most suspect patients receiving α1-blockers do not seem to benefit significantly from such a preventive measure. This fact has led specialists to suggest an additional mechanism through which α1-blockers could affect pupillary dilation [15, 16]. The long-term use of such agents has been found to induce alterations on the iris such as atrophy of the pupillary margin and the dilator muscle which are permanent and cannot be reversed with treatment discontinuation or other dilating agents [17].

The above-described mechanisms could also be partially applied to other agents predisposing to a floppy iris such as the intake of antipsychotics, benzodiazepines, or even several medications that treat arterial hypertension. However, the exact pathophysiology in such cases, as well as with other risk factors, has not been fully understood yet. Nevertheless, the association between floppy iris and other risk factors does not seem to be as strong as with tamsulosin [4, 5, 7]. Further research is required in order to shed light on the exact pathophysiology of IFIS and explain why some patients are more prone to its appearance than others.

Risk Factors

Medication

Tamsulosin

Tamsulosin is one of the most used α1 adrenergic receptor blockers for BPH and other urinary disorders. It was the first risk factor to be correlated with the appearance of IFIS and still remains the most predominant and well described [1, 5, 18]. This strong correlation could be attributed to the fact that tamsulosin's affinity to block α1 receptors and especially subtypes A and D is much higher than the one of other α1-blockers [19]. This has led to tamsulosin yielding a significantly increased odds ratio (OR = 206.5) and relative risk ratio (RR = 99.3) for IFIS development compared to other α1-blockers [20].

It is not clear whether the effect of tamsulosin in the appearance of IFIS is dose-dependent or not. Interestingly, the reported incidence of IFIS seems to be much higher in studies being conducted in Europe or the USA compared to studies originating from Japan where the recommended daily dosage of tamsulosin is half of the respective one in western countries [5, 21, 22]. These data could imply a possible positive correlation of IFIS incidence for patients on tamsulosin with its cumulative dosage. On the other hand, floppy iris has also been noted in cases receiving tamsulosin for as little as 2 days prior to surgery [23].

There is a long debate among cataract surgeons whether tamsulosin should be discontinued before phacoemulsification as a preventive measure for IFIS. As a matter of fact, some research results support its discontinuation for 4–7 days prior to surgery showing a lower incidence of IFIS [1, 13]. However, the cessation of tamsulosin does not entirely eliminate the risk of developing floppy iris, since cases of IFIS after years of tamsulosin discontinuation have been reported [24]. Consequently, it is suggested that urologists inform both patients and their ophthalmologists for the risk of IFIS before prescribing tamsulosin, when the patient is still phakic [25]. In cases of visually significant cataract, phacoemulsification prior to tamsulosin prescription is also an option. Alternatively, a non-selective α1-blocker could also be considered.

Other α1-Blockers

Alfuzosin, doxazosin, and terazosin are also commonly prescribed by urologists in order to deal with BPH and other lower urinary tract disorders. In contrast to tamsulosin, they are non-selective blocking equally all three α1-AR subtypes [19, 26–28]. Their lower affinity for the subtype A of α1 receptors could explain the much lower reported incidence of IFIS among patients receiving those medications in comparison to tamsulosin [2]. It is of note, that alfuzosin reduces the risk of IFIS development by almost 30 times in comparison to tamsulosin and is, therefore, preferred as first-line treatment in male phakic patients with BPH [2]. In a recent study, Dogan et al. compared the effects of systemic alfuzosin and tamsulosin on choroidal thickness and pupil diameter size, showing that alfuzosin was found to significantly decrease both, while, as expected, tamsulosin did not have any significant effect on the choroidal thickness [29]. Regarding pupillary dilation, patients on alfuzosin showed significantly smaller pupils than in the tamsulosin group. The authors suggested that alfuzosin leads to IFIS by blocking the α1 receptors, while tamsulosin induces additional atrophy of the pupil dilator muscle [29].

In recent years, two additional α1-blockers have been introduced in the treatment of BPH, *naftopidil* and *silodosin*. Naftopidil has been implicated in floppy iris syndrome, however at a slightly lower rate than tamsulosin [22]. Likewise, there are several reports in the literature of IFIS cases attributed to the systematic use of silodosin [16, 30–32]. However no large cohorts have been published so far and prospective randomized studies are expected to evaluate the exact hazard of developing IFIS with these agents.

Finasteride

Although α1-blockers are well established as the main risk factor for the development of IFIS, there are several other medications that have been implicated as causative agents. Finasteride is a drug commonly used to treat BPH and hair loss in men, as well as excessive hair growth in women. It is a specific 5a-reductase inhibitor and is generally considered an anti-androgen. It has been linked with cases of anterior subcapsular cataracts and IFIS, although no direct pathophysiologic mechanism has been found and it remains unknown whether finasteride has a direct effect on iris [5, 6, 32, 33]. Finasteride is supposed to have a short-term effect, and, consequently, its discontinuation prior to phacoemulsification could be of some benefit [6].

Neuromodulators

Since its original description, IFIS has been correlated with numerous neuromodulating agents including *benzodiazepines, donepezil, duloxetine, and mianserin* [5, 7, 34, 35]. Chatziralli et al. documented an increased occurrence of IFIS in patients receiving benzodiazepines in a large retrospective study, a correlation also verified in a univariate analysis by Kaczmarek et al. [5, 7]. In 2007, Papadopoulos et al. reported IFIS in a woman with a long history (8 years) of taking donepezil for Alzheimer's disease, while recently, González-Martín-Moro et al. reported a case of IFIS in a woman consuming duloxetine as an antidepressant for 3 years [34, 35]. Another antidepressant, mianserin, has been suggested as the causative factor for the appearance of IFIS in a woman receiving the abovementioned medication for 20 years prior to surgery [36].

It remains debatable whether the increased rate of IFIS in patients receiving the abovementioned medications is causative or coincidental. While mydriasis is understood to be opposed by cholinergic drugs, the precise pathogenetic process by which these drugs lead to the development of IFIS is less apparent and remains subject to future research [5, 7]. Nevertheless, it is advisable to include benzodiazepines, antidepressants, and anticholinergic drugs in the preoperative history taking and inform surgeons regarding the possibility of IFIS appearance.

Additionally, many antipsychotics have been implied to act as risk factors for the appearance of floppy iris during phacoemulsification. This list includes both typical and atypical antipsychotics, such as *quetiapine, chlorpromazine, zuclopenthixol, aripiprazole,* and *risperidone* [5, 37–42]. All these drugs, mainly used in the treatment of schizophrenia and other mental disorders, have a well-known blocking action against α-adrenergic receptors. As α1-antagonism is probably the causative mechanism to induce iris floppiness, the use of intracameral adrenaline or phenylephrine could possibly be beneficial as a preventive measure [38–42]. However, there are no large series or controlled studies on the effect of antipsychotics on the iris, and most data regarding possible correlations of IFIS and antipsychotics comes from case reports.

Antihypertensives

Beyond their main indication for the management of benign prostate hyperplasia, some non-selective α1-blockers are used as antihypertensives. *Doxazosin* has been reported to induce IFIS also in cases where it was systematically used to treat arterial hypertension [11, 43–45]. *Labetalol* has also been implicated in the appearance of IFIS [46]. Labetalol combines selective, competitive inhibition of alpha-1 adrenergic receptors and non-selective, competitive inhibition of beta-adrenergic receptors. Its α1-blocking effect is probably the one responsible for iris floppiness and poor pupillary dilation.

Angiotensin II receptor inhibitors have recently been suggested as a major risk factor for IFIS, especially in women [8]. However, it has not been clarified yet whether certain drugs such as losartan or arterial hypertension alone may be the key contributing factor to the development of floppy iris [8, 47].

Gender and Age

Gender has been reported as a risk factor for IFIS occurrence [7, 9, 48]. However, a reasonable argument could be whether the male gender is an independent risk factor for IFIS or if the reported correlation can be attributed to the significantly higher intake of α1-blockers by men for BHP treatment. Two studies that conducted multiple regression analysis, thus adjusting for covariates, reported adjusted risk ratios of 2.2 and 4.7 [5, 48]. Therefore, the male gender retained its positive correlation with IFIS. Females are not resilient to IFIS. Even though less commonly, IFIS could occur in females too. Females are also prescribed α1-blockers for detrusor underactivity and outlet obstruction, and other drugs correlated to IFIS development. However, this is often overlooked. As a result, when IFIS occurs in females since it is usually not anticipated, it is correlated with a higher incidence of postoperative complications. Specifically, nucleus drop, endothelial cell loss, vitreous loss, and posterior capsule rupture lead to a poor visual outcome [9]. Females should not be overlooked during the preoperative assessment. Clinicians should carefully document all factors predisposing IFIS to avoid an unanticipated IFIS, which could have severe consequences to the visual outcome.

Advanced age has been correlated with an increased tendency to IFIS development. Two mechanisms can explain this correlation: first, the progressive vasculature dysfunction, which has been demonstrated using fluorescein leakage as an indicator of vasculature dysfunction [49], and second, the progressive alterations of the synaptic transmission of norepinephrine that cause changes in the iris dilator muscle tone [50]. A study has found that with each 1-year that passes, the IFIS occurrence risk increases, with a proposed odds ratio (OR) of 1.09 (95% CI 1.03–1.16, $p = 0.006$) [7].

Arterial Hypertension

The role of arterial hypertension as a factor predisposing to IFIS development remains disputed. Except from the iris dilator muscle, $\alpha 1_A$ adrenergic receptors are found in the arteriolar muscularis of the human iris [51]. Various systemic diseases could also lead to endothelial dysfunction, increasing the iris dilator's resistance to epinephrine agonists [52]. Nevertheless, the existing results are conflicting, with several studies reporting no significant correlation between high blood pressure (HBP) and IFIS [7, 53], while others report significant results [5, 48]. Further studies are required to investigate the correlation among different HPB treatments and IFIS to determine whether HBP is an independent predisposing factor.

Dilated Pupil Diameter

The dilated pupil's preoperative diameter should be assessed since it has been reported as an independent factor for IFIS occurrence. A recent study reported that a well-dilated pupil preoperatively was a protective factor for IFIS development regardless of α1-blocker intake [54]. Similar studies report decreased preoperative dilated pupil as a predisposing factor for IFIS development [10, 55]. However, there is currently no consensus on a specific cut-off value, with studies using cut-offs ranging between 6.5 and 8 mm [2, 10, 55, 56]. Except for pupil diameter, the ratio between dilated pupil and the limbal diameter was proposed as a more reliable metric to assess IFIS risk, with the rationale that cornea and pupil sizes differ significantly among races and individuals [56, 57].

Preoperative Assessment and Prophylaxis

Surgical risk is not linear. Different risk factors impact on a different scale the surgical outcome, while combined risk factors could lead to an exponential increase of the surgical risk due to a synergistic effect. While several factors predisposing to IFIS have been investigated, a comprehensive tool that reliably assesses the risk for IFIS is not available. Such a tool could be developed using multiple regression models or even machine-learning methods such as Optimal Classification Trees [58]. Until a novel tool is developed, clinicians should carefully assess each patient for each factor predisposing to IFIS. Greater attention should be given to risk factors with high reported ORs such as α1-blockers, particularly tamsulosin, decreased dilated pupils, and medications such as specific antihypertensives, benzodiazepines, and antipsychotics.

As mentioned before, the cessation of drugs that predispose to IFIS prior to surgery does not fully eradicate the risk of IFIS, even though it could be helpful in some cases [1, 13]. Chang et al. had acknowledged in their initial study that a cessation of tamsulosin 4–7 days before cataract surgery decreased but did not eliminate the risk for IFIS development [1]. Many ophthalmologists anecdotally withdraw tamsulosin or alfuzosin shortly before surgery, even though there is currently in the literature no strong evidence that supports such a withdrawal [48]. Tamsulosin has a long half-life, and when taken for long intervals, it causes irreversible atrophy to the iris dilator. As a result, ceasing tamsulosin for few days could be inadequate.

There are currently no guidelines as to which patients are required a preoperative prophylactic strategy. The decision remains with the surgeon. Also, there is no consensus regarding which preventive measures are appropriate. Among these measures is the use of mydriatic regimens preoperatively. Topical atropine alone or with the addition of intracameral epinephrine has been reported to decrease IFIS rates in high-risk patients significantly [17, 59, 60]. Recently, an installation of atropine sulfate 1% 40 and 20 min prior to surgery was reported to decrease IFIS rates, particularly the severe forms [17].

Another group of agents used to facilitate pupillary mydriasis is the nonsteroidal anti-inflammatory drugs (NSAIDs), which block cyclooxygenase and inhibit the intraoperative pupillary miosis caused by prostaglandins. Ketorolac, which belongs to this group of drugs, was used in patients with a small dilated pupil (<5 mm) and was reported to decrease the need for iris rings to maintain pupil dilation to 0% compared to the control group (50%) ($p = 0.0034$) [61].

Surgical Management of IFIS

The use of intracameral mydriatics as an addition or even sometimes substitution of the preoperative mydriatics instillations has been widely adopted by many cataract surgeons. Direct contact of phenylephrine or epinephrine with the iris tissue has a beneficial effect on the pupil size and the tone of the iris dilatation muscle reducing the incidence and severity of IFIS. Some surgeons prefer to use intracameral mydriatics in combination with local anesthetic (lidocaine) or NSAID (ketorolac) [61, 62]. Intracameral epinephrine and phenylephrine promote pupillary dilation and reduce iris floppiness. Introduction of intracameral epinephrine/phenylephrine allowed to dramatically reduce the necessity to use pupil expansion devices both by experienced surgeons and residents in training [63, 64].

During surgery in anticipated IFIS cases, it is recommended to use anteriorly elongated corneal incisions; perform very gentle hydrodissection, lower fluidic parameters of the phaco machine; and keep the irrigation flow above the iris plane [65]. If the pupil starts to constrict, stretching of the pupil is ineffective, because the iris pupil margin remains elastic and the pupil immediately snaps back to its original size following attempts at stretching it.

Proper selection and use of ophthalmic viscosurgical devices (OVD) allow to stabilize the iris tissue and prevent iris billowing. There are several OVD techniques can be used to perform cataract surgery in patients taking tamsulosin. The combination of a soft-shell and ultimate soft-shell technique involves the use of different OVDs and adjustments to flow parameters. In the soft-shell bridge technique (SSB), dispersive OVD (Discovisc) is injected first coating the corneal endothelium and placed over the iris, visco-adaptive OVD (Healon5) is injected second in the center of the anterior chamber filling the space, and BSS is injected third over the anterior lens capsule. Then the surgeon performs phacoemulsification with very low fluidic parameters (flow less than 20 ml/min, aspiration 200 mmHg) to avoid OVD aspiration from the anterior chamber [66, 67].

When pharmacological approach does not provide sufficient pupil diameter, the use of mechanical pupil expansion devices is recommended [68, 69]. Flexible polymer iris hooks allow to expand the pupil and maintain its size throughout the procedure. The so-called "diamond" configuration of iris hooks placement (Fig. 27.2), when one of them is located closely adjacent to or even under the main cataract incision, helps to prevent iris incarceration into the wound and is considered especially useful in IFIS cases [70].

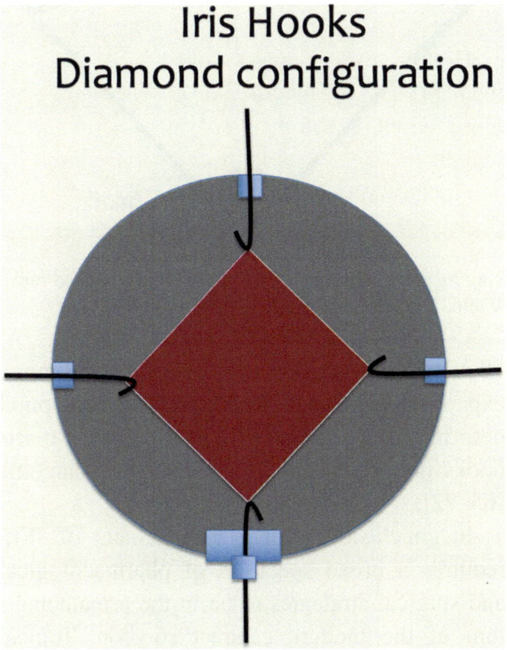

Fig. 27.2 Schematic view of iris hooks placement in a "diamond" configuration, with one of the hooks located adjacent to the main cataract incision

Pupil expansion rings in most cases are much easier to use; they require less operating time, do not require extra incisions, and provide a stable pupil during surgery minimizing postoperative pupil deformity [63, 71, 72]. David Chang was the first to report about the beneficial effects of the Malyugin Ring (Microsurgical Technology Inc., USA) in patients with IFIS [73].

Malyugin Ring is a device that can maintain a pupil in an extended position during phacoemulsification (Fig. 27.3). The ring has a plurality of loops that capture iris tissue. It is configured to extend the pupil when iris tissue is inserted into each loop having one-piece design with square shape and four equidistantly located circular loops [74]. The loops are located at each corner of the device utilizing the scroll principle of catching and holding the pupillary margin (Fig. 27.4). Each loop has a gap to accommodate the iris tissue. The triangular profile of the scroll gap adapts for various thickness of the pupillary margin in different individuals [68]. The device is made of 4-0 (Malyugin Ring version 1.0) or 5-0 (Malyugin Ring version 2.0) polypropylene and produced in two sizes: 6.25 mm and 7.0 mm. Malyugin Ring v1.0 (Classic) has thicker and stiffer thread and is, thus, theoretically better to use for very small and fibrotic pupils. Malyugin 2.0 is indicated in moderately dilated pupils and IFIS (there is no need to forcefully stretch the iris in these cases). The advantage of the 6.25 mm ring is that it is easier to insert and to remove. The advantage of the 7.0 mm ring is that it provides larger exposition of the lens and can be used if the pupil starts of bigger, especially in IFIS cases.

Theoretical mathematical modeling and computer simulations were used to assess billowing/buckling patterns of the iris under various loading pressures. This simulation demonstrates that pupil expansion device (such as the Malyugin Ring) effectively inhibits iris billowing even in the setting of floppy iris syndrome [75]. As a matter of fact, in patients prone to develop IFIS, when pupil expansion devices are utilized, they

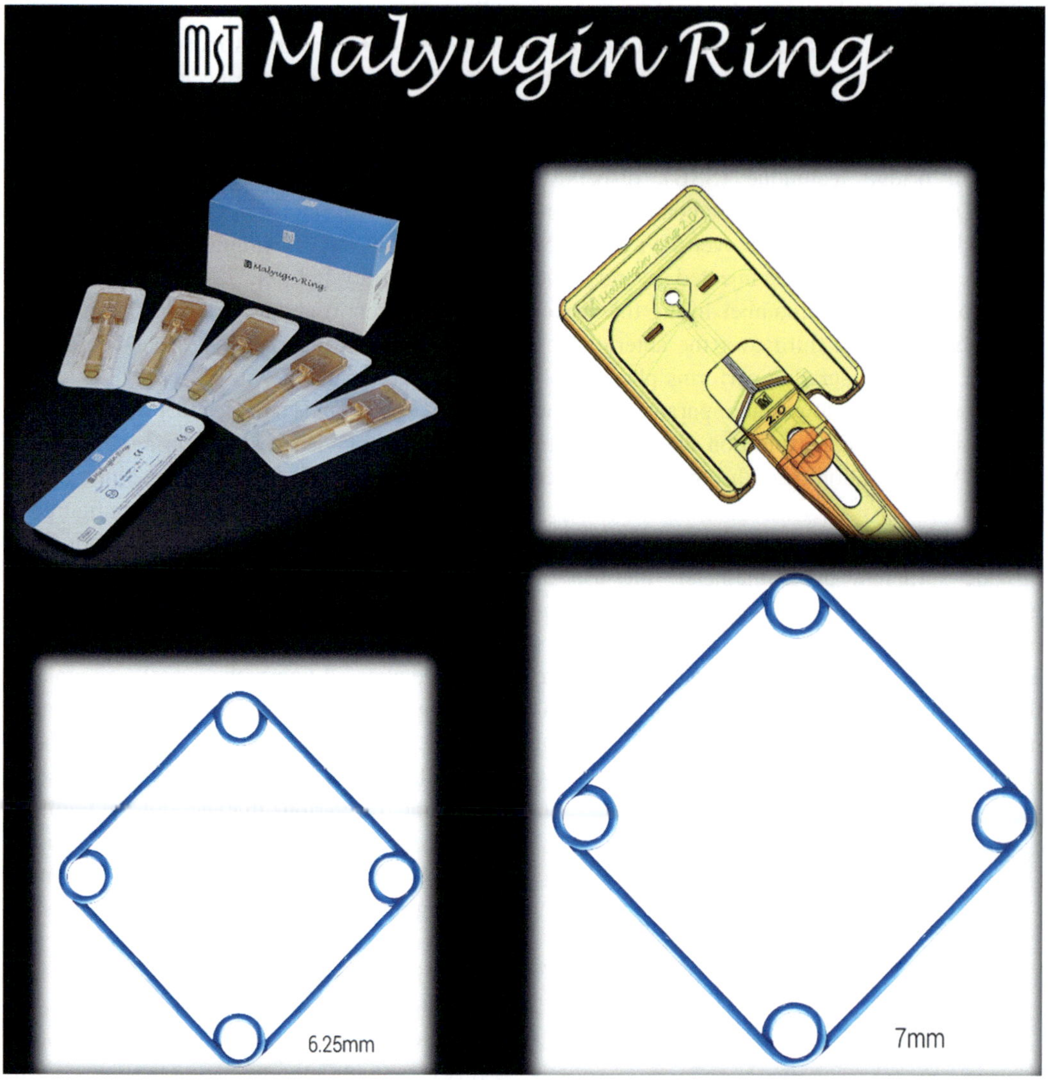

Fig. 27.3 Malyugin Ring System containing the Malyugin Ring located in the special holder with the attached injection device. Two sizes of the device are available: 6.25 and 7.0 mm. The latter is the best one to use in IFIS cases

should be employed as a prophylactic measure from the beginning of surgery rather than using them after floppy iris develops, which could eventually compromise the integrity of the capsulorhexis.

Iris hooks may be preferred by some surgeons, especially in cases with a shallow anterior chamber, as a safe and cheap alternative to rings. On the other hand, iris hooks are associated with an additional operating time. Notably, when compared with the Malyugin Ring, iris hooks took on average 10 min longer among consultants and 18 min longer among trainees [76]. Furthermore, expansion rings can significantly reduce pupil deformity and inflammation in comparison to iris hooks providing thus a better surgical outcome [63, 72].

In conclusion, proper management of IFIS requires a broad spectrum of pharmacological and surgical strategies to be in the armamentarium of the modern cataract surgeon. Topical medications augmented with intraocular mydriatic injections appear to be the mainstream providing success in the majority of cases. However, mechanical pupil dilation is very helpful in achieving and maintaining the mydriasis when all other strategies fail. Pupil expansion devices may cause pupil trauma to some extent. Some of these methods are associated with bleeding, loss of iris sphincter function, and abnormal pupil shape postoperatively. The easiness of manipulations and the final results vary significantly with different devices. Iris hooks and Malyugin Ring are the current standard of care for intraoperative mechanical pupil expansion in patients with IFIS. However, a variety of different devices were introduced into the clinical practice over the past years, some of them being currently under development (Fig. 27.5). In general, latest innovations significantly reduced the chance of complications and increased the success rate of cataract surgery in the setting of IFIS.

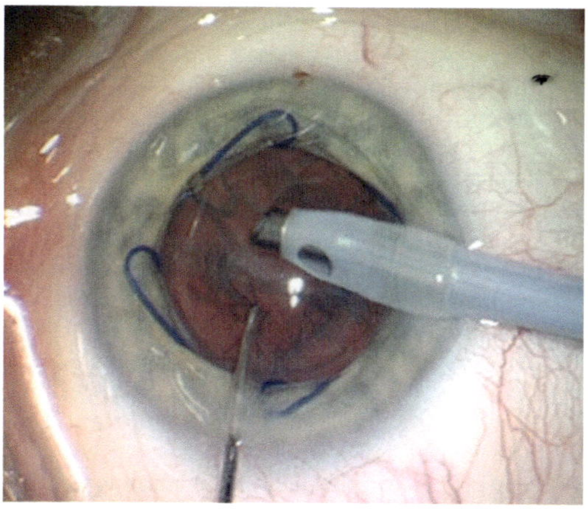

Fig. 27.4 Phacoemulsification in IFIS patient with the Malyugin Ring in place

Take-Home Notes

- Numerous studies have been published in the last 15 years proving that the appearance of IFIS significantly increases the risk of intraoperative complications, especially when not anticipated.
- Several risk factors, such as alpha1-blockers intake for benign prostate hyperplasia, have been linked to the

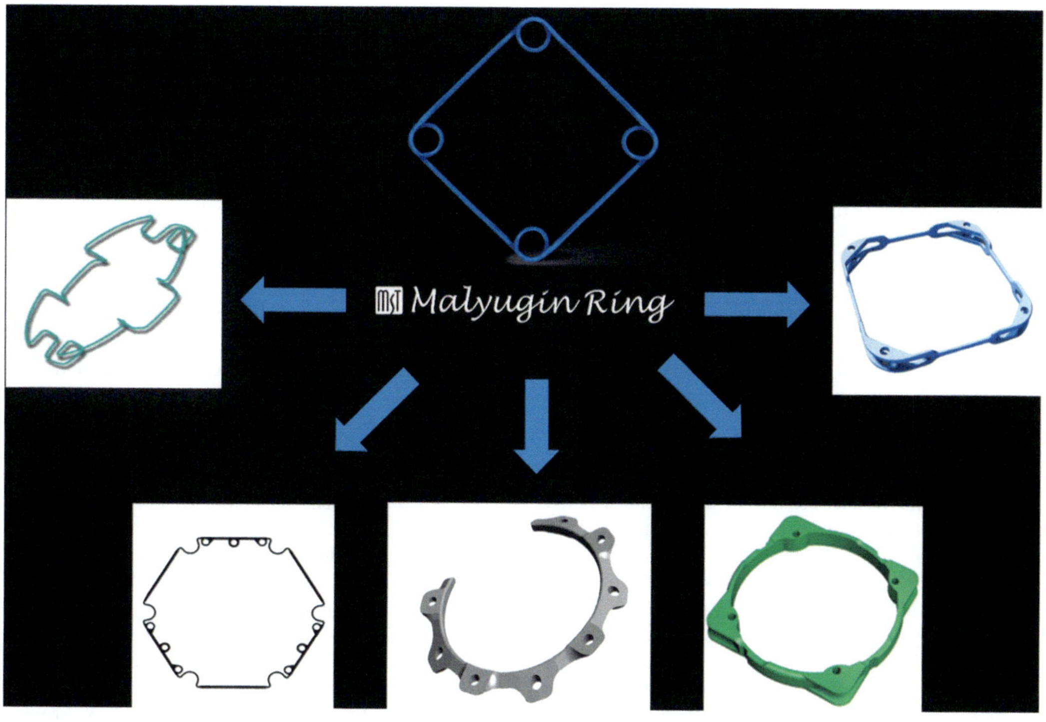

Fig. 27.5 Different pupil expansion rings currently commercially available

appearance of IFIS, predominantly in men, not exclusively though, as it may as well appear in female patients leading to vision-threatening complications.
- Therefore, it is critical for medical personnel being involved in the preoperative assessment of cataract patients to be able to identify high-risk cases and inform cataract surgeons accordingly.
- Patient data, including demographics, dilated pupillary size, and the intake of several medications such as alpha-1 blockers, benzodiazepines, antipsychotics, and antihypertensives, should always be reported in patients' records.
- The use of intracameral agents, such as epinephrine or phenylephrine, upon the beginning of surgery, as well as the employment of the newest, less traumatic pupillary expansion devices (such as the Malyugin Ring), can minimize most features of IFIS.

References

1. Chang DF, Campbell JR. Intraoperative floppy iris syndrome associated with tamsulosin. J Cataract Refract Surg. 2005;31(4):664–73.
2. Chang DF, Campbell JR, Colin J, Schweitzer C, Study Surgeon Group. Prospective masked comparison of intraoperative floppy iris syndrome severity with tamsulosin versus alfuzosin. Ophthalmology. 2014;121:829–34.
3. Cheung CM, Awan MA, Peh KK, Sandramouli S. Incidence of intraoperative floppy iris syndrome in patients on either systemic or topical alpha1-adrenoceptor antagonist. Am J Ophthalmol. 2007;143(6):1070.
4. Wahl M, Tipotsch-Maca SM, Vecsei-Marlovits PV. Intraoperative floppy iris syndrome and its association with various concurrent medications, bulbus length, patient age and gender. Graefes Arch Clin Exp Ophthalmol. 2017;255(1):113–8.
5. Chatziralli IP, Peponis V, Parikakis E, Maniatea A, Patsea E, Mitropoulos P. Risk factors for intraoperative floppy iris syndrome: a prospective study. Eye (Lond). 2016;30(8):1039–44.
6. Issa SA, Dagres E. Intraoperative floppy-iris syndrome and finasteride intake. J Cataract Refract Surg. 2007;33(12):2142–3.
7. Kaczmarek IA, Prost ME, Wasyluk J. Clinical risk factors associated with intraoperative floppy iris syndrome: a prospective study. Int Ophthalmol. 2019;39(3):541–9.
8. Tzamalis A, Malyugin B, Ziakas N, Tsinopoulos I. Angiotensin receptor inhibitors as main predisposing factor for intraoperative floppy iris syndrome in women. J Cataract Refract Surg. 2019;45(5):696–7.
9. Tzamalis A, Matsou A, Dermenoudi M, Brazitikos P, Tsinopoulos I. The role of sex in intraoperative floppy-iris syndrome. J Cataract Refract Surg. 2019;45(1):41–7.
10. Chen AA, Kelly JP, Bhandari A, Wu MC. Pharmacologic prophylaxis and risk factors for intraoperative floppy-iris syndrome in phacoemulsification performed by resident physicians. J Cataract Refract Surg. 2010;36(6):898–905.
11. Muqit MM, Menage MJ. Intraoperative floppy iris syndrome. Ophthalmology. 2006;113(10):1885–6.
12. Lim LA, Frost A. Iris tears secondary to intraoperative floppy iris syndrome associated with tamsulosin. J Cataract Refract Surg. 2006;32(10):1777.
13. Lunacek A, Mohamad Al-Ali B, Radmayr C, et al. Ten years of intraoperative floppy iris syndrome in the era of α-blockers. Cent European J Urol. 2018;71(1):98–104.
14. Schwinn DA, Michelotti GA. α1-adrenergic receptors in the lower urinary tract and vascular bed: potential role for the α1D-subtype in filling symptoms and effects of ageing on vascular expression. BJU Int. 2000;85(Suppl 2):6–11.
15. Zaman F, Bach C, Junaid I, et al. The floppy iris syndrome – what urologists and ophthalmologists need to know. Curr Urol. 2012;6(1):1–7.
16. Goseki T, Ishikawa H, Ogasawara S, et al. Effects of tamsulosin and silodosin on isolated albino and pigmented rabbit iris dilators: possible mechanism of intraoperative floppy-iris syndrome. J Cataract Refract Surg. 2012;38:1643–9.
17. Nuzzi R, Arnoffi P, Tridico F. Best prophylactic strategy in groups at risk of intraoperative floppy iris syndrome development: comparison between atropine instillation and adrenaline intracameral injection. Open Ophthalmol J. 2018;30(12):34–40.
18. Alio JL. Cataract surgery: from today's standards to future progress. Asia Pac J Ophthalmol (Phila). 2017;6(4):309.
19. Schwinn DA, Roehrborn CG. Alpha1-adrenoceptor subtypes and lower urinary tract symptoms. Int J Urol. 2008;15(3):193–9.
20. Keklikci U, Isen K, Unlu K, Celik Y, Karahan M. Incidence, clinical findings and management of intraoperative floppy iris syndrome associated with tamsulosin. Acta Ophthalmol. 2009;87(3):306–9.
21. González Martín-Moro J, Muñoz Negrete F, Lozano Escobar I, Fernández MY. Intraoperative floppy-iris syndrome. Arch Soc Esp Oftalmol. 2013;88(2):64–76.
22. Oshika T, Ohashi Y, Inamura M, Ohki K, Okamoto S, Koyama T, Sakabe I, Takahashi K, Fujita Y, Miyoshi T, Yasuma T. Incidence of intraoperative floppy iris

syndrome in patients on either systemic or topical alpha(1)-adrenoceptor antagonist. Am J Ophthalmol. 2007;143(1):150–1.
23. Shah N, Tendulkar M, Brown R. Should we anticipate intraoperative floppy iris syndrome (IFIS) even with very short history of tamsulosin? Eye (Lond). 2009;23(3):740.
24. Nguyen DQ, Sebastian RT, Kyle G. Surgeon's experiences of the intraoperative floppy iris syndrome in the United Kingdom. Eye (Lond). 2007;21(3):443–4.
25. Yaycioglu O, Altan-Yaycioglu R. Intraoperative floppy iris syndrome: facts for the urologist. Urology. 2010;76(2):272–6.
26. Wilde MI, Fitton A, Sorkin EM. Terazosin. A review of its pharmacodynamic and pharmacokinetic properties, and therapeutic potential in benign prostatic hyperplasia. Drugs Aging. 1993;3(3):258–77.
27. Fulton B, Wagstaff AJ, Sorkin EM. Doxazosin. An update of its clinical pharmacology and therapeutic applications in hypertension and benign prostatic hyperplasia. Drugs. 1995;49(2):295–320.
28. Wilde MI, Fitton A, Alfuzosin MTD. A review of its pharmacodynamic and pharmacokinetic properties, and therapeutic potential in benign prostatic hyperplasia. Drugs. 1993;45(3):410–29.
29. Dogan M, Kutluksaman B, Keles I, Karalar M, Halat AO. The effects of systemic alfuzosin and tamsulosin hydrochloride on choroidal thickness and pupil diameter sizes in cases with benign prostatic hyperplasia. Curr Eye Res. 2017;42(12):1638–43.
30. Ipekci T, Akin Y, Hoscan B, Tunckiran A. Intraoperative floppy iris syndrome associated with silodosin. Acta Ophthalmol. 2015;93(4):e306.
31. Chatterjee S, Agrawal D. Silodosin-associated intraoperative floppy iris syndrome. Indian J Ophthalmol. 2017;65(6):538–9.
32. Ozcura F, Irgat SG. Bilateral intraoperative floppy iris syndrome associated with silodosin intake. Eurasian J Med. 2020;52(1):100–2.
33. Wong AC, Mak ST. Finasteride-associated cataract and intraoperative floppy-iris syndrome. J Cataract Refract Surg. 2011;37(7):1351–4.
34. Papadopoulos R, Bachariou A. Intraoperative floppy-iris syndrome associated with chronic intake of donepezil. J Cataract Refract Surg. 2007;33(11):1997–8.
35. González-Martín-Moro J, González-López JJ, Zarallo-Gallardo J, Fernández-Miguel Y. Intraoperative floppy iris syndrome after treatment with duloxetine: coincidence, association, or causality? Arch Soc Esp Oftalmol. 2015;90(2):94–6.
36. Ugarte M, Leong T, Rassam S, Kon CH. Intraoperative floppy-iris syndrome, alpha1-adrenergic antagonists, and chronic intake of mianserin: is there an association? J Cataract Refract Surg. 2007;33(1):170.
37. Chatziralli IP, Sergentanis TN. Risk factors for intraoperative floppy iris syndrome: a meta-analysis. Ophthalmology. 2011;118(4):730–5.
38. Bilgin B, Ilhan D, Cetinkaya A, Unal M. Intraoperative floppy iris syndrome associated with quetiapine. Eye (Lond). 2013;27(5):673.
39. Pringle E, Packard R. Antipsychotic agent as an etiologic agent of IFIS. J Cataract Refract Surg. 2005;31:2240–1.
40. Unal M, Yucel I, Tenlik A. Intraoperative floppy-iris syndrome associated with chronic use of chlorpromazine. Eye (Lond). 2007;21:1241–2.
41. Matsuo M, Sano I, Ikeda Y, Fujihara E, Tanito M. Intraoperative floppy-iris syndrome associated with use of antipsychotic drugs. Can J Ophthalmol. 2016;51(4):294–6.
42. Ford RL, Sallam A, Towler HM. Intraoperative floppy iris syndrome associated with risperidone intake. Eur J Ophthalmol. 2011;21(2):210–1.
43. El-Ghatit AM. Association of IFIS and vasodepressor medication. J Cataract Refract Surg. 2006;32(4):546–7.
44. Herd MK. Intraoperative floppy-iris syndrome with doxazosin. J Cataract Refract Surg. 2007;33(4):562.
45. Dhingra N, Rajkumar KN, Kumar V. Intraoperative floppy iris syndrome with doxazosin. Eye (Lond). 2007;21(5):678–9.
46. Calotti F, Steen D. Labetalol causing intraoperative floppy-iris syndrome. J Cataract Refract Surg. 2007;33(1):170–1.
47. Altiaylik Ozer P, Altiparmak UE, Unlu N, Hazirolan DO, Kasim R, Duman S. Intraoperative floppy-iris syndrome: comparison of tamsulosin and drugs other than alpha antagonists. Curr Eye Res. 2013;38(4):480–6.
48. Neff KD, Sandoval HP, Fernández de Castro LE, Nowacki AS, Vroman DT, Solomon KD. Factors associated with intraoperative floppy iris syndrome. Ophthalmology. 2009;116(4):658–63.
49. Satoh K, Takaku Y, Ohtsuki K, Mizuno K. Effects of aging on fluorescein leakage in the iris and angle in normal subjects. Jpn J Ophthalmol. 1999;43(3):166–70.
50. Takayanagi I. Effects of aging on drug receptor mechanisms in smooth muscles. Nihon Yakurigaku Zasshi. 1994;104(3):163–75.
51. Panagis L, Basile M, Friedman AH, Danias J. Intraoperative floppy iris syndrome: report of a case and histopathologic analysis. Arch Ophthalmol. 2010;128(11):1437–41.
52. Schwinn DA, Afshari NA. alpha(1)-Adrenergic receptor antagonists and the iris: new mechanistic insights into floppy iris syndrome. Surv Ophthalmol. 2006;51(5):501–12.
53. Altan-Yaycioglu R, Gedik S, Pelit A, Akova YA, Akman A. Clinical factors associated with floppy iris signs: a prospective study from two centers. Ophthalmic Surg Lasers Imaging. 2009;40(3):232–8.
54. Mylona I, Dermenoudi M, Ziakas N, Tsinopoulos I. Increased pupil diameter is a protective factor against intraoperative floppy-iris syndrome. Clin Exp Optom. 2020;103(5):704–5.
55. Casuccio A, Cillino G, Pavone C, Spitale E, Cillino S. Pharmacologic pupil dilation as a predictive test for the risk for intraoperative floppy-iris syndrome. J Cataract Refract Surg. 2011;37(8):1447–54.

56. Terauchi Y, Horiguchi H, Shiba T. The pharmacological mydriatic pupil-to-limbal diameter ratio as an intuitive predictor for the risk of intraoperative floppy iris syndrome. J Ophthalmol. 2018;2018:2837934.
57. Blake CR, Lai WW, Edward DP. Racial and ethnic differences in ocular anatomy. Int Ophthalmol Clin. 2003;43(4):9–25.
58. Bertsimas D, Dunn J. Optimal classification trees. Mach Learn. 2017;106(7):1039–82.
59. Esen F, Bulut AE, Toker E. Efficacy and safety of low-concentration, bisulphite-containing, intracameral epinephrine and topical atropine treatments for the prevention of intraoperative floppy iris syndrome. Cutan Ocul Toxicol. 2018;37(3):286–90.
60. Bendel RE, Phillips MB. Preoperative use of atropine to prevent intraoperative floppy iris syndrome in patients taking tamsulosin. J Cataract Refract Surg. 2006;32(10):1603–5.
61. Visco D. Effect of phenylephrine/ketorolac on iris fixation ring use and surgical times in patients at risk of intraoperative miosis. Clin Ophthalmol. 2018;12:301–5.
62. Shugar JK. Use of epinephrine for IFIS prophylaxis. J Cataract Refract Surg. 2006;32:1074–5.
63. Bucci FA, Michalek B, Fluet AT. Comparison of the frequency of use of a pupil expansion device with and without an intracameral phenylephrine and ketorolac injection 1%/0.3% at the time of routine cataract surgery. Clin Ophthalmol. 2017;11:1039–43.
64. Wilson C, Hock L, Oetting T, et al. Pupil expansion device use and operative outcomes with topical dilation vs intracameral epinephrine in resident-performed cataract surgery. J Cataract Refract Surg. 2020;4:562–6.
65. Christou C, Tsinopoulos I, Ziakas N, Tzamalis A. Intraoperative floppy iris syndrome: updated perspectives. Clin Ophthalmol. 2020;14:463–71.
66. Arshinoff SA. Modified SST-USST for tamsulosin-associated intraoperative [corrected] floppy-iris syndrome. J Cataract Refract Surg. 2006;32(4):559–61.
67. Arshinoff SA, Norman RJ. Tri-soft shell technique. J Cataract Refract Surg. 2013;39(8):1196–203.
68. Malyugin B. Small pupil phaco surgery: a new technique. Ann Ophthalmol (Skokie). 2007;39(3):185–93.
69. Malyugin B. Cataract surgery in small pupils. Indian J Ophthalmol. 2017;65(12):1323–8.
70. Oetting TA, Omphroy LC. Modified technique using flexible iris retractors in clear corneal cataract surgery. J Cataract Refract Surg. 2002;28:596–8.
71. Chang D, Osher R, Wang L, Koch D. Prospective muticenter evaluation of cataract surgery in patients taking tamsulosin. Ophthalmology. 2007;114(5):957–64.
72. Enright J, Karacal H, Tsai L. Floppy iris syndrome and cataract surgery. Curr Opin Ophthalmol. 2017;28(1):29–34.
73. Chang D. Use of Malyugin pupil expansion device for intraoperative floppy-iris syndrome: results in 30 consecutive cases. J Cataract Refract Surg. 2008;34(5):835–41.
74. Malyugin B. Ring used in a small pupil phacoemulsification procedure patent US 8,323,296 B2. Filed: March 5, 2008.
75. Lockington D, Wang Z, Qi N, et al. Modelling floppy iris syndrome and the impact of pupil size and ring devices on iris displacement. Eye. 2020;34:2227–34.
76. Nderitu P, Ursell P. Iris hooks versus a pupil expansion ring: operating times, complications, and visual acuity outcomes in small pupil cases. J Cataract Refract Surg. 2019;45(2):257.

Iris Repair

28

Peter Szurman

Bullet Points

- Cataract surgery and iris repair can be combined well, but consider the increased risk of complications due to accompanying ocular comorbidities related to aniridia.
- Iris coloboma (sector defect) can be closed with primary sutures, mainly slipknots.
- Iridodialysis can be treated with iris base refixation via transscleral mattress sutures (U-suture).
- Persistent mydriasis is addressed with an iris cerclage suture (annular "tobacco-pouch" suture).
- Subtotal or total aniridia benefits from novel flexible iris prostheses with a custom-made iris drawing matching the color of the patient's natural iris.

Supplementary Information The online version contains supplementary material available at [https://doi.org/10.1007/978-3-030-94530-5_28].

P. Szurman (✉)
Eye Clinic Sulzbach, Knappschaft Hospital Saar, Sulzbach, Germany
e-mail: Peter.Szurman@kksaar.de

Introduction

The causes of partial or complete aniridia are diverse, but most cases occur after severe ocular trauma. The resulting pupil or iris defects can lead to visual impairment, discomforting glare, reduced contrast sensitivity, loss of depth of focus, and photophobia [1]. The cosmetic aspect should not be underestimated, either, because the mostly young (trauma) patients suffer from a considerably reduced quality of life. Surgical iris reconstruction can alleviate these symptoms.

In the past decades, numerous microsurgical techniques and prosthetic devices for iris repair have been developed. The various iris suturing methods, as well as alternative techniques including iris prosthetics, each have unique benefits, providing surgeons with a wide array of tools for iris reconstruction. Today, almost any complex situation can be met with good anatomical and functional results. However, due to the heterogeneity of the underlying pathology, iris reconstruction is individual, as is the surgical strategy. Therefore, the multitude of possibilities seems confusing at first glance. However, there are general rules that can help in choosing the correct strategy. This article aims to structure these variable pathologies and assign appropriate surgical techniques to them.

J. L. Alió et al. (eds.), *Cataract Surgery*, Essentials in Ophthalmology,
https://doi.org/10.1007/978-3-030-94530-5_28

Non-surgical and Alternative Approaches

Not every iris defect needs to be repaired. Patients with small sector defects may have little or no visual impairment. Superior defects may be well covered by the upper lid (Fig. 28.1a), and congenital iris colobomas usually cause no or surprisingly little discomfort despite the typical inferonasal localization. On the other hand, the lacrimal meniscus contributes a prismatic effect, which can turn even small iridectomies symptomatic. A meticulous patient history detailing complaints and expectations is mandatory. Also,

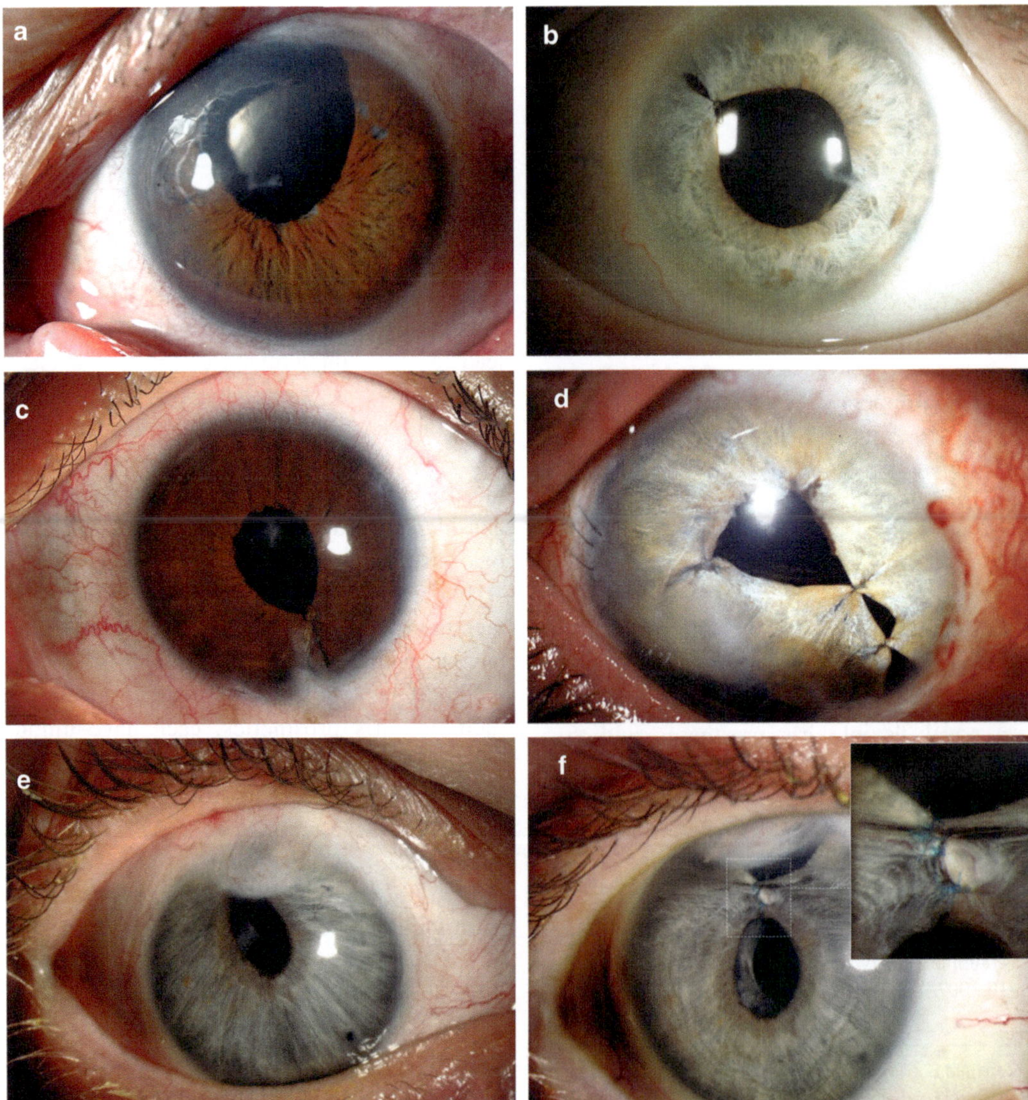

Fig. 28.1 Slit lamp photography of primary iris sutures: (**a**) superior coloboma covered by the upper eyelid; (**b**) McCannel suture for traumatic iris coloboma, together here with a scleral-fixated IOL; (**c**) pupilloplasty with light-tight sutures; (**d**) faulty pupilloplasty with a too-large seam distance, resulting in polycoria and disturbing double images; before (**e**) and after (**f**) primary iris sutures. Inlay: The sutures are under tension and have a tendency to pass through the atrophic iris stroma

tinted spectacles, iris-printed contact lenses, iris cauterization [2], and, with the utmost caution, corneal tattooing are part of the minimally invasive armamentarium.

Although corneal tattooing (keratopigmentation) has been around for many decades, it has only been sporadically used. Several techniques have been proposed, and, when performed correctly, good anatomical and cosmetic results have been reported [3, 4]. However, keratopigmentation may also increase rather than decrease photosensitivity, even when performed correctly [5]. Especially superficial manual micropunction with a non-confluent pattern can lead to a disastrous result with maximum glare (Fig. 28.2a, b). We recommend that unexperienced surgeons limit corneal tattooing solely to improve the cosmetic aspect of completely opaque eyes with corneal blindness (Fig. 28.2c).

Cataract Surgery Combined with Iris Repair: A One-Step or Two-Step Procedure?

When planning cataract surgery in an eye with additional iris pathology, the first question that arises is whether a combined or two-step procedure is appropriate. The answer is ambiguous.

On the one hand, if preexisting iris defects are not treated at the time of cataract surgery, an otherwise successful procedure will fail, and the patient will be dissatisfied. Remaining pupil or iris defects may impair visual quality by generating photic phenomena of the exposed IOL edge, double vision, polyopsia, and photophobia.

On the other hand, iris defects that occur during a complicated cataract surgery should instead be repaired later in an inflammation-free interval. Intraoperative iris damage such as phaco bites,

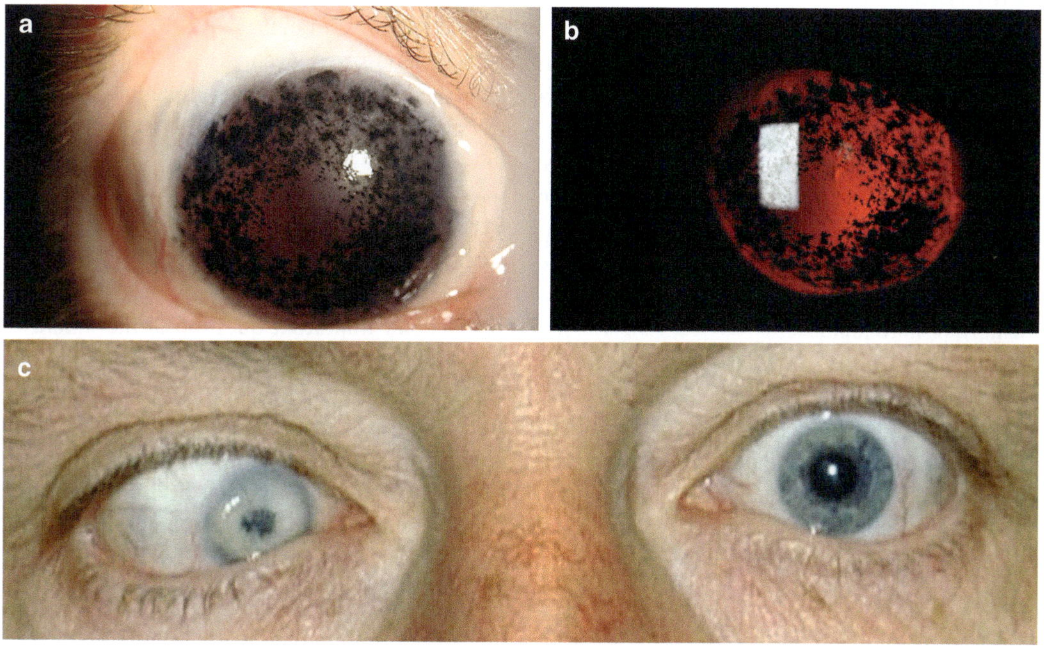

Fig. 28.2 (**a**) Faulty superficial manual micropunction with a non-confluent pattern. (**b**) Coaxial light discloses why the patient was highly disturbed by glare and double images and ended up in corneal transplantation. It is recommended to avoid turning one large pupil in a situation with a hundred small pupils! (**c**) Corneal tattooing for cosmetic purposes in corneal blindness

iris sphincter injuries, or iris prolapse typically occur in eyes where the iris is already the cause of the problem (e.g., narrow or atonic pupil, IFIS). Such complications are characterized by iris irritation, leaky tunnel incisions, hypotony, or a flat anterior chamber, resulting in significantly prolonged inflammation. In these cases, the most important measure is rapid completion of cataract surgery.

Even if there is a large iris defect or tissue loss, it is preferable to postpone the iris reconstructive procedure to a later date because iris injury and iris suturing act additively on inflammation. Furthermore, the exact extent of the damage as well as the resulting visual and cosmetic implications cannot be estimated at this time. Successful iris reconstruction always requires careful planning.

Comorbidities

The question of comorbidities is generally mandatory before every cataract surgery but is particularly important in combined iris pathology. Iris defects, depending on their cause, often have accompanying ocular comorbidities that can make cataract surgery considerably more difficult and increase the risk of complications. The causes can be traumatic, congenital (developmental), or iatrogenic:

1. Traumatic partial or complete aniridia usually has multiple pathologies such as zonular deficiency, primary capsule defects, vitreous prolapse, or compromised corneal endothelium. Postoperative complications such as retinal detachment, intraocular pressure increase, and corneal decompensation are common [6].
2. Congenital and developmental iris defects occur in a variety of conditions, including congenital aniridia, colobomas, iridocorneal endothelial (ICE) syndrome, Axenfeld–Rieger, and essential iris atrophy. Many of these patients have both zonular and capsular anomalies. Especially in congenital aniridia, the capsule may be thinned and rigid. Congenital iris colobomas may be associated with colobomas of the ciliary body and partial zonular deficiency (lens pseudo-coloboma), which may complicate cataract surgery.
3. Iatrogenic iris injuries in cataract surgery are often caused by complicative conditions, especially IFIS and vitreous pressure. In this case, iris reconstruction should only be performed in the inflammation-free interval under controlled conditions (e.g., under general anesthesia).

These comorbidities make the management of cataract patients with iris defects challenging, especially after trauma. Often, both anterior and posterior segments are likely to be damaged and need strategic planning. Retinal or vitreous pathology such as proliferative vitreoretinopathy (PVR) may require treatment with silicone oil tamponade. Therefore, whenever possible, iris reconstruction should be performed only after wound healing and management of other pathologies. This is also relevant in eyes with preexisting glaucoma because sulcus implantation might worsen this condition [7].

Strategic Considerations for Iris Reconstruction

The second important question is the nature of the iris defect. The highly variable iris pathology requires individualized surgical strategies. Accordingly, the multitude of iris reconstructive approaches and available techniques seem confusing at first glance. In real life, however, it is much simpler. It is extremely helpful to understand that all iris defects can be divided into four categories with defined strategic approaches:

1. Iris coloboma (sector defect)
2. Iridodialysis
3. Persistent mydriasis
4. Subtotal or total aniridia

The first three types of injuries can often be treated with special suturing techniques, which are described in detail below. However, one should be aware that only small-to-medium defects can be reconstructed with a primary suture.

As elastic as the iris tissue may appear during the process of pupil constriction/dilation, the iris stroma only allows a surprisingly limited gathering and stretching ability to bridge larger iris defects. In the long term, those sutures under tension often wander through the iris stroma with late reopening of the iris defect.

For larger defects, when the amount of iris remnants is insufficient to perform a suture pupilloplasty or the quality of the iris tissue is too poor to be repaired, prosthetic iris devices are preferred [7–9].

Defect Type 1: Traumatic Iris Coloboma (Sector Defect)

Traumatic colobomas are usually sector defects. Repair strategies depend largely on the extent of the lost or damaged iris and the health of the remaining tissue, but most cases can be easily treated with primary iris sutures. However, in iris surgery, it is important to proceed as minimally invasively as possible. Some basic considerations and rules must be followed:

- Sutured iris tissue never grows together. The closed defect must be held in place for life by the iris sutures.
- Only healthy iris stroma can be sutured; in atrophic stroma the suture thread passes through. Slit lamp examination in the coaxial position is helpful for evaluation.
- Iris tissue has limited elasticity. Therefore, only small-to-medium defects can be adapted up to a maximum of about 2 hours.
- Sutures must be sewn lightproof. If the seam distance is too far, the resulting polycoria will lead to very disturbing double or multiple images (Fig. 28.1d).

The following suturing techniques for iris reconstruction are suitable for repairing sector defects.

McCannel Suture

The McCannel suture is one of the earliest and simplest variants of the primary iris suture [10]. This technique allows direct suturing of the iris using three incisions and is suitable for small-to-medium sector defects (Fig. 28.1b).

The original McCannel technique involves passing a 10-0 polypropylene suture through two paracenteses created perpendicular to the iris defect (Fig. 28.3a). The suture needle will grab both iris edges. A third paracentesis is then created above the defect. A hook is used to externalize both ends of the suture through the paracentesis, where they are then tied externally, and the knot is allowed to slide back into the anterior chamber. Historically, this ab externo method has often been used as a pupil suture for closure of a preceding radial pupillotomy, performed to facilitate ICCE in small pupils.

Many modifications of the McCannel suture have been introduced [11, 12]. Nowadays, we mostly use a variation with only one paracentesis above the defect, where the needle is perpendicularly passed directly through the peripheral cornea without additional paracenteses. In peripheral defects, a complete ab externo suturing technique is also possible: the two iris edges are directly grasped with forceps via an enlarged paracentesis directly above the defect, externalized, sutured outside, and allowed to slide back into the anterior chamber.

In most cases, however, these techniques involve only one pupil suture and leave a triangular peripheral iridectomy. Therefore, this method is limited to superior defects.

Siepser Slipknot

In 1994, Siepser introduced a suturing strategy in which a surgeon can create a knot outside the eye and subsequently slide it into place atop the iris all while maintaining a closed chamber [13]. The sliding knot, an ab interno technique with even larger defects and multiple knots, can be adapted very accurately. The main advantage besides the closed chamber is that the edges of the iris are not moved during knotting, and thus an exact side-to-side connection is achieved (Video 28.1).

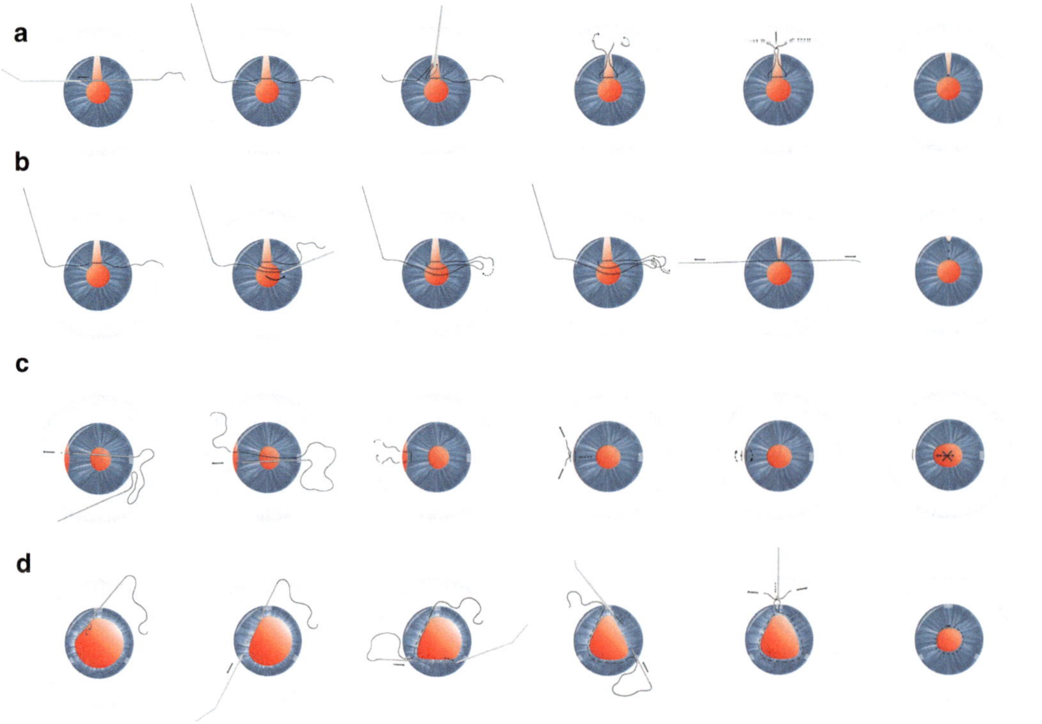

Fig. 28.3 Surgical steps for primary iris suturing: (**a**) McCannel suture, (**b**) Siepser knot, (**c**) iris base refixation in iridodialysis, (**d**) iris cerclage in chronic mydriasis

Numerous variations have been proposed [14] to facilitate locking the knot with [15, 16] or without [17] squaring, retrieval of the suture thread [18], or pushing the sliding knot into the anterior chamber [19].

The sliding knot, along with its variations, has become a basic technique for addressing a large number of iris pathologies. It is suitable for closing larger traumatic colobomas (Fig. 28.1c–f), sector iridectomies, iatrogenic iris defects (e.g., after the removal of iris tumors), or transillumination defects [20]. Variants are also used in complex maneuvers like pupilloplasty in corectopia, iridodialysis, and traumatic mydriasis.

Our current technique includes two paracenteses, a pressurized anterior chamber, a three-pass square knot, and an irrigation handpiece to retrieve and guide the needle (Fig. 28.3b). In brief, two paracenteses are created perpendicular to the iris defect. On the distal side, an irrigation handpiece is inserted to pressurize the anterior chamber; on the proximal side, a 10-0 polypropylene thread with a straight, 13 mm needle is inserted. Both iris edges are pierced, and the needle is inserted into the irrigation tip and guided outward. Next, a push–pull hook is used to guide a loop of suture from the opposite side of the anterior chamber out through the paracentesis. Then, a double-throw slipknot is tied, which is internalized by pulling both ends of the suture. The sutures are cut using a 23 g, curved vitreoretinal microscissor. The maneuver is repeated twice with single-throw slipknots to lock the knots.

An average of three sutures is required for a meticulous side-to-side closure of sector colobomas. It is important to strive for a complete, light-tight adaptation of the wound edges to avoid polycoria.

Bimanual Intraocular Microsuturing

An elegant alternative is the bimanual intraocular microsuturing (BIM) technique introduced by Hattenbach in 2016 [21]. Using a 25 gauge hybrid instrument set (Geuder, Heidelberg, Germany) consisting of a microneedle holder, thread forceps, and scissors, direct suturing within the anterior chamber is possible for the first time without the use of long needles, which had to be inserted and removed in the anterior chamber as part of conventional suturing techniques.

In combination with a microneedle (ONATEC, Neustadt, Germany), which is adapted to the instrument set, a completely new suture technique can be applied, with which almost any suture placement in the area of the anterior chamber or the anterior vitreous cavity is feasible. This allows intracameral sutures to be implemented in the smallest possible space. The 25 gauge format allows for a minimally invasive approach using small paracenteses while maintaining high anterior chamber stability.

Bimanual maneuvering of needle and suture is performed by a back and forth ("handshake") technique between two instruments. The suture material is guided inside and outside the anterior chamber ("in-out-in" technique) during knot tying. These microinstruments can be used not only for iris sutures at any point in the anterior chamber but also for suture fixation of dislocated intraocular lenses.

Pupilloplasty for Corectopia

Congenital, traumatic, or iatrogenic corectopia can also be treated with a newly formed, centered pupilloplasty by slipknots. In principle, surgical centering of the existing pupil is always preferable because even severely traumatized pupils often still show some sphincter activity, which is advantageous for the light-adapted visual quality. However, in the case of long-standing corectopia, shortened or scarred iris tissue often cannot be sufficiently mobilized from the periphery to achieve good centering of the existing pupil.

In these cases, a pupilloplasty can be performed by closing the decentered pupil with the slipknots described above and creating a new, centered artificial pupil with the vitrectomy cutter (Fig. 28.4). These results are cosmetically and optically excellent. However, this artificial pupil is not light reactive. Therefore, the decision should always be based on whether sufficient

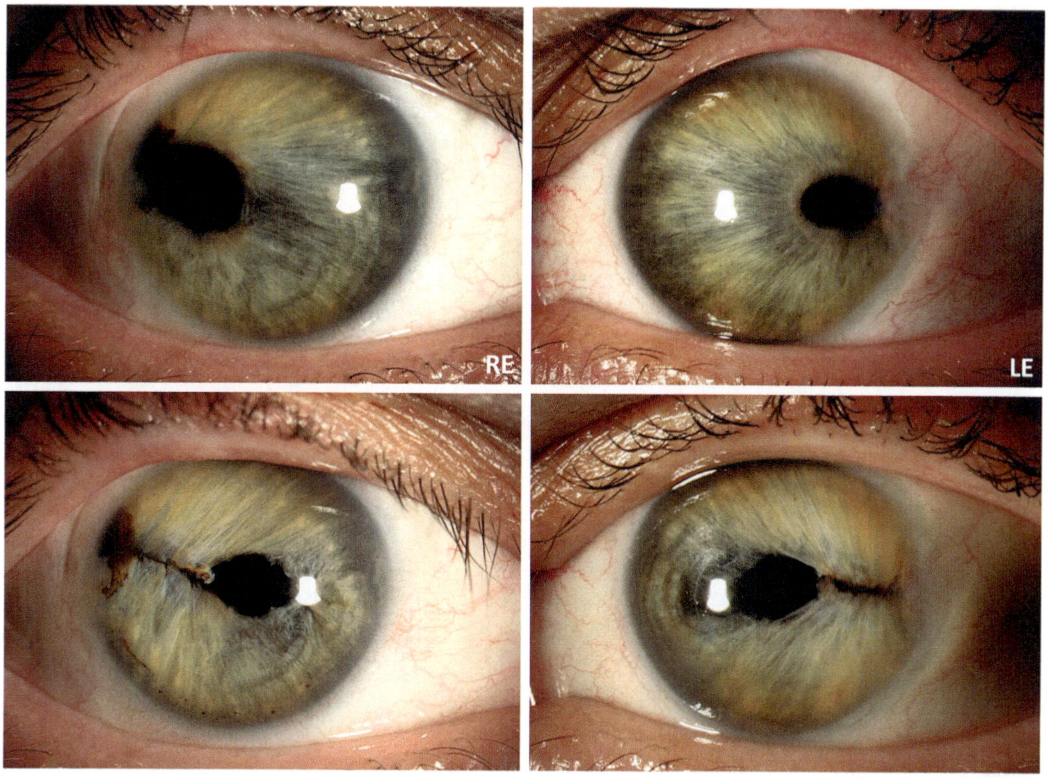

Fig. 28.4 Slit lamp photography of a corectopia due to an old iris prolapse into a temporal tunnel incision in a patient who underwent cataract surgery in childhood. Before (top) and after (bottom) pupilloplasty with newly formed pupil. After 30 years visual acuity increased from 0.2 to 0.5 (RE right eye, LE left eye)

pupil reactivity is still present or whether it seems worth preserving (Video 28.2).

Sector Iris Implants for Larger Iris Colobomas

For larger sector defects or transillumination areas that cannot be closed with primary iris sutures (>2 clock hours), sector implants may be an alternative. Whereas rigid poly(methyl methacrylate) (PMMA) segment rings were used in the past, flexible iris prostheses tailored to the appropriate size and shape are preferred now. Good cosmetic results can be achieved with individual choice of color. Detailed instructions are provided below.

Defect Type 2: Traumatic Iridodialysis

Iridodialysis, in which the iris root is torn off by the scleral spur (not to be confused with cyclodialysis), occurs most often due to trauma (Fig. 28.5a, b). Surgically induced iris base avulsion is also common, either as a result of a pro-

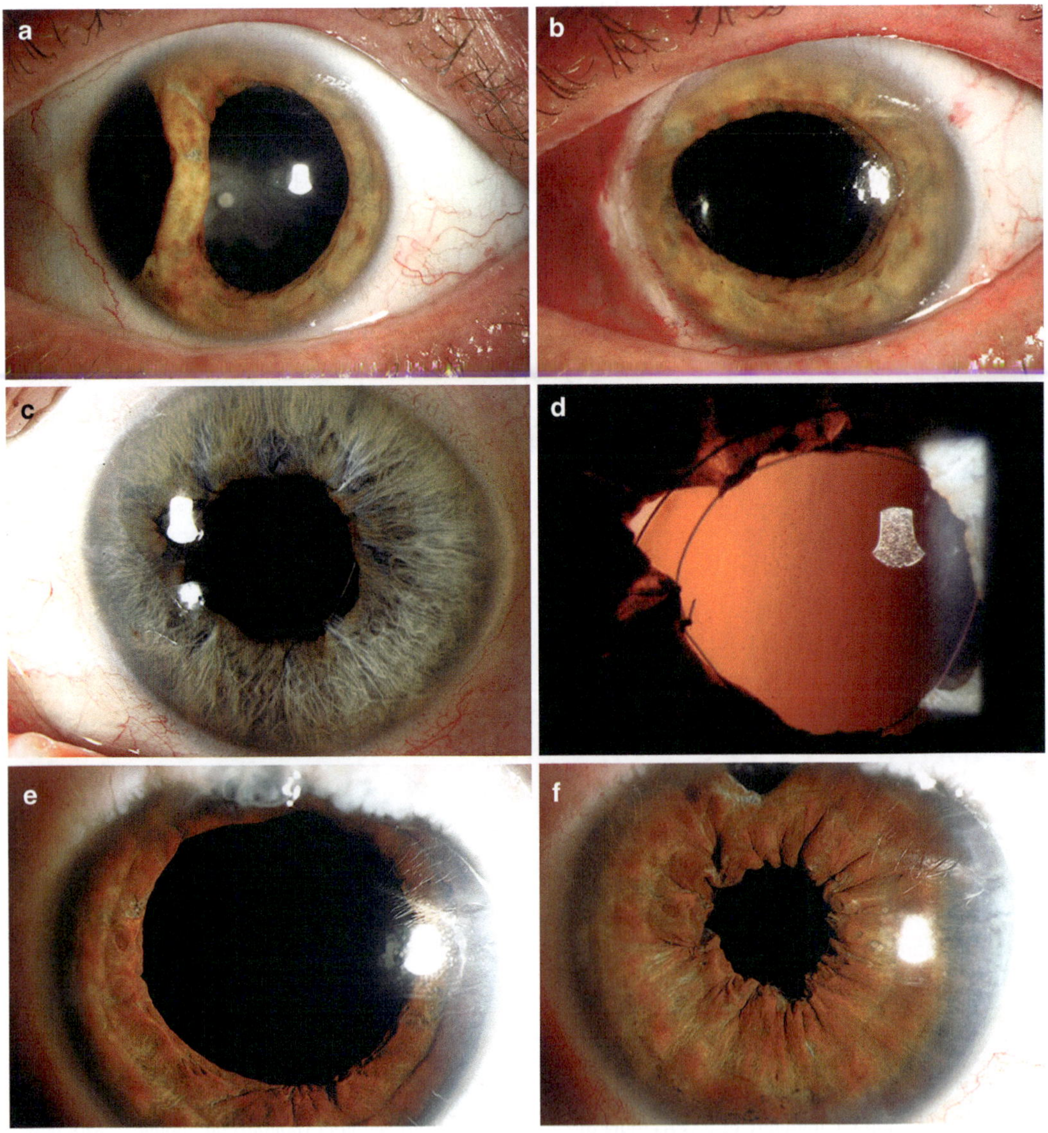

Fig. 28.5 Before (**a**) and after (**b**) iris base refixation (note the oval pupil). (**c**) Insufficient iris cerclage with too-few bites. (**d**) Same eye: the unsatisfactory result becomes particularly clear during coaxial light examination. Before (**e**) and after (**f**) regular iris cerclage. Note the jagged aspect of the pupil

nounced iris prolapse or inadvertent entanglement with a surgical instrument. Typically, this occurs when the phaco tip is inserted through a tunnel incision that is too narrow. Once the resistance is overcome, the phaco tip suddenly and uncontrollably penetrates the iris and tears off the iris base.

Iris base refixation can easily be achieved with transscleral mattress sutures (U-suture) [22, 23]. Alternatively, the iris base can be fixed with ab externo scleral sutures similar to ciliary body refixation, but this procedure is more complex and time-consuming.

In most cases, we use an ab interno transscleral mattress suture. In brief, the two straight 13 mm needles of a double-armed 10-0 polypropylene thread are inserted one after the other via an opposite paracentesis, pierced through the iris base at a distance of approximately one clock hour and then externalized through the sclera (transscleral ab interno technique). The needles are cut off, the two ends of the thread are knotted outside, and the knot is buried in the sclera by rotating the U-suture (Fig. 28.3c).

Caution is required during the technical maneuver: the surgeon must be aware that the iris base will be shortened by the sutures, causing the pupil to become decentered in the direction of the iridodialysis. To avoid an oval-shaped pupil, the sutures should only be loosely tightened. One has to keep in mind that the iris base does not grow together with the sclera and is held for life only by the mattress suture. Even when this rule is observed, these eyes often show oval mydriatic pupils postoperatively because tearing of the iris base leads to permanent denervation in this sector (Fig. 28.5b; Video 28.3).

Defect Type 3: Traumatic Mydriasis

Chronic mydriasis is the result of an atonic pupil (i.e., a permanent failure of the iris sphincter). The causes are manifold and most often caused by blunt trauma (traumatic mydriasis), acute glaucoma, or uveitis, but also after surgical dilation of narrow pupils (iris stretching, iris retractors, pupil expanders) (Fig. 28.5e).

Iris cerclage suture is the treatment of choice. This is a tobacco-pouch suture, in which small bites are taken around the pupillary circumference, and the annular suture is then knotted [24, 25] (Video 28.4). The iris cerclage technique has been particularly successful in treating traumatic mydriasis with good functional and cosmetic results [26]. Unlike any of the methods described above, this suture technique allows the surgeon to create a round pupillary aperture.

Because iris tissue is of limited elasticity, some rules must be observed when performing the iris cerclage (Fig. 28.3d). First, three paracenteses are applied at 120° intervals. A single-armed 10-0 polypropylene thread with a straight, 13 mm needle is inserted via the superior paracentesis and repetitively pierced through the pupillary margin at short intervals. The pupil should be threaded with approx. 5–6 bites per 120°. The bites can be supported with a manipulation instrument as an abutment. A blunt irrigation cannula is inserted via the next paracentesis to incorporate the needle and guide it outward. The needle is reinserted and threaded through the next 120°. After threading the entire circumference, the needle is externalized and cut off. The result is continuous bites encircling the pupillary margin with both suture ends exiting the 12 o'clock paracentesis. The suture can be tied externally, and the knot is slid back into the eye with a push–pull hook. The pupil size can be well dosed by the thread tension.

Note that the pupillary margin must be pierced sufficiently often (approx. 15–18 stitches) to avoid a jagged or squared pupil configuration (Fig. 28.5c). Also, sufficient iris tissue must be grasped with each bite to avoid cheese wiring. This is particularly important in view of the frequent posttraumatic iris stroma atrophy (Fig. 28.5d).

If the mydriasis is too pronounced or the iris stroma is very atrophic, iris cerclage is no longer feasible. Alternatively, a flexible iris prosthesis (fiber-free) can be implanted behind the iris remnants. Often the iris prosthesis does not require transscleral suture fixation because it is held in the sulcus by the iris remnants. For the implantation technique, see below.

There is one exception where iris cerclage is not the first choice of treatment: anterior PVR can also retract the iris into the chamber angle due to contractile myofibroblasts (up to pseudo aniridia). Similar to retinal surgery, these PVR membranes can be peeled off, allowing the iris to be mobilized again. For this purpose, an end-gripping or crocodile forceps is inserted into the pressurized anterior chamber. In many cases, the PVR membranes can be easily removed in large pieces. Bleeding usually does not occur because these membranes are only superficial. In contrast, mydriatic eyes in rubeosis iridis (e.g., in proliferative diabetic retinopathy) or after multiple silicone oil surgery are not suitable for iris peeling. These eyes show more adherent membranes and are prone to considerable bleeding, which can even worsen the condition.

Defect Type 4: Subtotal or Total Aniridia

All suturing techniques are limited to situations where sufficient vital iris tissue is available. In more complex cases, when the amount of iris remnants is insufficient to perform pupilloplasty or the quality of the iris tissue is too poor to be repaired, prosthetic iris devices are required [7, 8]. These prostheses play an important role in complex iris reconstruction, including partial aniridia (larger pupil defects that cannot be closed with sutures) as well as traumatic and congenital aniridia, especially albinism.

In the past, a number of technical options for iris replica have been developed, each with specific advantages and disadvantages [1]. Until the last decade, only iris implants made of rigid plastic were available because the material could be easily colored. These include iris diaphragm intraocular lenses and various segmental prosthetic iris systems. However, the major drawback of these early models was the need for large incisions of 10–13 mm [27]. In addition, the colors available for most of these prosthetic iris systems are not customized.

Today, a flexible artificial iris prosthesis that can be individually fabricated from photographs of the fellow iris and cut into the required shape is available, thus achieving excellent cosmetic and functional results [7].

Aniridia Iris Diaphragm Intraocular Lens

Black iris diaphragm intraocular lenses (Morcher; Stuttgart, Germany) have been available since 1991 [27]. These aniridia intraocular lenses are unique in that they contain a black iris diaphragm, thus combining the ability to correct both aniridia and aphakia (Fig 28.6a).

Essentially, the aniridia lens consists of a black, 10-mm-diameter PMMA plate that provides a central opening of variable diameter with or without the inclusion of an optically functional center. Since its first description, different models have been developed for different situations and needs. The aniridia lens is available for intracapsular and extracapsular implantation, with and without fixation loops on the haptics, and with different diameters of optic and pupil size to cope with partial and complete aniridia.

However, these PMMA implants are rigid and require a sclerocorneal incision of up to 14 mm in length, especially when transscleral fixation in the ciliary sulcus is required [28]. It should be noted that most eyes with complete aniridia are severely compromised due to either trauma or limbal stem cell deficiency associated with congenital aniridia. In these eyes, a very large corneoscleral incision can be detrimental. Although recent case studies show that glaucoma is common, serious complications attributable to the implant have not been reported [29, 30].

For several years these aniridia lenses have also been available with a color-printed aperture (type 308) instead of the black version, which improves the cosmetic aspect. However, they still appear unnatural because the color pigments are only printed on the lens. The missing 3D texture is especially noticeable in the side view, as we are accustomed to by natural iris crypts. A similar model is offered by Ophtec with various configurations and colors (Ophtec, Groningen, Netherlands).

Although new, flexible, and custom-made iris prostheses are gaining ground, iris diaphragm lenses still have application in total aniridia in combination with aphakia without capsule support. Here, the combined correction of aniridia and aphakia is still unique.

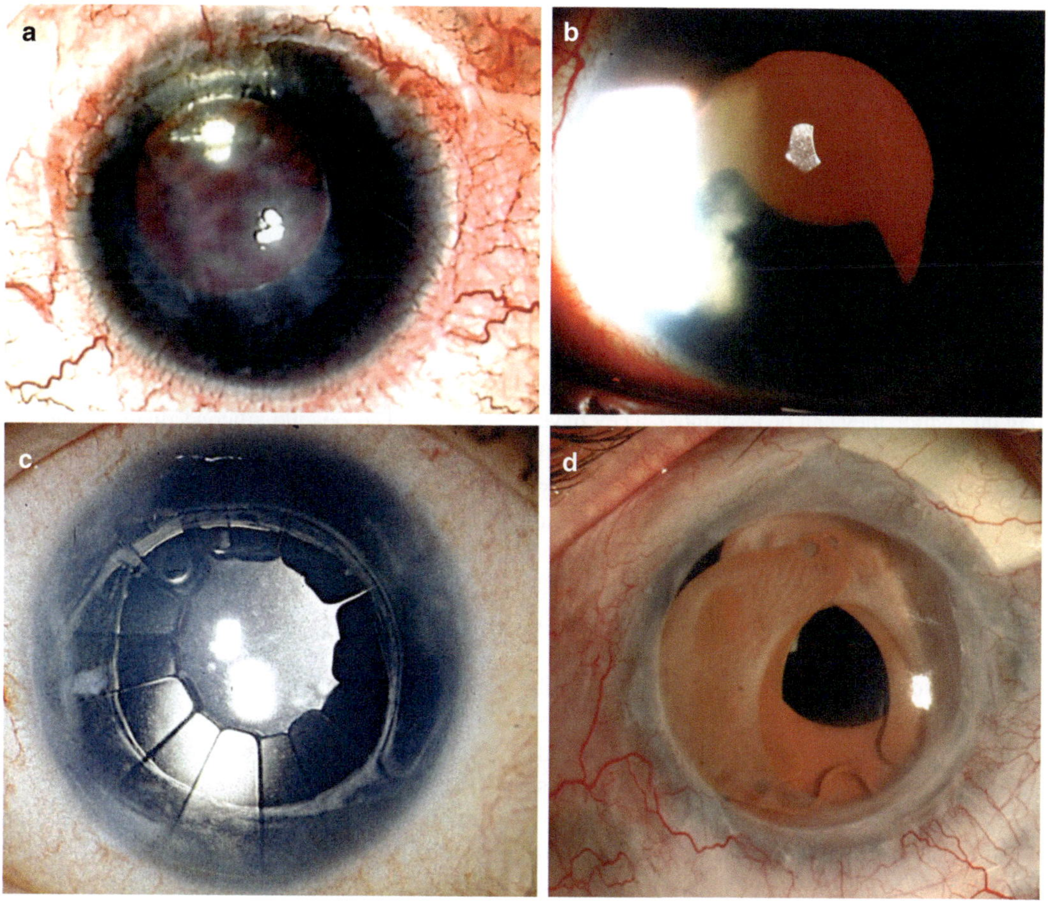

Fig. 28.6 Slit lamp photography of various rigid prosthetic iris systems: (**a**) Morcher Aniridia IOL, (**b**) Morcher segment rings leading to corneal decompensation, (**c**) Rosenthal–Rasch segment rings, and (**d**) assembled IPS® implants

Segmental Prosthetic Iris Devices

Another option for prosthetic restoration is the use of segmental prosthetic iris devices, which allow implantation through smaller incision sizes of around 3–4 mm. Segmental devices are based on two rationales: first, many cases disclose only partial aniridia or large sector defects that can be sufficiently covered with small-incision segmental devices, and second, they can be combined intraocularly to form a full diaphragm by implanting two or more small implants to cover complete aniridia without the need for a large incision. Three different systems are currently available:

1. Morcher Partial Aniridia Rings (types 94–96) are segmental prosthetic iris devices made of rigid black PMMA for sulcus or capsular bag implantation (Fig. 28.6b). They are designed to cover sector defects and large colobomas. Most models are brittle and prone to fracture. Similar models are available from Ophtec.
2. Morcher Aniridia Rings (type 50) consist of two overlapping, implanted aperture rings and are available in three pupil sizes (3.5, 4, and 6 mm). It is recommended to use the smallest pupil size (3.5 mm) to achieve a cosmetically acceptable result. Funduscopy and retina surgery are still possible. It should also be noted that the black PMMA material breaks very easily (Fig. 28.5c).
3. The Hermeking Iris Prosthetic System (IPS®) is a modular system from Ophtec with various elements, which are individually inserted into the anterior chamber and "plugged together"

intraocularly. The segments are intended for either intracapsular or sulcus implantation. Some "double" elements can be connected with a spring-action, flexible PMMA rod. Two double elements are needed for a full iris prosthesis. Additionally, a ring-clip element can be used to stabilize the modules. Suitable combinations of elements are used for partial prosthetic replacement (Fig. 28.6d).

In general, segmental prosthetic iris devices are best applied when there is an intact capsular bag into which they can be implanted. They have the advantage of being implantable through small incisions of 3–4 mm and can be individually selected according to the partial aniridia. Their possible disadvantage is dislocation, which leads to either insufficient overlapping of the elements or to ocular complications—mostly glaucoma and corneal problems [31, 32].

Our personal experience is that the majority of eyes with segmental iris prostheses develop corneal decompensation over time and are explanted on a long-term basis (Fig. 28.6b). Of course, it is not always possible to distinguish with certainty whether the underlying disease or the dislocated implant itself is the cause of the complications. Nevertheless, it is recommended to limit the implantation of segment prostheses to rather healthy eyes with localized segment defects and to suture them safely into the sulcus.

Artificial Iris Prosthesis

In 2008, the Customflex Artificial Iris® (HumanOptics; Erlangen, Germany) became the first foldable iris implant with a custom-made iris drawing matching the color of the patient's natural iris [33]. The multilayer implant consists of a silicone core matrix with integrated color pigment, coated with another layer of biocompatible medical-grade silicone. FDA approval has been granted in the meantime.

The color pigments are not printed on but applied three-dimensionally in depth, resulting in a three-dimensional effect of the iris crypts, similar to the natural iris. For this purpose, the iris prosthesis is individually fabricated for each patient according to a standardized photograph of the fellow eye and provides excellent cosmetic results. The latter point is important and legitimate considering that trauma patients are usually young and long for an acceptable aesthetic appearance.

The iris prosthesis is intended for implantation in the sulcus and is recommended only for pseudophakic or aphakic eyes. It has a diameter of 12.8 mm and an outwardly decreasing thickness of 0.4 mm at the pupillary ring and 0.25 mm in the periphery. The pupil diameter is fixed at 3.35 mm. The opaque silicone material and the selected pupil diameter create the best possible optical conditions for different light conditions. Funduscopic control of the retinal periphery is also possible without problems.

The implant is available with or without an embedded fiber mesh as a design variant.

1. Fiber-free implants are more flexible and thinner, can be easily folded and cut to size, and adapt well to the anatomical shape of the sulcus. They are preferred for full prostheses where transscleral suture fixation requires only a low holding function (Fig. 28.7b). Full prostheses can be easily combined with cataract surgery or scleral-fixed intraocular lenses.
2. Implants containing fiber have higher stiffness and offer more efficient suture holdability. This is particularly important for partial prostheses because additional, stable side-to-side connections are required (Fig. 28.7a). However, the primarily cast-in fibers are exposed during punching and cutting and have been shown to provoke a high rate of glaucoma and chronic anterior chamber irritation (Fig. 28.8d) [34].

Whenever possible, full prostheses (fiber-free) should be preferred over partial prostheses (containing fiber), even if there are still large iris remnants. Full prostheses are much more tissue-friendly and shorten the operation time, which is especially important for these severely traumatized eyes.

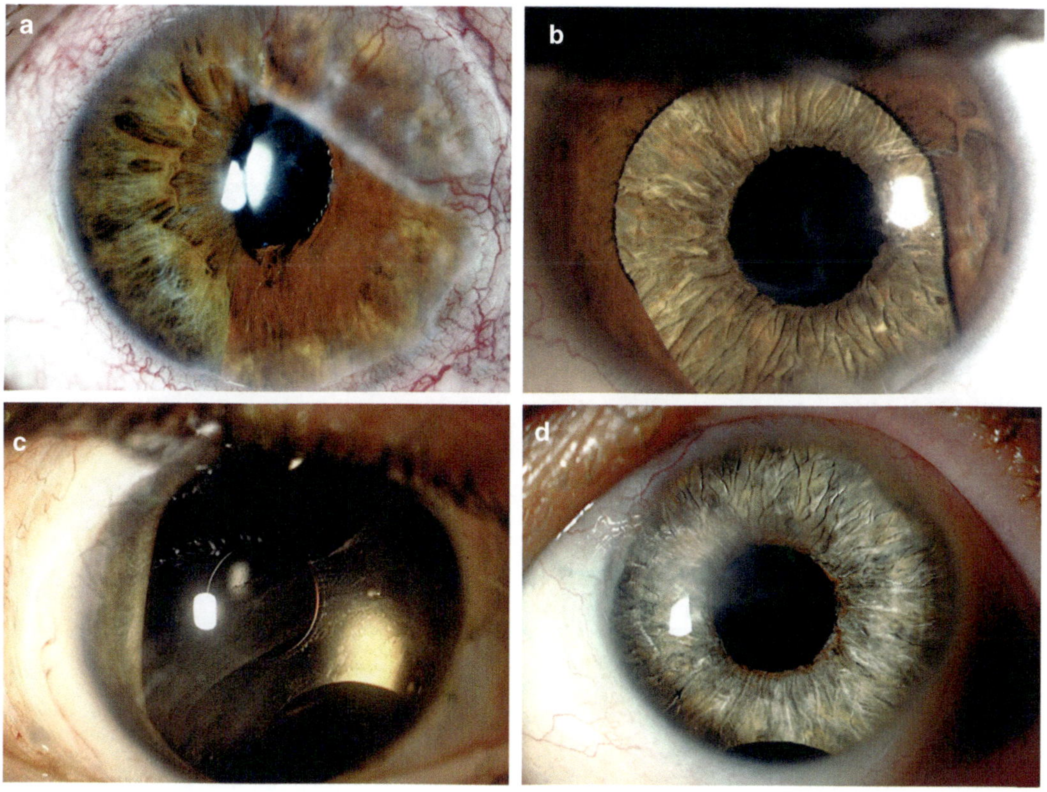

Fig. 28.7 (**a**) Flexible, partial iris prosthesis with side-to-side anastomoses. (**b**) Flexible, full iris prosthesis implanted behind iris remnants without transscleral suture fixation. (**c**) Open iris diaphragm with silicone oil in the pupillary plane. (**d**) Flexible iris prosthesis with additional inferior (Ando-) iridectomy in silicone oil surgery

Surgical Technique

All implants can be punched with a trephine and cut to size with scissors if only a segment is needed to close sector defects (Fig. 28.7a). Implants that are too large must be avoided, as they bulge in the eye and irritate the adjacent uveal tissue. The manufacturer's recommendation for optimal diameter size (using the vertical white-to-white distance) is not useful in practice because reliable limbal detection in these eyes is difficult. We instead recommend a simple rule that has been proven in a large series of case studies [34]. For all normally sized eyes (90% of cases), a full prosthesis with a diameter of 11 mm is perfect. A 12 mm and 10 mm iris should only be chosen for very large and very small eyes, respectively.

Partial prostheses have different advantages and disadvantages. On the one hand, they can be larger depending on their shape and; on the other hand, those containing fiber are stiffer and disclose sharp-edged polymer fibers, which, if the diameter is too large, leads to chronic irritation of the adjacent uveal tissue.

The prosthesis is foldable and can be implanted through a 3.5 mm incision either with forceps or with an IOL injector [35]. Detailed step-by-step instructions are available in previous literature [7, 34].

1. Full prostheses (fiber-free) can be implanted directly behind the residual iris tissue without suture fixation if sufficient supporting iris tissue is available (Fig. 28.7b). The implant can be placed in an IOL injector and implanted into the sulcus through a 3.2 mm, clear corneal incision. In most complex cases, however, transscleral fixation in up to three sites at 4, 8,

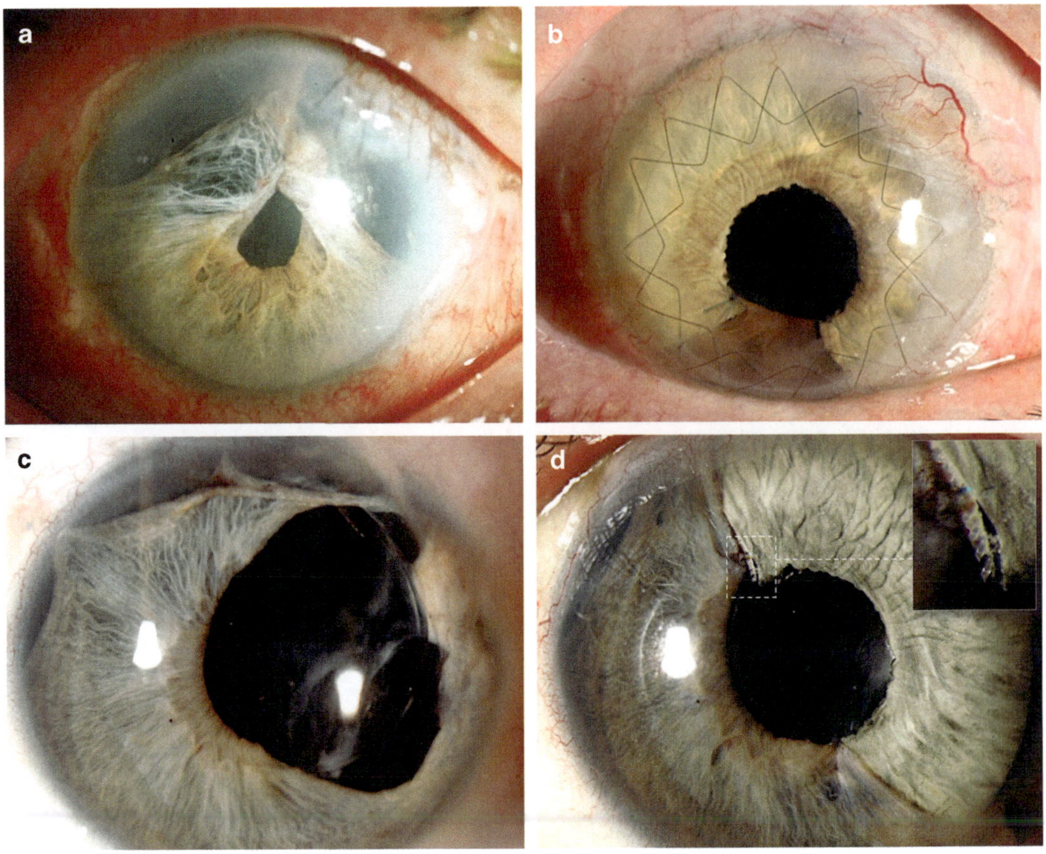

Fig. 28.8 Darkening of iris remnants in two patients after 17 and 12 months, respectively: Before (**a**, **c**) and after (**b**, **d**) implantation of punched and cut-to-size iris prostheses with exposed fibers due to chronic subclinical irritation caused by exposed tissue bases on uveal tissue. (**d**) Inlay showing the exposed fibers

and 12 o'clock is necessary [7]. After knot-free fixation of three single-armed 10-0 polypropylene loop threads with anchor stitches at the prosthesis edge, the needles are passed ab interno through the sulcus. The prosthesis is then double-folded and implanted with forceps. A controlled unfolding without endothelial contact is crucial. With fiber-free prostheses, the transscleral threads must be carefully tightened to prevent tearing. The sutures are fixed on the outside of the sclera with a Z-suture [36] (Video 28.5).

2. Partial prosthesis implantation is more complex because stable side-to-side connections are required (Fig. 28.7a). Therefore, implants with fibers are preferred because they ensure greater stiffness and suture holdability. First, the iris remnants are mobilized, and atrophic parts are excised. The transscleral fixation is performed analogously to full prostheses. Implantation is performed by rotating the implant lengthwise through the 3.5 mm tunnel and placing it securely in the sulcus under constant tension on the transscleral threads. The side-to-side connection is made with two sliding knots, as described above (Video 28.6).

The Customflex Artificial Iris® has no central optic, thus requiring an additional IOL implant if indicated. Full prostheses can be combined well with cataract surgery or more often with scleral-fixated intraocular lenses, since most eyes are aphakic. Two different techniques are possible.

Either the implantation is performed one after the other—first the scleral-fixated lens, then the iris prosthesis. In this case, the fiber-free version is preferable. The advantage is the small incision, and the disadvantage is the high number (up to 5) of transscleral sutures. Alternatively, the IOL can be fixed to the back of the prosthesis prior to implantation [37, 38]. Prostheses containing fiber are used for this purpose. The advantage is a shorter surgery time, and the disadvantage is the significantly larger incision of 7–8 mm [39].

Iris prostheses can also be combined with silicone oil surgery. For decades, an open iris diaphragm (PMMA) has been successfully used for keeping the oil behind the iris diaphragm (Fig. 28.7c) [40]. A flexible, full iris prosthesis with additionally punched inferior (Ando-) iridectomy (6 mm) is cosmetically much more appreciated (Fig. 28.7d). However, it is still under debate if the Customflex Artificial Iris® is suitable for this purpose because silicone oil sticks to the hydrophilic material and is more prone to enter the anterior chamber.

The complications are manifold, but it often remains unclear whether they are attributable to the underlying disease or the implant itself. Long-term studies have shown a complication rate of 25% [37], with the increase of intraocular pressure [41], corneal endothelial decompensation, and persisting inflammation being the most conspicuous [42]. A long-term study over 7 years [34] highlighted two important aspects in particular: first, the increased glaucoma rate and chronic anterior chamber irritation can be significantly reduced by the use of fiber-free prostheses, and second, a darkening of the iris remnants is observed in the long term, which leads to cosmetically relevant limitations (Fig. 28.8).

Conclusion

Cataract surgery can be combined well with iris repair. However, one should be aware of the increased risk of complications due to accompanying ocular comorbidities related to the underlying cause of the aniridia. With the iris reconstructive techniques presented here, most complex situations can be solved functionally and in a cosmetically satisfactory way. New iris prosthetic systems also allow the treatment of very large defects up to complete aniridia. In particular, the flexible Customflex Artificial Iris® is a valuable addition to the arsenal of available options for anterior segment reconstruction, when indicated. However, one should be aware of the risk of worsening preexisting pathologies that are common in these traumatized eyes, particularly glaucoma and endothelial problems. The goal is to proceed as minimally invasively and simply as possible. The combined treatment not only improves the quality of vision but also has a high cosmetic effect. Both improve the quality of life of these mostly young patients. The challenges of iris reconstruction may be great, but so is the resulting satisfaction of the surgeon and patient.

Take-Home Notes

- Only healthy iris stroma can be sutured; in atrophic stroma the suture thread passes through. Slit lamp examination in the coaxial position is helpful for evaluation.
- Sutured iris tissue never grows together. The closed defect must be held in place for life by the iris sutures.
- Iris tissue has limited elasticity. Therefore, only small-to-medium defects can be adapted up to a maximum of about 2 hours.
- Sutures must be sewn lightproof. If the seam distance is too far, the resulting polycoria will lead to very disturbing double or multiple images.
- Whenever possible, full prostheses (fiber-free) should be preferred over partial prostheses (containing fiber) to reduce the risk of glaucoma and inflammation.

References

1. Neuhann IM, Neuhann TF. Cataract surgery and aniridia. Curr Opin Ophthalmol. 2010;21:60–4.
2. Stopa M, Rakowicz P. Sutureless iris repair: cauterization technique. Retina. 2015;35:2647–9.
3. Rocher N, Hirst L, Renard G, et al. Corneal tattooing. A series of 14 case studies. J Fr Ophtalmol. 2008;31:968–74.
4. Hirsbein D, Gardea E, Brasseur G, Muraine M. Corneal tattooing for iris defects. J Fr Ophtalmol. 2008;31:155–64.
5. Alio JL, Al-Shymali O, Amesty MA, Rodriguez AE. Keratopigmentation with micronised mineral pigments: complications and outcomes in a series of 234 eyes. Br J Ophthalmol. 2018;102:742–7.
6. Burk SE, Da Mata AP, Snyder ME, et al. Prosthetic iris implantation for congenital, traumatic, or functional iris deficiencies. J Cataract Refract Surg. 2001;27:1732–40.
7. Szurman P, Jaissle G. Artificial iris. Ophthalmologe. 2011;108:720–7.
8. Mavrikakis I, Mavrikakis E, Syam PP, Bell J, Casey JH, Casswell AG, Brittain GP, Liu C. Surgical management of iris defects with prosthetic iris devices. Eye (Lond). 2005;19:205–9.
9. Srinivasan S, Ting DS, Snyder ME, Prasad S, Koch HR. Prosthetic iris devises. Can J Ophthalmol. 2014;49:6–17.
10. McCannel MA. A retrievable suture idea for anterior uveal problems. Ophthalmic Surg. 1976;7:98–103.
11. Pallin SL. Closed chamber iridoplasty. Ophthalmic Surg. 1981;12:213–4.
12. Shin DH. Repair of sector iris coloboma: closed-chamber technique. Arch Ophthalmol. 1982;100:460–1.
13. Siepser SB. The closed chamber slipping suture technique for iris repair. Ann Ophthalmol. 1994;26:71–2.
14. Lian RR, Siepser SB, Afshari NA. Iris reconstruction suturing techniques. Curr Opin Ophthalmol. 2020;31:43–9.
15. Engels T. Irisnähte in der geschlossenen Vorderkammer. Ophthalmo-Chirurgie. 1998;10:21–8.
16. Osher RH, Snyder ME, Cionni RJ. Modification of the Siepser slip-knot technique. J Cataract Refract Surg. 2005;31:1098–100.
17. Narang P, Agarwal A. Single-pass four-throw pupilloplasty knot mechanics. J Refract Surg. 2019;35:207–8.
18. Kim JH, Kang MH, Kang SM, Song BJ. A modified iris repair technique and capsular tension ring insertion in a patient with coloboma with cataracts. Korean J Ophthalmol. 2006;20:246–9.
19. Liu F, Zhou Q, Yu CQ, Guaiquil V, Geng Y, Chen X, Rosenblatt MI. Iris suture fixation: push-knot needle. J Cataract Refract Surg. 2017;43:456–8.
20. Snyder ME, Perez MA. Iris stromal imbrication oversewing for pigment epithelial defects. Br J Ophthalmol. 2015;99:5–6.
21. Hattenbach LO. May consultation #7. J Cataract Refract Surg. 2016;42:802–3.
22. Steinert RF. Minimally invasive iris surgery. In: Fine IH, Mojon DS, editors. Minimally invasive ophthalmic surgery. Berlin, Heidelberg: Springer; 2010. p. 153–9.
23. Tsao SW, Holz HA. Iris mattress suture: a technique for sectoral iris defect repair. Br J Ophthalmol. 2015;99:305–7.
24. Behndig A. Small incision single-suture-loop pupilloplasty for postoperative atonic pupil. J Cataract Refract Surg. 1998;24:1429–31.
25. Ogawa GS. The iris cerclage suture for permanent mydriasis: a running suture technique. Ophthalmic Surg. 1998;29:1001–9.
26. Frisina R, Parrozzani R, Tozzi L, et al. Pupil cerclage technique for treatment of traumatic mydriasis. Eur J Ophthalmol. 2020;30(3):480–6.
27. Sundmacher R, Reinhard T, Althaus C. Black-diaphragm intraocular lens for correction of aniridia. Ophthalmic Surg. 1994;25:180–5.
28. Thompson CG, Fawzy K, Bryce IG, Noble BA. Implantation of a black diaphragm intraocular lens for traumatic aniridia. J Cataract Refract Surg. 1999;25:808–13.
29. Aslam SA, Wong SC, Ficker LA, MacLaren RE. Implantation of the black diaphragm intraocular lens in congenital and traumatic aniridia. Ophthalmology. 2008;115:1705–12.
30. Roman S, Cherrate H, Trouvet JP, et al. Artificial iris intraocular lenses in aniridia or iris deficiencies. J Fr Ophtalmol. 2009;32:320–5.
31. Khng C, Snyder ME. Iris reconstruction with a multipiece endocapsular prosthesis in iridocorneal endothelial syndrome. J Cataract Refract Surg. 2005;31:2051–4.
32. Ozturk F, Osher RH, Osher JM. Secondary prosthetic iris implantation following traumatic total aniridia and pseudophakia. J Cataract Refract Surg. 2006;32:1968–70.
33. Koch HR. A new foldable artificial iris. Indications, surgical techniques and first results. Clin Exp Ophthalmol. 2008;36:A59.
34. Rickmann A, Szurman P, Januschowski K, Waizel M, Spitzer MS, Boden KT, Szurman GB. Long-term results after artificial iris implantation in patients with aniridia. Graefes Arch Clin Exp Ophthalmol. 2016;254:1419–24.
35. Ayliffe W, Groth SL, Sponsel WE. Small-incision insertion of artificial iris prostheses. J Cataract Refract Surg. 2012;38:362–7.
36. Szurman P, Petermeier K, Aisenbrey S, Spitzer MS, Jaissle GB. Z-suture: a new knotless technique for transscleral suture fixation of intraocular implants. Br J Ophthalmol. 2010;94:167–9.
37. Spitzer MS, Yoeruek E, Leitritz MA, et al. A new technique for treating posttraumatic aniridia with aphakia: first results of haptic fixation of a foldable intraocular lens on a foldable and custom-tailored iris prosthesis. Arch Ophthalmol. 2012;130:771–5.

38. Yoeruek E, Bartz-Schmidt KU. A new knotless technique for combined transscleral fixation of artificial iris, posterior chamber intraocular lens, and penetrating keratoplasty. Eye. 2019;33:358–62.
39. Mayer CS, Laubichler AE, Khoramnia R, Tandogan T, Prahs P, Zapp D, Reznicek L. Challenges and complication management in novel artificial iris implantation. J Ophthalmol. 2018;2018:3262068.
40. Heimann K, Konen W. Artificial iris diaphragm in silicone oil surgery. Fortschr Ophthalmol. 1990;67:329–30.
41. Jonsson NJ, Sahlmüller MC, Ruokonen PC, Torun N, Rieck P. Complications after cosmetic iris implantation. Ophthalmologe. 2011;108:455–8.
42. Spitzer MS, Nessmann A, Wagner J, Yoeruek E, Bartz-Schmidt KU, Szurman P, Szurman GB. Customized humanoptics silicone iris prosthesis in eyes with posttraumatic iris loss: outcomes and complications. Acta Ophthalmol. 2016;94:301–6.

29 Artificial Iris Implantation: Overview of Surgical Techniques

Vladimir Pfeifer, Miha Marzidovšek, and Zala Lužnik

Bullet Points
- Artificial iris (AI) can be implanted using four different surgical techniques.
- 8 years after anterior segment reconstruction, PKP, AI, and IOL implantation, the BCVA is 20/20.
- No CME up to 8 years after AI implantation when using four-floating suture technique.
- Modified Yamane AI and IOL implantation.
- 1.8 mm injector is used for AI implantation into the bag.

Introduction

Iris defects, either partial or total (aniridia), may be congenital or acquired. Congenital aniridia is most commonly caused by mutations in PAX6, FOXC1, PITX2, and CYP1B1 genes [1]. Acquired iris defects develop secondary to penetrating or blunt ocular trauma and iatrogenic trauma (e.g., due to iris tumor resections) or can be associated with iridocorneal endothelial (ICE) syndromes due to severe iris atrophy or other developmental ocular anomalies [2]. These patients present with several visual disabilities such as increased sensitivity to glare, reduced visual acuity, contrast sensitivity, lost depth of focus, and aberration errors. Moreover, aesthetic impairment can be considerable.

Although various conservative treatment approaches are available, such as tinted anti-glare spectacles, [3] colored contact lenses, [4] and lamellar intrastromal corneal tattooing, [5] they may yield insufficient functional and aesthetic results [3]. Surgical reconstruction of iris defects, on the other hand, can be challenging [6, 7]. In case of smaller circumscribed iris defects, pupil reconstruction can be achieved by direct iris suture placement [8]. However, if total aniridia or large and multiple complex iris defects exist, surgical reconstruction with an implantation of artificial iris prosthesis may be preferred. [6, 7] Currently, there are several implants available on the market such as Morcher (Stuttgart, Germany), which achieved good clinical outcomes, [6, 7] and Ophtec (Groningen, the Netherlands) artificial iris implants. Unfortunately, some of these systems usually require large corneal incisions of at least 10 mm [2]. Since 2002, a new foldable silicone-based custom-made iris prosthesis (Custom*flex*® Artificial*iris*; HumanOptics,

Supplementary Information The online version contains supplementary material available at [https://doi.org/10.1007/978-3-030-94530-5_29].

V. Pfeifer (✉) · M. Marzidovšek · Z. Lužnik
Eye Hospital, University Medical Centre, Ljubljana, Slovenia
e-mail: pfeifer@pfeifer.si

J. L. Alió et al. (eds.), *Cataract Surgery*, Essentials in Ophthalmology,
https://doi.org/10.1007/978-3-030-94530-5_29

Erlangen, Germany) [9] is available, and several novel surgical iris reconstruction techniques for medical and aesthetic rehabilitation were introduced with promising results [3, 8]. In addition to the silicone-based iris prosthesis, a hydrophobic acrylic foldable iris diaphragm either with or without optic which can be implanted in capsular bag or ciliary sulcus is also available on the market (Reper-NN LTD.; Russia) [10, 11]. In the following chapter, we will describe in a step-by-step fashion the major surgical approaches for artificial iris implantation and their advantages and disadvantages. In addition, most common surgical and postoperative complications as well as follow-up results will be discussed.

Artificial Iris Design

A Short History of Artificial Iris Devices

The first prosthetic iris device was implanted already in the 1960s by Peter Choyce [12]. The devices were made of polymethyl methacrylate (PMMA) and were implanted directly into the angle [12]. They were abandoned as they were likely to cause glaucoma and corneal failure [12]. In 1991, the next generation of prosthetic iris devices came on the market that were designed by Sundmacher et al. along with Morcher GMBH [12]. They were still made of PMMA optics with a black outer PMMA diaphragm, thus requiring extremely large incisions [12]. Subsequently, Volker Rasch and Morcher developed an injectable multipiece iris prosthesis that was a capsular tension ring-type device which was implanted in the capsular bag and was first implanted by Kenneth Rosenthal and then later by Robert Osher in 1996 [12]. In the following years, Morcher and Ophtec each developed several different artificial iris devices designed with or without optics offering also more color options, which improved cosmesis. However, they still did not exactly match the fellow eye, and some still required large incisions (Morcher) [12].

Custom-Made Silicon Iris Prosthesis

In the early 2000s, HumanOptics along with Hans Reinhard Koch started to design a silicone-based custom iris prosthetic device [9, 12]. In 2011, the new foldable and biocompatible custom-made silicon iris prosthesis was approved in the European Economic Area by Conformite Europeenne marking [8] and in 2018 by US Food and Drug Administration in the United States [3]. The surface of the hydrophobic-pigmented silicon artificial iris (Custom*flex*® Artificial*iris*; HumanOptics, Erlangen, Germany) is custom-made [9]. It consists of a black optically opaque posterior surface and a colored individually designed and hand-painted anterior surface based on patient's high-resolution photographs of his iris remnants and/or the healthy iris of the fellow eye. In case of intraoperative suture placement, it can be manufactured with an embedded fiber meshwork to prevent suture migration. The total artificial iris diameter is 12.8 mm, which can be trephined to custom dimensions during surgery. It has a fixed pupil diameter of 3.35 mm and is thicker at the pupillary margin (0.40 mm). The thickness decreases to 0.25 mm at the periphery. It is designed for posterior chamber implantation in pseudophakic or aphakic patients, alone or combined with an IOL. [9] On the horizon are also several other devices including a self-regulating artificial iris capable of self-changing pupil size [13, 14].

Preoperative Patient Evaluation

Artificial iris (AI) implants are indicated in patients with partial or complete aniridia in pseudophakic or aphakic eyes, either with or without remaining lens capsular support. As AI may induce cataract formation, it should not be used in phakic eyes [8, 15]. Table 29.1 summarizes most common indications for AI implantation such as traumatic aniridia due to penetrating eye injury, iatrogenic iris defects, traumatic mydriasis after blunt ocular trauma, congenital aniridia, Urrets-Zavalia syndrome, Axenfeld-Rieger

Table 29.1 Artificial iris implantation indications

Congenital:
Congenital aniridia
Axenfeld-Rieger syndrome
Acquired:
Posttraumatic:
1. Penetrating trauma
2. Blunt trauma (traumatic mydriasis)
Iatrogenic – surgically induced:
1. Intraoperative iris damage
2. Iris resection due to tumors
3. Urrets-Zavalia syndrome
Degenerative:
1. ICE syndrome: essential (progressive) iris atrophy

ICE syndrome iridocorneal endothelial syndrome

syndrome, and ICE syndrome [2]. The overall complexity of the anterior segment disease will determine which surgical approach the surgeon will use. Thus, to achieve the best postoperative results, careful preoperative planning and detailed patient history is required before iris reconstruction surgery is performed.

First, all patients should undergo precise clinical evaluation and several preoperative measurements, which include best corrected visual acuity, intraocular pressure measurement, endothelial cell density evaluation, axial length, keratometry, the white-to-white (WTW) diameter measured horizontally and vertically, and macular optical coherence tomography. In case of obscured optical clarity, an additional ultrasound examination should be obtained to exclude severe posterior segment disease. Second, to achieve the best postoperative aesthetic results, high-resolution true-color photographs of both eyes are mandatory. The surgeon needs to preoperatively decide if the AI will be fixated with sutures to order the appropriate design (with polymer fiber meshwork).

Surgical Techniques

In the past few years, several surgical techniques for AI implantation have been developed in regard to (a) size and extend of the iris defect, (b) the preoperative lens status (e.g., phakic, pseudophakic, aphakic), and (c) whether the lens capsular support is present or not. Based on these preoperative considerations, three major implantation techniques can be described: (1) partial AI implantation; (2) complete AI implantation into either capsular bag or into ciliary sulcus; and (3) complete AI implantation with scleral fixation.

Basic Surgical Considerations

In cases of sufficient capsular support, AI implantation should be performed through a small corneal incision (minimum 2.8 mm and maximum 7.0 mm) [8] using either forceps or an injector system. The foldable iris implant is then directly inserted into a capsular bag or ciliary sulcus (as discussed in more detail below), which can be additionally sutured to sclera or residual iris using Prolene sutures to achieve better implant position and stability. In aphakic eyes, this procedure can be combined with an IOL implantation as the total thickness of an artificial iris (0.25–0.4 mm), IOL (0.5–1.0 mm), and the residual iris tissue (about 0.5 mm) does not exceed the thickness of a natural human lens (3.5–5.0 mm) [8]. If necessary, the artificial iris can intraoperatively be trimmed with a trephine to the desirable diameter according to the patient's WTW measurements (approximately WTW distance minus 0.5 mm) [2, 3, 8].

Partial Artificial Iris Implantation

This technique may be suitable in selected cases of smaller iris defects affecting 1–3 clock hours [8]. First, the AI implant with a fiber meshwork is cut with scissors to the appropriate size and then inserted with forceps into the anterior chamber. The AI segment is then sutured in place to the patients' own iris remnant. This procedure is reported to be time consuming [8].

Complete Artificial Iris Implantation into Capsular Bag or Ciliary Sulcus

Sulcus-Fixation in Pseudophakic Eyes

This technique is used in preoperatively pseudophakic eyes with a stable IOL placed in the capsular bag with a large iris defects (> 2 clock hours) or with a persistent mydriasis. An injector system is used to implant the foldable artificial iris through a small corneal or scleral incision (2.8 mm) into the anterior chamber that is unfolded in the ciliary sulcus. This approach does not require suturing; thus it is quick and easy to perform. [8] However, as presented in Fig. 29.1, contact between the AI and intraocular structures

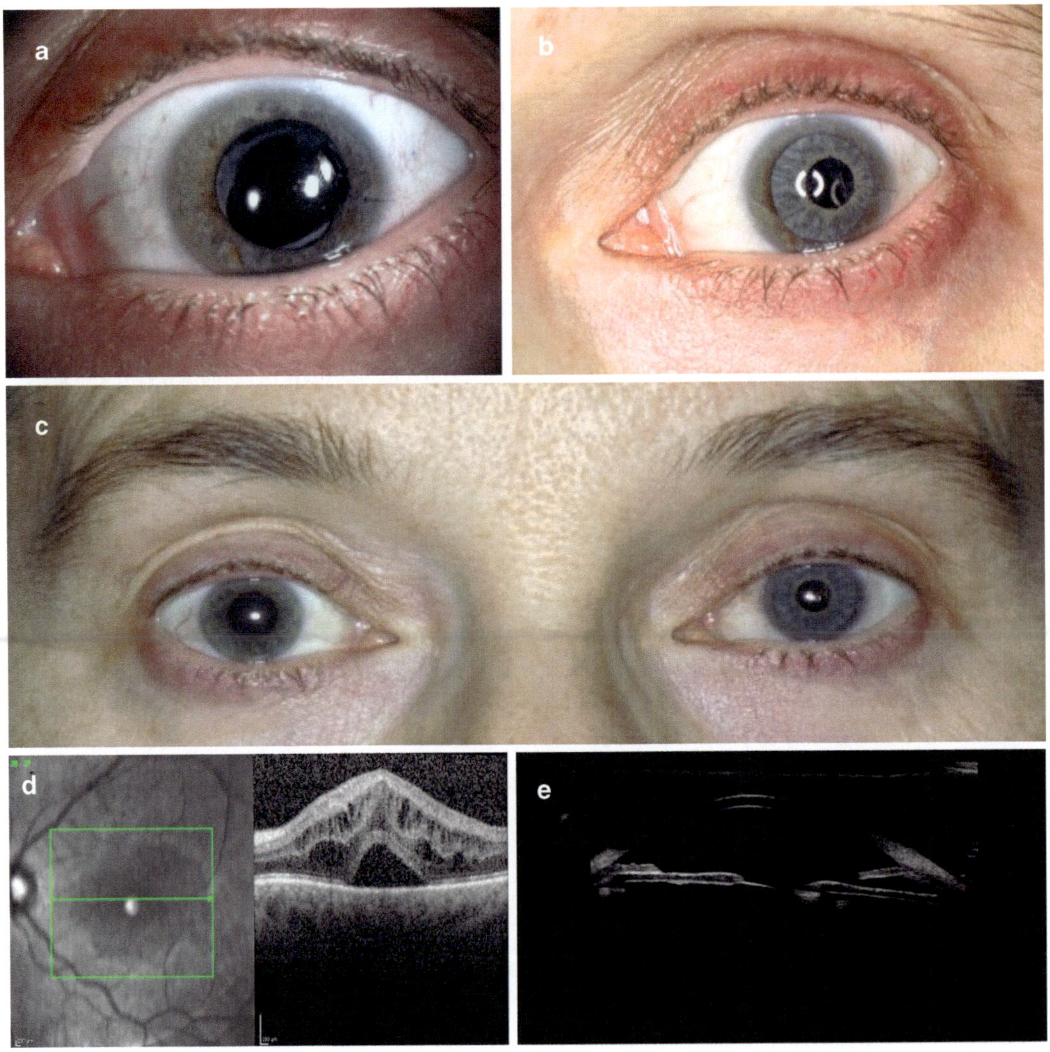

Fig. 29.1 Postoperative results of artificial iris implantation into sulcus. (**a**) Preoperative image of a patient that presented with posttraumatic mydriasis after blunt ocular trauma. First, we performed posttraumatic cataract extraction. At the time of surgery, capsular tension ring and intraocular lens were implanted into the capsular bag. The capsular tension ring was sutured to the sclera using 9.0 polypropylene suture. Due to posttraumatic mydriasis, we decided to implant an artificial iris. (**b**) Postoperative image of left eye 12 months after artificial iris implantation into the sulcus. (**c**) The aesthetic outcome was great, and the patient was very satisfied. Visual acuity was 20/20. However, 2 years later, her left eye became red and painful. Visual acuity dropped. On examination we found light anterior chamber inflammation. (**d**) Optical coherence tomography showed cystoid macular edema. (**e**) Ultrasound biomicroscopy revealed contact between the artificial iris and ciliary body and/or iris pigment epithelium, which might cause rubbing. She was started on topical corticosteroids and nonsteroidal anti-inflammatory drops, but the cystoid macular edema persisted; therefore intravitreal triamcinolone injections were started. Nevertheless, due to recalcitrant inflammation, we had to explant the artificial iris. We hypothesized that contact between the artificial iris and intraocular structures induced chronic inflammation resistant to medical treatment

might cause late and chronic intraocular low-grade inflammation recalcitrant to medical therapy, which resolved after AI was explanted. Similar to our surgical case presented in Fig. 29.1, we needed to explant AI implants from two other patients that underwent AI implantation into sulcus in another facility and presented to us with chronic low-grade inflammation. We hypothesized that in those cases, intraocular inflammation that occurred late after surgery might be a direct result of contact between AI and intraocular structures. Bahadur et al. also reported of required artificial iris exchange in five patients commonly due to corneal decompensation [16]. Original models included Ophtec, Morcher BrightOcular, and HumanOptics [16]. Three of the original artificial irises were passively placed in capsular bag or ciliary sulcus, and all five were exchanged with Morcher or HumanOptics, and all were implanted with suture fixation to sclera, although final visual acuity in most cases remained poor especially due to corneal decompensation and glaucoma [16]. However, recently in the US Food and Drug Administration (FDA) prospective, non-randomized, multicenter study, which determined the safety and effectiveness of the CustomFlexTM Artificial Iris for the treatment of eyes with congenital or acquired full or partial iris defects including 447 eyes, had zero cases that required device explant due to chronic inflammation [17, 18]. Although only 44 of 447 (9,84%) eyes underwent AI passive sulcus fixation without suturing with the last follow-up visit being scheduled 12 months postoperatively, [17, 18] it was speculated that inflammation incidence was lowered by modifying the device edge with circular trephination [17, 18].

Capsular Bag Implantation with a Combined Standard Cataract Surgery

This technique is safe and suitable if the patient has a preexisting cataract and a large iris defect (Video 29.1). In a large case series of 96 cases in the Figueiredo and Snyder study, 91% of artificial iris devices were implanted into the capsular bag [19]. Despite multiple ocular comorbidities, postoperative results showed no cases in which the iris device explant was required. [19] First, a standard cataract extraction is performed taking care to perform a minimal corneal incision of 2.2 mm and a planned capsulorhexis diameter of 6 mm. Phacoemulsification and implantation of an IOL is performed in a standard fashion (Figs. 29.2 and 29.3). It is mandatory to implant a capsular tension ring (CTR) to prevent future capsular shrinkage and decentration of the AI. Iridectomies are not necessary [8]. However, manipulation needs to be gentle to prevent rupture of continuous curvilinear capsulorhexis edge, as this would prevent from further artificial iris implantation into capsular bag.

Complete Artificial Iris Implantation with Scleral Fixation

If capsular support is compromised and extensive iris defects are present, scleral fixation can be used in several surgical variants.

Four-Floating Suture Technique (Pfeifer Technique)

To avoid contact with the AI and the intraocular structures, we modified previous fixation techniques. The four-floating suture technique enables AI implantation with no contact to the intraocular structures as it floats on the four sutures that are fixated to the sclera (Fig. 29.4, Video 29.2).

Thus, to avoid contact between AI and the intraocular structures, in this technique AI without meshwork is trimmed to 10.5 mm diameter using a trephine and sutured using four 9.0 polypropylene sutures. The sutures are tied to the artificial iris using a lasso technique (Fig. 29.4a). These sutures are attached to long-curved needles. Surgeon is sitting at the 12 o'clock position, where the main incision is performed. Anatomical center of the cornea is marked, and four additional points 2 mm behind the limbus that are 90 degrees apart are marked too. A 30 gauge thin-wall-needle is introduced from outside and through the sclera 2 mm behind the limbus near

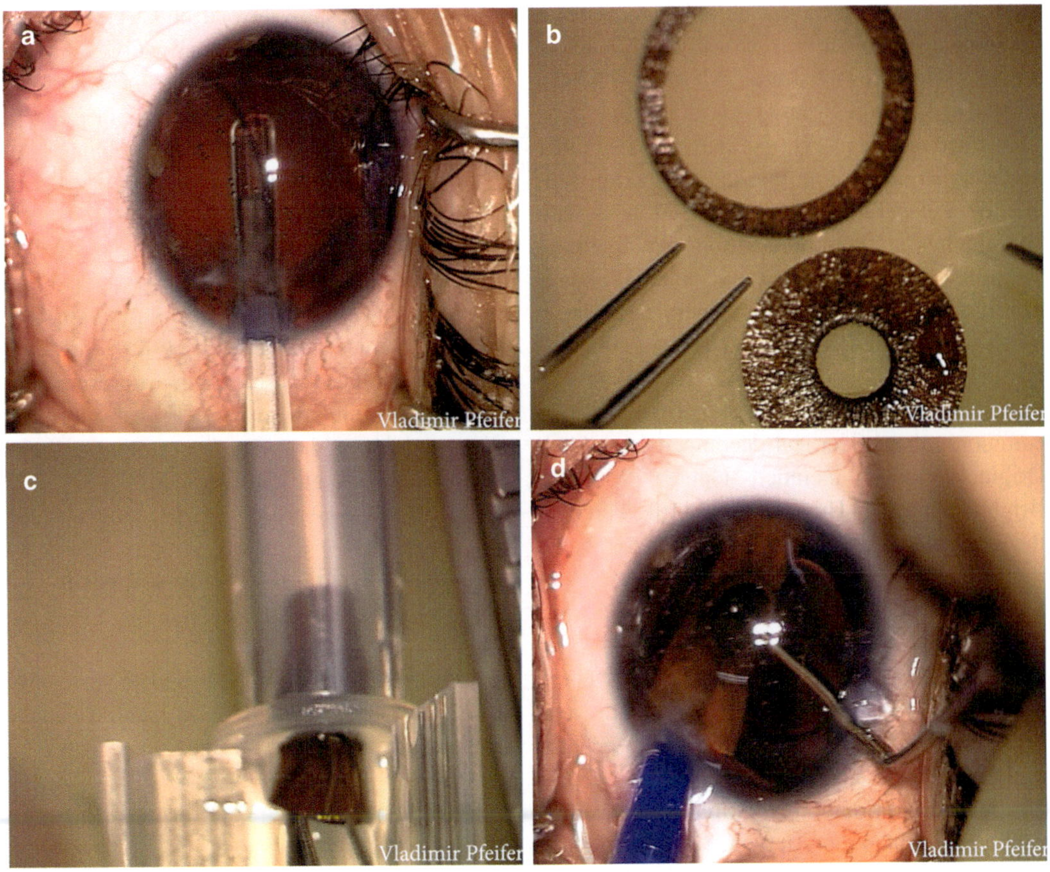

Fig. 29.2 Artificial iris implantation into capsular bag. In our opinion, the safest way to implant an artificial iris is implantation into capsular bag. Herein, we present a case of artificial iris implantation and cataract removal in a 20-year-old patient after penetrating eye injury to the left eye. (**a**) First, intumescent cataract extraction with a capsular tension ring (CTR) and IOL implantation was performed. Of note, if artificial iris will be implanted into a capsular bag, it is mandatory to insert a CTR into the capsular bag. Next, the capsulorhexis was enlarged. (**b**) The artificial iris was trephined to a 9.0 mm diameter, (**c**) folded, and bimanually inserted into a 1.8 mm injector. (**d**) The folded artificial iris was injected into the anterior chamber through a 2.2 mm incision and glided into the capsular bag using Ogawa hook as the second instrument. The artificial iris was unfolded bimanually. The periphery of the unfolded artificial iris is glided into the capsular bag by elevating the continuous curvilinear capsulorhexis (CCC) rim with one instrument and using the second instrument to glide it below. The manipulation needs to be gentle to prevent rupture of CCC edge, as this would prevent from further artificial iris implantation into capsular bag. Thus, the CCC should be big enough to allow artificial iris fixation into the bag

the 7 o'clock position. The 9.0 polypropylene suture on the long-curved-needle is introduced through the main incision at 12 o'clock and docked into the 30 gauge needle. The needle is brought out of the eye and left there. The same is done at the mark near the 4 o'clock position. Sutures are pulled until the AI is brought adjacent to the main incision. AI is folded and pushed through the main incision into the anterior chamber and unfolded. Two remaining needles are brought into the anterior chamber through the main incision and docked into the 30 gauge needles at 10:30 and 1:30 and pulled out of the sclera. The AI is centered by pulling the sutures and tightened to the sclera using Szurman zigzag suturing technique. At the end a knot is done, and conjunctiva is sutured or glued around the limbus. The incisions performed with a 30 gauge needle are watertight. If the incisions are done using a MVR knife, they should be sutured or

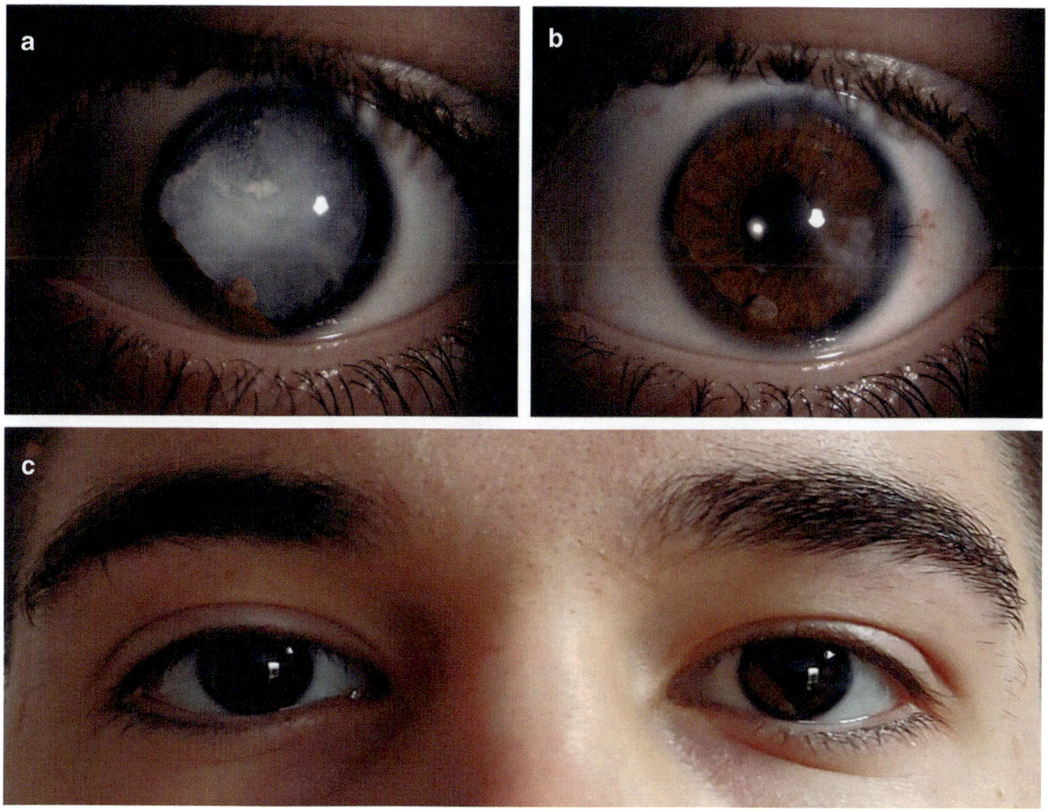

Fig. 29.3 Postoperative results of artificial iris implantation into capsular bag. Preoperative (**a**) and 10-month postoperative (**b, c**) images after artificial iris implantation into the capsular bag of the left eye of a 20-year-old patient with posttraumatic aniridia and cataract (the same patient as in Fig. 29.2) due to penetrating eye injury (perforation through cornea). (**a**) Patient presented with posttraumatic corneal leukoma, white cataract, and iris defect. (**b, c**) The postoperative cosmetic appearance was excellent with visual acuity of 20/20 10 months after surgery. No intraoperative or postoperative complications occurred

glued to be watertight. Care must be taken that the edge of the AI is not in contact with the pigment epithelium of the remaining iris or ciliary body (Fig. 29.4d). Ideally there should be a red reflex that is barely seen between the edge of the AI and the limbus (Fig. 29.4c, d). Using this technique, AI alone (Figs. 29.5 and 29.6) or attached to an IOL can be implanted (Video 29.3).

AI can also be implanted at the time of a penetrating keratoplasty (Figs. 29.7 and 29.8). Concomitantly, aphakia is treated by implanting an AI attached to an IOL (AI-IOL complex). Intraocular lens is sutured to the artificial iris through haptics using loop sutures, as presented in Fig. 29.7. This is done at four places. After artificial iris-IOL complex preparation, the cornea is trephined, and 30 gauge needles are introduced through the sclera 2 mm behind the limbus and docked with the needles of the sutures, which are brought out the eye on four places that were marked previously. Alternatively, the needles can penetrate the sclera 2 mm behind the limbus from inside out. The artificial iris-IOL complex is then pushed through the 8 mm opening in the cornea and centered by pulling the sutures. Finally, the sutures are secured into the sclera using the Szurman zigzag technique. The surgical technique is safe and reproducible, with good aesthetic and functional outcomes (Fig. 29.8).

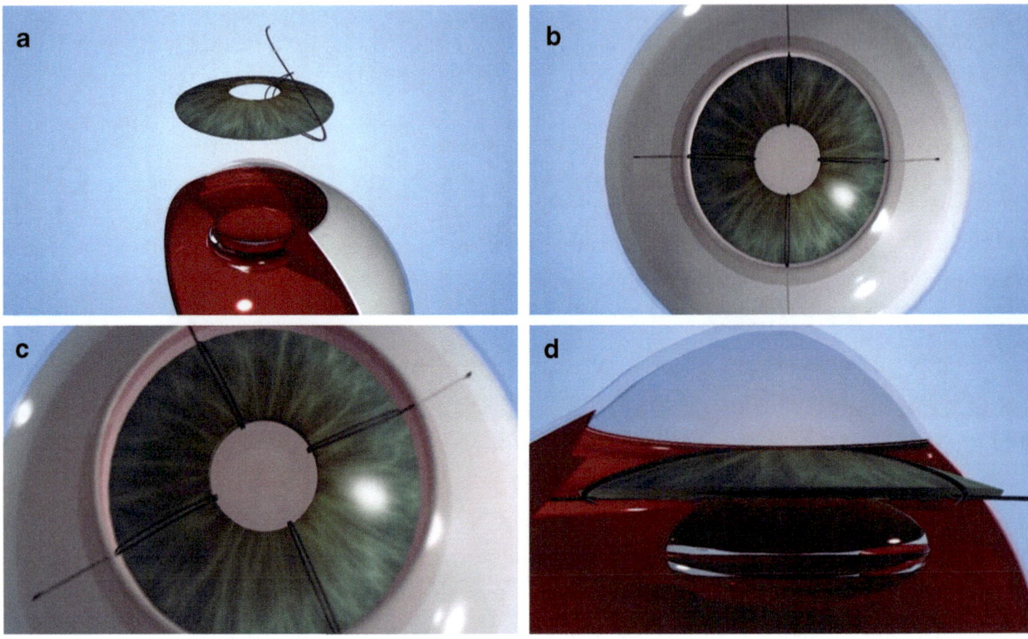

Fig. 29.4 Schematic representation of four-floating suture technique (Pfeifer technique). (**a**) The sutures are tied to the artificial iris using a lasso technique. (**b, c**) The artificial iris is centered with the four sutures that are fixated to the sclera. Care must be taken that the edge of the artificial iris is not in contact with pigment epithelium of the remaining iris or ciliary body (**d**). (**b, c**) Ideally, there should be a red reflex barely seen between the edge of the artificial iris and the limbus

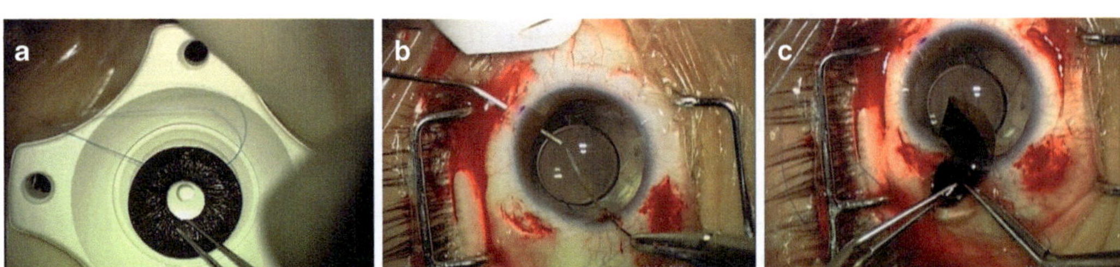

Fig. 29.5 Artificial iris implantation using four-floating sutures technique into a pseudophakic eye. When implanting the artificial iris into a pseudophakic eye, slight technique modifications are used. (**a**) First, artificial iris implant is trephined to diameter of 10.5 mm, and 9.0 polypropylene suture is used to do the lasso suture around the artificial iris four times. (**b**) The two needles are docked into the 26 gauge cannula or 30 gauge needle, which were introduced through sclera into posterior chamber 2 mm behind the limbus. The needles are pooled out the eye, and (**c**) artificial iris is folded and implanted into the anterior chamber. Docking is repeated. Two trailing sutures are placed at the proximal sites. The artificial iris is centered, and sutures are fixed to the sclera using the zigzag technique

Artificial Iris-IOL Complex Scleral Fixation Technique: The Modified Yamane Technique

In aphakic patients, AI can be implanted in combination with an intraocular lens using a modified Yamane technique (Video 29.4), as is step-by-step presented in Fig. 29.9. In short, AI of overall 12.8 mm in diameter is trimmed to 10.5 mm. Using a 30 gauge needle, tunnels on each side are made through the artificial iris 0.75 mm away from its edge. Next, each haptic of three-piece intraocular lens is introduced into

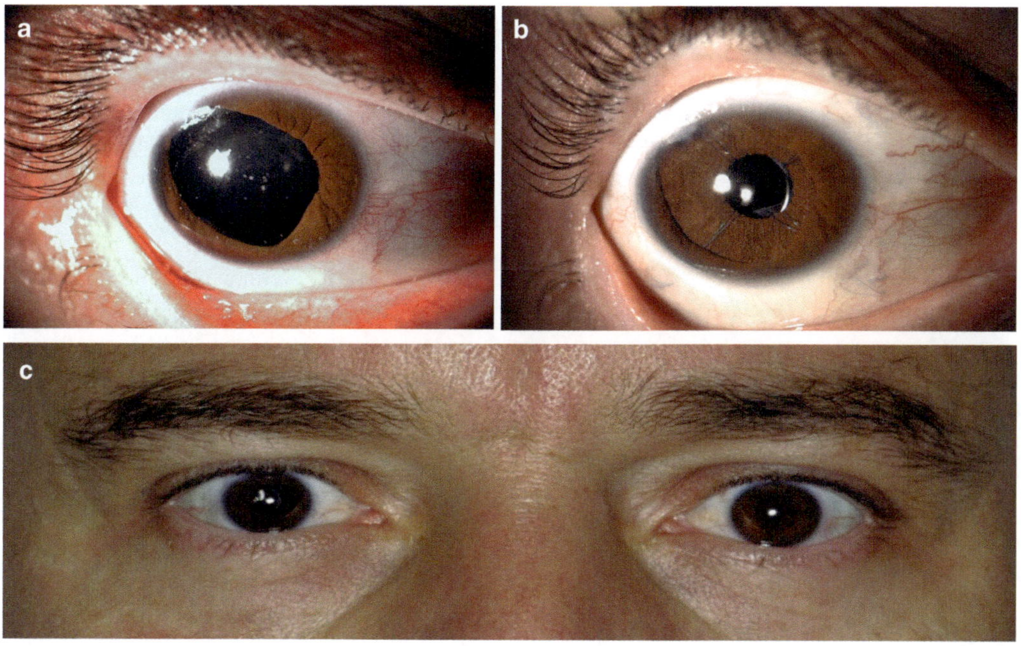

Fig. 29.6 Postoperative results of artificial iris implantation using four-floating suture technique. Preoperative (**a**) and 6-year postoperative (**b, c**) images after artificial iris implantation in the right eye of a 46-year-old patient with posttraumatic mydriasis after blunt ocular trauma (the same patient as in Fig. 29.5) using four-floating suture technique with visual acuity of 20/20 on last follow-up

the needle on each side, and the optics of an IOL are pushed to make contact with the center of an artificial iris. The center of the cornea and two points 2 mm behind limbus 180 degrees apart are marked (two marks on each side 2 mm apart). Anterior chamber maintainer is placed, set to 30 mmHg. With superior approach, the frown incision is done about 5.5 mm wide with diamond knife set to 250 microns, and next the stab incision is done. The safety suture is placed through the artificial iris. After that the complex of IOL/artificial iris is implanted into the anterior chamber. Scleral tunnel at markings 2 mm behind limbus in 10 degrees angle is made parallel to the limbus using 30 gauge needle, bent 45 degrees, and the haptic is docked into the lumen of a needle using 23 gauge forceps through side stab incision. The same is done on the other side, using 30 gauge needle bent 90 degrees and 23 gauge forceps, entering through the main corneal incision to dock IOL haptic into the needle's lumen. Both needles are pulled out simultaneously to externalize both haptics outside the sclera, then first haptic is grabbed with forceps, needle is detached, and haptic is flanged using cautery. Then the same is performed on the second haptic. Both haptics are pushed and buried into the sclera. Anterior chamber maintainer and safety suture are removed. Finally the incisions are sutured and hydrated. Good aesthetic and functional outcomes are achieved (Fig. 29.10).

Artificial Iris-IOL Complex Scleral Fixation Technique: Pfeifer-Canabrava Technique

The latest modification for AI implantation is the Pfeifer-Canabrava technique (Video 29.5, Fig. 29.11). Here the 6.0 polypropylene suture is used. Firstly, 4.5 mm frown incision is performed. Four points 2 millimeter behind the sclera are marked 90 degrees apart. The 6.0 polypropylene suture is brought into the anterior chamber and docked into the 30-gauge thin-wall-needle opposite the main incision 2 mm behind the limbus. Next, the second suture is done in a similar way.

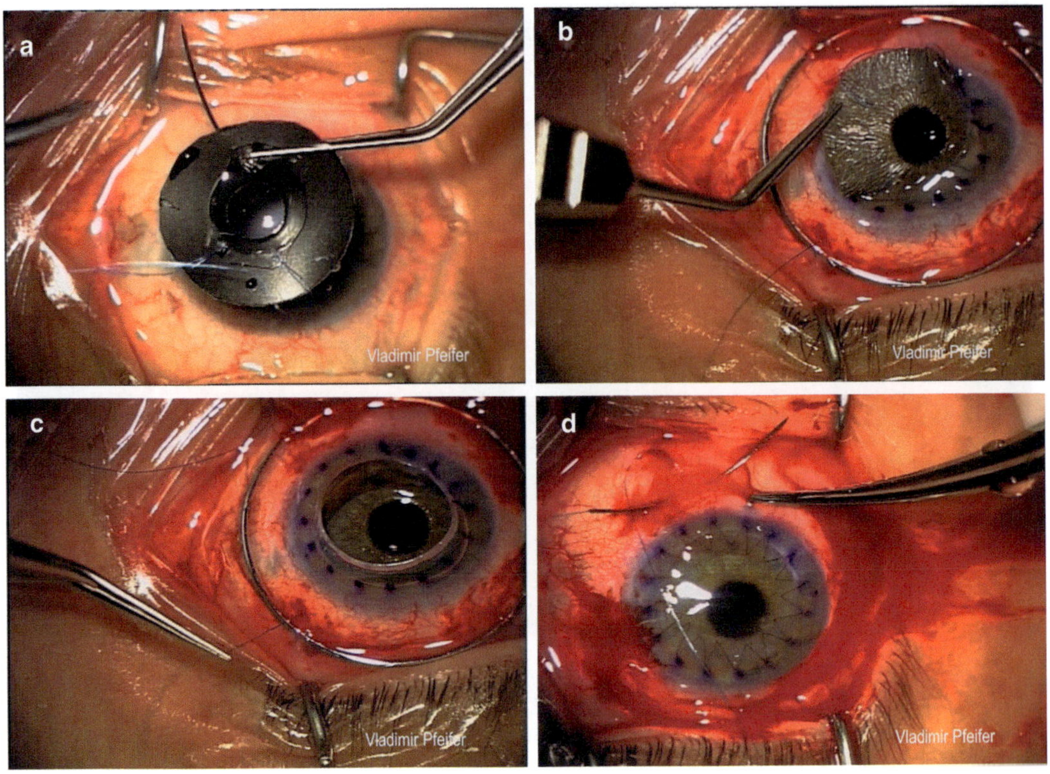

Fig. 29.7 Artificial iris-IOL complex implantation using four-floating suture technique combined with penetrating keratoplasty. (**a**) Intraocular lens is sutured to the artificial iris through haptics using a loop suture, which is done at four sites. After artificial iris-IOL complex preparation, the cornea is trephined, and 30 gauge needles are introduced through the sclera 2 mm behind the limbus and docked with the needles of the sutures, which are brought out the eye on four places that were marked previously. Alternatively, the needles can penetrate the sclera 2 mm behind the limbus from inside out. (**b**) The artificial iris-IOL complex is then pushed through the 8 mm opening in the cornea and (**c**) centered by pulling the sutures. (**d**) Finally, the sutures are secured into the sclera using the Szurman zigzag technique

The AI is trimmed to 10.5 mm, and a plate haptic IOL is centered onto the pupil of the AI. Then the 30 gauge needle is pushed through the leading haptic of the IOL and AI, and 6.0 polypropylene suture is docked into the lumen of the needle. The suture is brought out on the other side, and a flange is performed. Then the proximal sutures are placed 2 mm behind the limbus and guided out of anterior chamber through the IOL and AI using a 30 gauge needle. The next flange is created. The AI-IOL complex is implanted into the anterior chamber. By pulling on sutures the AI-IOL complex is centered. The sutures are cut and pulled, and four flanges are performed 2 mm behind the limbus. The AI is nicely centered, and the sutures are shortened using cautery. The conjunctiva is pulled so that the flanges jump under it. The main incision is sutured. Similarly, when performing this technique, the AI-IOL complex is postoperatively suspended in the anterior chamber. There is no contact between the AI and surrounding intraocular structures or tissues. Good aesthetic outcomes can be achieved (Fig. 29.12).

When using this surgical technique, care must be taken that there is always positive pressure in the anterior chamber. The pars plana infusion cannula is introduced into the anterior chamber perilimbal through the cornea. The intraocular pressure is set at 15 mm of mercury in all cases. When the 30 gauge needles are introduced through the sclera, IOP is raised to 30 mm of mercury.

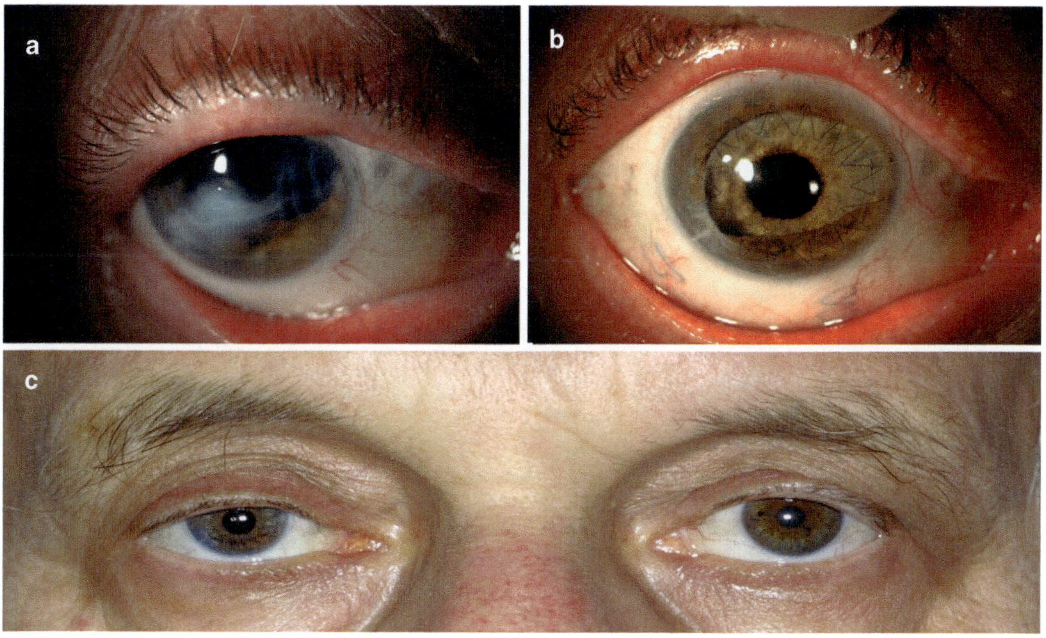

Fig. 29.8 Postoperative results of artificial iris-IOL complex implantation combined with penetrating keratoplasty. Preoperative (**a**) and 7-year postoperative (**b, c**) images after artificial iris-IOL complex implantation in the right eye of a 71-year-old patient with subtotal traumatic aniridia and aphakia after penetrating ocular trauma. The procedure was combined with penetrating keratoplasty (the same patient as in Fig. 29.7). Best spectacle corrected visual acuity was 20/32, and contact lens corrected visual acuity was 20/20, with no postoperative inflammation

Artificial Iris and Non-foldable IOL Implantation Sutured to Sclera

Mayer et al. [3, 8, 20] described a similar technique, where the AI and IOL were implanted and fixated to the sclera separately. The sutures of IOL and from the AI are placed before implantation. First, a non-foldable poly(methyl methacrylate) IOL (Morcher 81B) is implanted through 7.0 mm sclerocorneal incision and sutured to sclera with 10–0 polypropylene usually at 3 o'clock and 9 o'clock. In the same way the artificial iris is implanted and sutured to sclera at the 6 o'clock and 12 o'clock, thus reducing the axial tilt. The main incision is closed with 10-0 nylon sutures [8].

Artificial Iris and IOL Complex Implantation Sutured to the Sclera

Mayer et al. [8] also described alternative surgical techniques in which AI-IOL complex is implanted and sutured to sclera. First, the IOL is sewn on the back of an artificial iris implant through the haptics, near optic from posterior direction, and then turned around on the front side to go back through the iris. The complex is then implanted as a folded sandwich into the eye through a 5.5–6.0 mm sclerocorneal incision and sutured to sclera at 3 and 9 o'clock position. Prior to implantation, two concave iridectomies 180 degrees apart are cut with scissors, and distal haptics are cut off to reduce the size of the foldable complex, allowing smaller incisions and easier implantation. This technique includes only two scleral attachment points, which can be time sparing.

Another surgical approach so-called slip-and-slide technique was described, which allows implantation of artificial iris combined with an IOL through small incision (3.0 mm), thus reducing surgically induced astigmatism. The components of artificial iris and plate-haptic IOL are fixated with knotless sutures together at four points, but can be inserted separately and then assembled after implantation and finally sutured to sclera. It can be performed with a non-toric or toric IOL. [21]

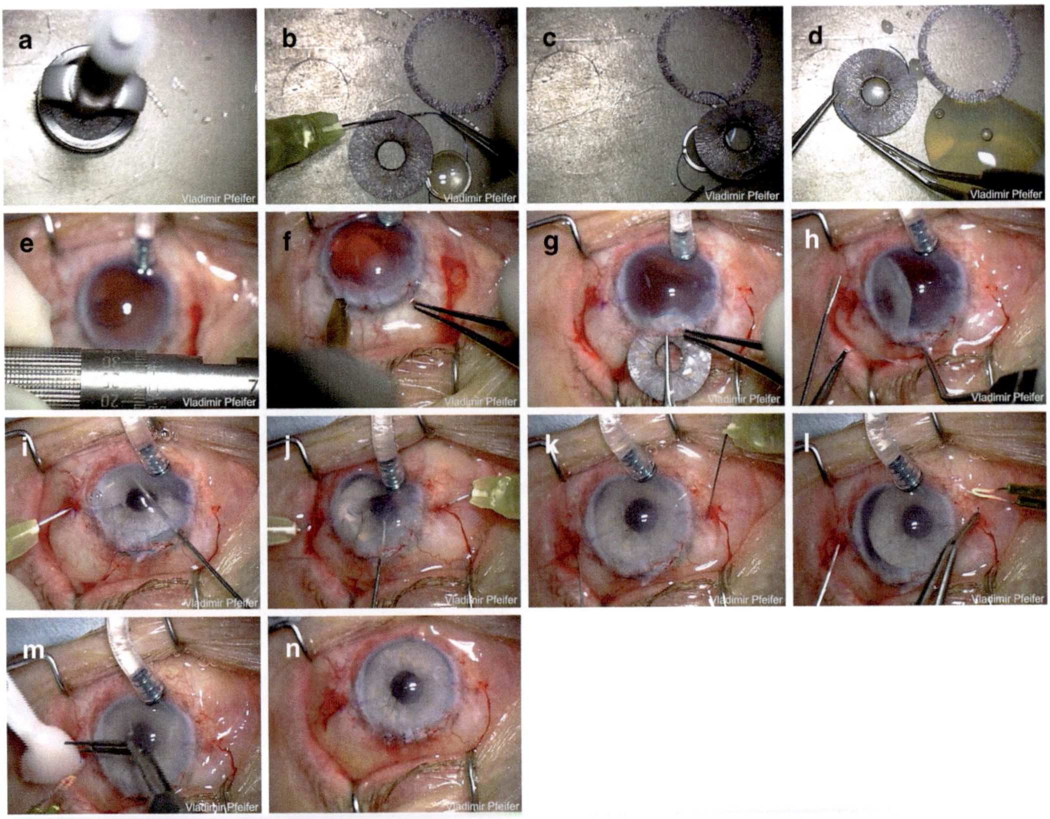

Fig. 29.9 Artificial iris-IOL complex implantation using Yamane technique into an aphakic eye. Artificial iris can be implanted in combination with an intraocular lens using Yamane technique in aphakic patients. (**a**) First, artificial iris is trephined to 10.5 mm. (**b**) The artificial iris is penetrated 0.75 mm from its edge in a 10 degree angle, and the haptic of the IOL is docked into a 30 gauge thin-wall-needle and (**c**) pulled out on the front side of the artificial iris. The same is done on the opposite side. (**d**) Artificial iris-IOL complex is ready for implantation. (**e**) The diamond knife is set at 0.25 mm. (**f**) The 4.5–5.0 mm frown incision is performed. Using bevel knife, the tunnel is performed, and entrance into anterior chamber is initiated using stiletto knife. (**g**) The artificial iris-IOL complex is grasped with a forceps and introduced into the anterior chamber. Care must be taken not to damage the haptics. If needed, the incision can be enlarged. (**h**) Safety suture placed near the edge of the artificial iris prevents slippage of the complex into the vitreous cavity. (**i**) The leading haptic is docked into the 30 gauge thin-wall-needle. (**j**) The needle is released, and the trailing haptic is docked into the needle on the opposite side. (**k**) Both needles are pulled out of the eye in the direction of the tunnel. The artificial iris-IOL complex centers nicely. (**l**) As the blue haptic is visualized on the left side, the needle is released, and the opposite haptic is grabbed using the forceps. After pulling it out of the needle, a flange is performed using cautery. (**m**) Then the leading haptic is grasped, pulled out of the needle, and another flange is created on the opposite side. (**n**) The haptics are pushed under the conjunctiva and slightly into the sclera. The bluish color should be visualized through the conjunctiva at the end of surgery if secondary centering of the artificial iris-IOL complex is needed

Other Surgical Approaches

Open-Sky Implantation During a Perforating Keratoplasty

Artificial iris implantation can be combined with a penetrating keratoplasty, as also in detail described above. In this case, the cornea is trephined, and AI with iridectomies is implanted directly through the corneal aperture into the ciliary sulcus or as presented also above with the four-floating sutures fixated into the sclera. Finally, a donor corneal transplant is sutured. [8]

A Sectoral Artificial Iris Implantation in Phakic Eye

The implant is cut according to the size of the iris defect and implanted through 3.5 mm sclerocorneal incision. Scleral side is sutured to the sclera

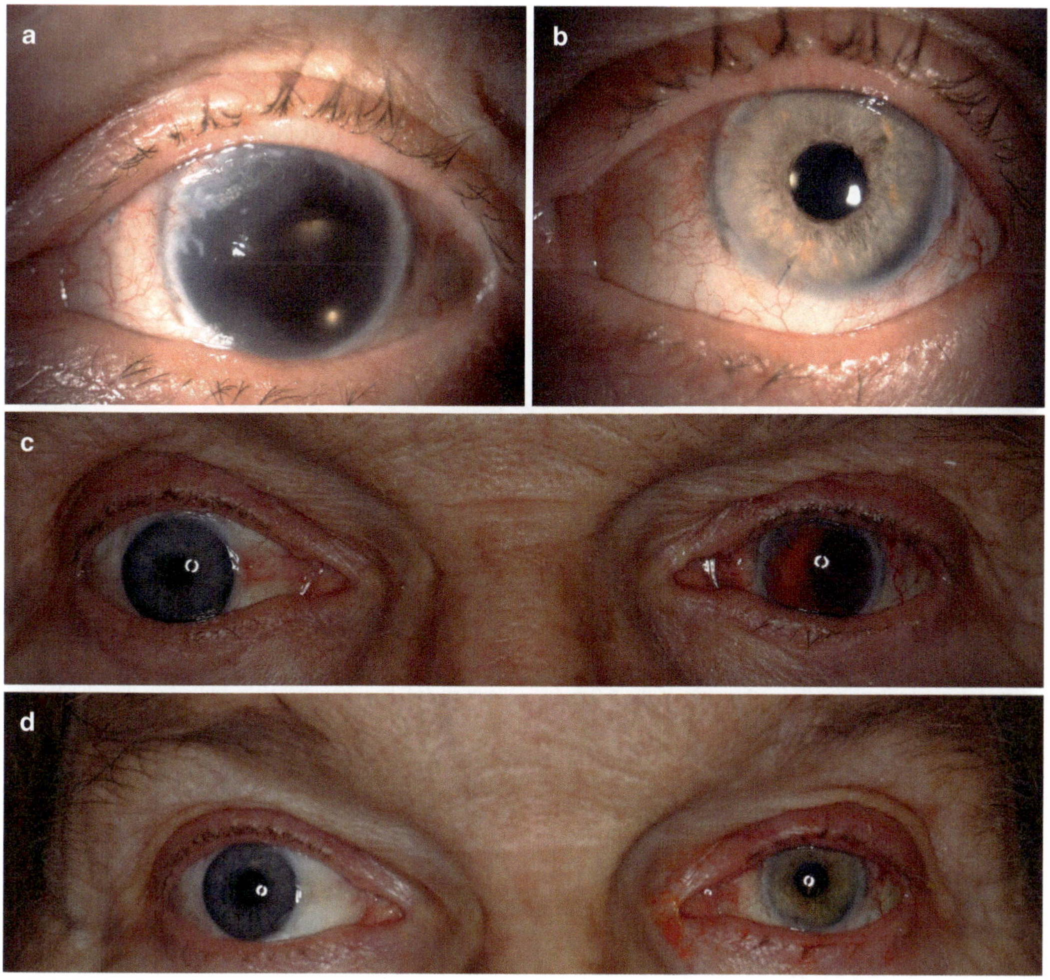

Fig. 29.10 Postoperative results of artificial iris-IOL complex implantation using Yamane technique into an aphakic eye. Preoperative (**a, c**) and 3-month postoperative (**b, d**) images after IOL explantation due to broken haptic and implantation of an artificial iris-IOL complex using Yamane technique into left eye of a patient (same patient as in Fig. 29.9) after globe rupture

with 10-0 polypropylene suture and remaining part to the natural iris tissue with Siepser slip-knot technique. This technique has proved to be successful. [22] In our case series, we have not used this technique.

Clinical Outcomes, Complications and Their Management

Significant advances in AI prosthesis development enabled new surgical approaches for anterior segment reconstruction in acquired or congenital iris defects, which already showed promising functional and aesthetic results. It needs to be emphasized that majority of patients present with complex eye comorbidities and other structural deformities (e.g., after trauma); thus postoperative functional outcomes can be importantly influenced by the preoperative posterior pole and overall eye health. Nevertheless, many patients report improvement in visual acuity and quality of vision (e.g., reduced glare, photophobia) [23]. In addition, most patients can achieve good cosmetic outcomes.

After AI implantation, there are several reported complications that need to be addressed medically or surgically and are often directly

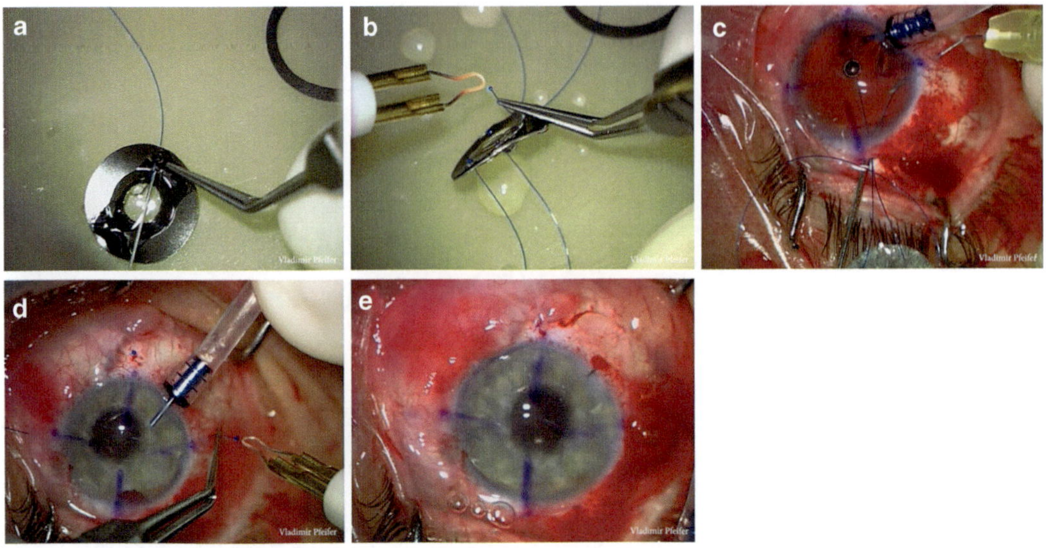

Fig. 29.11 Artificial iris-IOL complex implantation using Pfeifer-Canabrava technique. (**a**) The 6.0 polypropylene suture is introduced through the plate haptic IOL and AI. (**b**) Next, at one end of the suture, the flange is created using cautery. (**c**) The other end of the 6.0 polypropylene suture is brought into the anterior chamber and docked into the 30-gauge thin-wall-needle opposite the main incision 2 mm behind the limbus. (**d**) In this image the suture is brought out and a flange is performed. The AI is nicely centered, and the sutures are shortened using cautery. (**e**) The conjunctiva is pulled so that the flanges jump under it

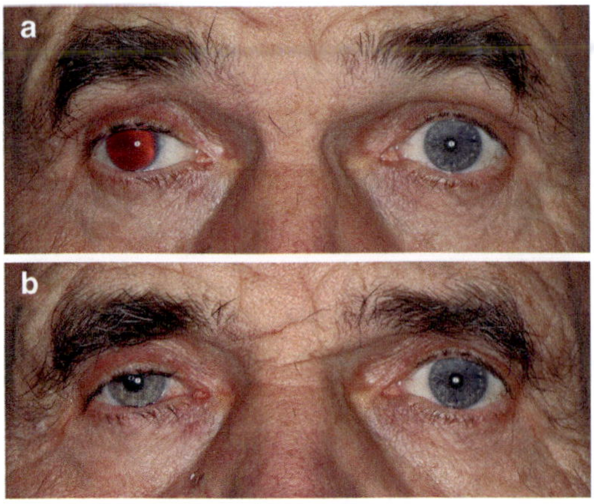

Fig. 29.12 Postoperative results of artificial iris-IOL complex implantation using Pfeifer-Canabrava technique into an aphakic eye. Preoperative (**a**) and 12-month postoperative (**b**) images after implantation of an artificial iris-IOL complex into the right eye of a 61-year-old aphakic patient (same patient as in Fig. 29.11) after globe rupture and anterior segment reconstruction with nice aesthetic appearance

related to other preoperative eye conditions (e.g., posttraumatic ocular hypertension or glaucoma) and/or to the surgical procedure itself rather than being caused by the intraocular device [24].

The most commonly reported complications in literature are (1) persistent intraocular inflammation and macular edema (21%), which was in majority successfully managed by continuous topical nonsteroidal therapy or parabulbar injection of betamethasone; (2) increased intraocular pressure (>20 mmHg) or glaucoma development (5.9–9%), which in most cases was sufficiently managed by topical antiglaucoma medications, some (3.9–15%) required further surgical management such as glaucoma valve implantation; (3) postoperative hypotony (9%) that was managed by at least one hyaluronic acid injection into the anterior chamber; (4) loss of endothelial cell count, which lead to corneal decompensation and required corneal transplantation (11–18%); and (5) artificial iris decentration or malposition (5.9–12%). Our surgical technique of AI repositioning is shown in Figs. 29.13 and 29.14 and Video 29.6.

Other rare but vision-threatening complications included retinal detachment (2%) and phthisis bulbi, which was probably due to severe preoperative trauma and endophthalmitis [20, 25]. Recently, Rickmann et al. [23] reported additional artificial iris-related complications

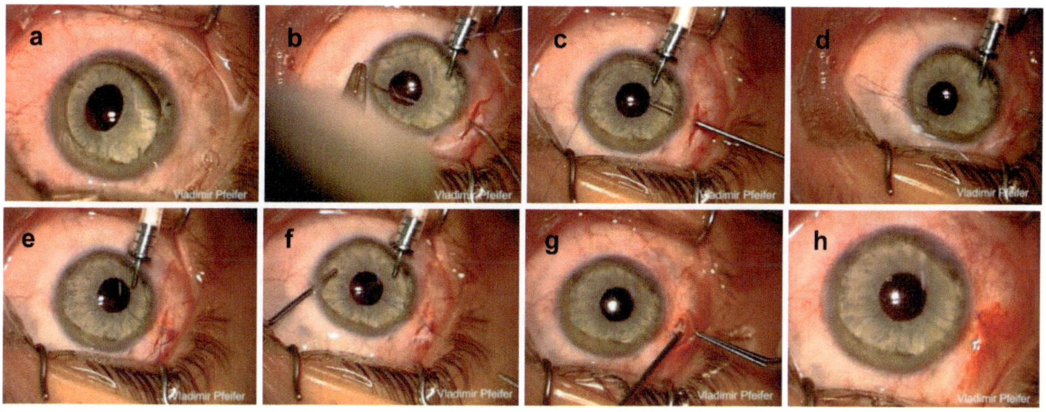

Fig. 29.13 Artificial iris repositioning. (**a**) AI is subluxated and slightly mobile. (**b**) The 9.0 polypropylene loop suture is docked into the 27 G cannula behind the AI and brought out of the sclera through 23 G incision 2 mm behind the limbus. (**c, d**) The loop of the distal part of the suture is pulled over the AI through the same incision. (**e, f**) The lasso is performed around the AI and tightened. The AI is centered by pooling the suture. Zigzag scleral fixation is performed. (**g**) Conjunctiva is glued using fibrin glue. (**h**) The AI is nicely centered

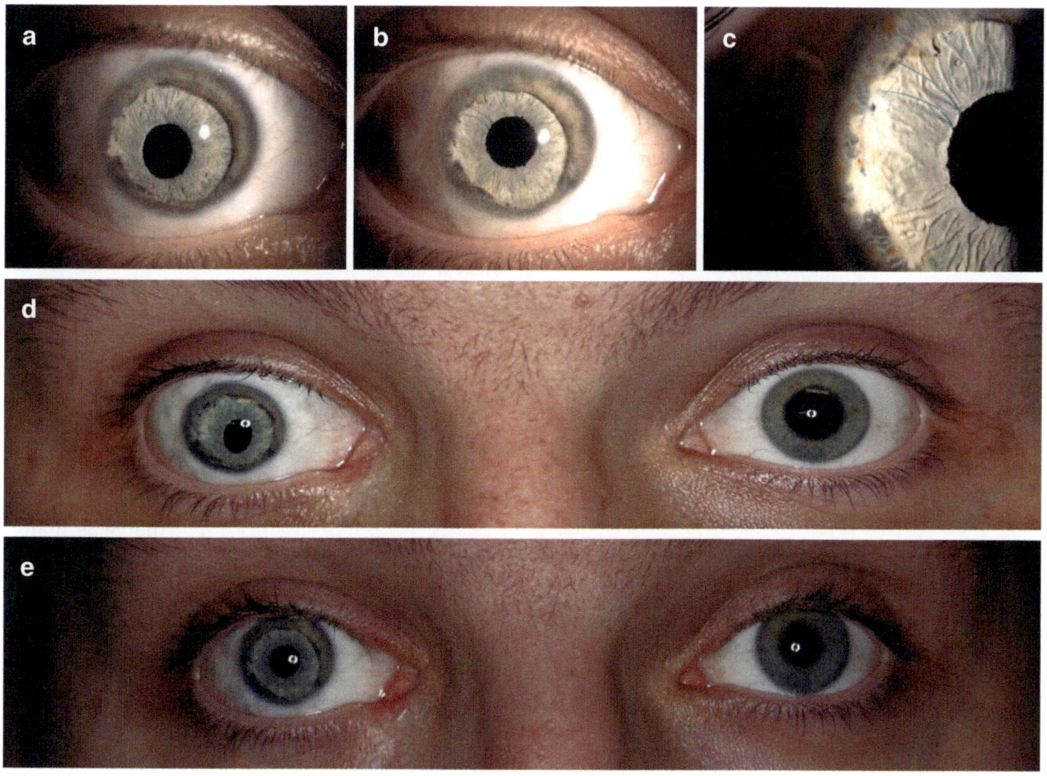

Fig. 29.14 Postoperative results of artificial iris repositioning. Preoperative (**a, d**) and postoperative (**b, c, e**) images after subluxated artificial iris repositioning (same patient as in Fig. 29.13)

such as darkening of the iris remnants and glaucoma development that were clearly associated with implants with integrated fiber mesh, but not to those without [23].

Table 29.2 summarizes our clinical outcomes in 18 consecutive patients, who underwent complex anterior segment reconstruction with the implantation of AI from 2013 to 2020. The majority of our patients (16/18) had posttraumatic aniridia or posttraumatic mydriasis with concomitant anterior segment injury, two presented with congenital aniridia. Three patients had an AI-IOL complex implantation with scleral fixation (modified Yamane technique). 12 patients had the AI implanted using four-floating suture technique. Two patients had AI implanted into the capsular bag and one AI-IOL complex implantation with modified Canabrava technique. Great aesthetic results were achieved in the majority of cases. Likewise, 2/3 of cases reported improvement in visual acuity. Importantly, except for the one patient (Fig. 29.1) that the AI was implanted into the sulcus, in our case series with a long follow-up period (first operation in 2013), no postoperative inflammation or macular edema was observed when there was correct AI placement without touching any eye structure. We can only speculate that this could be a direct reflection of our surgical technique which ensures floating AI or AI-IOL complex on suspension sutures or haptics without touching or rubbing against any other eye structure. The most common postoperative complications that occurred were elevated intraocular pressure (12%), artificial iris decentration (6%), corneal decompensation (6%), and phthisis bulbi in one patient. However, in this case this might be a consequence of severe eye trauma and multiple prior surgical interventions, which included corneal transplantation, vitrectomy due to retinal detachment, and several glaucoma procedures.

To sum up, iris defect reconstruction with an artificial iris implantation using described surgical approaches is safe; however due to the complex nature and concomitant eye diseases, close and long-term patient follow-up is essential to achieve best cosmetic and functional outcomes.

Table 29.2 Different surgical approaches and outcomes

Surgical technique	Number	Indication	Median age (min; max)	Median follow-up, mo. (min; max)	Outcome/complications
Implantation into capsular bag	2	Congenital aniridia (1), penetrating injury (1)	13.5 (7; 20)	23 (10; 36)	Post-op BCVA improved in both cases/ raised IOP (1)
4-floating sutures (Pfeifer technique)	12	Globe rupture (2), penetrating injury (2), blunt ocular trauma (6), iatrogenic – surgically induced (1), aniridia (1)	42.3 (18; 71)	64 (12; 85)	7/12 (58.3%) median postop BCVA increase of 0.6 (min. 0.13; max. 0.9) 2/12 (16.7%) no improvement in post-op BCVA due to preoperative retinal disease 3/12 (25%) median post-op BCVA decrease of 0.125 (min. 0.05; max. 0.2) due to corneal decompensation (2)[a]; enucleation (1)
AI-IOL (Pfeifer-Canabrava technique)	1	Globe rupture	61	12	Post-op BCVA decline/retinal disease; good aesthetic outcome
AI-IOL complex scleral fixation (modified Yamane technique)	3	Globe rupture	72 (67; 73)	24 (12; 24)	Pre- and post-op BCVA remained stable (2), post-op BCVA decline, ERM (1); significant aesthetic improvement

BCVA best corrected visual acuity, *CME* cystoid macular edema, *IOP* intraocular pressure, *IOL* intraocular lens, *ERM* epiretinal membrane, *Post-op* postoperative, *Mo* months
[a]waiting for EK (endothelial keratoplasty)

Conclusions

Iris defects can be successfully reconstructed with an AI implantation using various surgical approaches as presented in this chapter. The procedures are safe with good functional and aesthetic outcomes in majority of patients. However, even though postoperative complications are usually rare and related to concomitant eye diseases and/or direct surgical trauma rather than due to the device itself, surgeons need to be aware and know how to implant the AI and handle the most common postoperative complications. Therefore, proper surgical technique and close and long-term follow-up are mandatory for successful surgical outcomes.

Take-Home Message

- AI has to be implanted in the way it does not and will not come into the contact with intraocular tissue.
- AI must be trephined to 10.5 mm or less when implanted using four-floating suture technique (sulcus) or 9.0 mm when implanted into the capsular bag.
- If inflammation is present after AI implantation quick action should be taken to reposition the AI in the way it will not be in contact to intraocular tissue or explant it.
- Intracapsular AI implantation is the 1st choice technique if capsular bag is present.
- AI without meshwork is used in 100% of cases. When suturing the lasso is performed around the AI, or the IOL is being used as support. AI should float in anterior chamber fixed to the sclera using four sutures or IOL haptics if no capsular bag is present.

References

1. Samant M, Chauhan BK, Lathrop KL, Nischal KK. Congenital aniridia: etiology, manifestations and management. Expert Rev Ophthalmol. 2016;11:135–44.
2. Riedl JC, Schuster AK, Vossmerbaeumer U. Indications and surgical techniques for implantation of the Artificial Iris®. Ophthalmologe. 2020;117:786–90.
3. Yildirim TM, Khoramnia R, Masyk M, Son H-S, Auffarth GU, Mayer CS. Aesthetics of iris reconstruction with a custom-made artificial iris prosthesis. PLoS One. 2020;15:e0237616.
4. Jung JW, Han SH, Kim SA, Kim EK, Seo KY, Kim T-I. Evaluation of pigment location in tinted soft contact lenses. Cont Lens Anterior Eye. 2016;39:210–6.
5. Remky A, Redbrake C, Wenzel M. Intrastromal corneal tattooing for iris defects. J Cataract Refract Surg. 1998;24:1285–7.
6. Burk SE, Da Mata AP, Snyder ME, Cionni RJ, Cohen JS, Osher RH. Prosthetic iris implantation for congenital, traumatic, or functional iris deficiencies. J Cataract Refract Surg. 2001;27:1732–40.
7. Osher RH, Burk SE. Cataract surgery combined with implantation of an artificial iris. J Cataract Refract Surg. 1999;25:1540–7.
8. Mayer C, Tandogan T, Hoffmann AE, Khoramnia R. Artificial iris implantation in various iris defects and lens conditions. J Cataract Refract Surg. 2017;43:724–31.
9. Humanoptics. https://www.humanoptics.com/en/Humanoptics.
10. Pozdeyeva NA, Pashtayev NP, Lukin VP, Batkov YN. Artificial iris-lens diaphragm in reconstructive surgery for aniridia and aphakia. J Cataract Refract Surg. 2005;31:1750–9.
11. Https://www.reper.ru/irisReper.
12. Walter T. Parker, David R. Hardten MES (2019) Iris prosthesis implantation. Video atlas of anterior segment repair and reconstruction. https://doi.org/10.1055/b-0039-172073.
13. Na J-H, Park SC, Sohn Y, Lee S-D. Realizing the concept of a scalable artificial iris with self-regulating capability by reversible photoreaction of spiropyran dyes. Biomaterials. 2013;34:3159–64.
14. Shareef FJ, Sun S, Kotecha M, Kassem I, Azar D, Cho M. Engineering a light-attenuating artificial iris. Investig Ophthalmol Vis Sci. 2016;57:2195–202.
15. Koch KR, Heindl LM, Cursiefen C, Koch HR. Artificial iris devices: benefits, limitations, and management of complications. J Cataract Refract Surg. 2014;40:376–82.
16. Bahadur GG, Miller KM. Artificial iris exchange. J Cataract Refract Surg. 2020;46:1630–6.
17. https://clinicaltrials.gov/ct2/show/nct01860612. Safety and effectiveness of the customflex artificial iris prosthesis for the treatment of iris defects.
18. https://www.Accessdata.Fda.Gov/Cdrh_Docs/Pdf17/P170039b.Pdf. Safety and effectiveness of the customflex artificial iris prosthesis for the treatment of iris defects.
19. Figueiredo GB, Snyder ME. Long-term follow-up of a custom-made prosthetic iris device in patients with congenital aniridia. J Cataract Refract Surg. 2020;46:879–87.

20. Mayer CS, Laubichler AE, Khoramnia R, Tandogan T, Prahs P, Zapp D, Reznicek L. Challenges and complication management in novel artificial iris implantation. J Ophthalmol. 2018;2018:3262068.
21. Wolf A, Shajari M. Slip-and-slide technique for combined small-incision artificial iris and IOL implantation. J Cataract Refract Surg. 2020;46:1433–5.
22. Magnus J, Trau R, Mathysen DGP, Tassignon M-J. Safety of an artificial iris in a phakic eye. J Cataract Refract Surg. 2012;38:1097–100.
23. Rickmann A, Szurman P, Januschowski K, Waizel M, Spitzer MS, Boden KT, Szurman GB. Long-term results after artificial iris implantation in patients with aniridia. Graefe's Arch Clin Exp Ophthalmol. 2016;254:1419–24.
24. Bonnet C, Miller KM. Safety and efficacy of custom foldable silicone artificial iris implantation: prospective compassionate-use case series. J Cataract Refract Surg. 2020;46:893–901.
25. Spitzer MS, Nessmann A, Wagner J, Yoeruek E, Bartz-Schmidt KU, Szurman P, Szurman GB. Customized humanoptics silicone iris prosthesis in eyes with post-traumatic iris loss: outcomes and complications. Acta Ophthalmol. 2016;94:301–6.

Advanced Iris Repair

30

Gregory S. H. Ogawa

Interesting Aspects of the Chapter

In this chapter, you will find out the following:

- The use of globe pressurization modalities, sutures, and instrumentation for iris repair.
- The method to place a multibite interrupted iris suture.
- How to perform an exquisite congenital iris coloboma repair
- The ways to use iris diathermy to refine the shape and centration of the pupil
- How to tie intraocular knots in the iris, and the range of knot techniques

Supplementary Information The online version contains supplementary material available at [https://doi.org/10.1007/978-3-030-94530-5_30].

G. S. H. Ogawa (✉)
Eye Associates of New Mexico, Complex Anterior Segment, Cornea & Cataract, Medical Administration Officer, Albuquerque, NM, USA

University of New Mexico, Department of Ophthalmology, Albuquerque, NM, USA
e-mail: gogawa@eyenm.com

Introduction

A badly damaged or malformed iris can top a patient's ocular problem list due to things like photophobia, poor vision, and dysphotopsia. This chapter addresses the more advanced and complex aspects of iris repair – it is not intended to cover the subject starting from the very beginning. That said, much in the chapter will still prove useful for the surgeon starting out in the field of iris surgery. The improvement in patient quality of life from sound surgical management of iris abnormalities can, in some cases, be quite profound, making skill development in iris repair a worthy pursuit. In the following text, videos, and figures, the surgeon will learn about the preparation and instrumentation for iris surgery, as well as multiple iris repair techniques. One will also discover how to tie iris suture knots that are cinched inside the eye, as opposed to knots cinched outside the eye that can tear, damage, and deform the iris. An alternative to direct repair or replacement of the iris is the option of corneal tattooing.

Iris Repair Versus Iris Prosthesis

There exists a variety of procedures and techniques that may be performed to repair iris abnormalities, but in certain situations, there is just not enough iris to work with to make a repair. Iris

J. L. Alió et al. (eds.), *Cataract Surgery*, Essentials in Ophthalmology,
https://doi.org/10.1007/978-3-030-94530-5_30

may be stretched to a certain degree to suture it while closing a defect, but if it is pulled too tightly, then the iris may tear at the suture, iris root, or elsewhere. If the iris is over-tensioned, there is also the possibility of causing chronic inflammation. A useful guide is that if more than two wraps with a single throw in 10-0 polypropylene suture is required to hold the iris in the desired position, then it is likely being pulled too tightly. In these situations, one may need prosthetic iris for all of the treatment or as an adjunct to iris repair, depending on the type of prosthesis being used. The subject of surgery involving iris prostheses is covered in chapter IP elsewhere in this textbook.

Preparations for Iris Repair

Globe Pressurization

During iris repair, the globe needs to be pressurized in order to minimize bleeding and maintain a reasonably normal anatomic configuration of the eye.

- If the lens capsule diaphragm is intact, then an ophthalmic viscosurgical device (OVD) may be used for this purpose. A dispersive OVD more effectively holds iris tissue in place, but it is harder to remove. A cohesive OVD, at the other end of spectrum, is easier to remove, but does not hold iris in a given location as effectively, while a cohesive-dispersive OVD has some of the characteristics of both.
- If the lens diaphragm is not intact, then infusion should be used to keep the globe pressurized and formed. A 23 g high flow limbal infusion cannula works well by keeping the incision size small, yet allowing good fluid flow into the eye. If an infusion cannula is needed often, then a reusable model (e.g., D&K 8-616-1) is economical, while sporadic use may tend toward a variety of disposable models. The infusion can be provided from a machine with an active pump system, but the advantage of a gravity feed system is that it does not push fluid into the eye as aggressively if the IOP is temporarily decreased when fluid egresses through a paracentesis or other incision. There are also machines that can be set up with a gravity cassette or an active pressure cassette.
- With either type of infusion system, the IOP only needs to be at, or a little above, physiologic pressures. The high infusion pressures often used in phaco (phacoemulsification) surgery should be avoided for iris work – those elevated infusion pressures are needed for removal of cataracts because of the rapid rate at which fluid is removed from the eye during phaco.

Sutures and Needles

- The standard suture material for iris repair is 10-0 polypropylene. It offers an excellent combination of adequate strength and flexibility. Inside the eye, it degrades extremely slowly. It is only where it is within sclera that the degradation rate moves into the range of 1–2 decades, based on the author's experience. The fortunate thing with iris repair is that if 10-0 polypropylene passed through sclera does degrade to the point of breakage, it rarely creates a major problem, and if needed that area of iris may be resutured. These sorts of situations rarely occur, possibly because of the low tensile stress that the iris places on the sutures.
- Long curved transchamber needles (at least 13 mm long) make it easier to get from the limbus, down to the iris, and them back up to the limbus for needle passes through the iris. A fine spatula side-cutting needle (e.g. Ethicon CTC-6 L) has the advantage of being able to pass through sclera or corneal tissue without needing to go through a paracentesis and it makes the smallest orifice when passed through iris tissue; however, it may be more difficult for some surgeons to control inside the eye. A taper cut needle, with similar length and curvature, is typically more rigid (e.g., Ethicon CIF-4) making it easier to control inside the eye, but it needs to be passed through limbal paracentesis openings, and because of its continuous taper, it tends to

drag on iris tissue for much of the needle pass, and make a larger orifice in the iris. The author prefers the fine spatula needle type because of the much greater flexibility in entry-exit locations and the low drag coefficient on iris tissue. That said, there are excellent iris surgeons who use either of these types of needles or even both. Straight transchamber needles may also be used for iris suturing, but for the needle to exit the eye, the entire needle must come to the limbus plane, which automatically elevates the iris to that same plane. In some situations that does not cause problems, and in other situations it does because of iris deformation or even stress and tearing of iris root, or attenuated iris tissue.

Instrumentation

- An appropriate needle holder is essential for iris suturing. Because of how fine the needles are, a fine-tipped needle holder is needed, but because of how long the needles are, a holder with a stout hinge section is beneficial for being able to get a solid grasp of the needle. (e.g., Osher needle holder, Storz E3807 WO) One should avoid using a locking needle holder so as to increase the felicity with which one sutures. If one compares equivalently designed titanium and steel needle holders, the titanium needle holder grasps the stainless steel needles better because the physical properties of titanium allow it to have greater friction on the stainless steel needles. However, if one is choosing between a fine titanium needle holder and a robustly hinged, fine-tipped stainless steel needle holder (e.g., Osher), then the latter will generally be preferred by most surgeons. A pair of coaxial scissors to cut the suture tails allows the surgeon to cut the tails where the knot is located rather than dragging the knot, suture, and iris toward an incision where extraocular scissors can cut the tails. Cutting the knot "in situ" is critical for friable, attenuated iris and other situations. If one uniformly uses 23 g instrumentation and infusion cannula, then instruments and infusion may be switched around among the paracenteses as needed during the case. Of course, 25 g coaxial scissors may also be used for this purpose through a 23 g paracentesis.
- While any type of paracentesis blade may be used for these cases, an angled 23 g microvitreoretinal (MVR) type blade is very sharp and has the advantage of easily creating paracentesis of uniform size with the incision parallel to the iris.
- A range of instruments can be used to support the iris while passing the needle through iris tissue. Sometimes no support is required, but in other situations, a coaxial intraocular forceps, iris reconstruction hook, IOL manipulator, or other instrument may be needed to support the iris in order to avoid putting excessive stress on the iris tissue and the delicate iris root.
- For some versions of intraocular knots, one, or more, 23 or 25 g intraocular curved shaft forceps are required. Reusable forceps are available from several manufacturers, and disposable 25 g VR forceps may manually be bent in the shaft area to make them useable in the anterior chamber.
- Intraocular vitreoretinal (VR) bipolar diathermy probes can be extremely useful for adjusting pupil location and shape by contracting iris stroma, as described later in this chapter. This instrument is commonly used by VR specialists for cauterizing retinal vessels. With the shift to progressively smaller VR instrumentation, these probes are often available in 25 g size, although 23 g through 27 g should work equally well for iris shaping. The disposable versions have the added advantage of the surgeon being able to manually put a bend into the shaft of the probe for improved ergonomics and iris access.

Vitreous Removal

If vitreous is near or around the iris in need of repair, then it should be removed prior to commencing iris surgery in order to avoid vitreous traction and retinal tears. In some instances, the vitreous can be adequately removed through a limbal paracentesis with a guillotine-type vitreous suction cutter. In other situations, a single port pars plana approach may be necessary with the same type of cutter. The infusion in either case can be through the limbal infusion cannula, and illumination from the operating microscope is almost always adequate, so that it is the reason why only one port is needed if a pars plana approach is used. The pars plana access may be achieved with a trocar cannula (available in 23 g size and smaller) or with an incision created using a straight MVR blade of the appropriate width.

Pharmacologic Agents

If the iris work is to be done in isolation (not combined with cataract surgery), then avoiding preoperative dilating or constricting drops is typically advisable. Having an intraocular miotic agent available for during surgery is useful in almost all iris repair surgeries. Acetylcholine works more quickly and avoids excessively strong constriction of the sphincter muscle. It may be instilled more than once, if need be. Carbachol may also be used to achieve iris sphincter constriction, but should be used sparingly because of the tendency to produce exaggerated pupil constriction since it blocks acetylcholinesterase. Excessive sphincter contraction, from carbachol, may make it more difficult for the surgeon to intraoperatively assess the adequacy of iris repairs.

Crystalline Lens

Iris repair in the presence of a noncataractous crystalline lens is a high-stake endeavor. Even subtle bumps to the lens may cause a cataract to form. Additionally, dispersive OVD that is a mix of sodium chondroitin sulfate and sodium hyaluronate has an increased chance of causing a feathery subanterior subcapsular cataract to form even during the case, in the author's experience. This tendency is not as pronounced with an OVD that contains just sodium hyaluronate. All of that said, very experienced iris surgeons may offer iris reconstruction in situations where young patients with clear lenses have disabling symptoms from an iris defect. In these situations, using OVD to float the iris up away from the lens and also using intraocular forceps to stabilize the iris in a position well away from the lens during needle passes may be useful. For any patient considering iris repair with a clear crystalline lens, thorough counseling is mandatory including the potential that cataract surgery may be needed during the case, or soon after the case. Doing biometry and having the appropriate IOL options in the OR is recommended if one undertakes these sorts of cases.

Types of Iris Repair

Iridodialysis Repair

The iris root is the thinnest and also weakest part of the iris. It is prone to tears predominantly from external blunt trauma and also from intraocular surgery. Hyphema often accompanies the acute injury. Small tears, in the range of 1 clock hour, often do not need repair, but as the size increases, and traction on the iris toward the pupil from fibrotic surface bands increases, the iridodialysis becomes progressively more optically disabling. Additionally, if cataract surgery is performed and the resulting IOL optic edge is in the iridodialysis space, then glare and other dysphotopsias may occur. Because the dilator muscles are in the posterior portion of the iris stroma, the iris edge tends to roll posteriorly along the dialysis, making it harder to engage the iris with needle passes from the anterior surface of the iris.

- A conjunctival peritomy should be performed in the area where iridodialysis repair will be performed, with cautery to achieve hemostasis on the scleral surface. In instances where the pupil is moderate size to large, some acetylcholine should be injected into the anterior chamber so that the iris is not bunched toward the periphery. Globe pressurization with OVD or infusion should then be achieved. If there is a fibrotic surface band from the blood at the time of injury, then sometimes a "V" configuration will exist in the edge of the iridodialysis. Two intraocular forceps might be useful to lightly stretch the iris in a radial direction by grasping near the pupil and at the edge of the iridodialysis before gently pulling. (Video 30.1) Sometimes IOL manipulators may be used for this same purpose.

- An IOL manipulator or forceps may be used to help determine the number of fixation points that will be needed for the repair, and the location for each. It often requires fewer fixation points for an iridodialysis repair than one might initially imagine. (Fig. 30.1a, b, c, d).
- The primary way to manage iridodialysis is with horizontal mattress sutures. The double armed 10-0 polypropylene suture is passed: one needle at a time through a paracentesis about 180 degrees away from the desired suture location, then posteriorly through the pupil before catching the far periphery of the iris with the spatula curved transchamber needle, and then passing the needle out through sclera at about the level of the iris root. The surgeon passes the second needle through the same paracentesis, being certain to not catch corneal tissue, then posteriorly through the pupil and then anteriorly through the far

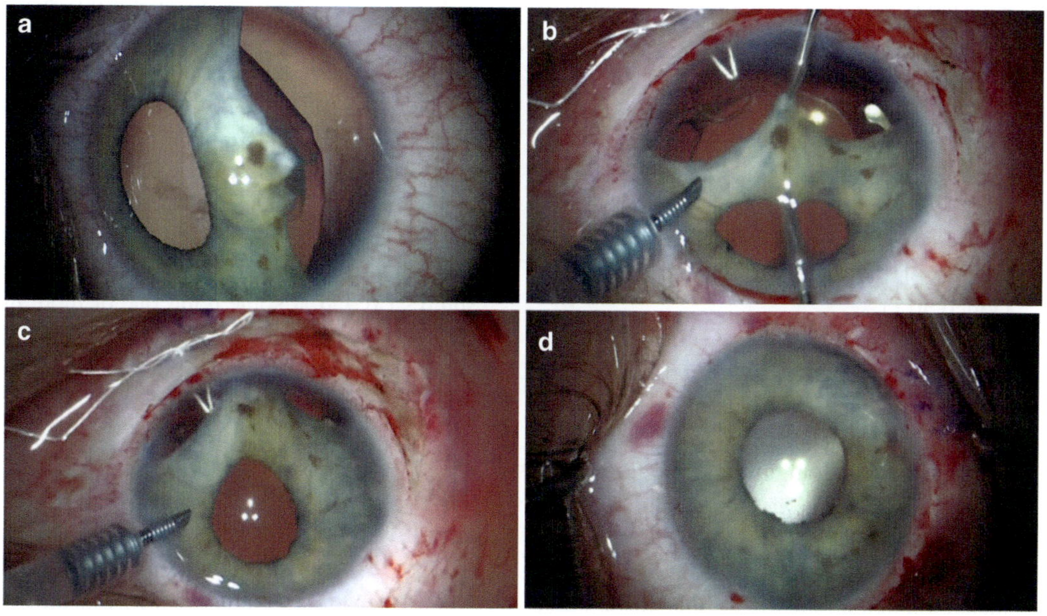

Fig. 30.1 (**a**) A 21-year-old male with a right eye large inferior iridodialysis, extensive zonular defect, vitreous prolapse, underdeveloped lens inferiorly, and a cataract from a fishing weight injury 13 years prior to surgery. (**b**) Stretching the contracted iris with coaxial forceps prior to suture repair of the dialysis. Anterior vitrectomy, cataract aspiration, and ePTFE (Gore-Tex) sutured capsular tension segment with acrylic IOL placement in the bag had already been completed. The ePTFE was tied with a two wrap throw and a half bow in order to adjust the bag/IOL position should it be needed after iris repair. A 23 g reusable titanium infusion cannula is shown for maintaining globe pressurization. (**c**) First mattress suture placed with 10-0 polypropylene double armed with 13 mm × 0.15 mm curved spatula needles in the middle of the iridodialysis defect. Needles were passed through the pupil, then anteriorly through the periphery of the iris, since the iris usually rolls or curves posteriorly. A small amount of hang back was utilized to achieve the desired pupil position. Typically, the 10-0 sutures are tied with a two wrap throw and a half bow in order to adjust tension prior to completion, but in this case, the knots were finalized as they were placed. (**d**) Completed repair after placement of three mattress sutures. It is worth noting that even with an iridodialysis this large, a relatively small number of fixation points can support the iris. The pupil is well centered and did not need iris sphincter sutures. Purkinje images 1, 3, and 4 are well lined up in the center of the cornea, indicating a flat and centered IOL

periphery of the iris, adjacent to the first pass, before passing the needle out through the sclera approximately 1.5–2 mm to the side of the first suture, again at the level of the iris root. The suture arms are trimmed outside the eye then a two wrap throw, with or without a half bow on top, will hold the suture and iris in place while the position is assessed. If only one mattress suture is placed, then the suture tension may be adjusted with the emphasis on an adequate closure of the iridodialysis and good pupil contour, rather than on complete closure of the iridodialys [1]. If more than one mattress suture is placed, then each one should usually be temporarily tied until the last is in position, then the tension of each can be adjusted before final tying the 2-1-1 knot with the knot and then buried inside the eye. A Sinskey hook may be useful for helping to push the knot in through the sclera or even for slightly enlarging the tract through the sclera as part of the process to get the knot inside the eye. It is important to get the knot actually inside the eye through the scleral wall to avoid erosion of the knot through the sclera [2]. (Video 30.1).

- In the situation of a clear crystalline lens being present, the author adjusts the approach to create a relatively peripheral corneal paracentesis in a "backward" configuration in the area of the iridodialysis, going from central to periphery of the cornea. The same double-armed suture is used through this single paracentesis with OVD, intraocular forceps, or other instrumentation to hold the iris off the lens in order to pass the needles through the iris and out through the sclera at the iris root level. The suture arms are managed in the same way as described above. In this setting, one should use the least number of mattress sutures needed to control the symptoms, not the number to get a nice cosmetic result. Again, this is a high stakes iris repair situation that requires very thorough patient counseling and precase preparation.
- There are a variety of iris-suturing techniques, including for iridodialysis repair, that fall under the heading of sewing machine techniques [3, 4]. Most of these involve scleral grooves or scleral flaps (with flap closure using other sutures) and hollow bore needles, all with diameters much larger than the 6 mil (0.15 mm) width of the spatula curved transchamber needle described above. Some of the sewing machine techniques are executed as a running suture, while others as interrupted sutures. Since iridodialysis repair does not need continuous peripheral iris support, a running suture is not needed, and in fact likely decreases the quality of the result because of decreased adjustability once the sutures are placed. There are probably surgeons in whose hands sewing machine techniques work well for iridodialysis repair, but in the author's experience, they complicate what is otherwise a straight-forward technique, do not readily allow for passing the needle from posterior to anterior allowing for suturing the peripheral edge of the posteriorly rolled iris, and create more iris tissue damage because of the larger diameter needles. Other fixation techniques for iridodialysis repair continue to emerge, for example, large diameter polypropylene sutures [5] and at some point one or more of them may have enough follow-up with good results to become a standard that replaces the mattress technique described above.

Multibite Interrupted Pupil Margin Suture

A common location for injury to the iris is the iris sphincter muscle along the pupil margin. These injuries may also include stromal tears and damage in the same area as the sphincter muscle damage. With focal injury a simple interrupted suture – one bite on each side of the defect – is all that is needed. In areas of more diffuse sphincter damage, one or more multibite interrupted sutures may be required. These are particularly useful when there is still sphincter function along part of the pupil margin, but multiple clock hours with no sphincter function. (If there is no sphincter function for 360 degrees, then that is the situation where an iris cerclage suture is appropriate, as described later in this chapter.) Since this chapter covers advanced repairs, the simple interrupted will not be described here, but a surgeon can understand the simple interrupted by cognitively deconstructing the multibite.

- The rationale for the multibite interrupted suture is that if one places a simple interrupted over an extended span of nonfunctioning sphincter, then the two sutured points will come together, but the intervening iris can readily pooch out, creating a radial opening in the iris at the location of the suture. Whereas if multiple bites are placed with the needle over that span, then all the pupil margins along that spread will be brought up into the suture.
- Placement of acetylcholine in the anterior chamber is highly useful in these cases to help demonstrate where the sphincter still functions and where it does not. Analysis of the radiality of the iris architecture can also help separate functioning sphincter (radial) from nonfunctioning sphincter (splayed) [6].
- The multibite interrupted starts with the standard pressurization of the globe and removal of any vitreous in the area. The needle on a single-armed 10-0 polypropylene is passed through the limbus, then posteriorly through the iris near the margin at, or close to, where there is some remaining sphincter function. The needle is then passed up through the iris adjacent to where it was passed posteriorly through the iris. Subsequent passes through the iris may continue in this basting stitch pattern, or convert to a whipstitch where the needle tip goes around the pupil margin, and then passes through the iris from posterior to anterior for all of the subsequent passes. The main advantage of switching to a whipstitch is that it is easier to get the needle passes closer together and decreases the chance of iris pooching peripherally, creating a radial opening once it is tied. The number of bites is dependent on the tissue need for support, but can vary from 3 bites all the way up to about 7 bites in the most extreme cases.
- Once the passes through iris are completed, then an intraocular knot is tied prior to trimming the suture tails with coaxial intraocular scissors. Later in the chapter, different categories and examples of intraocular knots are described. The author typically uses a knot in which the throws are formed outside the eye, and then an IOL manipulator functions as a pulley to take the throws inside the eye and cinch them [7]. This knot can also be seen in the video of this procedure and other procedure videos in this chapter where intraocular knots are needed.
- Having the first multibite interrupted suture completed makes it more obvious to the surgeon where subsequent multibite interrupted sutures need to be placed to achieve an appropriate pupil shape and size. The same procedural steps can be repeated as many times as needed to achieve an acceptable result. The author typically targets a pupil of about 4 mm (or a little smaller) in diameter as measured externally as a target when there is some acetylcholine in the AC. This simulates a relatively bright light situation and will typically be adequate to control photophobia. Patients with darker fundi (and irides) will often tolerate more light entering the eye, and those with lighter fundi (and irides) generally tolerate less light. (Video 30.2).

Iris Gathering Suture for Iris Transillumination Defects

During cataract, and other surgeries, it is not rare for iris to prolapse out through the main incision, or through a paracentesis. Often patients have no symptoms from the focal changes in the iris, but other times, they have significant dysphotopsia-type symptoms – particularly if the pigment epithelium is absent from that area. If the area of transillumination is large, an iris prosthesis may be required as described in the chapter on Iris Prosthesis. For more modest defects, "gathering" sutures may improve or resolve the symptoms. The concept is bringing tissue closer together to increase the optical opacity of the area, but in some instances, it requires frank imbrication [8].

- Acetylcholine should be injected into the anterior chamber, followed by the desired method to keep the globe formed. The 6 mil (0.15 mm) wide spatula long curved transchamber needle should be used for this, on 10-0 polypropylene since the iris is fragile enough in these areas that using the needle with the least amount of traction on the iris is desired. These suture passes need to start in an area of intact iris, then weave through the area of transilluminating iris (almost like blanket weaving), and then end with a bite in intact iris at the other side of the transillumination. When tying the intraocular knot for this section of iris work, it is not always necessary to fully compress all the tissues. The suture only needs to compress iris tissue enough to minimize the transillumination. The suture tails should be cut with coaxial scissors. Often two of these sutures are needed, one more central, and one more peripheral, to adequately control the light transmission issue.
- It is not unusual for the iris sphincter to also be damaged in these situations. If it is, then the surgeon should start with a simple or multibite interrupted suture at the pupil margin to repair that area. Doing so will often make a substantial improvement in the amount of light passing through the iris peripheral to the sphincter repair. If there is still too much light passing through the iris stroma, then one or two gathering sutures may be placed to treat the area. (Video 30.3).

Congenital Iris Coloboma Repair

The congenital iris coloboma is relatively unique among iris defects in that the iris was never normal. The individual was born without closure of the optic fissure during embryogenesis. The anterior segment coloboma can be as subtle as an area of abnormal looking iris stroma inferonasal to the pupil, to a radial iris defect going all the way to the periphery that includes the ciliary body with an absence of lens zonules. The form with absent lens zonules produces what is often referred to as a lens coloboma because the zonules are not present to provide traction on the lens equator to pull it out to the same level as the rest of the lens during lens development and growth. The reason for mentioning this in a chapter on iris repair is that in some situations, vitreous prolapses through that equatorial zonular defect and needs to be removed as part of the surgery repairing the iris. Of course, the posterior colobomas that typically accompany the anterior defects can create visual field defects and even have a devastating impact on vision if it involves the macula.

- Congenital iris colobomas rarely need repair before the time of cataract surgery. The reason is that the natural lens is roughly 12 mm in diameter, so an ectopic iris coloboma still has crystalline lens behind it, allowing for focusing of light. Most IOL optics are about 6 mm in diameter, so after cataract surgery, without addressing the coloboma, the IOL edge is often in the middle of the coloboma with an aphakic space more peripherally, and a pseudophakic space more centrally. The colobomatous pupil in this situation creates an optically poor space that can produce monocular diplopia, edge glare, decreased visual acuity, decreased contrast sensitivity, coma, etc.
- The fundamental thing for the surgeon to understand when repairing these defects is that the iris coloboma margin contains pupillary sphincter muscle. It is functionally an extension of the pupil. With larger iris colobomas that are fixed to the iris root area, the sphincter muscle in the coloboma pulls the colobomatous pupil inferonasally toward that fixation point. So the key to repair is to get rid of the sphincter muscle along the sides of the coloboma. Earlier techniques either did not address this or partially addressed this [9, 10]. The technique described here is for iris coloboma repair at the time of cataract surgery with PCIOL, or as a secondary procedure if the patient previously had cataract surgery without iris coloboma repair [11].
- After cataract surgery with placement of IOL is completed, acetylcholine should be injected into the anterior chamber while observing

how the colobomatous and noncolobomatous pupil respond. (Try to avoid phenylephrine or epinephrine in the infusion bottle during cataract surgery.) The superonasal location is generally a good position to place the 23 g limbal infusion cannula. If there is vitreous prolapse peripherally, then that should be addressed with standard vitreous removal settings for a 23 g vitrectomy probe. Then the vitrectomy machine setting should be lowered to a cut rate of about 1 cut per second with very low vacuum and aspiration flow rate settings. The vitrectomy port is then used to slowly remove the sphincter muscle by removing the coloboma sphincter margin. One can start peripherally first, or select the transition from the normal pupil margin to the coloboma, and begin there. As the colobomatous sphincter is removed, the surgeon may notice the relaxation of the stroma adjacent to the coloboma as it moves centrally. Start slowly, go slowly, and do not remove excess tissue since that makes it harder to close.

- Once the colobomatous sphincter is removed, then the suture repair begins. The sutures are placed as simple interrupted sutures, with the first one bringing together normal pupil sphincter from the nasal and temporal sides. An intraocular knot tied and trimmed holds the pupil margin sides together. [See intraocular knot tying section later in the chapter.] Additional interrupted sutures are sequentially placed, moving from central to periphery, bringing the two, now stromal sides, of the coloboma together. There is often a very small peripheral triangular defect, of no optical significance, that is best left unsutured to avoid tearing iris tissue. If there is an area back toward the pupil that does not seem to have come together adequately, then an additional suture may be placed at that location. Because the most peripheral sutures have the potential to stress/tear the iris, it is important to use a knot-tying technique that can tie the knot down in the iris plane, rather than needing to lift the iris to the limbus plane to cinch the knots. Those options would include the Ike Ahmed two intraocular forceps technique [12, 13], and the Ogawa intraocular knot [7] (Fig. 30.2a, b, c). Pupil shape and centration may be adjusted as needed by using intraocular diathermy as described later in this chapter. (Video 30.4).

Iris Cerclage for Permanent Mydriasis

Large pupils with no iris sphincter activity at all need extensive iris suturing, or an iris prosthesis. The prosthesis approach is described in the chapter on Iris Prosthesis (Chap. 29, Vladimir Pfeifer). Several of the multibite interrupted sutures may be used; however, this tends to put excessive stress on attenuated iris between the sutures and results in a polygonal-shaped pupil, like a square or a pentagon. For the atonic mydriatic pupil, an iris cerclage suture is effective, minimizes stress on the iris tissue, and produces a very good cosmetic and functional result [14].

- Injecting acetylcholine into the anterior chamber may help confirm that there is no sphincter activity. This can also be determined in the office before surgery by watching for iris movement at the slit lamp when shining light in through the pupil, presuming the retina and optic nerve have reasonable function. Next a globe pressurization method is selected and applied before creating several 23 g paracentesis openings around the periphery, each with their internal aspect flared parallel to the iris, to make it easier to pass needles in and out of the eye. If significantly wider paracenteses are created, then flaring may not be needed. For larger resting pupil diameters, it is helpful to have a greater number of limbal access points with a usual minimum for this surgery of 4. An incision for a cataract or IOL surgery can be used as one of the access points.
- One of the critical aspects of this procedure is to avoid catching corneal tissue in the corneal openings when passing the needle through. For going into the eye, a round cyclodialysis spatula, or even one side of a tying forceps, can gape the paracentesis while the needle tip is slid down the side of the instrument into the eye. For exiting the eye, the same maneuver

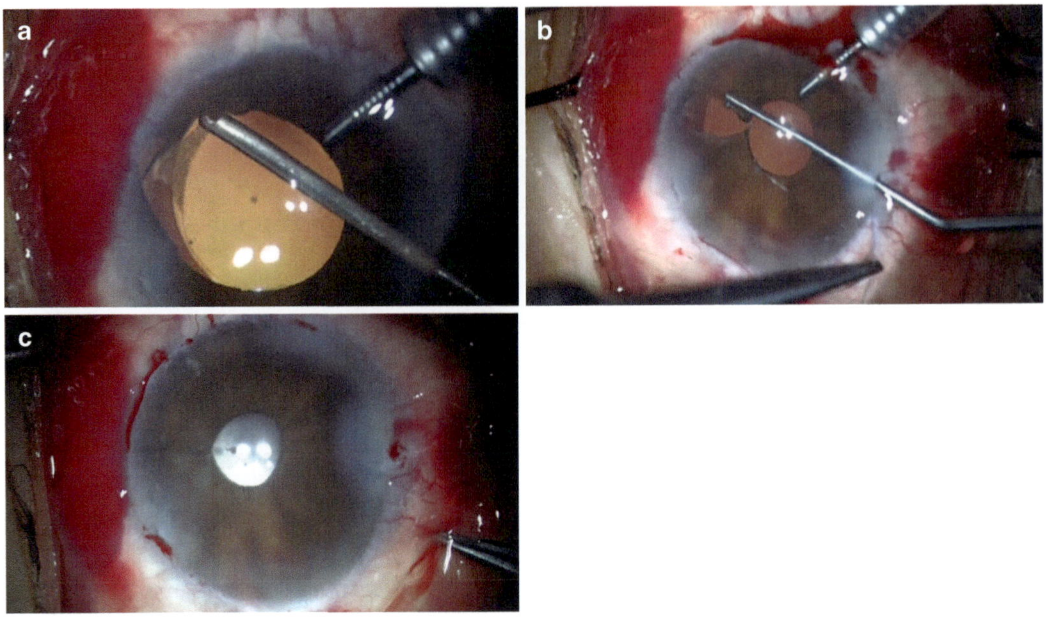

Fig. 30.2 (**a**) Patient with a left iris coloboma. The vitrector is being used at a rate of 1 cut per second, low flow, and low aspiration to trim the iris sphincter muscle off the sides of the colobomatous part of the pupil. A 23 g self-retaining limbal infusion cannula keeps the globe formed. Cataract removal with lens implantation had already been performed followed by instillation of acytelcholine to bring down the pupil size and make it clearer where the transition from coloboma to normal pupil occurs. (**b**) A suture was placed through the nasal and temporal aspects of the normal appearing ends of the pupil. Here the first throw of the first suture is being gradually tightened before the iris edges come together and the two wrap throw is cinched. An angled IOL manipulator functions as a pulley to provide tension on the throw 180 degrees away from the paracentesis. (**c**) After completion of the case, the resulting pupil appears centered and Purkinje images verify a well-positioned IOL. The iris stroma, without colobomatous sphincter, has been closed with interrupted 10-0 polypropylene sutures to almost the periphery of the iris

with the cyclodialysis spatula may be performed, or the needle tip may be docked into the tip of a 24 g plastic IV catheter (angiocath) or a 27 g steel cannula. The needle can sometimes penetrate through a wall of the angiocath, creating small challenges, and the needle tip can readily get dulled putting it into a steel cannula. Since none of these maneuvers are perfect, the surgeon should test at every paracentesis to be sure that corneal tissue has not been caught. This is done by moving the needle tip a few mm into the eye, or out of the eye, then grasping the needle to slide it side to side. If no corneal tissue was caught, then the needle shaft will move the full width of the incision. If corneal tissue has been caught, then the needle shaft will pivot with the tissue perforation site as a fulcrum.

- Using a 4″ long double armed 10-0 polypropylene with the long curved 6 mil spatula needles works well for this procedure. Keeping it double-armed gives the surgeon an "out" should something happen that stops progression in the first direction, or even for ergonomic convenience. In order to have this option available, the first needle pass must be done through a paracentesis as described above, not catching any corneal tissue in the incision. The location that the surgeon sits, and the starting place, can all be done as works best for the individual surgeon. One way that works well for the partially ambidextrous surgeon is to start sitting near the patient's left shoulder – regardless of whether it is a left or right eye – and enter the eye through an incision at about the 10:30 position. The suturing can progress in a counterclockwise fashion with the surgeon moving the operative chair position until the surgeon is positioned near the patient's right shoulder. At this time, if desired, the surgeon can shift up to the top of the patient's head, use the other needle, go through that 10:30 position incision, and go through the iris in a clockwise direction until reaching the point where suturing progress stopped in the counterclockwise direction before tying the intraocular knot, targeting a pupil size of approximately 4 mm as measured externally. (Fig. 30.3a, b, c).

- There are some tips on suturing the iris that can help yield a better result. In some situations, the needle may be woven through the iris near the pupil margin without supporting the iris, but in other situations, an IOL manipulator, iris reconstruction hook, or coaxial forceps may be useful. Coaxial forceps can control the iris well, although they seem to be a little rougher on the iris, due to the multiple forceps compressions, than using one of the other options for support. More bites, as opposed to fewer bites, gives a smoother pupil margin – 24 or more bites can be a good target. The first pass through the iris from a paracentesis is typically in an anterior to posterior direction, then the next is posterior to anterior creating the first two bites of a basting stitch. After that, switching to a whipstitch going posterior to anterior (or anterior to posterior if the surgeon prefers) with each pass allows the surgeon to get the bites closer together which aids in placing more bites for a smoother pupil margin. The most common location to have a suturing gap is at a paracentesis where the needle exited the eye and then re-entered. To

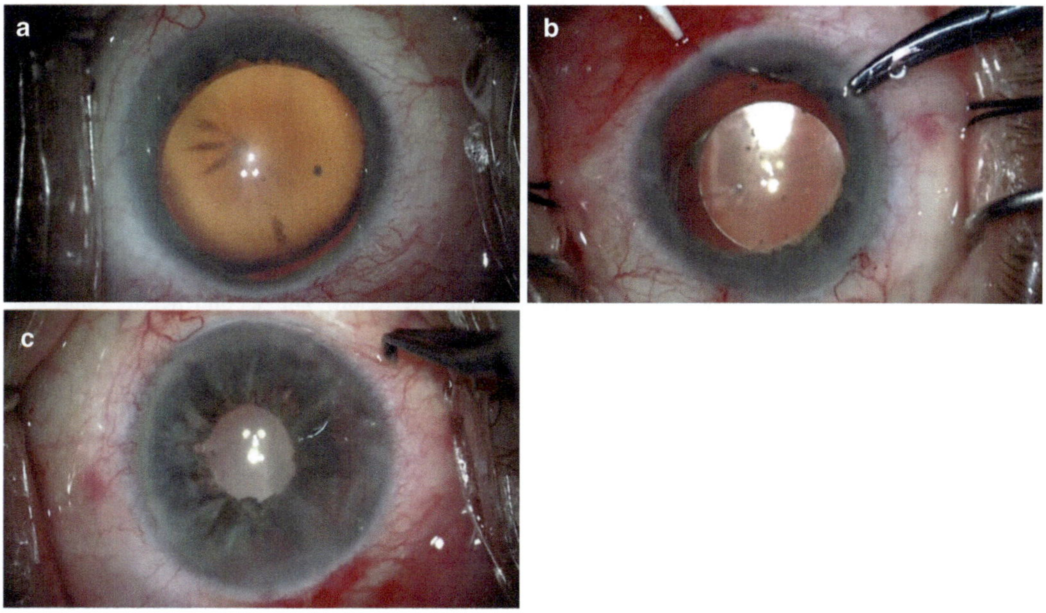

Fig. 30.3 (**a**) Trauma caused this large unreactive pupil. Essentially 360 degrees of absent pupil sphincter function is the situation in which it is appropriate to place a cerclage suture. The pupil is so large down and to the right in this image that one can see around the crystalline lens. (**b**) The 10-0 polypropylene cerclage suture placement started down and to the left in this image (10:00 position for the eye) and progressed in a counterclockwise direction going in through a paracentesis, weaving through the pupil margin, and exiting out the next paracentesis. Here the iris bites can be seen wrapped around the needle in a spiral resulting from whip-stitch style suturing. A 24 g plastic IV catheter (angiocath) was used to catch the needle tip inside the eye and guide it out through the paracentesis without catching corneal tissue, and not dulling the needle tip. (**c**) The completed case with a pupil size of about 4 mm as measured externally, and optimal Purkinje images indicating excellent IOL position. The small notch in the pupil margin on the left of the image occurred at the most common location – a site where the needle exited the eye and re-entered to begin suturing the iris again. It is visible under the microscope, but this size is not particularly visible to the naked eye

minimize the chance of a suturing gap in this location, the surgeon can visualize where the last suture pass exited the iris and try to start the next suture pass as close to that as possible. After the knot has been tied and trimmed, an IOL manipulator may be carefully used to slide the iris around a bit on the suture to optimize the iris position. Essentially, the iris is suspended off the cerclage suture like a curtain on a curtain rod, with the iris root providing the analogous function to gravity for a curtain.

"Coat Hanger" Repair for Large Iris Defects

There are situations where the best one can do with closing an iris defect still leaves a substantial size iris opening. An iris prosthesis may be a good option in these situations, but for various reasons, a prosthetic iris may not be available for the patient. In these cases, there are still suture options that can improve the situation. Various types of bridging sutures may be helpful. The author began using this "coat hanger" type of bridging suture roughly 2 decades ago and has found it to be of notable benefit to multiple patients.

- The location where a coat hanger suture tends to yield the most benefit is for large superior iris defects. The reason for this is that the upper lid usually covers part of the upper cornea, and then patients can also volitionally lower the upper lid further as needed. Often when a lot of superior iris is missing, the iris needs to be lifted superiorly and brought together horizontally toward the midline. This may be achieved with multiple bridging sutures, but the coat hanger configuration can generally achieve all of it with a single suture.
- The fundamental concept behind the coat hanger suture is to create suture force vectors that are not directly in line with the sutures themselves. At the iris, the two sides of the suture travel in different directions, so the force vector resulting from the suture is someplace in between the direction of the sutures. The actual direction of the iris movement depends not only on the direction that the suture sides are pulling, but also on the stretchiness of the iris material in the various directions. Because of this combination of forces, the iris moves along the suture to a position where the forces equilibrate. Hence, the iris does not simply move in the direction half way between the two sides of the suture.
- To create a coat hanger, the suture is kept double armed and the suture needles are passed through a single paracentesis incision about 180 degrees away from the defect. The setup for this suture technique is similar to the horizontal mattress described above for iridodialysis repair. After the first needle passes through the paracentesis, it needs to go through the particular part of the iris that will benefit from being pulled toward the midline and superiorly. Next the needle goes to a location at the plane of the iris root and out through the sclera at a point that will create the proper vector force for iris positioning. Using intraocular forceps or an IOL manipulator first to assess the iris deformability before selecting placement of the suture through the sclera may be useful for optimizing the result. The second needle enters the eye through the same paracentesis (being sure to not catch corneal tissue), then passes through the analogous iris material and sclera on the other side of the eye. The surgeon ties the suture arms outside the eye first with a two wrap throw, then proceeds to adjusting the suture tension to get the iris in the desired position. Sometimes intraocular forceps are useful for encouraging the iris to move to the desired position rather than putting all of that strain/stress on the suture and the iris at the point of the suture material passing through the iris. Once the desired tension is achieved, two single wrap throws are placed on the knot to lock it in place. After trimming the tails, the knot is placed inside the eye by either using a Sinskey hook to push the knot in through the sclera, or even by using a smooth jawed intraocular forceps to grasp the suture internally and pull the knot into the eye. (Fig. 30.4a, b).

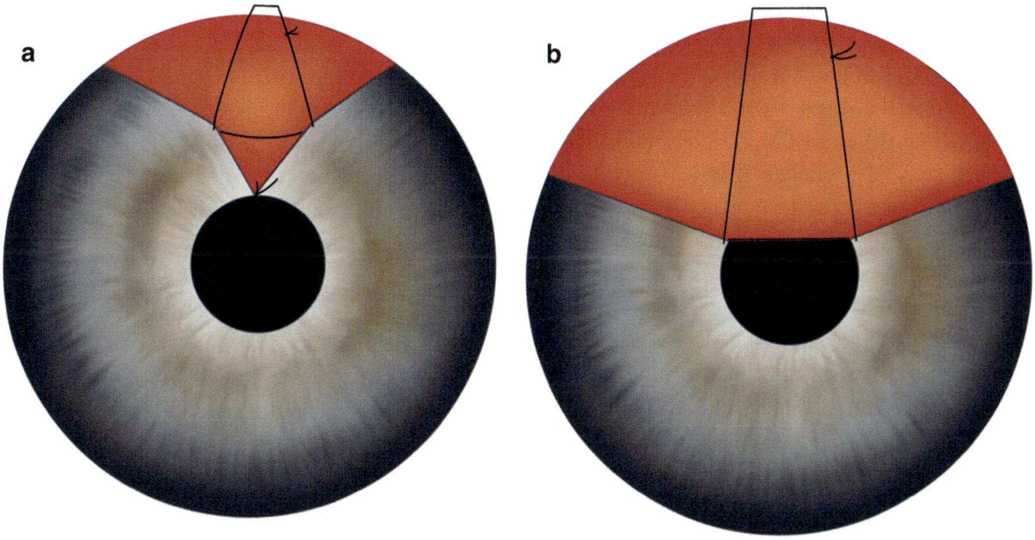

Fig. 30.4 (**a**) Schematic diagram of a "coat hanger" repair in a situation where it was possible to close the iris superiorly, but a large defect remained. The author calls this a coat hanger repair because of its shape. Where the suture passes through the iris, the vector force is between the two sides of the suture and hence both lifts the iris and brings the two sides together. The iris' resistance to stretching in any particular direction has an impact on how much and in which direction the iris actually moves. The 10-0 polypropylene knot is pushed into the eye with a Sinskey hook or pulled into the eye using coaxial forceps, grasping the suture inside the eye. (**b**) Schematic diagram of a "coat hanger" repair with superior pupil margin and a large area of superior iris missing. Without the suture, the iris would drape down inferiorly covering only about the lower 1/3 of the corneal area. While this repair is far from providing complete closure, it creates a much more manageable situation, especially when superior like this, since the patient may use the upper eyelid to help block some of the light that would otherwise go in through the upper section of absent iris

Diathermy Contouring of Pupil Shape and Position

There is a tremendous amount of iris repair that can be accomplished with suturing, but there are times when a bit of additional tuning may be useful. Intraocular diathermy application to the iris can provide that refinement in certain situations. The diathermy instrument is described above in the instrumentation section. Essentially, treatments with this instrument on the anterior surface of the iris cause focal shrinking [13, 15, 16]. One can start with low energy and increase it until the desired effect is seen. Fortunately, unpublished work by Michael E. Snyder, MD, has found that even with rather high diathermy energy, the iris does not suffer dramatic injury, so there seems to be a margin of safety on the settings. The treatments may darken moderate and lighter colored irides, so one should pay attention to this in order to try to make any color changes look as naturally positioned as possible.

- For shaping the pupil, one applies treatments on the side of the pupil that needs to be pulled peripherally. Treatments closer to the iris margin create more acute shaped changes in the pupil margin. Treatments applied a bit further from the pupil margin pull the pupil toward the treatment with a gentler curve. Treatments circumferentially adjacent to each other pull a larger arc of the pupil margin toward the treatments. Treatments applied radially adjacent to each other tend to have an additive effect along the meridian of the treatments.
- To shift the position of the pupil, the treatments should be performed on the side of the iris in the direction that the surgeon desires the pupil to move. The treatments are often applied in a "field" or larger area of iris to

avoid creating focal irregularities. The treatments may even be placed in the more peripheral sections of the iris, if need be. One should remember that even when the intention is to shift the position of the iris, the pupil margin shape may also change from treatments that are closer as opposed to further from the pupil margin.

- A balanced approach between shifting and shaping should be followed when one needs to accomplish both functions. The surgeon may wish to start with the function that is more greatly needed, and then shift to begin work on the other in case the second function affects the first. In other words, avoid getting the pupil shape perfect before starting moving the pupil position, since moving the pupil position may change the pupil shape.
- Caution should be exercised near areas of iris that have been sutured since the additional iris tension in those areas may pull open iris defects that appeared closed from suturing. Diathermy treatments may even create enough tension on the iris to strain the tissue at suture sites to enlarge the suture holes or worse.
- Even though thermal contraction in the cornea has been shown to relax over time regardless of the thermal device, [17] the contraction in the iris seems to be quite stable over time. It is not clear why the shape changes have been so stable, but so far, this is the observation of surgeons utilizing this sort of treatment. Applying diathermy treatments may be a little bit addicting because of the control and results available as the iris is treated. However, the surgeon should keep in mind that the view through the operating microscope is way beyond what the patient or others will have when viewing the iris, so it does not need to look perfect under the microscope. Additionally, even though this is performed in an aqueous environment, the diathermy treatments still create minor trauma sites to the iris, which has the potential to increase postoperative inflammation if more treatments than necessary are applied.

Intraocular Knots for Iris Suturing

- Intraocular knots are formed with throws, each with some number of suture wraps, just as with other surgical knots [18]. The standard shorthand for indicating number of throws and wraps is to indicate the number of wraps for the first throw, followed by a hyphen, then the number of wraps in the second throw, and so on. Using this notation, a knot with 3 wraps in the first throw, 1 wrap in the second throw, and 1 wrap in the third throw would be indicated as a 3-1-1 knot. The friction created by a knot is completely reliant on the knots internal friction if it is not compressing tissue (such as a knot for an iris cerclage suture), but does get some assistance in its frictional holding power if it is compressing tissue (such as when squeezing iris tissue together). If one is relying on the internal friction of the knot in 10-0 polypropylene, then a minimum knot configuration should be a 2-1-1 knot.
- The knot described by McCannel many decades ago [19] pulled the iris to the main wound at the limbus, which displaces and applies tension on the iris. While in some situations, this may still be appropriate, cinching knots at, or close to the final location of the knot is much less likely to damage or distort the iris. Table 30.1 lists many of the published and presented knots where the throws remain inside the eye as they are cinched, and to varying degrees, keep the iris in place as the knot is tied. The knots are divided into three categories based on where the throws are created and whether instruments are used inside the eye to tighten the knot. Macro videos of all the knots in the table are viewable in another publication [6], but here three of the knots will be described in some detail, with macro videos demonstrating each of the three. Video of the Ogawa Knot in the microscopic environment may be seen in multiple surgical videos for this chapter.

Table 30.1 Table of intraocular knots

Siepser style knot: Throws formed and tightened from outside the eye	Ogawa style knot: Throws created outside the eye, then taken inside the eye with an instrument to tighten the knot	Ahmed style knot: Two coaxial forceps used inside the eye to form and tighten the knot
Original Siepser (2-1) [20]	Original Ogawa (2-1-1) [7]	Ahmed (2-1-1) [12, 13]
Osher, Cionni Snyder variant (2-1) [21]	Ahmed variant (2-1-1) [22]	
Condon variant (2-1-1) [23]		
Ahmed variant (3-1-1) [24]		
Schoenberg, Price variant (2-1-1, knot behind iris) [25]		
Narang, Agarwal variant (4 wraps, 1 throw) [26]		

Osher, Cionni, Snyder Variant of the Original Siepser Knot – Throws Formed Externally and Tightened with no instrument inside the Eye

All of the Siepser style knots hook a loop of the suture from the far side of the iris and pull that loop out through a paracentesis opening on the side of the eye where the throws will be formed. The other suture end is passed through the loop (twice), and then both suture ends are pulled outside the eye to cinch the throw inside the eye. The same sort of loop is hooked out in the same fashion, but with this variant, the other suture end is passed through the suture loop (once) in the opposite direction as the first throw. In order to make this knot as a 2-1-1, the loop is hooked out a third time, and the other suture end is passed through the loop (once) in the same direction as the first throw. The reason for alternating the direction that the suture end is passed through the loop is to form the knot in a square configuration. Whether the throws lie down flat to create a true square knot configuration depends on whether the iris is free to turn back and forth since each suture arm is always pulled out of the same side of the eye, respectively, so that it is not possible to lay down the suture throws flat by alternating the direction that the arms are pulled [21]. (Video 30.7).

Ogawa Knot – Throws Formed Externally, Tightened with an Instrument Internally

For this knot, the throws are all formed outside the eye with tying forceps, in a conventional fashion, then the two suture arms are held in one forceps while an IOL manipulator functions like a pulley to take one arm into the eye, with the throw following. The IOL manipulator is moved past the knot location to cinch the throw with the tension of the arms at the knot oriented about 180 degrees apart. By creating the throws with wraps in alternating directions (using the long arm to do the wrapping each time) and alternating which suture arm is pulled into the eye with the IOL manipulator, the knot can be formed square and cinched down square, if the surgeon desires. When doing this procedure, one needs to make one suture arm loop a little longer outside the eye so that the IOL manipulator can go past the knot location. If the suture arm loops are of the same length, then the IOL manipulator will not be able to travel past the knot location, decreasing the ability to properly tighten the throws, and increasing the chance that the IOL manipulator knob could get caught in the throw [7] (Video 30.8).

Ahmed Knot – Two Intraocular Forceps

This intraocular knot requires two smooth platform intraocular forceps of 23 g or 25 g. These knots are formed and tied just like one would do outside the eye, but it is all done inside the eye. After passing the suture through the iris, one arm is left moderately long, and the other should be cut short just outside the globe. The longer suture is held inside the eye with one forceps and wrapped twice around the distal portion of the other forceps before that second forceps grasps the other suture, inside the eye, that was cut at the external surface of the eye. The sutures are then manipulated to tighten down the first throw. The forceps holding the longer suture is used to wrap the suture once around the distal portion of the second forceps in the opposite direction of the first wraps. The shorter tail is grasped inside the eye again with the second forceps with suture manipulation to tighten down the second throw, but pulling the sutures in the opposite direction so that the throw lies down square as it is cinched. The first forceps grasps the longer tail again and wraps the suture around the second forceps once, in the same direction as for the first throw, then the second forceps grasps the short arm again to form and cinch the final throw before trimming the suture ends [12, 13] (Videos 30.2 and 30.9).

Corneal Tattooing for Iris Abnormalities

In certain situations, a corneal solution to iris abnormality may be a more desirable route for the surgeon to pursue. An example of this category would be a phakic patient, with no cataract, who has disabling symptoms from essential iris atrophy (part of the Irido-Corneal-Endothelial Syndrome spectrum). In such situations, obstructing iris could be removed intraocularly, and then one of a variety of corneal tattooing techniques could be utilized to create a centered corneal pupil, and corneal iris peripherally [27]. This technique has other uses for both visual impairment situations and socially unacceptable ocular appearance situations [28, 29].

Conclusion

The decision of whether the patient has an iris abnormality that should be treated with an iris prosthesis is an important first decision when considering an iris abnormality. Not all patients will have access to an iris prosthesis, so that could limit the options in some situations. Advance iris repair surgery requires globe pressurization, sutures, and instrumentation that are generally not part of normal cataract surgery, so that should be thought through and arranged before undertaking these cases. The spectrum of advanced iris repair techniques described offer additional "tools" for the surgeon wishing to move into more advanced and complex iris surgery. Intraocular knots that are cinched in the vicinity of the final desired knot location are an important part of effective suture repair of the iris. Corneal tattooing should be kept in mind as an option for appropriate patient situations.

Take-Home Notes

- Globe pressurization is a critical part of iris repair surgery.
- Adjust the sutures of an iridodialysis repair with attention to the pupil shape/position and not to complete closure of the defect.
- Cataract surgery in a patient with congenital iris coloboma requires coloboma repair to achieve a good result from the cataract surgery.
- Iris cerclage surgery is only appropriate for eyes with absent iris sphincter function for essentially 360 degrees.
- Intraocular knots should be tightened inside the eye at the appropriate location to avoid damage to and distortion of the iris.

References

1. Snyder ME, Lindsell LB. Nonapposition repair of iridodialysis. J Cataract Refract Surg. 2011;37:625–8.
2. Kir E, Kocaturk T, Dayanir V, Ozkan SB, Dündar SO, Aktunç TO. Prevention of suture exposure in transscleral intraocular lens fixation: an original technique. Can J Ophthalmol. 2008;43:707–11.
3. Zeiter JH, Shin DH, Shi DX. A closed chamber technique for repair of iridodialysis. Ophthalmic Surg. 1993;24:476–80.
4. Ravi Kumar KV. Modified sewing machine technique for iridodialysis repair, intraocular lens relocation, iris coloboma repair, Cionni ring fixation, and scleral-fixated intraocular lens. Indian J Ophthalmol. 2018;66(8):1169–76. https://doi.org/10.4103/ijo.IJO_1320_17.
5. Kusaka. Iridodialysis repair by riveting. J Cataract Refract Surg. 2019;45:1531–34.
6. Foster GJL, Ayres B, Fram N, Khandewal S, Ogawa GSH, MacDonald SM, Miller KM, Snyder ME, Vasavada AR. Management of common iatrogenic iris defects induced by cataract surgery. J Cataract Refract Surg. 2021;47:522–32.
7. Ogawa GSH, O'Gawa GM. Single wound, in situ tying technique for iris repair. Ophthalmic Surg Lasers. 1998;29:943–8.
8. Snyder ME, Perez MA. Iris stromal imbrication over sewing for pigment epithelial defects. Br J Ophthalmol. 2015;99:5–6. https://doi.org/10.1136/bjophthalmol-2013-304437.
9. Blackmon DM, Lambert SR. Congenital iris coloboma repair using a modified McCannel suture technique. Am J Ophthalmol. 2003;135:730–2.
10. Cionni RJ, Karatza EC, Osher RH, Shah M. Surgical technique for congenital iris coloboma repair. J Cataract Refract Surg. 2006;32:1913–6.
11. Ogawa GSH. Congenital iris coloboma repair with excision of colobomatous sphinter muscle. J Cataract Refract Surg. 2020. https://doi.org/10.1097/j.jcrs.0000000000000440
12. Ahmed IK. Intraocular knot tying with two micro tying forceps. In: Cataract surgery, telling it like it is meeting. Sarasota: Circa; 2015.
13. Ahmed IK. More cautery – centration of an inferior iris defect. Video J Cataract Refract Glaucoma Surg. 2016;32:4, Iris Reconstruction. https://vjcrgs.com/volume32-issue4/more-cautery.
14. Ogawa GSH. Iris cerclage suture for permanent mydriasis: a running suture technique. Ophthalmic Surg Lasers. 1998;29:1001–9.
15. Ahmed IK. Iris and pupil shaping with intraocular diathermy. In: Cataract surgery, telling it like it is meeting. Sarasota, FL: Circa; 2015.
16. Snyder ME. Cautery shaping. Video J Cataract Refract Glaucoma Surg. 2016;32:4. https://vjcrgs.com/volume32-issue4/cautery-shaping.
17. Ogawa GSH, Azar DT, Koch DD. Laser thermokeratoplasty for hyperopia, astigmatism, and myopia. In: Azar DT, editor. Refractive surgery. Stamford: Appleton & Lange; 1997. p. 491–9.
18. Edlich RF, Long WB. Surgical knot tying manual. 3rd ed. Norwalk: Covidien; 2008. p. 22. http://www.covidien.com/imageServer.aspx?contentID=11850&contenttype=application/pdf
19. McCannel MA. A retrievable suture idea for anterior uveal problems. Ophthalmic Surg. 1976;7:98–103.
20. Siepser SB. The closed chamber slipping suture technique for iris repair. Ann Ophthalmol. 1994;26:71–2.
21. Osher RH, Snyder ME, Cionni RJ. Modification of the Siepser slip-knot technique. J Cataract Refract Surg. 2005;31:1098–100.
22. Ahmed IK. Forceps tightening modification of Ogawa in situ knot. In: Cataract surgery, telling it like it is meeting. Sarasota: Circa; 2015.
23. Condon GP. Modified siepser sliding knot demo. Available at: https://eyetube.net/video/rireg/ (requires registering for eyetube). Posted 2010. Accessed 10 Mar 2018.
24. Ahmed IK. The siepser sliding knot for iris repair. Available at: https://www.youtube.com/watch?v=4QipgGl1HTk. Posted July 21, 2013. Accessed 10 Mar 2018.
25. Schoenberg ED, Price FW. Modification of Siepser sliding suture technique for iris repair and endothelial keratoplasty. J Cataract Refract Surg. 2014;40:705–8.
26. Narang P, Agarwal A. Single-pass four-throw technique for pupilloplasty. Eur J Ophthalmol. 2017;27:506–8.
27. Alio JL, Rodriquez AE, Toffaha BT, Pinero DP, Moreno LJ. Femtosecond-assisted keratopigmentation for functional and cosmetic restoration in essential iris atrophy. J Cataract Refract Surg. 2011;37:1744–7.
28. Al-Shymalia O, Rodriquez AE, Amesty MA, Alio JL. Superficial Keratopigmentation: an alternative solution for patients with cosmetically or functionally impaired eyes. Cornea. 2019;38:54–61.
29. Balgos JD, Amesty MA, Rodriguez AE, Al-Shymali O, Abumustafa S, Alio JL. Keratopigmentation combined with strabismus surgery to restore cosmesis in eyes with disabling cornel scarring and squint. Br J Ophthalmol. 2020;104:785–9.

31 Correction of Severe Iris Defects and Cases of Traumatic Aniridia with Aphakia by Combined Scleral Fixated Intraocular Lens and Keratopigmentation

Jorge L. Alió, Ali Nowrouzi, and Jorge Alió del Barrio

Bullet Point

- The combined implantation of scleral fixated intraocular lens (IOL) and femtosecond-assisted keratopigmentation is an alternative surgical procedure for the treatment of the complications related to traumatic and congenital aniridia.
- Therapeutic, and cosmetic, keratopigmentation has been successfully utilized and reported in different cases of iris defects with lower complication rates such as early post-op light sensitivity and color fading and change in color.
- Keratopigmentation either for cosmetic or therapeutic purposes has been demonstrated to be safe during a 10-year follow-up.
- This technique aims to provide a surgical alternative to the intraocular iris implants, especially for those cases where such iris implants, with or without combined IOL optic, are not available.

Supplementary Information The online version contains supplementary material available at [https://doi.org/10.1007/978-3-030-94530-5_31].

J. L. Alió (✉) · J. Alió del Barrio
Cornea, Refractive and Cataract Surgery Unit, Vissum Miranza Alicante, Alicante, Spain

Division of Ophthalmology, School of Medicine, Miguel Hernandez University, Alicante, Spain
e-mail: jlalio@vissum.com

A. Nowrouzi
Cornea, Cataract and Refractive Surgery Unit, Department of Ophthalmology, Hospital Quironsalud Marbella, Alicante, Spain

Introduction

Patients with severe iris defects or full aniridia (either congenital, traumatic, and iatrogenic) usually complain about photophobia, glare, decreased contrast sensitivity, decreased depth of focus, and reduced visual acuity [1]. These patients are generally also dissatisfied because of their cosmetic appearance. Furthermore, iris atrophy and pupil size deteriorate the visual function due to degradation of the retinal image quality in this cases [2]. These symptoms can range from patient observations to life-altering distractions and disabilities. It is important for the surgeon to not dismiss patient concerns solely based on the size of a defect.

J. L. Alió et al. (eds.), *Cataract Surgery*, Essentials in Ophthalmology,
https://doi.org/10.1007/978-3-030-94530-5_31

Nowadays, there are several surgical and nonsurgical options to correct iris defects, such as cosmetic colored contact lenses, microtying suture techniques, and prosthetic iris implants for larger defects [1]. Different models of prosthetic iris implants are available for aniridia, such as IOL-iris combinations, capsular tension ring-based prosthetic iris devices, and foldable custom artificial iris [1]. Examples of such prosthetic iris devices are the Morcher (Morcher, Germany) iris IOL implants, the Ophtec BV implants (Ophtec, Schweitzerlad), and REPER implants (Reper-NN, Russia).

The artificial iris, Custom*Flex*® (HumanOptics, Germany), is another therapeutic approach approved by the US Food and Drug Administration for aniridia, which is a thin, foldable, prosthetic iris made of silicone diaphragm, with the option of an integrated polymer fiber meshwork to which an IOL can be sutured to correct both aniridia and aphakia [1–3]. It has a fixed pupil aperture of 3.35 mm and an overall diameter of 12.8 mm that can be sized with a trephine for each case the implant is individually custom-made to match the patient's natural iris color.

In recent years, therapeutic and cosmetic corneal keratopigmentation has emerged as an option for patients affected by severe iris defects or abnormal iris cosmesis [4, 5]. This surgical technique has been demonstrated to be safe and to provide good cosmetic results and patient satisfaction even in the long term [6]. This surgical approach can also be successfully associated with other procedures such as squint, cataract, or eyelid surgery [7].

In this context, the purpose of the current review is to describe a new surgical approach for the management of cases of aniridia associated with aphakia by a combined surgical procedure of sulcus sutured intraocular lens (IOL) with therapeutic keratopigmentation (KTP).

Surgical Technique

The summary of this new corneal surgical approach is as follows:

Femtosecond-assisted KTP is performed under topical anesthesia (tetracaine and oxibuprocaine) as described in the previous publications [4–6]. Briefly, an intrastromal tunnel is created using a femtosecond laser (Visumax, Zeiss, Germany) with the following parameters: depth of 250 μm, the inner diameter of 4 mm, the outer diameter of 9 mm, and energy of 2 mJ. Then, a lamellar dissector (Alio keratopigmentation corneal dissector, Epsilon, Irvine, California) is used to open the intrastromal femtosecond tunnel and to extend it to the external border of the cornea to reach a total diameter of 11.5 mm. Finally, the appropriate mineral micronized colour pigment previously selected based on fellow eye's color (Blue Green, Alicante, Spain) is injected into the stromal tunnel using a 27-gauge cannula. It is important to explain that the tunnel length is planed based on the size of the iris defect. It could be partial in partial aniridia or complete in complete aniridia.

In cases of aphakia combined with aniridia sulcus, fixated IOL surgery can be performed immediately after the lamellar stromal dissection as is explained previously in our case study.

Postoperative topical therapy included a combination of topical antibiotics (ofloxacin 0.3% [Exocin]) and steroid (dexamethasone 0.1% [Maxidex]).

Case Reports

Case 1

A 44-year-old man diagnosed with posttraumatic full aniridia and aphakia presented in our clinic with a past medical history of repaired rupture of the globe after an accident 1 year ago. Because of secondary retinal detachment, he previously underwent globe reconstruction followed by a vitrectomy. The corrected visual acuity (CDVA) was 20/200 with the refraction of +13.50 −3.50 × 130, and intraocular pressure (IOP) of 15 mmHg. Combined implantation of a sulcus fixated IOL (MN60MA of 24 diopters) with femtosecond-assisted keratopigmentation was performed as described above.

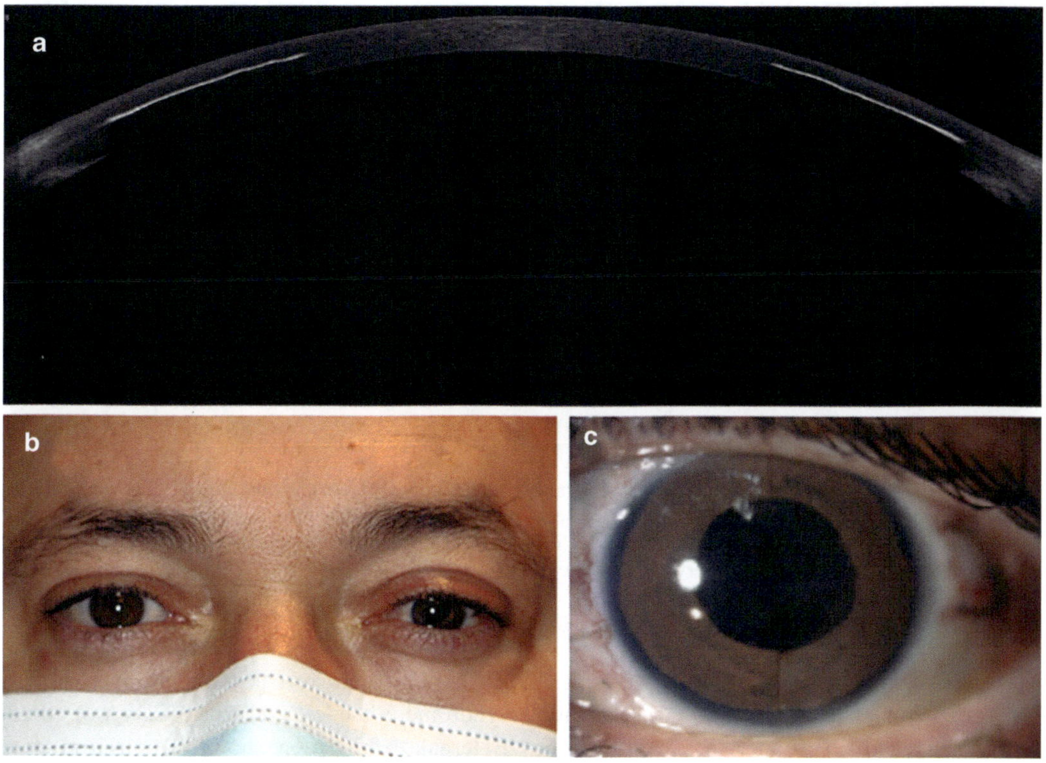

Fig. 31.1 (**a**) Optical coherence tomography (OCT) of femtosecond assisted-KTP. Intrastromal keratopigmentation at depth of 250 μm. (**b**, **c**): Binocular appearance 3 months after the surgery with the same color of the contralateral eye

Outcome

Follow-up at 6 months was unremarkable. The CDVA was 20/25 with the refraction of +2 −2 × 160 and IOP of 20 mmHg. No complications were reported during the follow-up period. The cosmetic appearance was acceptable (Fig. 31.1a, b, c). A highly significant reduction of glare and other visually disturbing phenomena was confirmed compared with preoperative symptoms.

Case 2

An 80-year-old woman diagnosed with posttraumatic full aniridia and aphakia after an accident 1.5 years ago presented in our clinic. The CDVA was 20/800 with the refraction of +13.00 −3.00 × 85 and IOP of 15 mmHg. Endothelial cell dysfunction was diagnosed with a central corneal thickness of 680 microns preoperatively. Combined implantation of a sulcus fixated IOL (MN60MA of 22 diopters) and femtosecond-assisted KTP was performed as described previously. Three months after the initial surgery, descemet stripping automated endothelial keratoplasty (DSAEK) was performed. (Fig. 31.2a, b, c).

Outcome

At the third postoperative month, CDVA was 20/63 with the refraction of +3 −1.75 × 30 and an IOP of 16 mmHg. She suffered from episodic macular edema, which responded to the implantation of dexamethasone. No complications were reported during the follow-up period. The cosmetic appearance was acceptable. A highly significant reduction of glare and other visually disturbing phenomena was confirmed. (Fig. 31.2b, c).

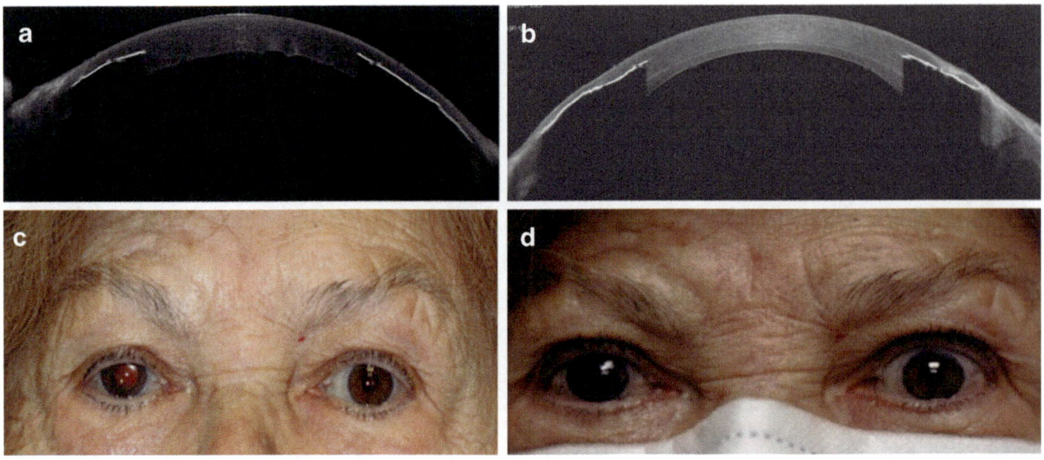

Fig. 31.2 (**a**): OCT of femtosecond assisted-KTP at depth of 250 μm of corneal stroma. (**b**): OCT of femtosecond assisted-KTP and DSAEK of 7.5 mm diameter. (**c**): Binocular appearance before the surgery with right eye complete post traumatic aniridia. (**d**): Binocular appearance 3 months after the surgery, femtosecond assisted-KTP eye with the same color of contralateral eye

Case 3

A 59-year-old man diagnosed with posttraumatic full aniridia and aphakia after a car accident 1.5 years ago underwent vitrectomy surgery and extraction of his displaced IOL in the vitreous cavity presented in our clinic.

His best CDVA was 20/160 with the refraction of +12.50 −3.50 × 85. Combined implantation of a sulcus fixated IOL, and femtosecond-assisted keratopigmentation, was performed as explained previously.

Outcome

At the third postoperative month, CDVA was 20/25 with the refraction of +2 −3 × 80 and IOP of 16 mm Hg. No complications were reported during the follow-up period. The cosmetic appearance was acceptable. Light sensitivity, glare, and other visually disturbing phenomena disappeared almost completely, as confirmed by the questionnaire postoperatively.

Case 4

A 23-year-old woman was referred to our clinic with complaints of severe light sensitivity and cosmetic deformation of the iris in her left eye. The examination revealed the presence of ICE syndrome in the left eye, with a CDVA of 20/25. External examination showed a piriform oval pupil pattern in the eye. Slit-lamp examination revealed advanced iris atrophy (Fig. 31.3a). The endothelial guttata-like changes were confirmed by specular microscopy with a low cell count (1225 cell/mm [2]). The IOP was normal, and the gonioscopy showed no abnormality in angle. No other pathologic finding was detected in the anterior chamber, retina, and optic nerve. Examination of the right eye was normal; the CDVA was 20/20. The patient complained of photophobia and blurred vision while reading. On the follow-up visit 3 months later, she complained of fluctuating vision and poor tolerance while wearing the cosmetic contact lens. The examination revealed that the iris defect had progressed, affecting a larger area with corectopia and polycoria, resulting in monocular diplopia (Fig. 31.3b). After obtaining adequate informed consent from the patient, the KTP was performed, assisted by the femtosecond laser.

Outcome

At the third postoperative date, minimal conjunctival injection and ocular discomfort had

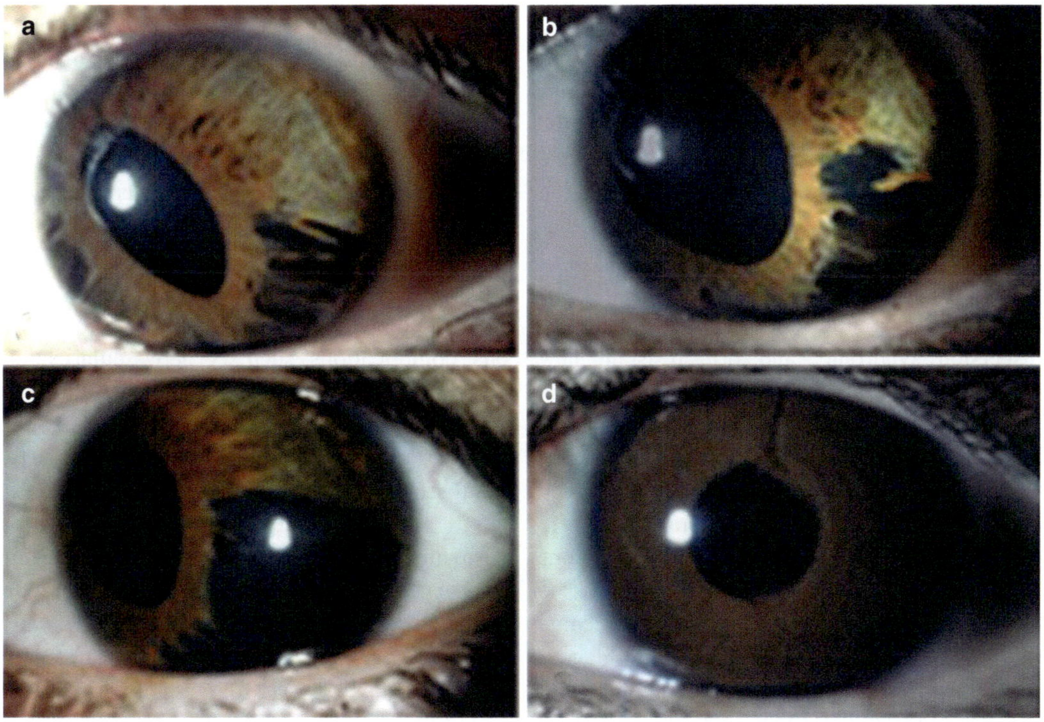

Fig. 31.3 (**a**): Frontal image obtained with a slit-lamp biomicroscope of the essential iris atrophy. (**b**): Second visit, 3 months later (larger irregular pupil and more atrophic areas). (**c**): Third visit, 3 months later (typical polycoria and corectopia). (**d**): Postoperative visit, 3 days after femtosecond-assisted KTP

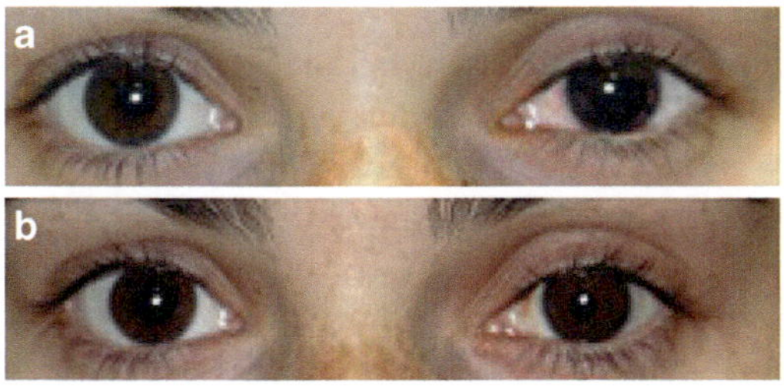

Fig. 31.4 (**a**): Binocular cosmetic appearance before surgery. (**b**): Binocular cosmetic appearance 3 months after surgery

disappeared completely. No intraoperative or postoperative adverse events were seen during the follow-up. Three months after the procedure, the CDVA was 20/20 and complete elimination of photophobia and diplopia was achieved with an excellent cosmetic result (Fig. 31.4a, b). Follow-up of 12 months was unremarkable.

Discussion

For conventional surgical approaches to correct aniridia, intraocular surgical devices such as the Morcher (Morcher, Germany) iris IOL implants and the Ophtec BV implants (Ophtec, Schweitzerlad) offer correction for aniridia. However, they require a large corneal incision (150–180°) and the iris color is pure black in Morcher iris implants and just provides 3 types of colors in the Ophtec BV implants, which is not ideal cosmetically. However, the newest foldable REPER implant (Reper-NN, Russia) does not need a large corneal incision as it is a foldable implant, and it provides more colors with better cosmetic results. One of the postoperative complications that are related to devising implantation is the rotation of the occlude paddle [8].

It is important to take into consideration, although good functional and cosmetic outcomes were reported for prosthetic iris [9], the complications associated with the implantation of the artificial iris are a concern [9–12]. Severe complications are classified as severe dislocation of artificial iris with the necessity of surgical revision and refixation of the implant, formation of posterior synechiae requiring synechiolysis, severe ocular hypertension with severe pigment dispersion syndrome, and drug-resistant new onset of glaucoma, which requires shunt surgery with glaucoma valves [13]. Corneal decompensation, which needed lamellar or perforating keratoplasty, and the retinal detachment, which needed vitrectomy, are also reported as severe complications. Other less severe complications are sutures cutting through the residual iris tissue forming a secondary pupil, the onset of glaucoma that could be controlled with topical antiglaucomatous medication, and the formation of cystoid macular edema requiring intravitreal steroid treatment. Transient ocular hypotension after surgery is also reported in some cases. Recurrent bleeding, stable artificial iris deviation, and capsular fibrosis are other complications. Furthermore, loosening of the sutures can cause a dislocation. The reasons for the early subluxations were pre-existing scars, synechiae, adhesions at the implantation site, or loose structures resulting from any previous trauma. This may lead to unstable artificial iris fixation. Exemplary, postoperative eye movement or gravity can force the artificial iris to leave its intended position, forming a "slide-off phenomenon." In some cases, the artificial iris tilts to one side of the suture axis heading toward the vitreous with the risk of causing severe mechanical retinal damage.

Regarding artificial iris implantation, Bonnet et al. studied the preliminary safety and efficacy of custom silicone artificial iris implantation in 19 eyes, one year after implantation. They found very mixed safety data in 19 eyes. Eight eyes experienced postoperative complications. There were 4 IOP elevations, 2 corneal decompensations, 1 case of cystoid macular edema, and 1 device dislocation. Four eyes underwent secondary surgical interventions including 2 adverse events (1 glaucoma surgery, 1 device dislocation) [14].

Therapeutic and cosmetic keratopigmentation has been successfully utilized and reported in different cases of iris defects with lower complication rate such as early post-op light sensitivity, which resolves automatically in around 90% of cases in 6 months postoperatory and then color fading and change in color and some more serious complications such as neovascularization and visual field limitations [13]. Its use can be combined with the implant of the intraocular lens as described in this report. Previously, femtosecond-assisted corneal KTP has been proposed for the treatment of opaque corneas for cosmetic purposes as well [15–17]. Based on our experience using cosmetic keratopigmentation either for cosmetic or therapeutic purposes, this therapeutic approach has been demonstrated to be safe during a 10-year follow-up [5, 6, 18, 19].

D'Oria et al., in a study showed the safety and effectivity of this surgical approach in a group of 79 eyes of 40 patients, femtosecond-laser-assisted intrastromal keratopigmentation was performed in 39 patients, and superficial automated keratopigmentation in 1 patient. The follow-up time was between 6 and 69 months (mean follow-up was 29 months). Patient satisfaction was excellent, respectively, in 90% and 92.5% of cases. After the retreatments in just 9 cases, all the patients were satisfied with the cosmetic aspect [18].

Balgos et al. also from our clinical research group confirmed good cosmetic results of combined corneal KTP with strabismus correction surgery for patients with corneal scarring and strabismus in a total of 72 consecutive patients and 73 eyes with the mean follow-up time of 2.5 ± 3 years. Cosmesis was good for all patients, even in those who required repeat KTPG or strabismus surgery, or in those whom orthotropia was not totally restored [7].

In this report, we show cases of traumatic aniridia as examples of the applicability of KTP for the restoration of functional problems created by iris defects as a combination approach with IOL scleral fixation [7]. In our cases, femtosecond-assisted KTP proved to be effective in solving patient's visual symptoms while providing excellent cosmetic results. KTP also would be an appropriate therapeutic approach for severe symptomatic iatrogenic aniridia.

In summary, the femtosecond-assisted KTP technique combined with scleral IOL fixation could be a good solution for the functional eye disability related to congenital, and traumatic aniridia as a combination treatment with scleral fixated IOL implant.

This technique aims to provide a surgical alternative to the intraocular iris implants, especially for those cases where such iris implants, with or without combined IOL optic, are not available. Femtosecond-assisted KTP offers a surgically straightforward technique to restore iris function and cosmetics, requiring a short learning curve and low complication rate.

Take Home Message

Therapeutic keratopigmentation is an acceptable therapeutic approach for traumatic aniridia with or without aphakia with a low complication rate. This technique aims to provide a surgical alternative to the intraocular iris implants, especially for those cases where such iris implants, with or without combined IOL optic, are not available. Femtosecond-assisted KTP offers a surgically straightforward innovative accessible alternative approach to the already proposed surgical techniques for the correction of these complex situations to restore iris function and cosmetics.

References

1. Weissbart SB, Ayres BD. Management of aniridia and iris defects: an update on iris prosthesis options. Curr Opin Ophthalmol. 2016;27(3):244–9.
2. Mavrikakis I, Mavrikakis E, Syam PP, Bell J, Casey JH, Casswell AG, Brittain GP, Liu C. Surgical management of iris defects with prosthetic iris devices. Eye (Lond). 2005;19(2):205–9.
3. Rickmann A, Szurman P, Januschowski K, Waizel M, Spitzer MS, Boden KT, Szurman GB. Long-term results after artificial iris implantation in patients with aniridia. Graefes Arch Clin Exp Ophthalmol. 2016;254(7):1419–24.
4. Alió JL, Rodriguez AE, Toffaha BT, Piñero DP, Moreno LJ. Femtosecond-assisted keratopigmentation for functional and cosmetic restoration in essential iris atrophy. J Cataract Refract Surg. 2011;37:1744–7.
5. Alio JL, Sirerol B, Walewska-Szafran A, et al. Corneal tattooing (keratopigmentation) with new mineral micronised pigments to restore cosmetic appearance in severely impaired eyes. Br J Ophthalmol. 2010;94:245–9.
6. Alio JL, Al-Shymali O, Amesty MA, Rodriguez AE. Keratopigmentation with micronised mineral pigments: complications and outcomes in a series of 234 eyes. Br J Ophthalmol. 2018;102:742–7.
7. Balgos JD, Amesty MA, Rodriguez AE, Al-Shymali O, Abumustafa S, Alio JL. Keratopigmentation combined with strabismus surgery to restore cosmesis in eyes with disabling corneal scarring and squint. Br J Ophthalmol. 2020;104(6):785–9.
8. Date RC, Olson MD, Shah M, Masket S, Miller KM. Outcomes of a modified capsular tension ring with a single black occluder paddle for eyes with congenital and acquired iris defects: report 2. J Cataract Refract Surg. 2015;41(9):1934–44.
9. Koch KR, Heindl LM, Cursiefen C, Koch HR. Artificial iris devices: benefits, limitations, and management of complications. J Cataract Refract Surg. 2014;40(3):376–82.
10. Mayer CS, Reznicek L, Hoffmann AE. Pupillary reconstruction and outcome after artificial iris implantation. Ophthalmology. 2016;123(5):1011–8.
11. Rickmann A, Szurman P, Januschowski K, et al. Long-term results after artificial iris implantation in patients with aniridia. Graefes Arch Clin Exp Ophthalmol. 2016;254(7):1419–24. *Ophthalmology = Albrecht von Graefes Archiv fur klinische und experimentelle Ophthalmologie*. 2016;254(7):1419–1424.
12. Spitzer MS, Nessmann A, Wagner J, et al. Customized humanoptics silicone iris prosthesis in eyes with post-traumatic iris loss: outcomes and complications. Acta Ophthalmol. 2016;94(3):301–6.
13. Forlini C, Forlini M, Rejdak R, et al. Simultaneous correction of post-traumatic aphakia and aniridia with the use of artificial iris and IOL implantation. Graefes Arch Clin Exp Ophthalmol. 2013;251(3):667–75.
14. Bonnet C, Miller KM. Safety and efficacy of custom foldable silicone artificial iris implantation: prospective compassionate-use case series. J Cataract Refract Surg. 2020;46(6):893–901.
15. Kim J-H, Lee D, Hahn T-W, Choi S-K. New surgical strategy for corneal tattooing using a femtosecond laser. Cornea. 2009;28:80–4.
16. Kymionis GD, Ide T, Galor A, Yoo SH. Femtosecond-assisted anterior lamellar corneal staining-tattooing in a blind eye with leukocoria. Cornea. 2009;28:211–3.
17. Alio JL, Rodriguez AE, Toffaha BT, El Aswad A. Femtosecond-assisted keratopigmentation double

tunnel technique in the management of a case of Urrets-Zavalia syndrome. Cornea. 2012;31(9):1071–4.
18. D'Oria F, Alio JL, Rodriguez AE, Amesty MA, Abu-Mustafa SK. Cosmetic Keratopigmentation in sighted eyes: medium- and long-term clinical evaluation. Cornea 2020. 29.
19. Alio JL, Al-Shymali O, Amesty MA, et al. Keratopigmentation with micronised mineral pigments: complications and outcomes in a series of 234 eyes. Br J Ophthalmol. 2018;102:742–7.

32 Cataract Surgery in the Traumatized Anterior Segment

Victoria Liu, Siddharth Nath, and George H. H. Beiko

Bullet Points

- The risk of amblyopia in young children following traumatic cataract remains a concern; however, staged cataract surgery followed by aggressive amblyopia therapy may still be a feasible option leading to good visual outcomes (issue of interest: Timing to surgical repair in children, combatting amblyopia).
- Ocular Trauma Scores may help to predict visual outcomes following open- and closed-globe trauma in both adults and children; however, there is limited difference in visual outcomes following primary and secondary intervention and varying findings regarding visual outcome following repair after open-globe and closed-globe trauma (issue of interest: predicting visual outcomes).
- Causes of injury vary based on population affected and may have cultural associations. In the adult population, blunt globe trauma tends to be more prevalent and this may be associated with specific complications and management consideration (damage to angle structures) (issue of interest: causes of injury).
- Trauma to the anterior segment and capsular support proves challenging for many surgeons. Choice for fixation of

Supplementary Information The online version contains supplementary material available at [https://doi.org/10.1007/978-3-030-94530-5_32].

V. Liu
University of Ottawa Eye Institute, Ottawa Hospital Research Institute, University of Ottawa, Ottawa, ON, Canada

Division of Ophthalmology, Department of Surgery, Faculty of Health Sciences, McMaster University, Hamilton, ON, Canada
e-mail: Victoria.liu@medportal.ca

S. Nath
Department of Ophthalmology and Visual Sciences, McGill University, Montréal, Québec, Canada
e-mail: Siddharth.nath@medportal.ca

G. H. H. Beiko (✉)
Division of Ophthalmology, Department of Surgery, Faculty of Health Sciences, McMaster University, Hamilton, ON, Canada

Department of Ophthalmology and Vision Sciences, University of Toronto, Toronto, ON, Canada

J. L. Alió et al. (eds.), *Cataract Surgery*, Essentials in Ophthalmology,
https://doi.org/10.1007/978-3-030-94530-5_32

the intraocular lens may vary based on the support available, and this may augment visual outcomes and complication rates. Capsular tension rings may be a useful device when lacking zonular support and may be used in cases of severe zonulolysis (greater than 6 clock hours) and zonular dialysis with success (issue of interest: IOL implantation).
- Unconventional techniques including the use of femtosecond laser for the creation of capsulorhexis, or vitrector for the creation of a vitrectorhexis, can be included in management options for the cataract surgeon (issue of interest: Unconventional techniques).

Definitions

Open- Versus Closed-Globe Injury

The Birmingham Eye Trauma Terminology System, which was developed in 1996 (Fig. 32.1), is a standardized system used to define ocular trauma [1]. It defines ocular traumatology terms including eye wall, closed-globe injury, open-globe injury, rupture, laceration, penetrating injury, intraocular foreign body (IOFB) injury, and perforating injury [1]. This terminology has been used extensively in studies undertaken in the last decade, and these definitions will be used throughout this chapter.

Closed-globe injuries are categorized into zones based on the anatomic location of injury (Fig. 32.2a) [2]. Zone I injuries are limited to the bulbar conjunctiva, sclera, or cornea and can include but are not limited to corneal abrasions or foreign bodies [2]. Zone II involves other structures in the anterior segment; [2] this may include the lens and zonules. Zone III injuries are the most posterior and may involve the retina, vitreous, or optic nerve [2].

In open-globe injuries, zones of injury are classified according to the location of the most posterior full-thickness globe opening (Fig. 32.2b) [2]. Zone 1 injuries are full-thickness cornea or corneoscleral limbus openings; zone II openings involve the anterior 5 mm of the sclera, at the area of the pars plana; and zone III includes openings that are more than 5 mm posterior to the corneoscleral limbus [2]. Zone III injuries include injuries to the retina and posterior segment.

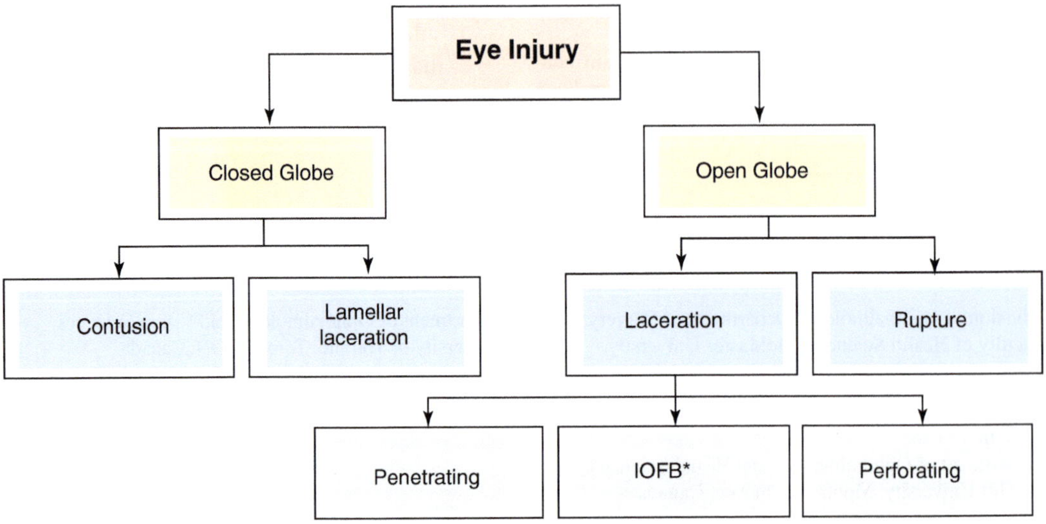

Fig. 32.1 Ocular trauma classification using the Birmingham Eye Trauma Terminology System [1]
*Intraocular foreign body (IOFB)
Adapted from: Classification of injury types: Kuhn et al. [1]

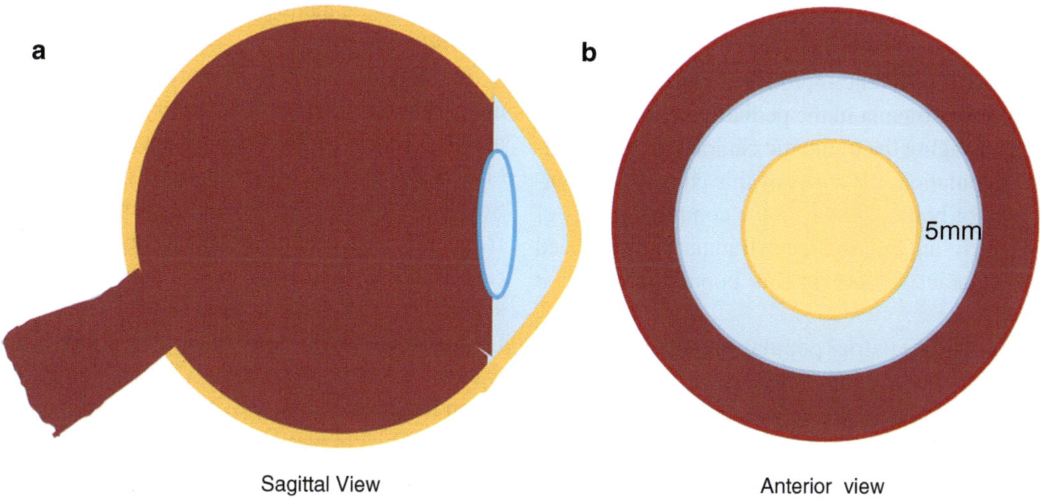

Fig. 32.2 Ocular trauma zones in closed- and open-globe trauma [2]. (**a**): Zones of injury in closed-globe trauma. Zone I (yellow): external injury to the bulbar conjunctiva, sclera, or cornea. Zone II (blue): anterior segment injury including the posterior lens capsule and pars plicata. Zone III (red): injury to posterior segment structures including the optic nerve and retina. (**b**): Zones of injury in open-globe trauma. Zone I: penetrating wounds to the cornea (yellow). Zone II (blue): full-thickness wounds to the sclera from the limbus to 5 mm posteriorly. Zone III (red): full-thickness wound posterior to 5 mm from the limbus. (Adapted from: Pieramici et al. [2])

Interventions for Traumatic Cataract: Primary Versus Secondary Procedure Timing

Options for the management of traumatic cataracts include the following: primary wound closure from a penetrating injury, primary lensectomy with intraocular lens (IOL) implantation, primary lensectomy without IOL implantation, secondary surgery with lensectomy and IOL implantation following primary closure, and secondary IOL implantation following primary lensectomy. In a review of the literature from the last 10 years, many studies did not define the timing interval between primary and secondary surgery. Definitions of early secondary surgery varied between within 72 hours of primary wound closure for vitrectomy, or within 1–8 weeks following the primary closure of a penetrating injury for secondary cataract surgery with IOL implantation [3–5]. For the purposes of this chapter, secondary interventions will be categorized into early (less than 1 week) or late (greater than 1 week) from primary wound closure or primary surgery, if specified.

Traumatic Cataract Surgery in the Pediatric Population

Pediatric

For the purposes of this chapter, the term "pediatric patients" will refer to all individuals under the age of 18, similar to the definition of age included in the literature related to pediatric cataract management. Traumatic cataracts, especially if accompanied by delayed cataract surgery, pose the risk of visual deprivation for children. The critical period for the development of amblyopia (amblyogenic age) is usually defined as up until 7–8 years of age; thus, this may lead to different intervention choices due to higher risk for the development of amblyopia in younger children [6]. Some recommendations for cataract intervention acknowledge the amblyogenic age; however, they suggest similar interventions to prevent amblyopia in older children as well. For example, one study recommends the induction of amblyopia therapy in a timely manner for children even older than 8 years [7]. This will be commented on throughout the chapter.

Causes of Pediatric Ocular Trauma

Although different approaches exist for managing ocular trauma in the pediatric population and for managing the traumatic cataract in the pediatric population, the focus of this chapter is a synthesis of both – exploring the common causes of pediatric anterior segment trauma and the need for cataract surgery in this population when it arises.

In the pediatric population, ocular trauma tends to occur more frequently in males, at a male-to-female ratio as high as 12:1; other studies have reported lower ratios of 5:1 and 4:1 [7–9]. This ratio decreases significantly with age [8]. A majority of studies demonstrate that most ocular traumatic cataracts present unilaterally [7, 10]. Traumatic cataracts can occur in children of all ages; however, in children of a young age, lack of adult supervision has been found to contribute to an increased incidence of ocular trauma [11].

Socioeconomic factors of ocular injuries have been studied in populations in India. Results from one clinic in New Delhi found that ocular injuries affect middle class (70%) and rural populations (58%) most commonly, whereas results from a tertiary care center in Western India determined that 74.5% of injuries occurred in those of lower socioeconomic status, and 92% were from rural areas [9, 12].

The causes of injury differ depending on country or region and may have cultural associations. Many studies focusing on the Indian population found that the most common cause of traumatic ocular injuries was a wooden stick or wooden splinters, and bow and arrow [12, 13]. Although wooden splinters accounted for a large number of penetrating injuries (30.8%) in a study in Northern India, it was found that the use of firecrackers was the most common cause of closed-globe injuries (34.3%) [13]. Cultural associations might explain the trends in the causes of injury. Dussehra and Diwali are Indian festivals where children commonly play with burning firecrackers, and bow and arrows, agents that can lead to ocular trauma [13]. One study reported that a common mode of injury was also "Gulli danda," a game played with wooden sticks by children in India [7].

In Shanghai, it has been reported that the most frequent causes of injury were sharp metal objects (40.2%), followed by toys (16.5%) and then wooden sticks (11.2%) [8]. Scissors, needles, and knives were the most frequently encountered sharp objects. With respect to toys, toy bullets, plastic toys, and slingshots were most frequently cited [8]. Likewise, a study set in Victoria, Australia, found that sharp pointed objects including sharp metal, scissors, knives, glass bottles, and wooden objects were the most common causes of penetrating ocular trauma [11].

In a study from the Children's hospital in Colorado, the majority of ocular trauma was peer-inflicted (68%): 18% of ocular trauma was chronic self-injury and 14.5% was a single self-inflicted event [10]. All of the cases with chronic self-injurious cataracts (eleven) had a diagnosis of autism spectrum disorder, chromosomal imbalances, developmental delay, or intellectual disability [10]. The mechanisms of injury reported from most prevalent to least prevalent included: chronic self- hitting (18%), knife (10%), BB gun (10%), and stick (8%) [10].

Open Eye Injuries with Traumatic Cataracts

The timing of traumatic cataract extraction and IOL implantation is highly debated in the literature. There are many advantages and disadvantages to immediate repair and late repair of open eye injuries with traumatic cataracts. In addition, there is no agreement on which procedures are most effective at reducing complication rates.

The options for surgical intervention for pediatric traumatic cataracts after open-globe injuries include the following: primary wound closure from a penetrating injury, primary lensectomy with IOL implantation, primary lensectomy without IOL implantation, secondary surgery with lensectomy and IOL implantation following primary closure, and secondary IOL implantation following primary lensectomy.

Closure with Primary Lensectomy

The argument used in the literature to recommend primary lensectomy if the anterior capsule is breached is that lens material may leak into the anterior chamber, leading to inflammation and/or increased intraocular pressure (IOP) [3, 4, 14, 15]. Furthermore, lens retention and elevated IOP may increase the risk of endophthalmitis [15]. However, a retrospective study by Yardley et Al. in 2017 found that out of 106 patients with ocular trauma, deferring lensectomy, and/or IOL placement after initial globe repair, did not negatively affect outcomes or complication rates including glaucoma and inflammation [16]. Five percent of children developed glaucoma, while three percent needed surgical glaucoma management [16]. It should be remembered that increased IOP in these cases may also be a result of the initial trauma causing angle recession [17].

Immediate Repair – Primary Closure with Lensectomy and IOL Placement

It is unclear in open-globe trauma whether primary wound closure with primary lensectomy and IOL implantation should be performed, or if primary closure with lensectomy should be followed by a deferred secondary IOL implantation.

In the older literature, some studies have supported primary IOL implantation at the time of corneal repair [17–19]. Advantages to this approach include the avoidance of multiple operations with general anesthesia, and faster visual rehabilitation to prevent the development of amblyopia, provided that it is anticipated that the visual prognosis is good [3].

However, in the more recent literature, a retrospective case series including 139 patients with corneal lacerations, primary globe repair with IOL implantation versus secondary IOL implantation was compared [15]. Options for surgical treatment were determined by the degree of trauma and the size of corneal lacerations [15]. In eyes with appropriate visualization, smaller corneal lacerations (<5.0 mm), or large peripheral lacerations not involving the cornea, primary IOL implantation was performed, and found to have good visual outcomes [15]. Of the 61 patients (49%) that received primary closure, lensectomy, and IOL implantation, 30 achieved a corrected distance visual acuity (CDVA) of 20/40 or better, whereas 47 of 78 patients (60%), who received secondary IOL implantation, achieved a CDVA of 20/40 or better. For patients in both groups who did not achieve a CDVA of better than 20/40, the visual outcomes were otherwise similar [15].

Thus, primary IOL implantation at the time of repair can decrease the risk of developing amblyopia or strabismus due to high anisometropia, and overcome the delay for visual rehabilitation [15]. However, other studies by Hilely et al. and Yardley et al., demonstrated that the interval between trauma and IOL implantation was independent of visual outcome for both open- and closed-globe traumas [16, 20].

Therefore, although primary IOL implantation provided good visual outcome, delaying the surgery if indicated due to the presenting circumstances would not compromise the final outcome [16, 20].

Late Repair, Staged Procedures

There is currently no consensus on the optimal time gap between primary closure and secondary cataract extraction in pediatric ocular trauma [3]. In adults, staged procedures, which may take up to 4 months, can ensure stabilization of the globe [3]. A lengthy time period to ensure globe integrity is not acceptable for children due to the risk of developing amblyopia [3]. One recent study investigated visual and refractive outcomes after secondary cataract extraction 1–8 weeks (mean 5 weeks) after primary corneal wound repair in the pediatric age group after penetrating open-globe trauma [3]. Seventy-six percent of eyes in the study achieved a best corrected visual acuity (BCVA) of 20/40 or better [3]. Final refraction in the eyes varied; however, mean postoperative spherical equivalent was −1.80 diopters (D), and 54% of eyes had a refractive outcome of less than

1.00 D from emmetropia [3]. This study considered the time to secondary repair at a shortened interval, and did not experience a high degree of amblyopia in their population, mostly related to aggressive visual rehabilitation and management [3]. The most common long-term postoperative complication with this management strategy was posterior capsular opacification in approximately 40% of patients.

Studies by Yardley et al. and Hilely et al., found no difference in visual outcome of open-globe trauma with increased intervals between trauma and IOL implantation [16, 20]. These studies recommend that secondary, or staged, IOL implantation may increase stability of the globe, improve surgical view, and allow for accurate biometry measurements for IOL implantation [16].

Certain patients may benefit from staged surgery with secondary IOL implantation. Cases with posterior segment pathology are better candidates for staged procedures as the visual prognosis is unknown upon initial wound repair [15]. One study achieved good visual outcome from staged surgery in eyes with large lacerations (>5.0 mm), central corneal involvement, poor visualization, or other anterior or posterior segment conditions that may have provided complications during surgery, including retinal detachments, vitreous hemorrhage, endophthalmitis, or intraocular foreign bodies [15].

Anterior and posterior reconstruction may include the removal of blood from the anterior chamber, reconstruction of the iris, removal of lenticular remnants, foreign body removal, retinotomies, and laser treatments [4]. Although primary internal reconstruction may be performed, for complex open-globe injuries, internal reconstruction is usually delayed as a secondary procedure 7–10 days after trauma when the risk of intraoperative hemorrhage is reduced [4].

Challenges of pediatric cataract surgery, and management of pediatric cataracts, includes choosing the appropriate IOL power [16]. In cases of ocular trauma, this challenge is further increased by difficulties such as a hypotony, corneal lacerations that result in unreliable biometric measurements, or refractive surprise when biometry from the contralateral eye is used as an estimate [15]. A secondary IOL implantation may provide the benefit of more accurate preoperative biometry measurements and calculation of IOL powers [3, 16].

Closed Eye Injuries with Traumatic Cataracts

As with injuries to the open eye, techniques for repair of traumatic cataracts induced from closed eye injuries are varied and include primary surgery with lensectomy and IOL implantation (classified as "immediate repair") or primary lensectomy with secondary IOL implantation (classified as "late repair"). Within the literature, there remains less debate about timing of lens implantation as closed eye injuries are overall more manageable. In fact, Yardley et al. have shown that in patients with closed-globe trauma, there is no difference in visual outcomes when comparing timing of IOL placement following lensectomy [16].

Closed eye injuries are typically easier to manage than open -globe injuries. Blunt trauma to the eye may be managed conservatively initially, by medical intervention to stabilize IOP and reduce inflammation, and then completion of lensectomy and IOL placement in a single surgery. In a study of 100 children, Ram et al. obtained favorable visual outcomes with this approach, and visual rehabilitation was often better following blunt trauma in comparison to penetrating traumatic injuries [13].

When considering placement of an IOL following closed eye injuries, the literature suggests that in-the-bag placement is more commonly achievable following blunt trauma [12, 21]. In a study of 14 closed eye injuries by Khokhar et al., a significant majority of blunt traumatic injuries allowed for in-the-bag placement of an IOL, while penetrating injuries required IOL placement into the ciliary sulcus [12]. IOL placement remains an important consideration when managing the traumatic cataract as sulcus or bag-sulcus positioning of an IOL can increase the potential for iris chafing and uveitis-glaucoma-hyphema (UGH) syndrome [22, 23].

Special Techniques

Noted in the literature are special techniques used in the management of pediatric traumatic cataracts.

A surgical technique called "optic buttonholing" is recommended in traumatic cataracts where there is capsular support but the IOL cannot be implanted in the capsular bag. The haptics are placed in the sulcus, and the optic is positioned posterior to the capsular remnants. Sen. et al. found this approach to be advantageous in secondary IOL implantation if scarring and fusion of the anterior and posterior capsule existed [15]. This technique allowed for stabilization of the IOL when placed in the sulcus, and prevented decentration and posterior capsular opacification [15].

A banded technique was described in a 2019 study by Chowdhary and Nischal in situations where part of the anterior capsule had been ruptured [24]. The approach as described aims to reduce or prevent pupil-lens capture and decentration of the IOL [24]. Two microvitreoretinal blade stab incisions are made at the limbus entering the anterior chamber at 100 degrees apart [24]. The anterior chamber is filled with an ophthalmic viscosurgical device, and the anterior capsule is stained using trypan blue 0.06% solution [24]. In the area of the intact anterior capsule, a capsulorhexis is created using 2 incision push-pull techniques [24]. The vitrector, without cutter, is used to aspirate lens material [24]. A 2-incision push pull capsulorhexis is also created in the posterior capsule, and then an anterior vitrectomy is performed. The results of this technique include a smaller anterior capsulorhexis, and band between the newly created capsulorhexis and anterior capsule tear [24]. This technique was used in 5 children, and no yttrium aluminum garnet (YAG) capsulotomy was needed for the band. The banded technique was successful in keeping the IOL posterior, and away from the iris [24]. An image of this technique in surgery is shown in Fig. 32.3.

The use of intracameral triamcinolone injections has been evaluated in a prospective study from 2016. In children, with an average age of 6, authors compared the use of subconjunctival injection of gentamicin and dexamethasone 4 mg, with postoperative prednisolone drops, cycloplegic and antibiotic drops, versus this regimen plus the use of an intracameral triamcinolone acetonide injection [25]. It was found that triamcinolone decreased inflammation in the anterior segment, including reduced cellular

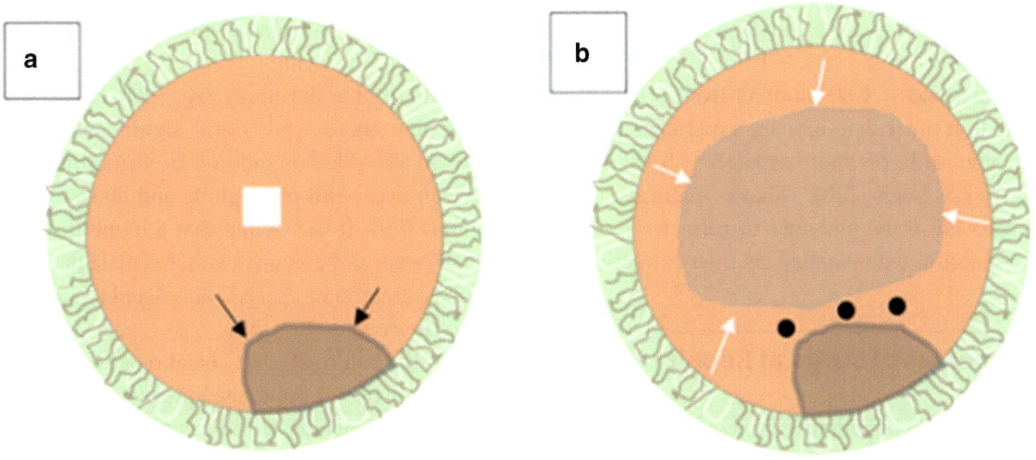

Fig. 32.3 Banded technique for cases of anterior capsule rupture in traumatic cataract surgery [24]. (**a**): Anterior capsule tear (black arrows). Intact anterior capsule (white square). (**b**): Anterior capsulorhexis created (white arrows), with "band" between anterior capsular tear and capsulorhexis (black dots). (Adapted from: Chowdhary ans Nischal [24])

deposits, reduced posterior synechiae and reduced visual axis obscuration for children with previous surgery for traumatic cataracts [25]. It is important to note that all children in the study had an anterior vitrectomy and primary posterior capsulotomy (PPC) at the time of surgery, and none of the children in the study had significant elevation of IOP post-operatively [25].

Special Concerns

Choosing the IOL power in repair of ocular trauma is difficult in the setting of adults and provides even greater challenges in the pediatric population. As previously discussed, performing biometric measurements on the affected eye prior to IOL implantation is a benefit of a staged procedure. In cases where this is not possible, studies have measured the fellow or unaffected eye to estimate the IOL power needed with varying success [15, 16, 26].

Specifically, in the pediatric population, IOL calculations are further complicated by the dynamic growth of the eye, especially in infancy [27]. A study involving 83 eyes of 81 infants and children, with 32 cataracts as a result of trauma, found that a myopic shift occurs following IOL implantation in pediatric patients [28]. This shift is greater in the younger age group and over a 2–3-year time period approximates −3.00 diopters from 0 to 2 years, −1.5 diopters from 2 to 6 years, and − 1.80 diopters from 6 to 8 years. Children older than 8 years experienced a mean myopic shift of approximately −0.38 diopters over 1.8 years [28]. These findings can be employed in the planning of refractive outcome for children with planned cataract extraction.

Outcomes of Surgical Repair

The majority of pediatric eyes in both penetrating and blunt eye trauma can achieve significant visual gain after repair and visual rehabilitation [12, 13, 29]. Closed or blunt eye trauma has been found to have better visual outcomes after repair as compared to open eye or penetrating injuries [8, 13, 16, 29]. A study by Ram et al. compared visual outcomes of children with traumatic cataracts suffering blunt trauma and those suffering perforating globe injuries and found that 57.62% of the penetrating trauma group had a best corrected visual acuity (BCVA) of ≥20/40, whereas a BCVA of ≥20/40 was achieved in 71.42% of the eyes in the blunt trauma group [13]. Amblyopia was found as a complication of almost 30% of patients in both groups [13]. The difference in visual outcomes was thought to be associated with factors including corneal scarring, posterior synechiae contributing to optic capture of the PCIOL and complications in the eyes with penetrating trauma [13]. Shah et al. reported a smaller magnitude of significant difference in the two groups with BCVA >20/60 in 55.3% of open-globe eyes, and 56.3% in closed-globe groups [29]. However, BCVA between 20/40 and 20/20 was achieved by 41.7% of patients in the closed-globe groups versus 33.8% of patients in the open-globe group [29]. Similarly, Yardley et Al. reported a CDVA of 20/40 or better among 63% of closed-globe injuries and 38% of patients with open-globe injuries [16]. This study noted an amblyopia complication rate in approximately 40% of children, which may have been due to the inclusion of younger children [16]. Other studies reported no significant differences in visual acuity between the open-globe and closed-globe groups following surgical intervention [7, 12, 30].

Furthermore, the study by Shah et al. also found that there were other significant differences in variables in addition to visual outcome between eyes with open-globe and closed-globe traumas [29]. It was found that a higher proportion of open-globe injuries affected male patients, involved trauma in Zones 2 and 3 and resulted in two or more surgeries [29].

It is difficult to predict visual outcomes based on the statistics as previously presented. Cataract formation in ocular trauma can impede visual acuity; however, other structures in the eye can also be damaged during trauma, leading to poorer visual outcomes. In adults, the ocular trauma score (OTS) has been used as a predictor of visual outcomes after ocular trauma [31, 32]. The score developed by the Ocular Trauma Classification Group, Kuhn et al., includes the initial visual acuity post trauma, as well as comorbidities at presentation including globe rupture, endophthalmitis, perforating injury, retinal detachment, or relative afferent pupillary defect [32, 33]. The OTS has a predictive accuracy of approximately 80% [33].

The calculation method and estimated visual outcomes of the OTS are shown in Tables 32.1 and 32.2. Using Table 32.1, for example, an individual presenting with a globe rupture and vision of 20/80 would have a score of 90–23 = 67. Inputting this score into Table 32.2 would predict a 44% chance for a vision of 20/40 or better at 6 months.

Table 32.1 Ocular trauma score (Kuhn et al., [32]). Deriving the OTS [34]

Variables at Presentation	Points
A: Visual Acuity	NLP[a] = 60
	LP[b] or HM[c] = 70
	1/200 to 19/200 = 80
	20/200 to 20/50 = 90
	≥ 20/40 = 100
B: Globe Rupture	– 23
C: Endophthalmitis	– 17
D: Perforating Injury	– 14
E: Retinal Detachment	– 11
F: Relative Afferent Pupillary Defect (RAPD)	– 10
Total = Sum of Points	

Table adapted from: Unver et al. [34]
[a]*NLP* No Light Perception
[b]*LP* Light perception
[c]*HM* Hand Motion

Previously, this score was used in adults; however, a 2012 study evaluated its use in the pediatric population [31]. In this study, certain conditions for repair were met, including eyes needing corneal wound repair that had IOL implantation during a secondary procedure; hazy ocular medium requiring a pars plana vitrectomy and capsulectomy; children younger than 2 years had secondary IOL implantation after the age of 2; all children were rehabilitated by an orthoptist for amblyopia therapy; and any further strabismus therapy was provided by a pediatric ophthalmologist if needed [31]. The predicted OTS calculated at the initial presentation was found to be a reliable predictor of final visual outcomes in traumatic cataract cases in children [31].

The pediatric ocular trauma score (POTS) was developed and validated in 2016 by Shah et al., and found to be a more sensitive and specific score to predict visual outcomes of pediatric ocular trauma with traumatic cataract [9]. The proposed POTS added 2 additional variables to the initial OTS as shown in Table 32.3.

Table 32.3 Additional variables for the pediatric ocular trauma score (POTS) [9]

Additional Variables at Presentation	Points
G: Age (years)	0 – 5 = – 10
	6 – 10 = – 7
	11 – 15 = – 5
H: Wound location	Zone I = 0
	Zone II = – 5
	Zone III= –10

Table adapted from: Shah et al. [9]

Table 32.2 Six-month follow-up visual acuity probabilities based on the OTS [32]

Total Points	OTS Score	Estimated Follow-up Visual Acuity at 6 months				
		NLP[a]	LP[b]/HM[c]	1/200 to 19/200	20/200 to 20/50	≥ 20/40
0 – 44	1	73%	17%	7%	2%	1%
45 – 65	2	28%	26%	18%	13%	15%
66 – 80	3	2%	11%	15%	28%	44%
81 – 91	4	1%	2%	2%	21%	74%
92 – 100	5	0%	1%	2%	5%	92%

Table adapted from: Kuhn et al. [32]
[a]*NLP* No Light Perception
[b]*LP* Light perception
[c]*HM* Hand Motion

Complications and Other Ocular Manifestations

Management of the traumatic cataract in the pediatric population is uniquely challenging not only because of the surgical approach, but also because of postoperative complications. In children, the most common and significant complications include amblyopia, posterior capsular opacification (PCO), and fibrinous uveitis. Other complications include retinal detachment, malignant glaucoma, and endophthalmitis. Complications occur at different time points in the postoperative period and differ in rates depending on the type of trauma sustained (blunt or penetrating) and the surgical approach implemented. Early complications and ocular manifestations include endophthalmitis, inflammatory reactions including fibrinous uveitis, and intraocular pressure increases, which can be sustained due to anterior segment structural damage. Corneal scarring, uveal prolapse, and other structural damage may complicate surgical management and compromise vision gain in the postoperative course. Amblyopia and PCO can be encountered as late complications in the pediatric population, although early visual rehabilitation and early interventions should be considered to lessen their burden. Retinal concerns including retinal detachment may occur during the trauma, surgical repair, and in the late postoperative period. These complications and ocular manifestations will be further discussed in the following paragraphs.

Structural Damage

Corneal involvement in penetrating trauma may complicate the course of repair; however, primary or secondary cataract extraction and IOL implantation may be possible in these situations. Postoperatively, corneal scarring may contribute to visual axis opacification, and astigmatism and refractive error among patients. Rates of corneal scarring in children have been noted to range from 9.5% to 28% [7, 13]; eyes with penetrating trauma were more often affected [13].

In the case of open-globe trauma, uveal prolapse presents an additional management consideration. A study of open-globe trauma found that 5 of 47 or 11% of children had associated uveal prolapse [3]. Similarly, Sen et al. found uveal tissue prolapse rate of approximately 57%, or 80/139 patients, following open-globe trauma. In the cases of closed-globe injuries, Khokhar et al. identified 56% of eyes with iris atrophy or distortion [12, 15]. In the context of primary closure, and subsequent cataract removal and IOL implantation, these iris issues require an additional management consideration [15].

Anterior capsule and posterior capsule tears may also occur with injury; it is important that surgeons are aware of these structural changes prior to surgery as they may increase the potential for ocular inflammation, compromise in-the-bag implantation of the IOL or increase the risk of intraoperative complications. Sen et al. found that anterior capsule tear and posterior capsule tear occurred in 70% and 25% of open-globe trauma, respectively, whereas lower rates of 15% anterior capsule rupture and 2–3% posterior capsule rupture (PCR) have been reported elsewhere [7, 13, 15]. Identification and implications of PCR are discussed later in the chapter.

Amblyopia

Amblyopia presents one of the most significant challenges following traumatic injury to the pediatric anterior segment as it may not reveal itself clinically until after the injury has happened. Rates of amblyopia following trauma remain variable, although in a study by Yardley et al., 39% of patients suffered from the complication, [16] and another study including 147 traumatic cataracts in the pediatric age group (under the age of 15) found that amblyopia therapy was needed in almost 30% of patients during follow-up [7]. In the latter study, the need for amblyopia therapy varied among age groups and included 51.21%, 26.02%, and 12.12% of patients in age groups 1–5, 6–10, and 11–15, respectively [7]. A higher-than-average rate may be due to the inclusion of a younger patient population, although the numbers presented in studies reinforce the need for urgent repair of the traumatic injury and aggressive management of refractive error to minimize the incidence amblyopia later in life, even in children older than 8 years [16].

Meier et al. also propose silicone oil tamponade as a predisposing factor for amblyopia [4].

Posterior Capsule Opacification

Of all complications following traumatic injury to the pediatric eye, posterior capsule opacification remains the most common. Within older literature, PCO is documented to occur in 21–100% of eyes post pediatric cataract surgery and presents a unique challenge as it may not be readily treatable in the clinic [13]. In a recent study regarding pediatric traumatic cataract, it was found that the rate of PCO was relatively similar between open- and closed-globe traumas at a rate of approximately 30% [13].

PCO is a cause of visual axis opacification (VAO), which may lead to vision deprivation and amblyopia if left untreated. VAO is more prevalent in children after ocular surgeries due to greater postoperative inflammation in this population [12]. As such, it is suggested that children of younger age receive a primary posterior continuous circular capsulorhexis (PCCC) with anterior vitrectomy during traumatic cataract surgery. In a study by Khokhar et al., children under the age of 6 received PCCC and 23-G anterior vitrectomy, leading to reduced rates of VAO following open-globe and closed-globe traumatic cataract surgeries at rates of 8.5% and 3.5%, respectively [12]. The VAO that occurred affected 12% of children between the ages of 6 and 10 years who had not received PCCC and anterior vitrectomy [12]. Thus, their study recommended performing PCCC until at least 10 years of age [12]. Another study taking place at a tertiary care center in northern India agreed that due to good outcomes in reducing VAO in children receiving PCCC and anterior vitrectomy, this approach may be recommended even in children older than 8 years if there is a posterior capsular plaque or thickening detected at the time of surgery [7]. Likewise, studies by Shah et al. and Jinagal et al. found that eyes having PCCC and anterior vitrectomy had better visual outcomes during follow-up [7, 29].

As children are not typically cooperative patients, PCO cannot be managed easily in the clinic with neodymium yttrium aluminum garnet (NdYAG) capsulotomy. Thus, given the potential for reduced visual rehabilitation and the difficulty in clinical management, there is consensus within the literature for primary capsulotomy and anterior vitrectomy in the pediatric population following traumatic injury requiring lensectomy and IOL placement.

Fibrinous Uveitis

Along with PCO, fibrinous uveitis is debated as being one of, if not the most common complication following lensectomy and IOL placement in the traumatized pediatric eye. In a study by Sen et al., fibrinous uveitis was observed to occur in 31% of patients following primary repair and IOL implantation and in 32% of patients following primary repair and secondary IOL placement [15]. Older literature finds rates as high as 40% following traumatic cataract surgery [13, 15]. The use of topical and systemic steroids may help to decrease the inflammatory response, especially in primary surgical repair following open-globe trauma [15].

Glaucoma

Trauma to the anterior segment may also result in glaucoma, postulated to be secondary to damage to the iridocorneal angle. This may create a pseudo-angle closure scenario in which intraocular pressure increases resulting in glaucomatous changes [4, 13]. Management of glaucoma in the postoperative setting should be sequential, beginning initially with topical medications and advancing to surgical intervention only if IOP remains uncontrolled [4]. Within the literature, surgical management largely involves conventional glaucoma surgeries and there is no evidence for the use of microinvasive glaucoma surgery (MIGS) in this population.

Other Complications

In addition to the above complications, cataract surgery in the traumatized pediatric eye may also be associated with strabismus, retinal detachment, or endophthalmitis. These complications are postulated to occur from heterogeneous mechanisms, both from the initial trauma and from iatrogenic injury encountered during the repair itself [10]. Management of such complications should follow the gold standard of care for repair of the specific pathology. Strabismus and retinal detachment may be managed by surgical repair and endophthalmitis should be aggressively treated with intravitreal antibiotics, or prophylactic antibiotics if the patient is deemed at high risk. This is further discussed later in the chapter. Within the literature, it is recommended that retina specialists be involved in management of retinal detachments early-on in the treatment of the traumatized pediatric eye as these cases require particular surgical planning and intervention [10].

Traumatic Cataract Surgery in the Adult Population

Causes of Injury

Ocular trauma and traumatic cataracts, especially open-globe injuries, have been found to affect male patients of younger ages [35, 36]. Also in agreement with this are studies of populations including parts of Nigeria, Northern India, Central China, Finland, Turkey, Australia, and United Arab Emirates (UAE), which found that males were more affected by ocular trauma and traumatic cataracts [35–42]. A study of penetrating ocular injury from Pakistan found that the male-to-female ratio was approximately 1.6:1 during the first decade of life, but increased to 10:1 after the first decade [38].

In higher age groups, age 15 years and older, there appears to be a greater incidence of blunt trauma, as compared to younger populations [35, 40]. In an elderly population in Nigeria, aged 65 and older, closed-globe injuries comprised the majority of injuries at 85.9%; the majority of these occurred on the farm, or at home [39]. A study set in India found that patients having traumatic cataracts tended to be from poor class (83%), and live in a rural area (94%); however, these demographic factors did not affect final visual outcomes [43]. Among all ages, the most common activities at the time of injury included playing (26.8%), house work (25.9%), and occupation related activities (18.9%) [43]. In a population of adults at a referral center in Mexico City, common causes included a blow (16.2%), rocket (7.5%), car accident (6.2%), or a metal rod or tube (6.2%) [44]. The majority of the traumatic events were described as being an "accident" in 23.8% of individuals, or occurred while working (13.8%), playing (7.5%), or fighting (7.5%) [44]. A Chinese study presented similar trends, with the most common agents of trauma being firecrackers (24.5%) and metal/knife/scissors (21.4%) [37]. The most common victims of ocular trauma were males aged 30–59 years, who typically were the breadwinners of the family; thus, their injury and absence from employment may contribute to the economic and psychological burden [37]. One study examining trends in the high-income developing country of the United Arab Emirates (UAE) in the city of Abu Dhabi found that the majority, or approximately 70 percent, of injuries in adults occurred at work, and only affected males, with only 13.9% of injuries occurring at home [42]. Sharp objects caused the majority of injuries [42].

Recent results from a tertiary referral center in Sydney, Australia, and another from Southern Finland provide insight into trends in the developed world. A retrospective case series of open-globe injuries over a 5-year period found that falls were the most common cause of open-globe injury in older aged individuals [36]. Across all age categories, working with metal was a common cause of both penetrating eye injuries and intraocular foreign bodies (IOFBs) and, thus, highlights the importance of wearing protective eyewear [36]. A moderate amount of cases were also associated with the use of alcohol, with 52%

of assault cases involving its use [36]. In the Finnish working-age population, open-globe injuries were predominantly caused by work tools, and 3 of 9 injuries were associated with alcohol use [40]. Contusions in this population were mainly caused by sports equipment, contact with body parts, sticks, and tools [40].

Although closed-globe and open-globe injuries comprise a significant portion of ocular trauma, other ocular injuries including chemical burns, fractures, eyelid wounds, optic nerve injuries, and other minor injuries have been reported in the literature, with a subset of the trauma population forming traumatic cataracts.

Anatomical Surgical Approach

Lens injury and traumatic cataracts typically are associated with damage to other structures of the eye. Damage can include capsular rupture, zonular dialysis, trauma to the iris, angle structures, posterior segment, and more. Upon receiving a case of trauma, damage to other structures of the eye may be apparent, or only discovered during or after surgery.

The degree of capsular bag support available after trauma may guide surgical techniques for intraocular lens implantation at primary or secondary repair. Various lens options and techniques can be used for fixation in the angle, to the iris, sclera, or ciliary sulcus [45]. Options for lens fixation based on capsular support are shown in Fig. 32.4.

Open Eye Injuries with Traumatic Cataracts

The options for surgical intervention in open-globe trauma remain similar to those in the pediatric population; however, the risk of amblyopia does not factor into the timing of the surgical repair. Options for repair include primary wound closure from a penetrating injury, primary lensectomy with IOL implantation, primary lensectomy without IOL implantation, secondary surgery with lensectomy and IOL implantation following primary closure, and secondary IOL implantation following primary lensectomy.

Closure with Primary Lensectomy

Closure with primary lensectomy, or lensectomy during an early procedure, remains a recommendation in the adult population in cases of capsular or lenticular trauma. Lens proteins released into the anterior chamber can lead to intraocular inflammation, increased intraocular

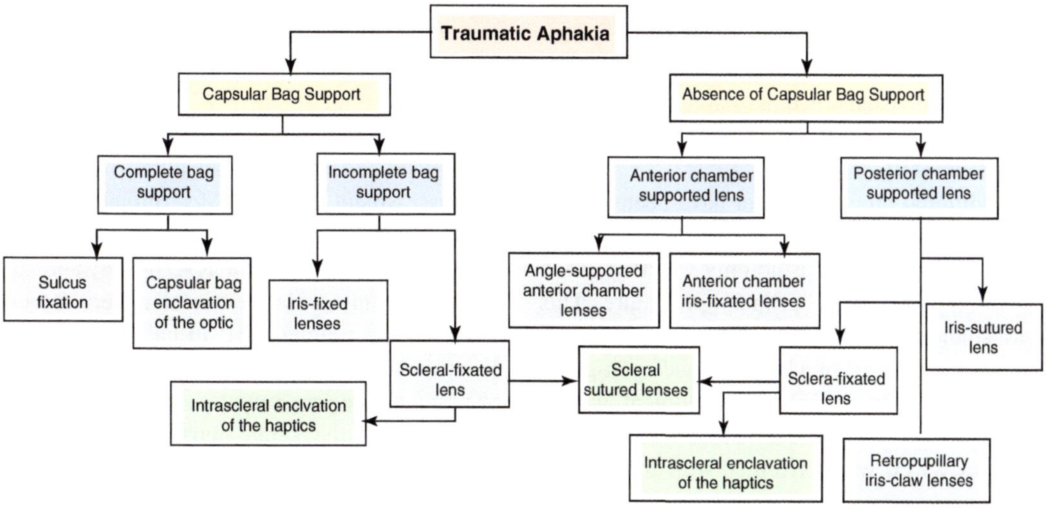

Fig. 32.4 Approach to surgical repair of aphakic eyes secondary to trauma. Options for fixation of the intraocular lens based on anatomic infrastructure in the anterior segment [45]. (Adapted from: Fiorentzis et al. [45])

pressure, and increased risk of endophthalmitis [46, 47]. Furthermore, in significant lens trauma, fragments of the lens can mix with the vitreous to create a "vitreous-lens admixture," a potential inciting factor for proliferative vitreoretinopathy [47].

Immediate Repair – Primary Closure with Lensectomy and IOL Implantation

Similar to the pediatric population, it is also unclear in open-globe trauma whether primary wound closure with primary lensectomy and IOL implantation offers advantages as compared to a deferred secondary IOL implantation. Visual outcomes of both procedures in open-globe trauma have been shown to be similar.

Benefits of a primary procedure include earlier vision rehabilitation (especially in the younger age group, or young men), decreased cost, decreased loss of employment, avoidance of an additional surgery and additional use of anesthesia, and avoidance of problems of secondary IOL insertion (such as poor iris dilation and posterior synechiae) [46, 48]. A 2017 study to determine the optimum time for traumatic cataract surgery found that there was no difference in 6-month visual outcomes between early and late interventions. There was also no difference in intraoperative and postoperative complications between these two groups [48]. Furthermore, a retrospective study including 151 eyes suffering open-globe injury and traumatic cataracts secondary to combat trauma found no significant difference in visual outcomes based on the timing of implantation, suggesting either approach is acceptable [49].

Additional procedures that have been recommended to improve visual outcome include a primary posterior capsulotomy (PPC) and vitrectomy during the primary procedure. This was studied in a cohort of 555 patients with traumatic cataracts, of which 394 had open-globe injuries [43]. In eyes needing corneal wound repair and with increased inflammation with hazy medium, a PPC was performed with anterior vitrectomy during the primary surgery, with IOL placement performed in a staged manner [43]. Another study examining all age groups also found visual outcome benefited from PPC and anterior vitrectomy in both open- and closed-globe traumas [50]. Thus, a PPC procedure appears to lead to a significant improvement in visual acuity as compared to those that did not receive the procedure [43, 50].

Implantation of the IOL during a primary procedure in open-globe and closed-globe traumas is found to result in better visual acuity if the IOL is placed in the capsular bag, as opposed to the ciliary sulcus. Although Serna-Ojeda et al. identified this trend, however, it was acknowledged that there may be other factors that were not analyzed that led to this difference in visual acuity [44]. Potential reasoning for this may include changes in refraction if the IOL is placed in different locations in the eye, or increased inflammation induced by sulcus implantation [44].

Late Repair, Staged Procedures

Secondary procedures are also found to be safe and provide good visual outcomes following initial repair [46, 49]. A study of open-globe injuries found no difference in outcomes between early procedures, or late procedures performed after 1 month following trauma [48]. However, this study outlined strict exclusion criteria such as patients with trauma and released lens materials in the anterior chamber [48]. Secondary procedures may be advantageous in cases of severe corneal injury, or in cases where there may be poor visualization due to the trauma [51]. After a primary procedure, time can allow for a thorough assessment of the eye, determination of the visual potential for visual rehabilitation, for more accurate planning of IOL power, and the treatment of any ocular injuries that were associated with the trauma [46]. In cases of corneal lacerations, a secondary procedure can allow for the removal of corneal sutures, and a more stable assessment of the keratometry for IOL power needed in surgery [46].

Closed Eye Injuries with Traumatic Cataracts

The literature also presents similar visual outcomes among immediate repair and late repair of closed eye injuries with traumatic cataracts. A study by Rumelt and Rehany tried to identify if the time to cataract extraction and IOL implantation affected visual outcomes [46]. They classified eyes into the primary group (patients receiving surgery within 24 hours from trauma), or secondary group (patients receiving surgery at least 1 week after trauma) [46]. The visual outcomes following surgery (BCVA of 20/40 or better) were similar in both primary and secondary surgeries following closed-globe injuries; however, this study also included children in their analysis [46]. Similar findings regarding traumatic cataracts secondary to ocular trauma also found no difference in visual outcomes between eyes receiving primary or secondary IOLs [49]. Since amblyopia is not a concern in older individuals, the surgery can be dictated by a physician's findings at presentation and a surgeon's preferences [46]. In choosing surgical options, a patient's situation may also recommend choices; for example, a monocular patient experiencing trauma may benefit from a primary procedure that would expedite the recovery time. The advantages of immediate and late repair remain similar to that previously described for open-globe injuries.

Other factors including patient reporting time may influence the time to intervention following ocular trauma. A study in 2011 by Shah et al., examined ocular trauma reporting trends in a cohort of 687 patients presenting to a Tertiary care center in Western India [52]. A significant portion of patients with closed-globe injuries reported more than 30 days after trauma (104 of 191 patients), while only 40 patients reported from 0 to 1 days [52]. In contrast to this, open-globe trauma patients reported earlier, with 132 of 496 patients reporting within 1 day, and 132 of 496 patients reporting more than 30 days following injury [52]. It was found that the patients who presented earlier appeared to have worse visual outcomes, although it was hypothesized that this may be due to a higher incidence of open-globe injuries reporting earlier and closed-globe injuries of lesser severity presenting later after the traumatic insult [52].

Pediatric Closed-Globe Injury Case (Surgical Video is Included)

In September of 2016, 15-year-old male presented with a blunt trauma to the right eye. Three hours earlier, he was walking past his father who was cutting the lawn with a motorized lawn mower. He was struck by a rock, which was propelled by the mower.

Examination revealed vision of hand motions (barely). There was a central corneal epithelial defect, corneal edema, the anterior chamber was formed with a dense hyphema; iris trauma and traumatic mydriasis was present, and the IOP was 16 mm Hg by applanation. No further details of the lens or posterior segment could be ascertained. Ultrasonography (U/S) revealed that the retina was flat.

The diagnosis was a blunt closed-globe injury with hyphema. The management that was initiated was that which is recommended for a traumatic hyphema: 1% atropine drops, topical steroids, and limited physical activity.

Daily visits to monitor inflammation and IOP was instigated. By Day 5, the epithelial defect had resolved, the hyphema measured 3 mm, IOP was 11 mm Hg, the lens was white, and the retina was flat. By Day 17, a superior blood clot overlying an area of presumed iridodialysis remained; the lens was white, there was no inflammation, and IOP was 17 mm Hg. By Day 40, the hyphema had resolved, the blood clot had resolved, the IOP was 10 mm Hg, no inflammation was present, a white cataract was present, and the flat retina on ultrasound.

Discussion to address the white cataract was explored with the parents and the patient; the decision was made to defer the surgery until the school break. Delayed surgery was feasible in this case as the risk of amblyopia was low, there was no inflammation, the IOP remained in range without treatment, and U/S did not reveal any significant retinal pathology.

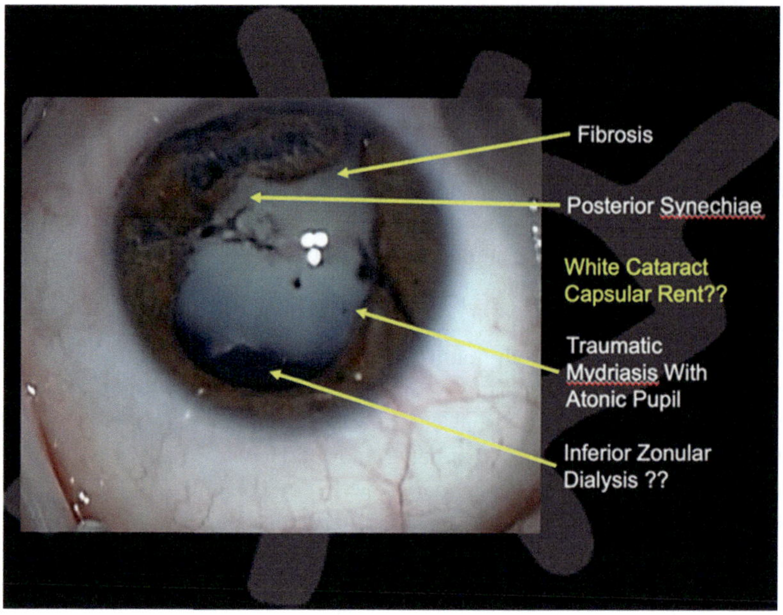

The photograph above demonstrates the eye at surgery. Traumatic mydriasis, posterior synechiae, white cataract due to presumed capsular rent, and likely inferior zonular dialysis. The surgical plan was to use vision blue to assist with the capsulorhexis, perform pupilloplasty to deal with the traumatic mydriasis, and to use a 3 piece IOL (as this would enable the most options for IOL placement whether in the bag, in the sulcus, sutured to iris, or fixated to sclera). A vitrector was at the ready as a capsular rent was suspected.

Special Techniques

In addition to surgical timing decisions, traumatic cataract surgery provides other challenges that should be tackled using a variety of surgical techniques. Novel techniques have been reported in the literature to manage complicated cases and augment visual outcomes.

Foreign Body Removal

Lacerations with IOFB are one of the categories of open-globe injuries. Previous review of the literature has shown IOFBs account for 18–41% of all open-globe injuries, and 58–88% reside in the posterior segment [53]. The majority of IOFBs are metallic and may contain ferromagnetic particles [53]. IOFB is typically removed at the time of primary repair, either by pars plana vitrectomy (PPV) or with other special techniques [53–56]. Early removal is recommended to prevent inflammatory response and development of endophthalmitis. With respect to lenticular surgery at the time of IOFB removal, studies have shown cataract surgery and IOL implantation can be performed in primary surgery or secondary surgery depending upon other factors [53]. Posterior segment IOFBs, intravitreal foreign bodies (IVFB) are typically removed via pars plana vitrectomy [53, 55].

The recent literature reports the use of magnets for the removal of metallic/ferromagnetic foreign bodies. A pars plana approach and use of a magnet through the sclerotomy site to remove the IVFB, with IOL implantation and cataract surgery performed at a second operation, have been shown to be safe and to result in good visual outcomes, without the need for PPV at the second surgery [54].

In certain patients, primary IOL implantation with cataract and vitreoretinal surgery has also been found to be a safe option. Another study presented the results of small incision cataract surgery with PPV in which the IOFB was removed through the sclerocorneal tunnel using a magnet. These procedures were performed prior to IOL implantation in 18 patients. It was ensured that prior to magnetic removal of the foreign body, the foreign body was detached from the surrounding vitreous. The majority of patients had satisfactory visual outcomes following surgery, although late-onset RD occurred in 5 out of 18 cases [56].

An additional study reported a novel technique, the "magnet handshake," which appeared to be useful in removing large, irregular IOFBs of more than 5 mm, or when forceps grasp would not be possible. After anterior continuous circular capsulorhexis and removal of the lens, the retinal surgeon frees the IOFB with vitrectomy, and an intraocular magnet (IOM) is introduced through the vitrectomy port. The IOFB is lifted to the iris plane, and a second IOM is introduced through the scleral tunnel to meet the first, in an interaction deemed the "magnet handshake." The IOFB could then be extracted through the scleral tunnel securely, with no slippage. Final BCVA of 20/60 or better was achieved in 70% of patients with large IOFBs using this technique, with no intraoperative complications. This technique can be used for larger IOFBs, for removal through the sclerocorneal tunnel instead of sclerotomy, and provides good visual and anatomic outcomes [55].

Vitrectorhexis

Creating a capsulorhexis after an open-globe injury can be challenging due to the disturbed anatomy and a poor view of the anterior segment. Vitrectorhexis, the creation of anterior capsulorhexis using a vitreous cutter, has been a technique typically used in the pediatric population to cut through softer lens material. In a study by Resch et al., a vitrectorhexis was performed in 8 eyes after penetrating mechanical corneal trauma. To create the anterior capsulorhexis using a vitrector, a 23 G vitreous cutter and standard 23 G infusion cannula were placed through side ports, with the cut rate set at 500 cuts per minute. The rhexis was performed starting at the site of anterior capsule rupture. Hydro-delineation, without hydro-dissection, and cautious removal of the lens was performed in the case of a posterior capsular rent. The case series found that this technique could be used safety in adult eyes following open-globe injury and with complex anterior segment trauma [57].

Capsular Tension Rings

In the presence of zonular weakness, or capsular instability, a capsular tension ring (CTR) implant can be used to allow for in-the-bag IOL implantation. A study of 6000 cataract cases, not specifically related to trauma, found that 0.75% of the time a CTR was used, with 6 of these cases being due to blunt trauma [58]. The CTR, modified CTRs, or capsular tension segments (CTS) help to maintain the shape of the capsular bag, and redistribute force from the areas of weakness, to stronger zonules [58, 59].

Timing of insertion of the CTR in a case of traumatic cataract with zonular dialysis is preferable after lens extraction since inserting the CTR before phacoemulsification was found to put more stress on the intact zonules in situations of dense cataracts [59]. Modified CTRs (Cionni 1 L, 13.0 mm diameter, Morcher GmbH, or Cionni 2 L, 13.0 mm diameter Morcher GmbH) have also led to successful visual outcomes with low complication rates in traumatic zonulopathy and cataract surgery [60]. In a study of 16 eyes following traumatic cataract, modified CTRs were placed after phacoemulsification and were effective in preserving the capsular bag for PCIOL placement [60].

In the older literature, CTRs have been found to provide stability and lens centration in eyes with less than 6 clock hours of zonular loss; yet, further research has shown that modified CTRs can be used with more than 6 clock hours of damage [61]. Cionni 1 L, Cionni 2 L. CTR and CTS used alone or in combination were used in eyes with more than 6 hours of zonulolysis, achieving good visual outcome in 92.7% of traumatized eyes with severe lens subluxation [61]. Double eyelet modified CTRs were also successfully used in a study of 16 traumatic cataract cases with greater than 7 clock hours of zonular loss or weakness [60]. Results demonstrated no cases of IOL or capsular bag decentration [60].

Overall, the literature recommends the use of CTR devices in cases of subluxated cataracts, or zonular weakness, to allow for in-the-bag IOL implantation in traumatic cataract surgery. These rings should be implanted after phacoemulsification and may be used successfully in cases with greater than 6 clock hours of zonular loss or weakness.

Femtosecond Laser

Although not typically used in trauma cases, multiple reports have demonstrated the applications of femtosecond lasers in the management of traumatic cataracts. As in surgery of nontraumatic cataracts, a femtosecond laser can be used to create a consistent capsulorhexis in traumatic cataract surgery, especially in the presence of radial tears, and anterior or posterior capsule tears [62–64]. The femtosecond laser can also be used for liquefaction and fragmentation of the lens, applying less energy to traumatize the endothelial cells of the cornea, which may already be injured due to trauma [65].

Special Concerns

IOL Calculations

As previously stated, the ability to perform preoperative biometry for patients with traumatic cataracts is one of the benefits of performing a secondary procedure after primary repair with or without lensectomy. IOL power calculations can be difficult in cases with open-globe injuries, and often power calculations are performed using the contralateral unaffected eye [46]. Secondary procedures offer more accuracy in lens power calculation as compared to this method and may take into account additional scarring and changes in astigmatism [66]. Older literature previously documents the inaccuracies involved in estimating IOL power from the unaffected eye following open-globe trauma in a patient with a corneal laceration. In the reported case, refractive surprise measuring 4.00 D was the result of measurements taken from the contralateral eye [26].

Posterior Capsule Rupture (PCR)

Traumatic cataracts are often associated with other ocular injuries, including PCR. It is beneficial to identify PCR prior to surgical intervention as it can complicate cataract extraction and IOL implantation. Different techniques have been outlined in the literature to best detect PCR in eyes with traumatic cataract in preoperative examinations. Echography with a 20 MHz probe has been studied in cases of traumatic cataract and has been found in one study to be an accurate imaging modality for the detection of PCR with sensitivity and specificity values of 93% and 86%, respectively [67]. The use of other frequencies in echography such as 10 MHz or 50 MHz is possible; however, these result in lower resolution, or less penetration to investigate the posterior capsule, respectively. In one case, the use of 35 MHz ultrasound biomicroscopy (UBM) was reported for the detection of PCR with some success at higher resolution [68]. Larger studies would be needed to confirm the use and accuracy as compared to the more tested 20 MHz frequency method.

Other modalities, including anterior segment optical coherence tomography (AS-OCT), and Scheimpflug imaging using Pentacam were used in comparison to 20 MHz echography in 21 eyes to evaluate the posterior lens capsule in traumatic cataract in a 2014 study. It was found that 20 MHz echography had a higher accuracy than AS-OCT and Scheimpflug imaging [69].

Identifying PCR or capsular abnormalities after traumatic injury to the lens is important in lens surgery for surgical planning to prevent intraocular complications. Although some tears may be identifiable on slit-lamp examination, another imaging modality, specifically 20 MHz echography, may provide better visualization.

Outcomes: Visual and Anatomic

Visual outcomes following cataract surgery in the traumatized anterior segment may be favorable; however, there remains considerable debate within the literature regarding the timing and technique of surgery as well as the prognostic value of the nature of the injury [35, 44, 46, 48, 49, 52, 70].

In a large retrospective investigation of both children and adults, Shah et al. compared the visual outcomes of cataract surgery from both open- and closed- globe injuries as well as early and delayed treatment [52, 70]. In their study, favorable visual outcome was defined as >20/60 by the Snellen chart; they observed 58% of open-globe injuries to achieve this recovery in comparison to only 39.1% of closed-globe injuries [52]. In contrast, a prospective study by Sharma et al. found the blunt trauma group to have more favorable visual outcomes; however, their study only enrolled 48 patients [35]. Multiple other investigations have found no significant difference in visual outcomes between open- and closed-globe traumas, with favorable outcomes achievable in both groups. A study by Smith et al., however, has found prognostic value in the ocular trauma score discussed previously, in estimating final visual recovery [49].

Timing and technique of surgical intervention remain hotly debated. There are theoretical benefits and drawbacks to both early and late interventions and much of the literature fails to reach consensus on which approach may be better. In adults, it is thought that early intervention may be beneficial to stabilize an eye in which lens material has entered the anterior chamber and resulted in uveitis and increased IOP [48]. Early procedures often suffer, however, from being reliant on the unaffected eye for IOL biometry. Drawbacks and inaccuracies of this method have been discussed previously in this chapter. Late procedures allow for operation within a quiet eye and may often permit more accurate biometry.[5,6] In a randomized controlled trial of 60 patients, Tabatabaei et al. found no difference between early and late interventions. This trend was also observed by Rumelt et al. in a retrospective study of 69 cases and Smith et al. in a retrospective case series of 181 cases [46, 48, 49]. In assessing the timing of surgery, Shah et al. found that treatment of patients between 2 and 30 days after injury resulted in the most optimal visual outcome in comparison to treatment within the first 24 hours or treatment beyond the first month [70]. Their reasoning for this centered on the nature of the ocular injury – considering that patients who present in the first 24 hours are likely to have the most severe injuries (and thus have the poorest initial prognosis), while those who present beyond 30 days after injury may have already sustained long-term sequelae from the initial ocular insult [52, 70].

In addition to the timing of surgical intervention, IOL positioning may also affect final visual outcome. In a retrospective study of 80 patients, Serna-Ojeda, et al. found that in-the-bag placement of an IOL was associated with significantly better visual outcomes in comparison to placement in the ciliary sulcus or iris-fixation [44]. Aphakia was almost universally associated with poor visual outcome [44, 46]. Importantly, in their study, Serna-Ojeda, et al. noted that although only 66.25% of patients had IOL placement in-the-bag, 73.5% of patients overall achieved a visual outcome of 20/60 or better by the Snellen chart, and 42.5% of patients had vision of 20/25 or 20/20, reaffirming the potential for favorable visual recovery after traumatic cataract surgery [44].

Complications and Other Ocular Manifestations

Complications and other ocular manifestations may occur as a result of trauma, during surgical intervention and at later time points in adults. Many studies in the recent literature have reported common complications including but not limited to corneal opacities and damage, increased IOP, zonular dialysis, PCR, and endophthalmitis. In this section, these ocular manifestations and complications will be discussed. These complications are discussed generally as affecting the adult population, although some studies included younger patients.

Corneal Involvement

Corneal involvement, scarring and edema, is a vision limiting complication that can occur as a result of trauma, especially in open-globe and penetrating injuries. Many studies have reported the rates of this complication in the postoperative period ranging from 12% to 38% of patients [35, 44, 71]. A study by Serna-Ojeda et al., found that of 14 patients who did not achieve vision of 20/200 or better, 5 had corneal scarring among other complications [44]. Trauma to the anterior segment has the potential to harm corneal endothelial cells and cause edema following repair. There is the potential of corneal edema following traumatic cataract surgery, and one study in an African population documented 2 cases of corneal decompensation, among 59 cases of mild-to-moderate corneal edema for 2 weeks postoperatively [71].

Posterior Capsule Rupture

As previously mentioned, PCR may occur as a result of trauma and can be identifiable on preoperative imaging used to plan surgical intervention. Large or significant PCRs may prevent implantation of the IOL in the capsular bag. This has been documented in 21–23% of patients following trauma, more frequently in open-globe trauma, although one study did not find a significant difference [44, 48].

Zonulolysis and Lens Subluxation

Zonular dialysis, weakness of the zonules, can increase risk of lens subluxation and complicate the management of traumatic cataracts. Studies have reported options for in-the-bag IOL implantation using modified CTRs, CTRs, and CT segments, [60, 61] with good success; yet, these still remain challenging cases. The management of traumatic cataract with zonulolysis using these devices allows for greater control and can help to minimize further complications associated with anterior chamber intraocular lenses (ACIOLs), retinal complications, and increased intraocular pressure [61]. In open-globe injuries, zonulolysis was found to affect approximately 13% of individuals; this was managed using the aforementioned methods [48]. Other studies report zonular dialysis and lens subluxation in adults occurring at rates of approximately 18–23% and 8%, respectively [35, 44].

IOP Elevation

Similar to pediatric cases, elevated IOPs following traumatic cataracts remain a significant complication occurring as a result of trauma and may remain following surgical repair. Intraocular pressure was found to be increased more frequently following blunt trauma as a possible result of angle recession. Sharma et al. reported a rate of increased IOP of 36% following blunt trauma, with no cases within the open-globe trauma group, with rates of angle recession and glaucoma ranging from 23% to 36% [35, 44, 71]. Serna et al., also reported 5 cases of vision less than 20/200 being attributable to glaucoma among other complications. Typically, increased IOP can be well managed medically as per standard procedures; however, some patients require glaucoma drainage devices (tubes, shunts) to control elevated IOP [71].

Inflammatory Sequelae

Studies have reported other complications and ocular manifestations as a result of inflammation and trauma in the eye including but not limited to anterior chamber inflammation, posterior synechiae, and iridocyclitis [35, 48]. Sharma et al. found that posterior and anterior synechiae occurred more frequently in open-globe trauma; of patients with open-globe trauma in a 2017 study, inflammation and posterior synechiae affected a minority of patients [35, 48].

Structural Damage

In addition to lens subluxation, and corneal perforations associated with trauma, the iris and the uvea may also be damaged. Uveal prolapse and traumatic mydriasis are found to occur in both open and closed traumas [35].

Severe damage to the iris and lens concurrently can be repaired in a variety of ways. In the case of significant iris trauma or traumatic aniridia, a patient's quality of vision can be reduced, due to light sensitivity and glare. In a secondary surgery, artificial iris and lens complexes can be fixated in the eye. The Customflex Artificial Iris (Dr. Schmidt Intraocularlinsen GmbH, distributed by HumanOptics AG) has been found to provide customizable cosmetic results for the treatment of traumatic aniridia [72, 73]. Intraocular lenses fixated to custom silicone iris prosthesis have also been reported as a novel method of repairing traumatic aniridia and aphakia; using the iris prosthesis can aid in posttraumatic situations in which there is a lack of structural anatomic support for the IOL [73].

Retinal Involvement

In addition to anterior segment injury and formation of traumatic cataract, the posterior segment including the retina may be severely damaged by ocular injury. In two studies, varying rates of retinal detachments were reported. In the first, 13% and 17% of patients had complications of vitreous hemorrhage, and retinal detachment, respectively [35]. Patients with open-globe and closed-globe injuries were reviewed, with no significant differences between groups [35]. However, another study by Serna-Ojeda et al. only identified 1 of 64 individuals with retinal detachment, vitreous hemorrhage, and choroidal neovascular membrane postoperatively, causing poor visual outcome [44].

Macular commotio retinae can be associated with blunt traumatic injuries, causing visual impairment. Blanch et al. identified 53 cases of blunt ocular trauma with macular commotio retinae, causing reduced visual acuity with 74% of patients recovering better than 20/30 vision [74]. Extramacular commotio retinae affected 117 patients, with 55 of 58 (95%) followed recovering greater than 20/30 visual acuity. Although the reduction in vision is minimal, this could potentially be a significant change in vision for patients as a result of trauma [74].

Endophthalmitis

Endophthalmitis is another potential complication of ocular trauma, with the risk being increased by lens fragments remaining in the anterior chamber and vitreous following trauma. Endophthalmitis has been reported as a complication of open-globe trauma in low rates, especially with early intervention and repair within the first 24 hours [75]. Zhang et al. reviewed records of open-globe injury cases in a 5-year period in the setting of China. This study found a rate of endophthalmitis in this population of approximately 12%, with other values in the literature ranging from 3% to 30% after open-globe injury [76, 77]. After IOFB, there has been a reported incidence of up to 48% [76]. A study by Essex et al., suggests that dirty wounds, delay in primary repair, and lens rupture increase the incidence of endophthalmitis [77].

In cases of open-globe trauma, prophylactic intravitreal antibiotics at the time of primary repair reduces the risk of endophthalmitis, particularly in high-risk patients [78]. High-risk patients include patients with delayed presentation after injury of more than 24 hours, rural setting, dirty wound, retained IOFB, and/or ruptured lens capsule [78].

Thus, recommendations for risk management after open-globe trauma include early primary repair and intravitreal antibiotics for those at high risk of intraocular infection.

Take-Home Notes

- Early presentation and management of traumatic cataracts are essential for good visual outcomes, and the ability to manage complications.
- For complex cases, an experienced team may be necessary to manage other sequelae. Appropriate imaging needs to be done prior to surgical intervention to identify additional damage from the traumatic insult. This may include the management of retinal detachments with retinal specialists, or anticipating posterior capsule rupture through imaging prior to surgical intervention.
- Secondary IOL implantation, or staged procedures, can be used successfully for both children and adults to lead to good visual outcomes following open or closed trauma. However, aggressive visual rehabilitation and amblyopia therapy is needed for the management of amblyopia in children (even older than the age of 8).

- PCCC is a necessary technique for children, even in older children (8–10 years of age) to avoid visual axis opacification and risk of amblyopia. Similarly, this should be a consideration in inflamed eyes in the adult population.
- The best option for visual outcomes and minimizing complication is fixation of the IOL in the capsular bag; however, options for IOL implantation may change based on other trauma to the anterior segment. Helpful devices for IOL implantation in anterior segment trauma are CTRs or modified CTRs, which can be used even in greater than 6 hours of zonular weakness to allow for implantation in the capsular bag.

References

1. Kuhn F, Morris R, Witherspoon CD, Heimann K, Jeffers JB, Treister G. A standardized classification of ocular trauma. Ophthalmology. 1996;103(2):240–3.
2. Pieramici DJ, Sternberg P, Aaberg TM, Bridges WZ, Capone A, Cardillo JA, et al. A system for classifying mechanical injuries of the eye (globe). Am J Ophthalmol. 1997;123(6):820–31.
3. Arora K, Arora P, Ganesh S, Gupta S, Das RR. Visual and refractive outcomes of children after early secondary cataract extraction following wound repair for penetrating ocular trauma. J Pediatr Ophthalmol Strabismus. 2018;55(2):122–7.
4. Meier P. Combined anterior and posterior segment injuries in children: a review. Graefes Arch Clin Exp Ophthalmol. 2010;248(9):1207–19.
5. Mittra RA, Mieler WF. Controversies in the management of open-globe injuries involving the posterior segment. Surv Ophthalmol. 1999;44(3):215–25.
6. Papageorgiou E, Asproudis I, Maconachie G, Tsironi EE, Gottlob I. The treatment of amblyopia: current practice and emerging trends. Graefes Arch Clin Exp Ophthalmol. 2019;257(6):1061–78.
7. Jinagal J, Gupta G, Gupta PC, Yangzes S, Singh R, Gupta R, et al. Visual outcomes of pediatric traumatic cataracts. Eur J Ophthalmol. 2019;29(1):23–7.
8. Du Y, He W, Sun X, Lu Y, Zhu X. Traumatic cataract in children in Eastern China: Shanghai pediatric cataract study. Sci Rep. 2018;8(1):2588.
9. Shah MA, Agrawal R, Teoh R, Shah SM, Patel K, Gupta S, et al. Pediatric ocular trauma score as a prognostic tool in the management of pediatric traumatic cataracts. Graefes Arch Clin Exp Ophthalmol. 2017;255(5):1027–36.
10. Qiu H, Fischer NA, Patnaik JL, Jung JL, Singh JK, McCourt EA. Frequency of pediatric traumatic cataract and simultaneous retinal detachment. J Am Assoc Pediatr Ophthalmol Strabismus. 2018;22(6):429–32.
11. Staffieri SE, Ruddle JB, Mackey DA. P- Rock, paper & scissors? Traumatic paediatric cataract in Victoria 1992–2006. Clin Experiment Ophthalmol [Internet]. 2010 Feb [cited 2020 Jun 2]. Available from: http://doi.wiley.com/10.1111/j.1442-9071.2010.02236.x.
12. Khokhar S, Gupta S, Yogi R, Gogia V, Agarwal T. Epidemiology and intermediate-term outcomes of open- and closed-globe injuries in traumatic childhood cataract. Eur J Ophthalmol. 2014;24(1):124–30.
13. Ram J, Verma N, Gupta N, Chaudhary M. Effect of penetrating and blunt ocular trauma on the outcome of traumatic cataract in children in northern India. J Trauma Acute Care Surg. 2012;73(3):726–30.
14. Agrawal R, Shah M, Mireskandari K, Yong GK. Controversies in ocular trauma classification and management: review. Int Ophthalmol. 2013;33(4):435–45.
15. Sen P, Shah C, Sen A, Jain E, Mohan A. Primary versus secondary intraocular lens implantation in traumatic cataract after open-globe injury in pediatric patients. J Cataract Refract Surg. 2018;44(12):1446–53.
16. Yardley A-M, Ali A, Najm-Tehrani N, Mireskandari K. Refractive and visual outcomes after surgery for pediatric traumatic cataract. J Cataract Refract Surg. 2018;44(1):85–90.
17. Lamkin JC, Azar DT, Mead MD, Volpe NJ. Simultaneous corneal laceration repair, cataract removal, and posterior chamber intraocular lens implantation. Am J Ophthalmol. 1992;113(6):626–31.
18. Bienfait MF, Pameijer JH, de Blécourt-Devilee MW. Intraocular lens implantation in children with unilateral traumatic cataract. Int Ophthalmol. 1990;14(4):271–6.
19. Moisseiev J, Segev F, Harizman N, Arazi T, Rotenstreich Y, Assia EI. Primary cataract extraction and intraocular lens implantation in penetrating ocular trauma. Ophthalmology. 2001;108(6):1099–103.
20. Hilely A, Leiba H, Achiron A, Hecht I, Parness-Yossifon R. Traumatic cataracts in children, long-term follow-up in an israeli population: a retrospective study. 6.
21. Xu Y-N, Huang Y-S, Xie L-X. Pediatric traumatic cataract and surgery outcomes in eastern China: a hospital-based study. Int J Ophthalmol. 2013;6(2):160–4.
22. Chang DF, Masket S, Miller KM, Braga-Mele R, Little BC, Mamalis N, et al. Complications of sulcus placement of single-piece acrylic intraocular lenses: recommendations for backup IOL implantation following posterior capsule rupture. J Cataract Refract Surg. 2009;35(8):1445–58.
23. Zhang L, Hood CT, Vrabec JP, Cullen AL, Parrish EA, Moroi SE. Mechanisms for in-the-bag uveitis-

glaucoma-hyphema syndrome. J Cataract Refract Surg. 2014;40(3):490–2.
24. Chowdhary S, Nischal KK. Banded technique for pediatric traumatic cataract surgery. J Cataract Refract Surg. 2019;45(1):8–10.
25. Mohamed TA, Soliman W, Fathalla AM. Effect of intracameral triamcinolone acetonide on postoperative intraocular inflammation in pediatric traumatic cataract. Eur J Ophthalmol. 2016;26(2):114–7.
26. Cohen KL. Inaccuracy of intraocular lens power calculation after traumatic corneal laceration and cataract. J Cataract Refract Surg. 2001;27(9):1519–22.
27. Khokhar S, Pillay G, Dhull C, Agarwal E, Mahabir M, Aggarwal P. Pediatric cataract. Indian J Ophthalmol. 2017;65(12):1340–7.
28. Enyedi LB, Peterseim MW, Freedman SF, Buckley EG. Refractive changes after pediatric intraocular lens implantation. Am J Ophthalmol. 1998;126(6):772–81.
29. Shah MA, Shah SM, Gosai SR, Gupta SS, Khanna RR, Patel KB, et al. Comparative study of visual outcome between open- and closed-globe injuries following surgical treatment of traumatic cataract in children. Eur J Ophthalmol. 2018;28(4):406–11.
30. Shah MA, Shah SM, Appleware AH, Patel KD, Rehman RM, Shikhange KA. Visual outcome of traumatic cataract in pediatric age group. Eur J Ophthalmol. 2012;22(6):956–63.
31. Shah MA, Shah SM, Applewar A, Patel C, Patel K. Ocular trauma score as a predictor of final visual outcomes in traumatic cataract cases in pediatric patients. J Cataract Refract Surg. 2012;38(6):959–65.
32. Kuhn F, Maisiak R, Mann L, Mester V, Morris R, Witherspoon C. The ocular trauma score (OTS). Ophthalmol Clin N Am. 2002;15(2):163–5.
33. Scott R. The ocular trauma score. Community Eye Health J. 2015;28(91):44–5.
34. Unver YB, Kapran Z, Acar N. Ocular trauma score in open-globe injuries. J Trauma 2009;3.
35. Sharma AK. Visual outcome of traumatic cataract at a tertiary eye care centre in North India: a prospective study. J Clin Diagn Res. 2016;10(1):NC05–8.
36. Beshay N, Keay L, Dunn H, Kamalden TA, Hoskin AK, Watson SL. The epidemiology of open globe injuries presenting to a tertiary referral eye hospital in Australia. Injury. 2017;48(7):1348–54.
37. Qi Y, Zhang YF, Zhu Y, Wan MG, Du SS, Yue ZZ. Prognostic factors for visual outcome in traumatic cataract patients. J Ophthalmol. 2016;2016:1–6.
38. Malik IQ, Ali Z, Rehman A, Moin M, Hussain M. Epidemiology of penetrating ocular trauma. Pak J Ophthalmol. 2012;28(1):14–6.
39. Onakpoya OH, Adeoye A, Adeoti CO, Ajite K. Epidemiology of ocular trauma among the elderly in a developing country. Ophthalmic Epidemiol. 2010;17(5):315–20.
40. Sahraravand A, Haavisto A-K, Holopainen JM, Leivo T. Ocular traumas in working age adults in Finland - Helsinki Ocular Trauma Study. Acta Ophthalmol. 2017;95(3):288–94.
41. Soylu M, Sizmaz S, Cayli S. Eye injury (ocular trauma) in southern Turkey: epidemiology, ocular survival, and visual outcome. Int Ophthalmol. 2010;30(2):143–8.
42. AlMahmoud T, Al Hadhrami SM, Elhanan M, Alshamsi HN, Abu-Zidan FM. Epidemiology of eye injuries in a high-income developing country: an observational study. Medicine (Baltimore). 2019;98(26):e16083.
43. Shah M, Shah S, Shah S, Prasad V, Parikh A. Visual recovery and predictors of visual prognosis after managing traumatic cataracts in 555 patients. Indian J Ophthalmol. 2011;59(3):217.
44. Serna-Ojeda JC, Cordova-Cervantes J, Lopez-Salas M, Abdala-Figuerola AC, Jimenez-Corona A, Matiz-Moreno H, et al. Management of traumatic cataract in adults at a reference center in Mexico City. Int Ophthalmol. 2015;35(4):451–8.
45. Fiorentzis M, Viestenz A, Heichel J, Seitz B, Hammer T, Viestenz A. Methods of fixation of intraocular lenses according to the anatomical structures in trauma eyes: fixation of intraocular lens following trauma. Clin Anat. 2018;31(1):6–15.
46. Rumelt S, Rehany U. The influence of surgery and intraocular lens implantation timing on visual outcome in traumatic cataract. Graefes Arch Clin Exp Ophthalmol. 2010;248(9):1293–7.
47. Kuhn F. Traumatic cataract: what, when, how. Graefes Arch Clin Exp Ophthalmol. 2010;248(9):1221–3.
48. Tabatabaei SA, Rajabi MB, Tabatabaei SM, Soleimani M, Rahimi F, Yaseri M. Early versus late traumatic cataract surgery and intraocular lens implantation. Eye. 2017;31(8):1199–204.
49. Smith MP, Colyer MH, Weichel ED, Stutzman RD. Traumatic cataracts secondary to combat ocular trauma. J Cataract Refract Surg. 2015;41(8):1693–8.
50. Shah M, Shah S, Patel K, Shah A, Pandya J. Maximizing the visual outcome in traumatic cataract cases: the value of a primary posterior capsulotomy and anterior vitrectomy. Indian J Ophthalmol. 2014;62(11):1077.
51. Agarwal A, Kumar DA, Nair V. Cataract surgery in the setting of trauma. Curr Opin Ophthalmol. 2010;21(1):65–70.
52. Shah MA, Shah SM, Shah SB, Patel CG, Patel UA, Appleware A, et al. Comparative study of final visual outcome between open- and closed-globe injuries following surgical treatment of traumatic cataract. Graefes Arch Clin Exp Ophthalmol. 2011;249(12):1775–81.
53. Loporchio D, Mukkamala L, Gorukanti K, Zarbin M, Langer P, Bhagat N. Intraocular foreign bodies: a review. Surv Ophthalmol. 2016;61(5):582–96.
54. Su Z, Ye P, Lin J, Zhang L, Huang X. Minimal surgery achieved good visual acuity in selected patients with magnetic intravitreal foreign body and traumatic cataract. BMC Ophthalmol. 2019;19(1):54.
55. Dhoble P, Khodifad A. Combined cataract extraction with pars Plana vitrectomy and metallic intraocular foreign body removal through sclerocorneal tunnel

using a novel “magnet handshake” technique. Asia-Pac J Ophthalmol. 2018;7:114–8.
56. Mahapatra S, Rao N. Visual outcome of pars plana vitrectomy with intraocular foreign body removal through sclerocorneal tunnel and sulcus-fixated intraocular lens implantation as a single procedure, in cases of metallic intraocular foreign body with traumatic cataract. Indian J Ophthalmol. 2010;58(2):115.
57. Resch MD, Balogh A, Sándor GL, Géhl Z, Nagy ZZ. Vitrectorhexis in penetrating eye injuries in adults. Eur J Ophthalmol. 2019;29(6):689–93.
58. Rai G, Sahai A, Kumar PR. Outcome of capsular tension ring (CTR) implant in complicated cataracts. J Clin Diagn Res. 2015;9(12):NC05–7.
59. Ma X, Li Z. Capsular tension ring implantation after lens extraction for management of subluxated cataracts. 6.
60. Buttanri IB, Sevim MS, Esen D, Acar BT, Serin D, Acar S. Modified capsular tension ring implantation in eyes with traumatic cataract and loss of zonular support. J Cataract Refract Surg. 2012;38(3):431–6.
61. Chee S-P, Jap A. Management of Traumatic Severely Subluxated Cataracts. Am J Ophthalmol. 2011;151(5):866–871.e1.
62. Grewal DS, Grewal SP. Femtosecond laser-assisted cataract surgery in pre-existing posterior capsule rupture following closed globe injury. Clin Exp Ophthalmol. 2015;43(5):478–80.
63. Prager AJ, Basti S. Femtosecond laser-assisted cataract surgery in management of posterior capsule tear following blunt trauma: case report and review of literature. Am J Ophthalmol Case Rep. 2020;19:100742.
64. Nagy ZZ, Kránitz K, Takacs A, Filkorn T, Gergely R, Knorz MC. Intraocular femtosecond laser use in traumatic cataracts following penetrating and blunt trauma. J Refract Surg. 2012;28(2):151–3.
65. Szepessy Z, Takács Á, Kránitz K, Filkorn T, Nagy ZZ. Intraocular femtosecond laser use in traumatic cataract. Eur J Ophthalmol. 2014;24(4):623–5.
66. Shah AS, Turalba AV. Intraocular lens implantation in penetrating ocular trauma. Int Ophthalmol Clin. 2010;50(1):43–59.
67. Tabatabaei A, Kiarudi MY, Ghassemi F, Moghimi S, Mansouri M, Mirshahi A, et al. Evaluation of posterior lens capsule by 20-MHz ultrasound probe in traumatic cataract. Am J Ophthalmol. 2012;153(1):51–4.
68. Kucukevcilioglu M, Hurmeric V, Ceylan OM. Preoperative detection of posterior capsule tear with ultrasound biomicroscopy in traumatic cataract. J Cataract Refract Surg. 2013;39(2):289–91.
69. Tabatabaei A, Hasanlou N, Kheirkhah A, Mansouri M, Faghihi H, Jafari H, et al. Accuracy of 3 imaging modalities for evaluation of the posterior lens capsule in traumatic cataract. J Cataract Refract Surg. 2014;40(7):1092–6.
70. Shah MA, Shah SM, Shah SB, Patel UA. Effect of interval between time of injury and timing of intervention on final visual outcome in cases of traumatic cataract. Eur J Ophthalmol. 2011;21(6):760–5.
71. Rogers G, Mustak H, Hann M, Steven D, Cook C. Sutured posterior chamber intraocular lenses for traumatic cataract in Africa. J Cataract Refract Surg. 2014;40(7):1097–101.
72. Rana M, Savant V, Prydal JI. A new customized artificial iris diaphragm for treatment of traumatic aniridia. Contact Lens Anterior Eye. 2013;36(2):93–4.
73. Spitzer MS, Nessmann A, Wagner J, Yoeruek E, Bartz-Schmidt KU, Szurman P, et al. Customized humanoptics silicone iris prosthesis in eyes with post-traumatic iris loss: outcomes and complications. Acta Ophthalmol. 2016;94(3):301–6.
74. Blanch RJ, Good PA, Shah P, Bishop JRB, Logan A, Scott RAH. Visual outcomes after blunt ocular trauma. Ophthalmology. 2013;120(8):1588–91.
75. Zhang Y, Zhang MN, Jiang CH, Yao Y, Zhang K. Endophthalmitis following open globe injury. Br J Ophthalmol. 2010;94(1):111–4.
76. Bhagat N, Nagori S, Zarbin M. Post-traumatic infectious Endophthalmitis. Surv Ophthalmol. 2011;56(3):214–51.
77. Essex R, Yi Q, Charles P, Allen P. Post-traumatic endophthalmitis☆. Ophthalmology. 2004;111(11):2015–22.
78. Abouammoh MA, Al-Mousa A, Gogandi M, Al-Mezaine H, Osman E, Alsharidah AM, et al. Prophylactic intravitreal antibiotics reduce the risk of post-traumatic endophthalmitis after repair of open globe injuries. Acta Ophthalmol. 2018;96(3):e361–5.

Traumatic Cataract

33

Thomas A. Oetting

Key Issues
- If vitreous is present, deal with it first.
- Capsule and zonular issues complicate nuclear disassembly.
- Strategy for zonular support depends on extent of zonular damage.
- Repair traumatized iris after lens removal and placement of intraocular lens.
- Practice surgical techniques on simulated eyes.

Briefly

Traumatic cataract present interesting challenges to the cataract surgeon. The cataract can present immediately after trauma with capsule rupture or years later. The traumatic cataract is associated with zonular, capsular, and iris issues, which must be addressed during the surgery. Vitreous prolapse around loose zonules can be particularly difficult and may require consultation with a vitreoretinal surgeon. The capsular and zonular issues lead to more deliberate and careful nuclear disassembly techniques. The typical steps for traumatic cataract are (1) attend to any vitreous, (2) anterior capsulotomy recognizing the need for possible capsule support, (3) support zonules with capsular rings or retractors for surgery, (4) careful nuclear disassembly; (5) support IOL for long-term stability, and finally (5) repair any iris injuries. Close follow-up with attention to possible glaucoma and retina sequelae is critical to long-term visual rehabilitation.

Supplementary Information The online version contains supplementary material available at [https://doi.org/10.1007/978-3-030-94530-5_33].

T. A. Oetting (✉)
University of Iowa, Department of Ophthalmology, Iowa City, IA, USA
e-mail: thomas-oetting@uiowa.edu

Mechanism of Lens Trauma

Blunt trauma is more common than open globes and both can cause traumatic cataract. In adult patients, falls (older adults) and workplace injuries (younger adults) are the most common causes of open globe injury [1, 2]. Blunt trauma is often associated with assault, and Shriver has shown particularly in women that blunt trauma can be associated with Intimate Partner Violence [3].

Blunt trauma is associated with cataract often complicated by weakened zonules (Table 33.1). A sector of weakened zonules can allow vitreous to prolapse into the anterior chamber. Rarely, blunt trauma alone can cause a rupture of the capsule [4]. The cataract from blunt trauma can present years later or within days of the trauma.

J. L. Alió et al. (eds.), *Cataract Surgery*, Essentials in Ophthalmology,
https://doi.org/10.1007/978-3-030-94530-5_33

Table 33.1 Trauma Mechanism

Mechanism	Cataract surgery issues	Common issues
Blunt	Weak zonules Vitreous Prolapse Torn capsule (rare)	Hyphema Iridodialysis Retinal dialysis Commotio Retina Ocular hypertension
Open globe		
Anterior penetration	Torn anterior capsule Weak zonules Analogous to radial tear	Ocular hypertension Infection Lens-induced inflammation
Posterior penetration	Torn posterior capsule Weak zonules Analogous to posterior polar	Ocular hypertension Infection Lens-induced inflammation Retinal dialysis Iatrogenic after vitrectomy and intravitreal injection
Perforating Lens	Torn anterior and posterior capsule Weak zonules Displaced lens material Vitreous prolapse Consider pars plana lensectomy	Ocular hypertension Infection Lens-induced inflammation Retinal dialysis

Often, the cataract from blunt trauma progresses slowly and, even if immediate, can be usually removed when convenient.

Open globes are associated with traumatic cataract either due to blunt injury of the lens or penetration of the capsule (Table 33.1). Capsule injuries, either anterior or posterior, can make nuclear disassembly difficult particularly when hydro-dissection or rotation of the nucleus is required. Ocular Coherence Tomography and ultrasound can be useful to evaluate the status of the lens capsule [5, 6]. Penetrating lens injuries can be either anterior or posterior or in perforating injuries of the lens, both capsules can be ruptured [7] Inflammation or glaucoma from lens particles can accelerate the need for removal of the traumatic cataract. However, waiting for traumatic corneal edema to resolve is often the best strategy for a definitive lens procedure. Often, with severe capsule trauma and especially with posterior lens material, the best strategy is a pars plana vitrectomy and lensectomy.

Iatrogenic lens trauma from past ocular surgery or intravitreal injections is increasingly common [8–10]. Injury to the posterior capsule from intravitreal injection or from past pars plana vitrectomy can be difficult to detect but should be suspected in any rapid cataract following a retinal procedure. Laser vitreo-lysis procedures for symptomatic floaters have also been associated with capsular injury and cataract formation [11].

Vitreous First

The first step when approaching a traumatic cataract is to detect or prevent vitreous prolapse. Staining vitreous in the anterior chamber is possible with triamcinolone, typically preservative-free [12, 13]. Removing the prolapsed vitreous can be done with an anterior approach, but the technique is most complete when the vitreous cutter is more posterior using a pars plana approach [14].

Sequestering the vitreous in areas of weakened zonules can be helpful in traumatic cases. Arshinoff described a technique using both cohesive and dispersive ophthalmic viscoelastic devices (OVD) to protect the cornea [15]. Fig. 33.1 shows a modification of his technique called the "sideways" Arshinoff shell. In this technique, a viscous dispersive OVD is first placed over an area of weak zonules (Fig. 33.1a) and the cohesive OVD is placed across from the weak zonules (Fig. 33.1b), which forces the dispersive OVD into the area of weak zonules, hopefully sealing off the vitreous from the anterior chamber.

Another nice technique to sequester the vitreous is early placement of a capsular tension ring when you have a sector of zonular damage. Fig. 33.2 shows how early placement (before nuclear removal) can recenter the lens, helping to block the vitreous from coming forward. In Fig. 33.2a, the lens is clearly decentered with a sector of zonular weakness, but after placement

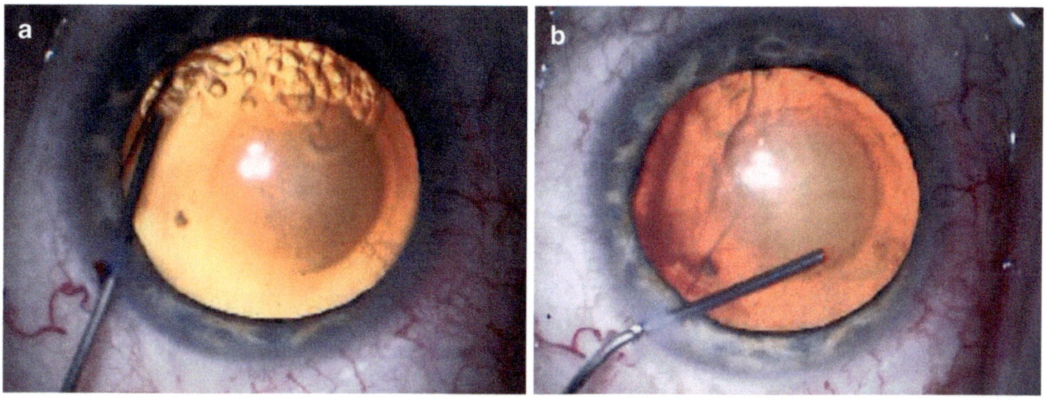

Fig. 33.1 Sideways Arshinoff Shell. (**a**) first place dispersive OVD over the area of zonular weakness. (**b**) second place cohesive OVD across from area of weakness to wedge dispersive OVD into area of zonular weakness

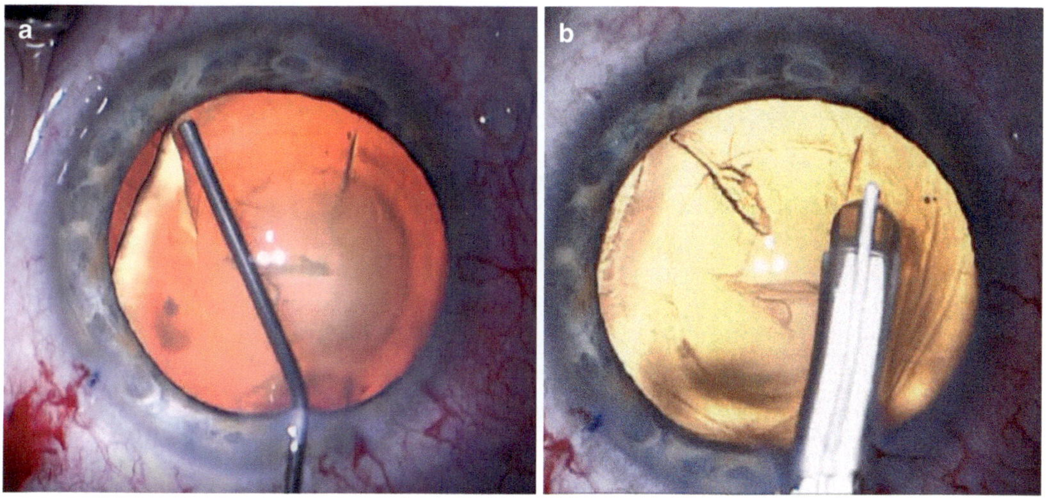

Fig. 33.2 CTR moves lens. (**a**) position of lens with weak zonules. (**b**) position of lens after placing the CTR

of the capsular tension ring (Fig. 33.2b), the lens is centered, reducing the risk of vitreous prolapse.

Capsulotomy

When the traumatized anterior capsule is already torn, creating a capsulotomy large enough for nucleus removal is difficult. A perfect capsulotomy is centered and round [16]. A good capsulotomy in a traumatic case is at least continuous, and centration and roundness are less important. Trypan blue and indocyanine green stain increases the capsule contrast by staining only the capsule and not the lens material [17, 18]. If the traumatic tear is central, then include that area in a larger continuous capsulotomy. Often the traumatic tear is peripheral, and the case is analogous to having a radial tear in a nontraumatic case where gentle techniques are used for nuclear disassembly.

When the capsule is intact, but the zonules are damaged, the capsulotomy can be difficult. It is important to center the capsulotomy on the lens and not on the pupil when the zonules are weak (Fig. 33.3). When the zonules are very weak, the capsule may not tear and the additional support of an iris hook (or several) for countertension can aid the capsulotomy (Fig. 33.4). The Femtosecond

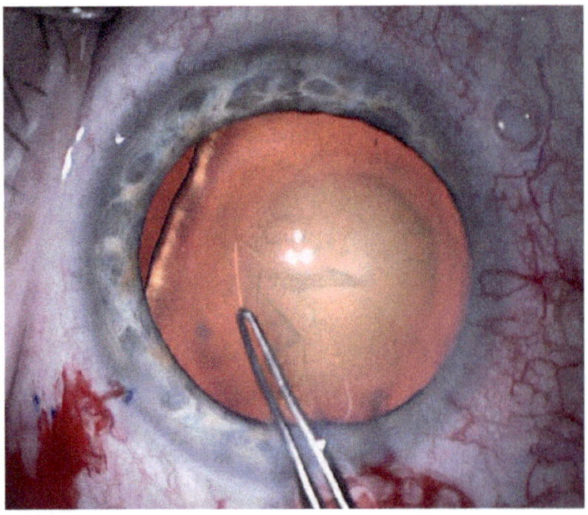

Fig. 33.3 Center the capsulotomy on the lens and not the pupil

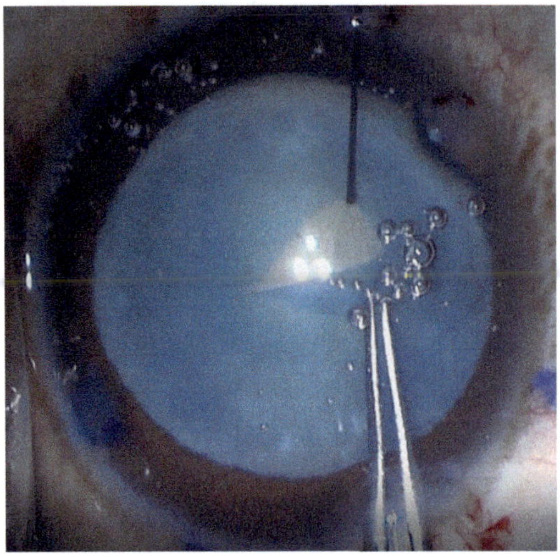

Fig. 33.4 An iris hook is used to apply countertraction during capsulotomy

laser can quickly create a capsulotomy with little zonular stress in traumatic cases [19].

Supporting the Zonules for Surgery

Following a continuous anterior capsulotomy, the anterior capsule can be used to support the lens during nuclear disassembly. The amount of support that is required depends on the amount of zonular loss (Table 33.2).

Table 33.2 Supporting the bag during nuclear disassembly

Supporting the bag for nucleus disassembly	Zonular loss
Early capsular tension ring (CTR) Cohesive OVD dissection Toward weak zonules	Up to 2–3 clock hours
Early capsular tension segment Support with iris hook Suture early	Up to 4–5 clock hours
Capsule retractors Place 1–4 Remove before placing IOL	Up to 12 clock hours

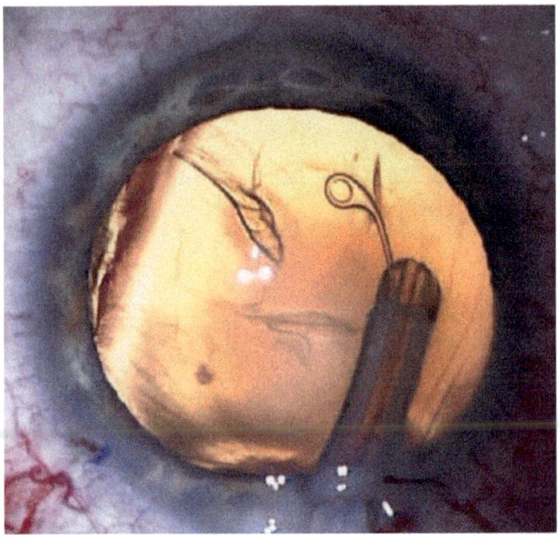

Fig. 33.5 Aim the leading eyelet of the CTR toward the area of weak zonules

One of the most effective techniques for minor loss of zonular support is early placement of a capsule tension ring (CTR) [20]. The CTR distributes the support from the weak to stronger zonules and can center the lens. The CTR is particularly useful when the zonulopathy is not progressive and when only a sector of zonules is damaged. The primary concern with placing the CTR early is that the CTR can trap cortical material and make cortical removal difficult. A key to early placement of the CTR is to use cohesive OVD dissection to create a space just under the capsule to place CTR (Fig. 33.2a) and not trap cortical material. Additionally, try to aim the leading CTR eyelet toward the weak area of zonules to further reduce zonular stress (Fig. 33.5).

Capsule retractors can fully or partially replace the zonular support to facilitate cataract surgery (Fig. 33.6). These devices are supported by a paracentesis and angle into the capsular bag to support the lens when the anterior capsule is intact. The surgeon can place only one or several to fully support the lens. While they only provide temporary support, they can be used during nuclear disassembly and then replaced with permanent support such as a CTR (Fig. 33.6). An alternative is to use a Capsular Tension Segment (CTS) held temporarily by an iris hook during surgery and then permanently attach the CTS following lens removal (Fig. 33.7).

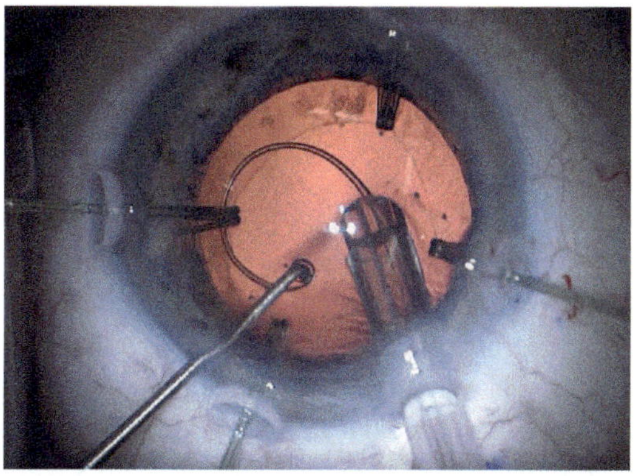

Fig. 33.6 Capsule retractors hold the capsule in place during lens removal and while placing the CTR

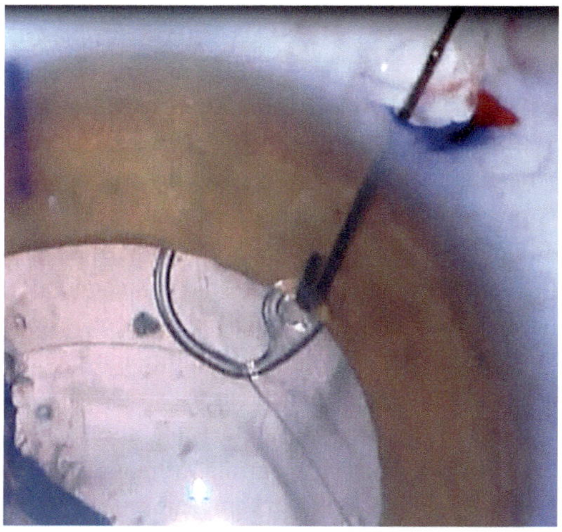

Fig. 33.7 An iris hook temporarily holds a CTS in place during lens removal

After the zonules are supported with an intact capsulotomy, proceed with gentle nuclear disassembly. The bottle height, vacuum, and flow rate of the pump should be lowered to allow slow and safe nuclear removal [21]. Surgeons should use the nuclear disassembly technique they are most comfortable with when zonules are loose. However, some surgeons feel that chopping techniques place less stress on the zonules assuming that they are proficient with this technique [22–26].

Nuclear Disassembly with Capsular Tears

Traumatic capsular tears make nuclear disassembly difficult. The primary concern is that any pressure against the capsule will extend the existing tear, allowing nuclear material to fall posteriorly. Also, additional tearing of the capsule can make subsequent capsular support of the IOL impossible. Avoiding hydro-dissection in these cases is important as this step creates pressure between the nucleus and the partially torn capsule. Nuclear disassembly techniques that do not require hydro-dissection or those that allow for a more controlled dissection between the capsule and nucleus are preferred when the capsule is potentially deficient (Table 33.3).

Traumatic capsular tears are analogous to other situations cataract surgeons face. Techniques for a traumatic anterior capsule tear are like commonly used strategies for errant radial tears when a routine capsulotomy does not go well. Surgical strategies for the weakened capsule of the posterior polar cataract are useful when we encounter a traumatic posterior tear [27, 28].

The strategy for traumatic nuclear disassembly with a tear depends on the density of the lens (Table 33.3). If the lens is very dense and capsule support is compromised, consider conversion to an extracapsular surgery technique. Similarly, if the capsule is tentative and some nuclear material has likely already fallen posteriorly, then referring the patient for a pars plana vitrectomy with lensectomy is reasonable. Most of the cases with

Table 33.3 Techniques for nuclear disassembly with capsule tears

Technique	Strategy	Advantages	Disadvantages
Bowl then collapse	No hydro-dissection Sculpt out large bowl Gentle dispersive OVD dissection Remove lens with I/A or anterior vitrector	No hydro-dissection or rotation, so less likely to expand tear Nice for soft lenses	Difficult with even moderate density lenses
Modified stop and chop	No hydro-dissection Sculpt long deep groove Gently divide into 2 pieces Hydro-delineation Careful rotation and chopping Low bottle height and vacuum	No hydro-dissection, so less likely to expand tear Familiar	Difficult with soft or hard lenses
V groove	Sculpt two long grooves join in subincisional area forms V shape Gently divide into 3 pieces	No hydro-dissection or rotation, so less likely to expand tear Nice for dense lenses	Difficult with soft lenses V grooves can be hard to produce
Pars plana Vitrectomy Lensectomy	Pars plana vitrectomy Lens removal	No capsule required for lens removal	Big setup May need retina surgeon

existing traumatic capsule tears can be handled with anterior segment approaches that vary depending on lens density.

When the lens is soft with a capsular tear present, the surgeon can simply sculpt out a central bowl with the phacoemulsification handpiece. The remaining material can then be removed after gentle hydro-delineation or OVD dissection. This allows the lens material to prolapse on itself with less outward pressure against the weakened capsule.

When the lens is of medium density, the surgeon should first sculpt a central deep groove and then divide the lens into two pieces without rotation or hydro-dissection. Hydro-delineation is then directed into the side of the groove, possibly freeing the central nucleus. Because the lens is already cracked centrally, fluid that inadvertently tracks into the subcapsular area can vent through the divided lens, reducing pressure on the weakened capsule. The space formed by the groove allows the two halves to fold inward, which creates less pressure on the weakened capsule.

When the traumatic cataract is very dense, consider pulling out an old but robust technique. Dr. Charles Kelman described the "V groove" technique also sometimes referred to as the Victory groove in 1994 [27]. The surgeon sculpts two grooves that intersect in the subincisional space to form a V or lambda shape (Fig. 33.8a). The V groove separates the nucleus into three pieces. The three pieces are divided with instruments as in Gimbal's divide and conquer [22]. The separation of the entire nucleus occurs without rotation and without dissection (Fig. 33.8b). This technique is ideal for dense lenses with a suspected capsular tear such as in posterior polar cataract [28].

Supporting the Intraocular Lens

After the traumatic cataract is removed, the IOL is placed using the remaining capsule if present. Table 33.4 summarizes IOL placement depending on the amount of capsule and zonular support that remains. Rarely, the IOL placement is done at a subsequent procedure if additional devices are needed for IOL placement.

Using only an IOL and a CTR, the surgeon can handle a broad spectrum of zonular deficiency (Table 33.4). With only minimal zonular loss, a simple 3 piece can be oriented so that the haptics axis provides maximum centration. Implanting a CTR gives even more support. A

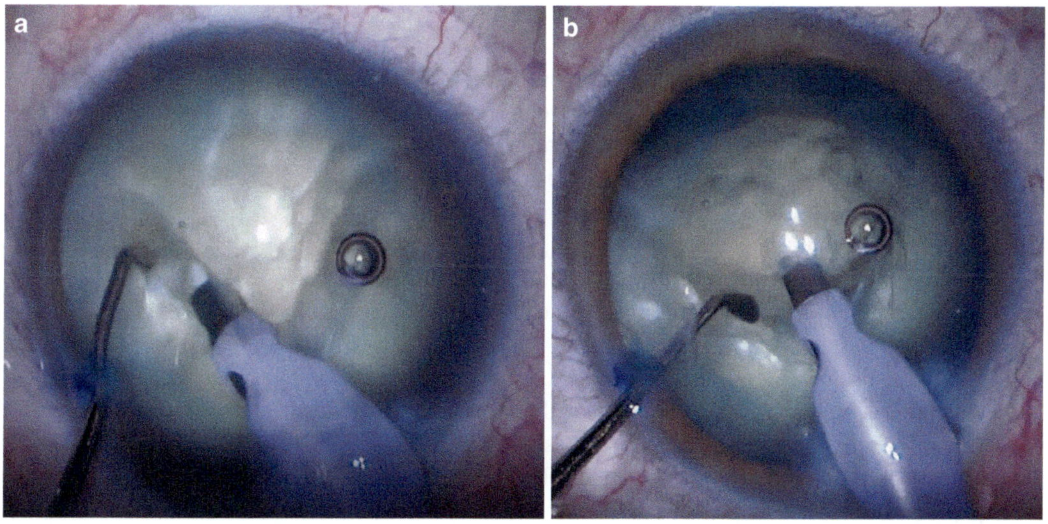

Fig. 33.8 V groove technique. (**a**) make 2 grooves that intersect in the subincisional space. (**b**) break the nucleus into 3 pieces with the grooves without rotation or hydro-dissection.

Table 33.4 Supporting the intraocular lens (IOL)

Supporting the IOL	Zonular Loss
3-piece IOL Haptic toward weak zonules Gentle placement	Up to 1 clock hour
Capsular tension ring (CTR) IOL in bag Haptic location not important	Up to 2–3 clock hours
CTR with capture Traditional optic capture Haptics in sulcus, optic in bag	Up to 4–5 clock hours
CTR and capsular tension segment (CTS) IOL in bag Many fixation techniques	Up to 6–8 clock hours
CTR and 2 CTS May need to place CTS first IOL in bag	Up to 12 clock hours
Intra scleral haptic fixation (IHSF) Yamane Agarwal Glued IOL *Sutured IOL* Scleral Iris *Anterior chamber IOL* Angle supported Iris clip supported	No Capsule

very interesting option is to use a CTR and a 3 piece IOL in the traditional optic capture configuration [29, 30]. Traditional optic capture is very stable with the haptics in the sulcus and the optic in the bag (Fig. 33.9). The haptics in the sulcus give immediate support, and the captured optic help prevent phimosis, which can cause subsequent decentration.

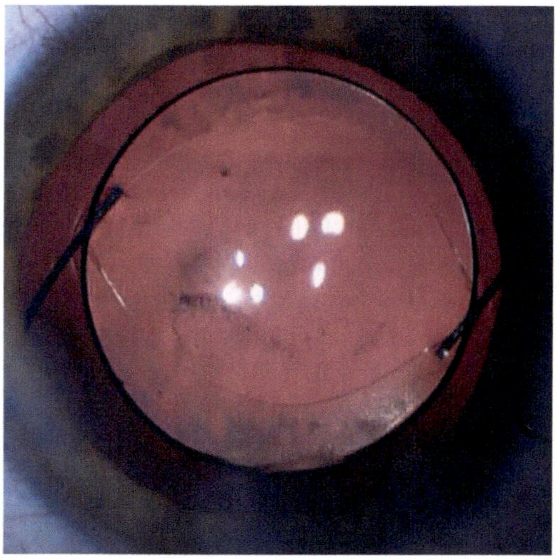

Fig. 33.9 Traditional optic capture with the haptics in the sulcus and the optic in the bag

In the setting of an intact anterior capsule and posterior capsule tear, optic capture is useful. Traditional optic capture with 3-piece haptics in the sulcus and the optic posterior and captured by the capsule is more stable than simply placing the entire IOL in the sulcus [29]. Reverse optic capture with haptics in the compromised bag and the optic captured anteriorly is another option even for single piece acrylic IOLs [31].

The CTS adds additional support when attached to the sclera [32]. Many techniques have been described to attach this device to the sclera including prolene and gortex suturing techniques [32–34], sliding suture techniques [35], and using the Canabrava double flange technique [36]. When 2 CTS are used together with a CTR, an IOL can be supported in the bag with no real zonular support [32].

When the capsule does not support an IOL, there are many techniques to support an IOL with iris or scleral tissue (Table 33.4). Wagoner's classic study [37], recently confirmed by Shen's task force paper [38], does not support using one technique over another. The surgeon should use the technique they are most comfortable with when faced with no capsular support.

Repair the Iris Last

The techniques for repairing traumatic iris damage are outside the scope of this chapter. The iris damage should be repaired after the lens is removed and the IOL is placed. An iris hook can be used to hold damaged iris away from the operative field until the end of the case when the surgeon is ready for iris repair. The iris can also be repaired in a subsequent procedure if the surgeon is not experienced with iris repair techniques.

Practicing These Techniques

Simulation techniques have dramatically improved with the advent of very realistic artificial eyes. Rogers showed that practicing techniques with structured simulation can shift the learning curve and lessen complications of early cases [39]. Practicing on artificial eyes in the operating room is a high-fidelity simulation as the surgeon uses the same microscope and phacoemulsification machine used for patients (Fig. 33.10).

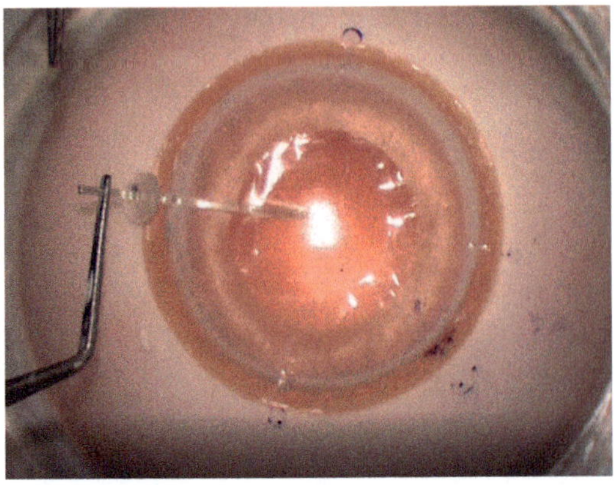

Fig. 33.10 Phillips PS35 artificial eye to practice placement of capsular retractors

Take-Home Points

- Traumatic cataract can come from blunt injury or open globe.
- The first step is to attend to traumatic vitreous prolapse.
- Support for weakened zonules is facilitated by a continuous anterior capsulotmy.
- The CTR is a useful device for traumatic cataract.
- The nucleus disassembly technique depends on the capsule status and the density of the lens.
- The surgeon should be familiar with different methods to fixate an IOL when capsular support is compromised."

References

1. Beshay N, Keay L, Dunn H, Kamalden TA, Hoskin AK, Watson SL. The epidemiology of Open Globe Injuries presenting to a tertiary referral eye hospital in Australia. Injury. 2017;48(7):1348–54.
2. Bauza AM, Emami P, Soni N, Holland BK, Langer P, Zarbin M, Bhagat N. A 10-year review of assault-related open-globe injuries at an urban hospital. Graefes Arch Clin Exp Ophthalmol. 2013;251(3):653–9.
3. Cohen AR, Renner LM, Shriver EM. Intimate partner violence in ophthalmology: a global call to action. Curr Opin Ophthalmol. 2017;28(5):534–8.

4. Mangan MS, Arıcı C, Tuncer İ, Yetik H. Isolated anterior lens capsule rupture secondary to blunt trauma: pathophysiology and treatment. Turk J Ophthalmol. 2016;46(4):197–9. https://doi.org/10.4274/tjo.85547.
5. Pujari A, Sharma N. The emerging role of anterior segment optical coherence tomography in cataract surgery: current role and future perspectives. Clin Ophthalmol. 2021;15:389–401.
6. Perry LJ. The evaluation of patients with traumatic cataracts by ultrasound technologies. Semin Ophthalmol. 2012;27(5–6):121–4.
7. Razeghinejad R, Lin MM, Lee D, Katz LJ, Myers JS. Pathophysiology and management of glaucoma and ocular hypertension related to trauma. Surv Ophthalmol. 2020;65(5):530–47.
8. Miller DC, Christopher KL, Patnaik JL, Lynch AM, Seibold LK, Mandava N, Taravella MJ. Posterior capsule rupture during cataract surgery in eyes receiving intravitreal anti-VEGF injections. Curr Eye Res. 2020;23:1–6.
9. Hahn P, Yashkin AP, Sloan FA. Effect of prior anti-VEGF injections on the risk of retained lens fragments and endophthalmitis after cataract surgery in the elderly. Ophthalmology. 2016;123(2):309–15.
10. Lee AY, Day AC, Egan C, Bailey C, Johnston RL, Tsaloumas MD, Denniston AK, Tufail A. United Kingdom age-related macular degeneration and diabetic retinopathy electronic medical records users group. Previous intravitreal therapy is associated with increased risk of posterior capsule rupture during cataract surgery. Ophthalmology. 2016;123(6):1252–6.
11. Sun IT, Lee TH, Chen CH. Rapid cataract progression after Nd:YAG Vitreolysis for vitreous floaters: a case report and literature review. Case Rep Ophthalmol. 2017;8(2):321–5.
12. Kasbekar S, Prasad S, Kumar BV. Clinical outcomes of triamcinolone-assisted anterior vitrectomy after phacoemulsification complicated by posterior capsule rupture. J Cataract Refract Surg. 2013;39(3):414–8. https://doi.org/10.1016/j.jcrs.2012.10.042. Epub 2013 Jan 18. PMID: 23337526.
13. Burk SE, Da Mata AP, Snyder ME, Schneider S, Osher RH, Cionni RJ. Visualizing vitreous using Kenalog suspension. J Cataract Refract Surg. 2003;29(4):645–51.
14. Arbisser LB, Charles S, Howcroft M, Werner L. Management of vitreous loss and dropped nucleus during cataract surgery. Ophthalmol Clin N Am. 2006;19(4):495–506.
15. Arshinoff SA. Dispersive-cohesive viscoelastic soft shell technique. J Cataract Refract Surg. 1999;25(2):167–73. https://doi.org/10.1016/s0886-3350(99)80121-7. PMID: 9951659.
16. Gimbel HV, Neuhann T. Continuous curvilinear capsulorhexis. J Cataract Refract Surg. 1991;17(1):110–1. https://doi.org/10.1016/s0886-3350(13)81001-2.
17. Newsom TH, Oetting TA. Indocyanine green staining in traumatic cataract. J Cataract Refract Surg. 2000;26(11):1691–3.
18. Kazem MA, Behbehani JH, Uboweja AK, Paramasivam RB. Traumatic cataract surgery assisted by trypan blue. Ophthalmic Surg Lasers Imaging. 2007;38(2):160–3.
19. Prager AJ, Basti S. Femtosecond laser-assisted cataract surgery in management of posterior capsule tear following blunt trauma: case report and review of literature. Am J Ophthalmol Case Rep. 2020;19:100742.
20. Price FW Jr, Mackool RJ, Miller KM, Koch P, Oetting TA, Johnson AT. Interim results of the United States investigational device study of the Ophtec capsular tension ring. Ophthalmology. 2005;112(3):460–5.
21. Osher RH. Slow motion phacoemulsification approach. J Cataract Refract Surg. 1993;19(5):667. https://doi.org/10.1016/s0886-3350(13)80025-9. PMID: 8229730.
22. Gimbel HV. Divide and conquer nucleofractis phacoemulsification: development and variations. J Cataract Refract Surg. 1991;17(3):281–91.
23. Pacifico RL. Divide and conquer phacoemulsification. One-handed variant. J Cataract Refract Surg. 1992;18(5):513–7.
24. Nagahara K. "Phaco Chop," presented as a video at the 1993 ASCRS symposium on cataract, IOL and refractive surgery. Seattle; 1993; "Phaco-Chop Technique Eliminates Central Sculpting and Allows Faster, Safer Phaco," Ocular Surgery News, international edition, October 1993, pages 12–13.
25. Can I, Takmaz T, Cakici F, Ozgül M. Comparison of Nagahara phaco-chop and stop-and-chop phacoemulsification nucleotomy techniques. J Cataract Refract Surg. 2004;30(3):663–8.
26. Pandit RT, Oetting TA. Pop-and-chop nucleofractis. J Cataract Refract Surg. 2003;29(11):2054–6.
27. Kelman CD. V Groove phaco technique: fast, easy, safe: interview with Dr. Kelman. Ophthalmol Times 1994;19:12.
28. Malhotra C, Dhingra D, Nawani N, Chakma P, Jain AK. Phacoemulsification in posterior polar cataract: experience from a tertiary eye care Centre in North India. Indian J Ophthalmol. 2020;68(4):589–94.
29. Kemp PS, Oetting TA. Stability and safety of MA50 intraocular lens placed in the sulcus. Eye (Lond). 2015;29(11):1438–41.
30. Chang DF, Masket S, Miller KM, Braga-Mele R, Little BC, Mamalis N, Oetting TA, Packer M. ASCRS Cataract Clinical Committee. Complications of sulcus placement of single-piece acrylic intraocular lenses: recommendations for backup IOL implantation following posterior capsule rupture. J Cataract Refract Surg. 2009;35(8):1445–58.
31. Jones JJ, Oetting TA, Rogers GM, Jin GJ. Reverse optic capture of the single-piece acrylic intraocular lens in eyes with posterior capsule rupture. Ophthalmic Surg Lasers Imaging. 2012;43(6):480–8.
32. Hasanee K, Ahmed II. Capsular tension rings: update on endocapsular support devices. Ophthalmol Clin N Am. 2006;19(4):507–19.

33. Kirk TQ, Condon GP. Simplified ab externo scleral fixation for late in-the-bag intraocular lens dislocation. J Cataract Refract Surg. 2012;38(10):1711–5. Erratum in: J Cataract Refract Surg. 2013 Mar;39(3):489. PMID: 22999598.
34. Hoffman RS, Fine IH, Packer M. Scleral fixation without conjunctival dissection. J Cataract Refract Surg. 2006;32(11):1907–12.
35. Oetting TA, Tsui JY, Szeto AT. Sliding internal knot technique for late in-the-bag intraocular lens decentration. J Cataract Refract Surg. 2011;37(5):810–3.
36. Canabrava S, Canedo Domingos Lima AC, Arancibia AEL, Bicalho Dornelas LF, Ribeiro G. Novel double-flanged technique for managing Marfan syndrome and microspherophakia. J Cataract Refract Surg. 2020;46(3):333–9.
37. Wagoner MD, Cox TA, Ariyasu RG, Jacobs DS, Karp CL; American Academy of Ophthalmology. Intraocular lens implantation in the absence of capsular support: a report by the American Academy of Ophthalmology. Ophthalmology. 2003.
38. Shen JF, Deng S, Hammersmith KM, Kuo AN, Li JY, Weikert MP, Shtein RM. Intraocular lens implantation in the absence of zonular support: an outcomes and safety update: a report by the American Academy of ophthalmology. Ophthalmology. 2020;127(9):1234–58.
39. Rogers GM, Oetting TA, Lee AG, Grignon C, Greenlee E, Johnson AT, Beaver HA, Carter K. Impact of a structured surgical curriculum on ophthalmic resident cataract surgery complication rates. J Cataract Refract Surg. 2009;35(11):1956–60.

34 Femtosecond Laser in Complex and Complicated Cases

H. Burkhard Dick and Ronald D. Gerste

Bullet Points

- Laser cataract surgery has proved to be safe and effective in many cases of ocular comorbidities; the procedure, however, might be off-label in such complex situations.
- In intumescent cataract, a minicapsulotomy prior to the "real" one reduces intralenticular pressure and helps avoid the so-called Argentinian flag syndrome.
- Miosis caused by laser-induced prostaglandin release can be prevented by a speedy procedure and by preoperative application of NSAID (nonsteroidal anti-inflammatory drug) eye drops.
- Since there is some indication of a lower probability of postoperative cystoid macular edema than after standard cataract surgery, laser cataract surgery (LCS) may be preferable to conventional phacoemulsification in retinal disease where any (additional) inflammatory stimulus has to be avoided.
- Contraindications against the use of the femtosecond laser in cataract surgery are most of all: certain facial features that prevent proper docking, obesity that makes lying on the treatment bed impossible, tremors like in Parkinson's disease, claustrophobia and other forms of anxiety, severe deformations of the spine.

Introduction

Femtosecond laser cataract surgery is an established procedure whose precision, safety, and predictability have proven extremely valuable in countless surgeries all over the world. It is particularly benefitting for patients who will receive an innovative intraocular lens (IOL) like, for instance, a toric IOL, a bag-in-the-lens IOL, a potentially accommodative IOL, a multifocal IOL. But laser cataract surgery (LCS) is not just for the healthy, uncomplicated patient without any noteworthy medical history, without any ocular comorbidity. The technology has by now time

Supplementary Information The online version contains supplementary material available at [https://doi.org/10.1007/978-3-030-94530-5_34].

H. B. Dick
Ruhr University Eye Clinic, Bochum, Germany
e-mail: burkhard.dick@kk-bochum.de

R. D. Gerste (✉)
Ophthalmologist and Science Publicist,
North Potomac, MD, USA

J. L. Alió et al. (eds.), *Cataract Surgery*, Essentials in Ophthalmology,
https://doi.org/10.1007/978-3-030-94530-5_34

and again been successful in cases that pose a challenge for the surgeon and usually comes with significant risk for the patient. This is reflected less in studies but rather in case reports and small series, particularly when rare conditions are concerned. In the hands of an experienced surgeon, the femtosecond laser offers chances for patients that have often been deemed problematic. It has to be noted, however, that some if not most of these interventions are considered off-label, in particular since the manuals provided by the manufacturer are in general quite restrictive when it comes to indications and quite generous with alleged contraindications.

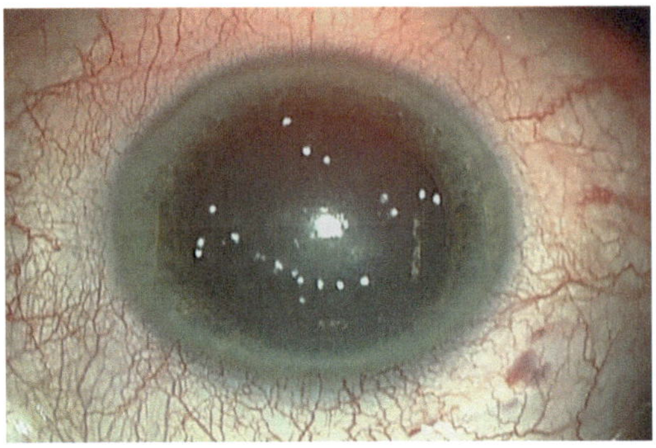

Fig. 34.1 Corneal scars (after keratitis epidemica) marked using chalk for LCS

In the following, we will review the use of the femtosecond laser in the cataract surgery of patients that come with pathologies beyond a simple lens opacification. This chapter does in no way claim completeness – some challenging cases like pediatric cataracts are featured in other chapters – and rather strives to give an impression of the possibilities offered by LCS. It is still an evolving technology, and its limits have not been reached yet.

Corneal Pathologies

While laser application is rightfully excluded in cases of severe corneal opacifications and massive corneal opacities, in eyes with a paracentral opacity where preoperative imaging can demonstrate that the extent of the scar lies outside the laser delivery zone, the femtosecond laser may be used (Figs. 34.1, 34.2, 34.3, and 34.4). The location of the capsulotomy and the depth and energy

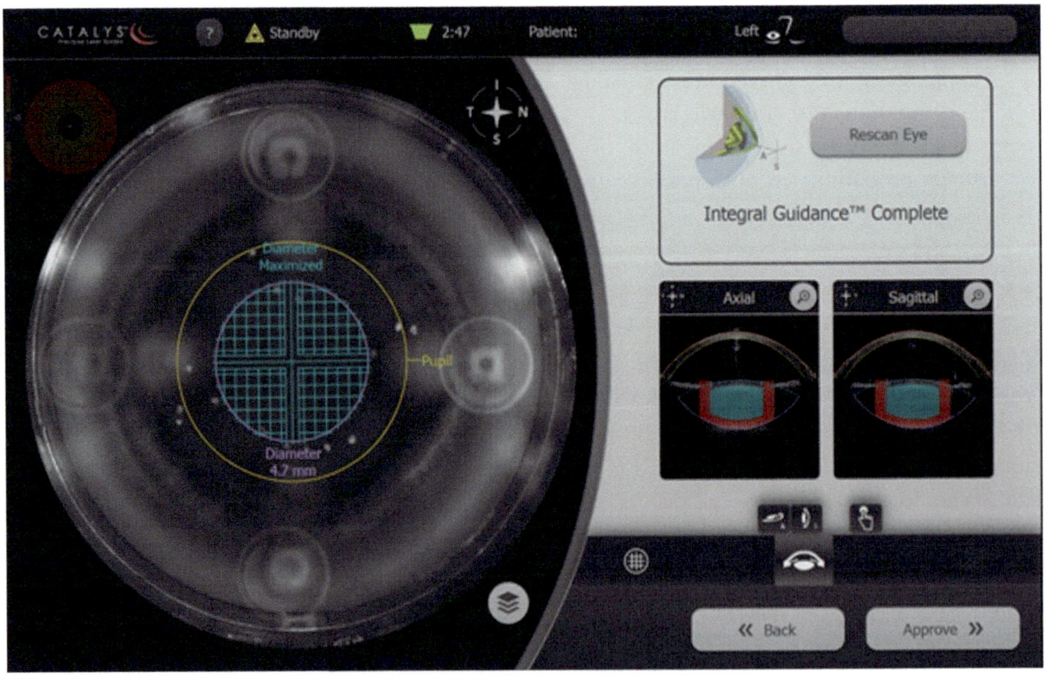

Fig. 34.2 Fitting and adjusting the capsulotomy according to the marked scars (laser monitor view)

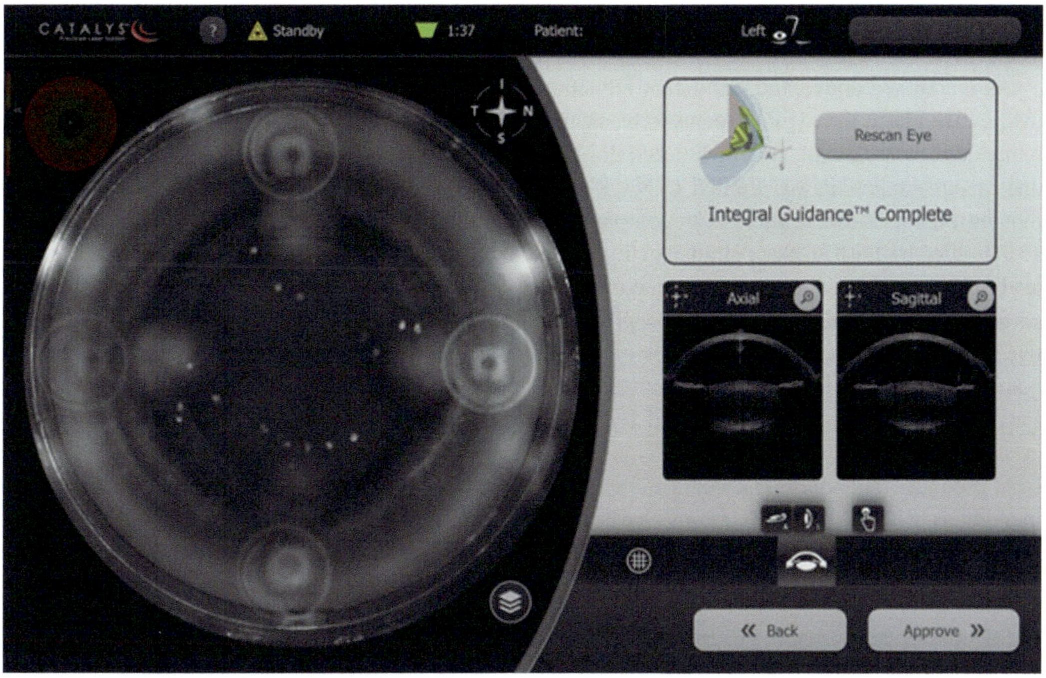

Fig. 34.3 Lasing the capsulotomy after capsulotomy adjustment (laser monitor view; infrared camera)

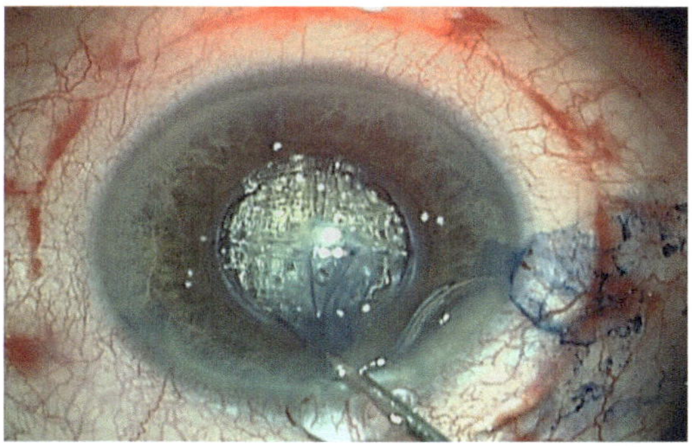

Fig. 34.4 View through OR microscope after laser capsulotomy has been performed

parameters can be modified to successfully perform a capsulotomy while avoiding the area of the corneal scar as delineated by intraoperative imaging. [1] Grewal et al. described a case where the ability to customize the laser to treat through central and paracentral clear cornea permitted a perfect though slightly smaller (4.7 mm) than usual capsulotomy and the surgery was successfully completed. [2] The intraoperative OCT provided by some laser platforms has been described by Hou et al. as very helpful in customizing the position and tilt of the capsulotomy in eyes with a distorted anterior capsule, which they encountered in a patient with Peters' anomaly type 2, a condition with central corneal opacification and often corneolenticular adhesions. In this case, the customization of the laser settings led to a well-centered capsulotomy and the intervention resulted in a (given the severity of the disease) good visual acuity [3].

There is, under the right circumstances, no need to refrain from LCS in patients who had previously undergone penetrating keratoplasty. Martin et al. reported treating 12 postpenetrating keratoplasty patients with LCS. Docking in all cases was successful. The authors suggested increasing the energy level if required, due to reduced corneal clarity. Their initial settings were between 10 and 12 μJ with final settings reduced to 6 μJ. [4] Nagy et al. reported a 33-year-old man who underwent laser cataract surgery following penetrating keratoplasty. Intraoperative OCT identified the scar at the graft-host junction, and the scar did not interfere with the laser capsulotomy. This group required no ultrasound to remove the lens; the endothelial cell count remained unchanged up to a year after surgery [5].

As mentioned above, the significant reduction in effective phaco time (EPT) seems to result in a remarkable decrease of endothelial cell loss: in one of our studies, it was limited to 8.1% three months postoperatively after LCS compared to 13.7% after traditional phacoemulsification. This leads to the conclusion that the technique might be particularly beneficial in eyes with a low preoperative endothelial cell count like in cases of cornea guttata and Fuchs dystrophy [6]. Patients with Fuchs dystrophy have been identified by Hatch et al. as those – together with patients suffering from pseudoexfoliation, brunescent cataracts, and individuals with a history of trauma – who may particularly benefit from this technology. [7] This was reinforced by a study from Singapore that focused on the postoperative loss of endothelial cell density (ECD) in 140 eyes with Fuchs endothelial dystrophy of which 68 underwent femtosecond laser cataract surgery and 72 underwent standard phacoemulsification. Eyes with mild cataract in the phacoemulsification group had a mean ECD loss of 10.7% and those with moderate or hard cataract of 19.5%. This loss was significantly smaller following LCS with a mean of 0.9% in mild and 8.2% in moderate and hard cataracts, leading the authors to conclude that there is less risk of corneal decompensation to these vulnerable eyes if they are exposed to reduced ultrasound energy due to the laser procedure. [8]

Brunescent and Intumescent White Cataracts

Brunescent cataracts, for instance, usually require an increased phacoemulsification time and are at higher risk for thermal and mechanical injuries to the cornea and corneal edema. In a study on 240 eyes, LCS was more effective than phacoemulsification in fragmenting the advanced cataract in so far as requiring far less effective phacoemulsification time (EPT). In eyes with LOCS III grade 3 cataracts, EPT ranged from 0.46 to 3.10 seconds (mean 1.38) in the phacoemulsification group, while it was zero in the LCS group. In eyes with grade 4 brunescent cataracts, EPT was 2.12 to 19.29 seconds (mean 6.85) in the phacoemulsification group and 0 to 6.75 seconds (mean 1.35) in the LCS group. [9]

A comparable situation exists with intumescent cataracts – described in more detail in another chapter – which usually pose a challenge to the surgeon since they tend to have increased intralenticular pressure due to liquefication of the cortex. This often comes along with a swelling and consecutive thickening of the intumescent white lens as well as a flat anterior chamber. (Fig. 34.5) To release this pressure, a minicapsulotomy technique where a smaller capsulotomy is initially performed to release the intralenticular pressure (Video 34.1). With a diameter of 2.0 mm and 4 μJ pulse energy, this treatment usually leads to the discharge of lens material into the anterior chamber. This first step to release the pressure is followed by redocking to the laser and a second larger capsulotomy, usually with a diameter of 4.5 to 5.1 mm. If any capsule bridges remain, homogenous injection of ophthalmic viscosurgical device (OVD) in the anterior chamber and the dimple-down maneuver followed by the use of a microforceps to ensure complete capsular dissection through a paracentesis is performed. Identification of the anterior capsule by the laser platform's imaging system has been possible in all of our cases. [10] This procedure seems to render operating on intumescent cataracts relatively safe – and probably more so than manual capsulorhexis with its potential for complications. [11]

Small Pupil – Primary or Laser Induced

A small pupil is a problem in conventional cataract surgery and it is not much different in LCS: if the pupil is smaller than the intended diameter of the laser-guided capsulotomy, the procedure is no longer possible in the normal way. It is important – particularly in how this problem is going to be solved – to distinguish between a preexisting small pupil (after application of mydriatics and before the laser is docked and employed) and a small pupil following laser treatment. [12] A

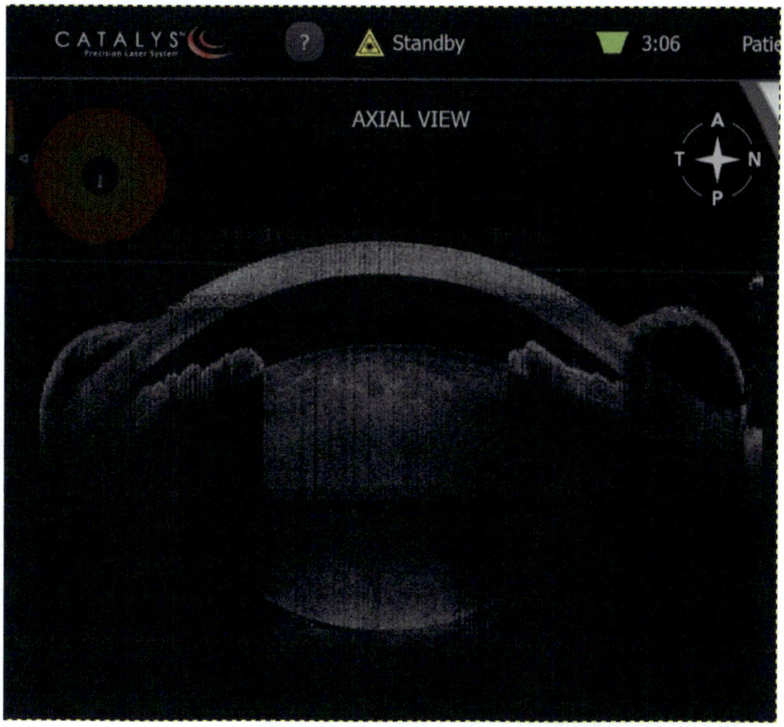

Fig. 34.5 Spectral-domain-assisted optical coherence tomography demonstrating a thick lens and a flat anterior chamber (intraoperative LCS view)

small pupil can make not only conventional cataract surgery but also laser cataract surgery more difficult. Most laser platforms have a capsulotomy diameter of 5.0 mm as a default setting, which means that a pupil size at least slightly larger would be desirable. Of course, the surgeon can choose a smaller capsulotomy, but the risk of capsular phimosis is reported to increase with diameters below 4.0 mm [1].

A poorly dilated pupil can be expected in eyes with comorbidities like pseudoexfoliation, glaucoma, chronic uveitis, and zonular dehiscence as well as after previous surgery and in eyes with floppy iris syndrome. A first step to resolve that problem would be the intracameral application of epinephrine. If this turns out to be unsuccessful, an OVD combined with a mydriatic drug will be given. There are a number of devices available that provide a pupil large enough to safely and effectively perform laser cataract surgery if these pharmacological options do not lead to the desired result. Iris retractors, for instance, can be used with or without ophthalmic viscosurgical devices (OVDs) (Fig. 34.6a, b, c). In the former case, the laser settings should be adjusted due to the presence of OVD in the anterior chamber. In these cases, a higher pulse energy (like 10 μJ) is recommended. The Malyugin ring is another device that helps in cases of preoperatively small pupils. Complete OVD removal is recommended, since more small adhesions of the anterior capsulotomy were observed when the anterior chamber was still filled with the viscoelastic [13] (Figs. 34.6 and 34.7).

Soon after the introduction of the femtosecond laser into cataract surgery, first reports of intraoperative miosis in some patients surfaced. [14] The cause of this problem – and it can be a problem since small pupils can increase the difficulty of the surgery and lead to higher complication rates during lens removal – was soon identified: it is the release of prostaglandins by the laser treatment, as is described in another chapter of this book. It has been well known for some time that prostaglandins appear in the aqueous humor following different mechanical or thermal stimuli. The principal source for prostaglandins in the eye is the nonpigmented epithelial layer of the ciliary body. In 113 patients aqueous humor was collected during cataract surgery right

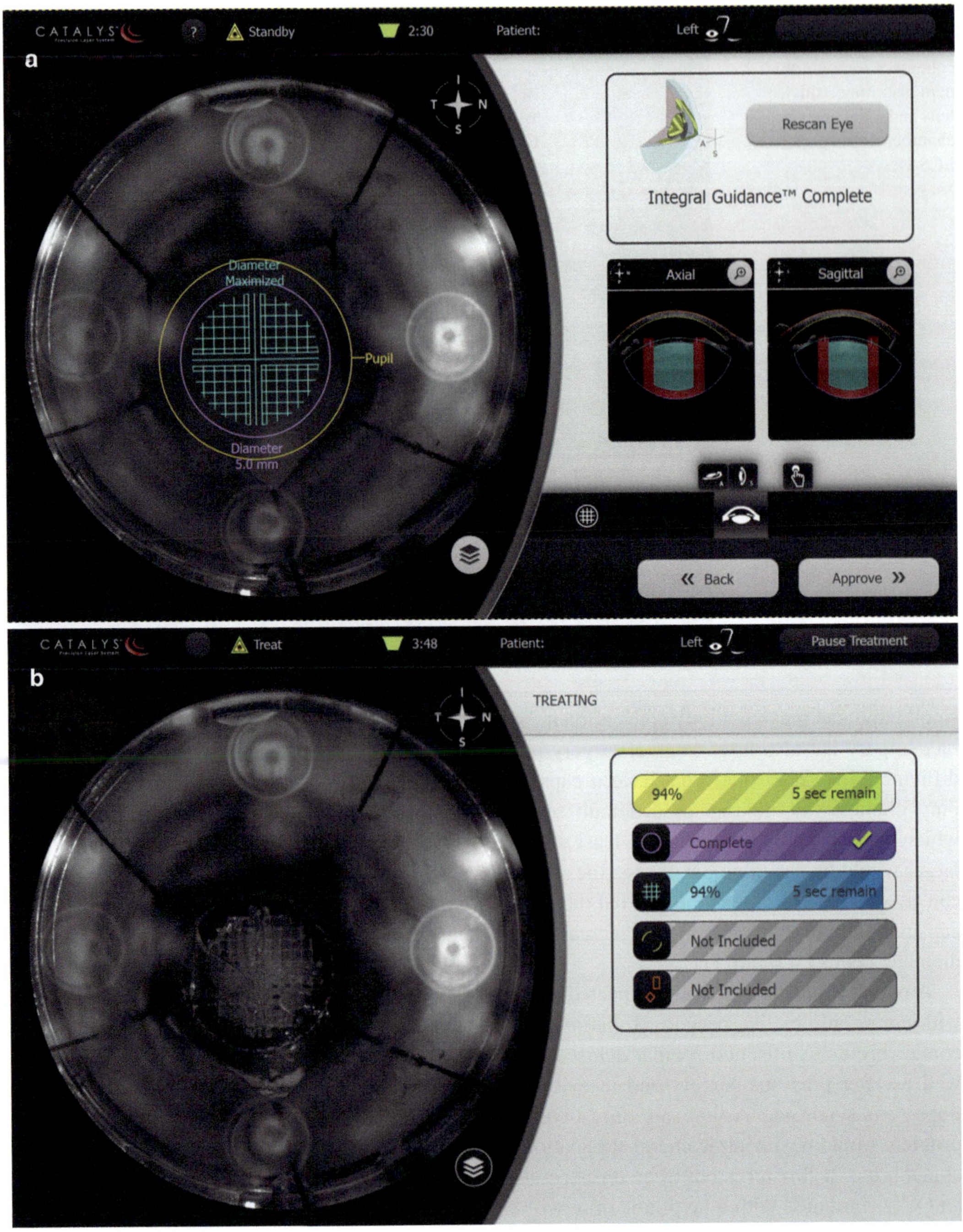

Fig. 34.6 (**a**) Treatment planning overlay for LCS in a small pupil dilated by iris retractors. (**b**) Laser treatment of an advanced cataract in a pupil dilated using iris retractors. (**c**) Laser fragmentation is completed in an eye with a small pupil and advanced a small pupil and advanced cataract dilated using iris retractors

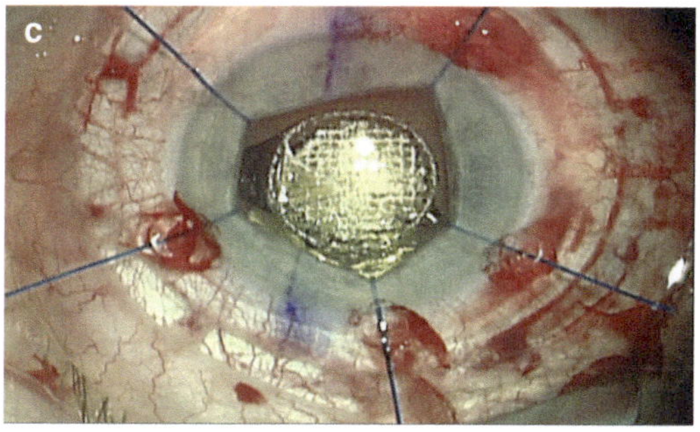

Fig. 35.6 (continued)

after femtosecond laser treatment; in the control group of 107 eyes samples were taken just before commencing conventional phacoemulsification. These probes showed significant differences. In the femtosecond laser group, the average level of prostaglandin E_2 in one part of the study was 182 pg/ml – more than tenfold the concentration of PGE_2 in the control group, which was 17.3 pg/ml. [15] Besides a speedy transition from laser treatment to the manual conclusion of the procedure, administering nonsteroidal anti-

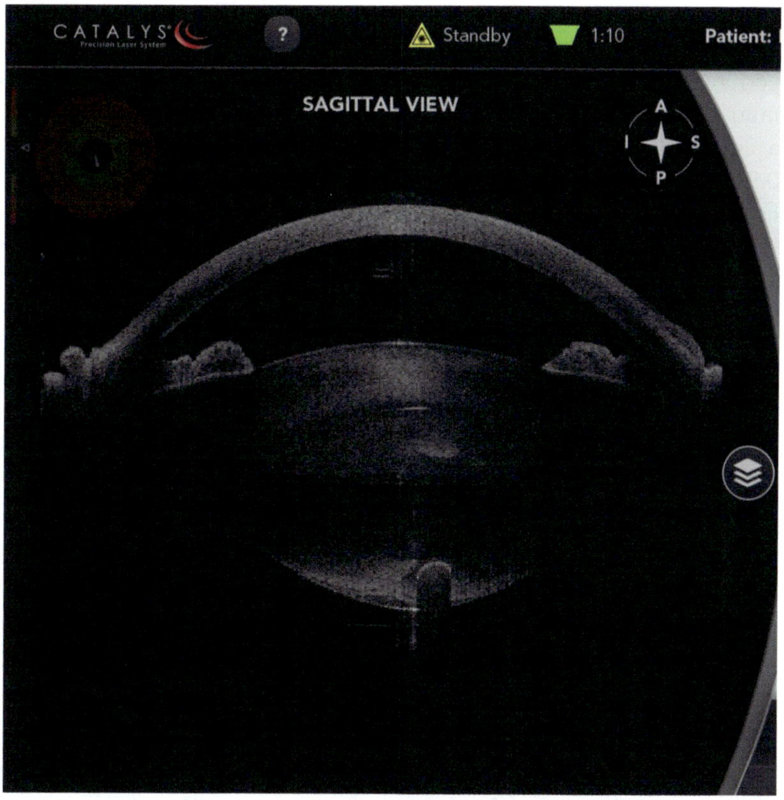

Fig. 34.7 Preoperative posterior capsular rupture induced by inadvertent injection of a corticosteroid carrier into the lens: intraoperative SD OCT verifies the intralenticular position and rupture (sagittal view)

inflammatory drugs (NSAID), one eye drop three times on the day of surgery before initiating treatment, has proven to reliably prevent miosis. [16]

Posttraumatic Cases

The Hungarian group that first introduced the femtosecond laser into cataract surgery performed LCS successfully on a 38-year-old man who suffered a penetrating eye injury while working with wire. The corneal laceration was sutured immediately after the trauma; the cortical cataract that developed soon after was operated upon in a second session with the laser performing a relatively small capsulotomy (4.5 mm). One month postoperatively, the patient had a corrected distance visual acuity (CDVA) of 0.9. [17] A completely different approach was used by our team in treating a 39-year-old patient who had suffered a penetrating injury of both the cornea and the anterior capsule with an intralenticular foreign body. A large capsulotomy diameter of 6.7 mm was chosen (with a dilated pupil diameter of 7.6 mm) to include the foreign body area and the break in the anterior capsule. The procedure (which needed no lens fragmentation) proved what a safe method the femtosecond laser can be to open the capsule precisely and gently, particularly under such delicate circumstances. One week postoperatively, the CDVA had already improved to 0.8 (logMAR +0.1). In a larger number of cases like that, it might be feasible that the complication rate turns out to be lower than after conventional lens removal due to less mechanical manipulation. [18] In an even more severe case, femtosecond laser cataract surgery was successful in a posttraumatic cataract with lens subluxation and vitreous in the anterior chamber, which did not hamper the effect of the laser. Here the option to customize capsulotomy and fragmentation settings once again proved valuable and despite the severity of the case, postoperative uncorrected visual acuity of 20/20 and a flawless positioning of the IOL were achieved. [19]

If a capsular rupture already occurred making lens/cataract surgery necessary, the femtosecond-laser-assisted capsulotomy (e.g., in Nd:YAG vitreolysis, intravitreal drug injection) is very helpful because it offers a perfectly centered and sized anterior capsulotomy for subsequent optic capture of the three-piece intraocular lens placed into the ciliary sulcus (Figs. 34.8 and 34.9).

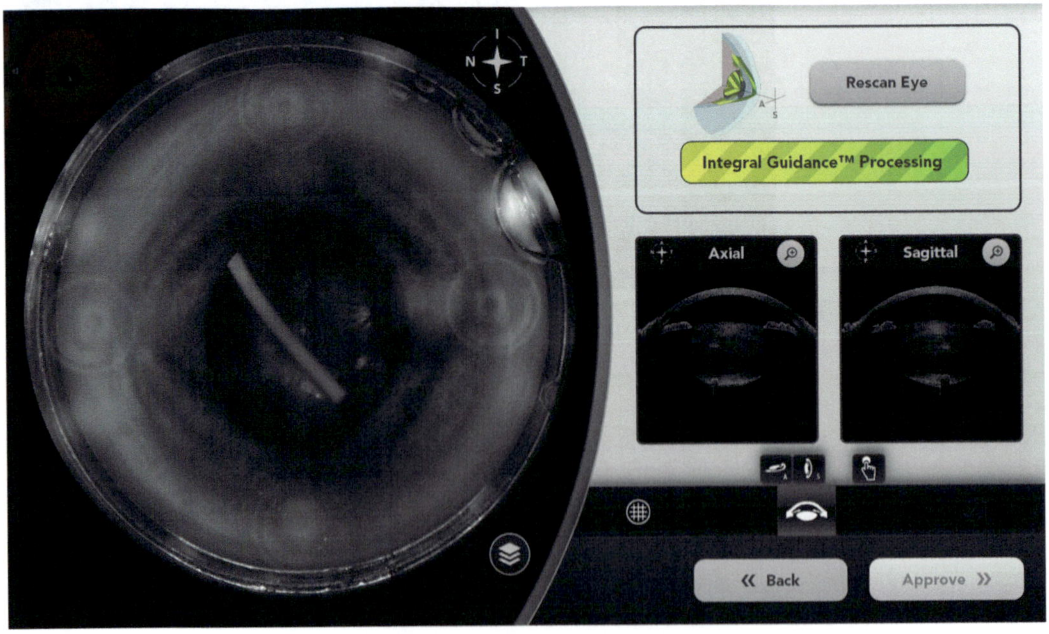

Fig. 34.8 Intraoperative camera view of the steroid in the lens before activation of the laser-assisted capsulotomy

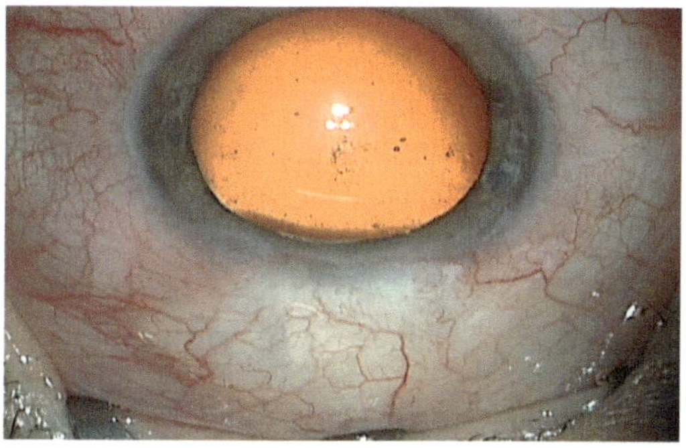

Fig. 34.9 Filter bleb at 12 o'clock after trabeculectomy with mitomycin C before docking the laser system to the eye

Zonular and Capsular Instability

Zonular weakness is associated with an increased likelihood if complications occur in cataract surgery. Clinical signs that point to this condition are lens subluxation, straightening of the lens equator, and irododonesis or phacodonesis. Since there is less tension in the anterior capsule, the force that has necessarily to be applied to perform capsulorhexis or, in the case of the laser, capsulotomy is larger than usual. Since the laser does not – unlike manual capsulorhexis – depend on zonular countertraction during this step, it offers significant benefit for these patients among whom Marfan syndrome is a classic example of a condition with zonular weakness. [1] We could prove this superiority of the laser in a 10-year-old boy with Marfan syndrome and associated ectopia lentis in both eyes who underwent successful LCS under general anesthesia in the right eye. In this case, the laser was not employed for lens fragmentation but rather to perform a relatively small (4.1 mm) capsulotomy. A foldable plate-haptic IOL was implanted in the young patient. There were no complications within the 10 weeks of follow-up; the CDVA was 0.8. [20]

Sometimes after cataract surgery, capsular bag fibrosis can lead to capsule contraction syndrome, also known as capsule fibrosis, which may cause a dislocation of the IOL or even retinal detachment. Manual widening of the capsule requires considerable surgical skills and may result in additional trauma in eyes with weakened zonular fibers. While applying a Nd:YAG laser might be effective, in eyes with dehiscent zonular fibers, the relatively high laser energy may further weaken the zonula fibers and destabilize the IOL position. With the femtosecond laser-emitting pulse energies in range of several microjoules, a contracted capsule can easily and safely be employed to extend a capsulorhexis even in eyes with severe fibrosis. In 3 patients, the laser capsulotomy was performed with diameters between 4.4 and 5.0 mm and pulse energy of 15 mJ. After laser treatment, the dense ring of fibrotic tissue was removed with a microforceps through a 1.2 mm incision. [21]

Retinal Disease

The last thing that patients suffering from AMD and other retinal diseases need is an additional inflammatory stimulation as it is an almost unavoidable consequence of cataract surgery. Inevitably, inflammatory mediators are released by the trauma of the intervention. According to existing studies on that matter, LCS might not do worse and may be even better than traditional phacoemulsification. Abell et al., for instance, demonstrated that postoperative aqueous flare was significantly greater in eyes that had undergone manual cataract surgery at 1 day and at 4 weeks postoperatively than in eyes after LCS. [22] Conrad-Hengerer et al. published similar results: when comparing 104 eyes that underwent laser cataract surgery with 104 fellow eyes, which had manual phacoemulsification, laser flare photometry showed higher levels in the standard group at the first postoperative visit 2 hours after surgery compared with the laser group. In the same study, retinal thickness was measured by spectral-domain optical coherence tomography. No significant differences could be detected, indicating that LCS did not obviously influence the incidence of postoperative macular edema. [23] Indeed, in a meta-analysis by Day et al., LCS was associated with a lower probability of postoperative cystoid macular edema than standard cataract surgery (odds ratio, OR: 0.58) with the reduced exposure to ultrasound energy as one likely aspect for explanation. [24]

A group from Switzerland has investigated whether there are differences in postoperative macular thickness, central macular volume, best-corrected visual acuity, and the number of anti-VEGF injection in patients with exudative age-related macular disease depending on the mode of cataract surgery, that is, laser-assisted compared to standard phacoemulsification. In none of these parameters was a significant difference found in 140 eyes over a mean follow-up of 619 days. More striking was the fact that in 33 eyes with "wet" AMD that had OCT measurements within 2 weeks of cataract surgery, the central macular volume was significantly lower in those eyes that had received laser treatment. [25]

Glaucoma

In some laser systems, a slightly curved transparent window is pressed against the cornea. This potentially strong deformation of the eye during docking can result in a significant rise of intraocular pressure (IOP). Particularly in elderly patients with ocular comorbidities, a major IOP elevation can restrict retinal blood flow, which poses a risk for optic nerve damage. Peer-reviewed data has shown that systems with a fluid-filled interface are safe for most glaucoma patients. A liquid immersion interface is an alternative solution for reducing eye deformation and the associated IOP elevation. [26] When these precautions are taken, it seems unlikely that the relative short time of docking could contribute in any way to glaucoma progression. Structural changes to the optic nerve head as a result of LCS have been ruled out by Renones et al.; the group in which they examined parameters like retinal nerve fiber thickness, macular thickness, and Bruch's membrane opening-minimum width rim by spectral-domain optical coherence tomography (SD-OCT) preoperatively and one month as well as six months after surgery consisted, however, of healthy, nonglaucomatous eyes. [27]

Uncontrolled IOP was described in 0.2% of 2,814 patients (of which 4% were labelled as glaucoma patients) undergoing LCS by Manning et al. [28]. In a Cochrane review comparing postoperative elevated intraocular pressure one day to one week after surgery, LCS was in comparison to standard phacoemulsification awarded an odds ratio (OR) of 0.57 with statistically 11 cases per 1000 compared to 20 cases per 1000 following phacoemulsification. [24]

Concerns about any negative effect of LCS on glaucomatous eyes have probably been laid to rest by the study published by Shah et al. in 2019. In this retrospective case series, 278 eyes diagnoses with glaucoma or suspected of glaucoma and 226 nonglaucomatous eyes in a control group underwent laser cataract surgery. On the first postoperative day, the mean IOP had risen in the glaucoma group more (by 3.4 mm Hg versus 2.0 mm Hg) than in the control group. At one week, the IOP had returned to baseline; after a month, there was a distinct IOP reduction that was sustained through 3 years in the glaucoma/glaucoma suspect group. [29]

Docking the laser might seem hazardous in an eye that earlier had undergone trabeculectomy (Fig. 34.10). Some laser systems list this condition as a contraindication against LCS; checking the laser platform's manual, therefore, is recommended when planning an operation in a patient with a history of filtering glaucoma surgery. Indeed, there is an increased risk of bleeding when the interface touches the bleb area. In our experience – this precaution has to the best of our knowledge currently not been evaluated in the literature – it has been proven to be extremely help-

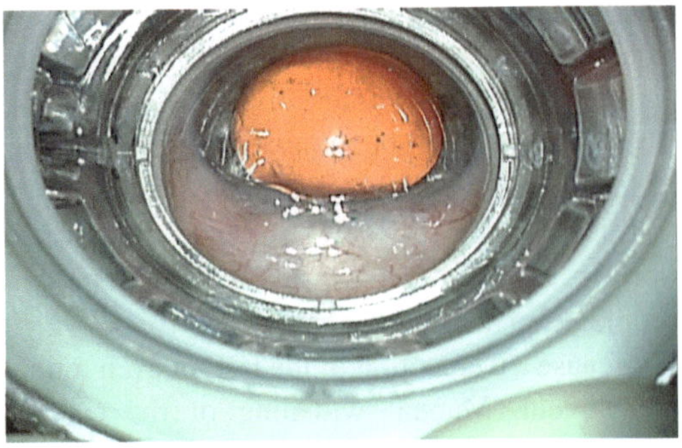

Fig. 34.10 Intentionally decentered docking of the same eye keeping the filtering bleb area free

ful to administer brimonidine eye drops prior to the intervention to prevent or minimize any bleeding. Furthermore, when gently and slowly lowering the interface during the docking process, we aim at a decentralized area of contact to avoid the segment of the surface where the bleb is located (Figs. 34.11 and 34.12). Some laser systems then allow a careful realignment to have the interface positioned correctly without touching the bleb and its surrounding conjunctiva. It works well in the hands of an experienced surgeon but is definitely a challenge (Figs. 34.13 and 34.14).

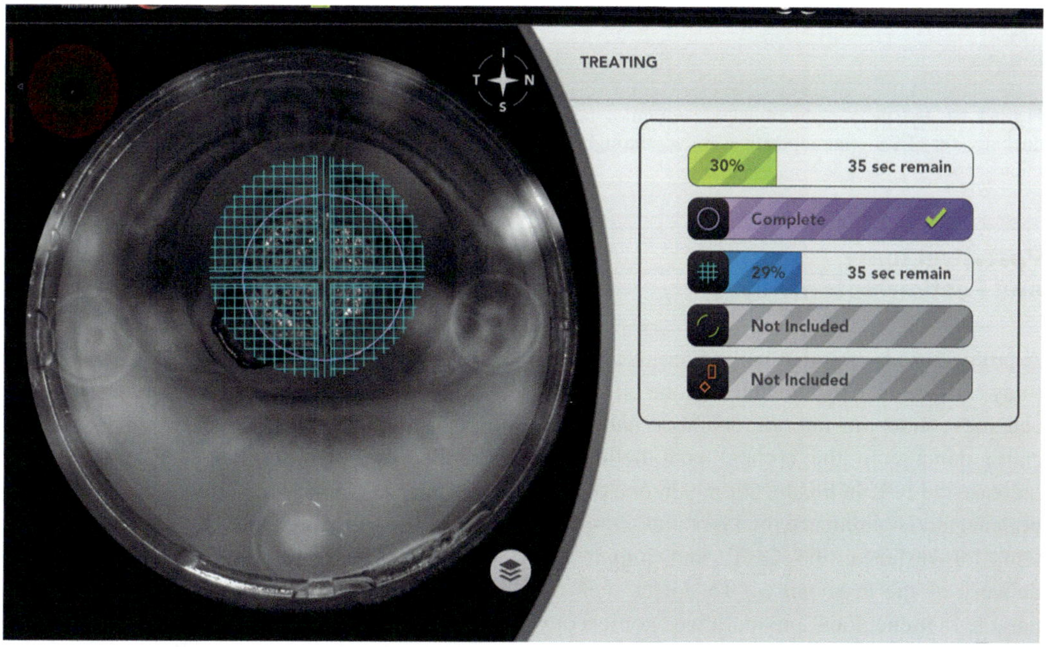

Fig. 34.11 Intraoperative view of the laser system monitor with an intentionally decentered eye because of a preexistent bleb

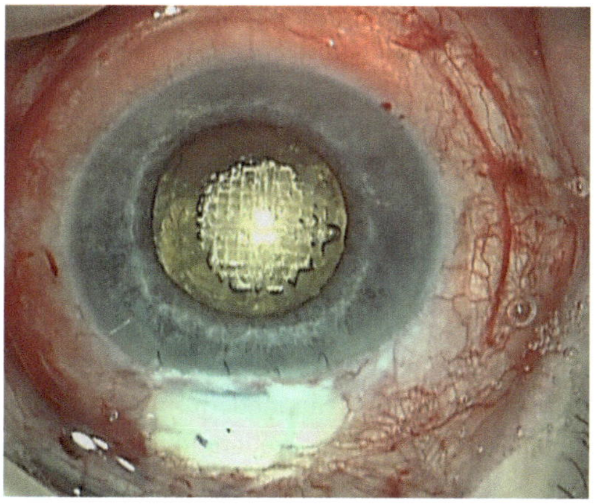

Fig. 34.12 Intraoperative situs after laser fragmentation and undocking showing slight bleeding of the conjunctiva in an eye with a filtering bleb after trabeculectomy (without preoperative administration of brimonidine)

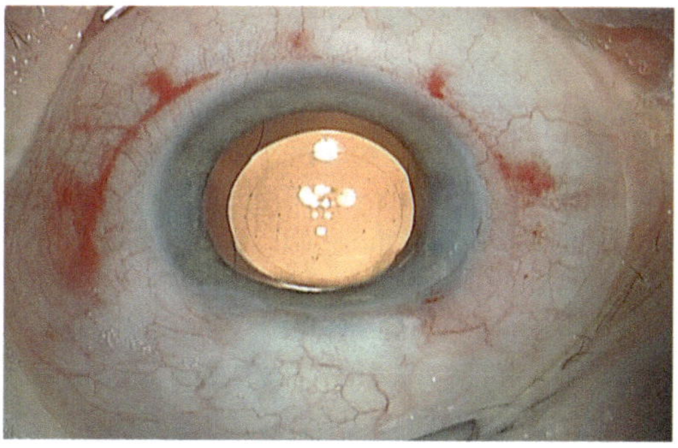

Fig. 34.13 Intraoperative situs after laser capsulotomy and undocking showing minimal bleeding of the conjunctiva in an eye with a filtering bleb after trabeculectomy (with the preoperative use of brimonidine)

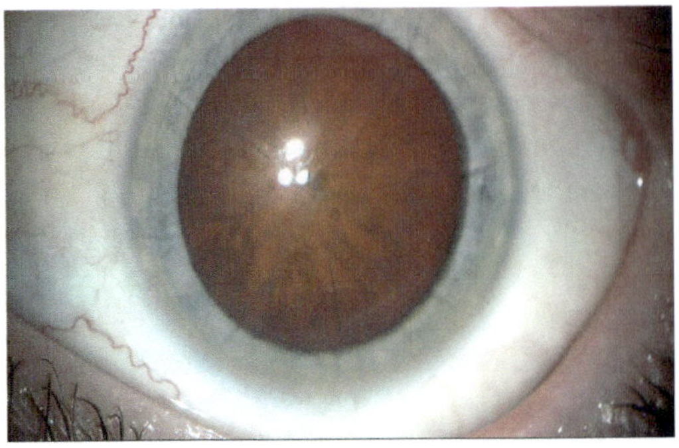

Fig. 34.14 Eye with eight radial keratotomies before docking for LCS (intraoperative view through the microscope)

Postvitrectomy and Postkeratotomy Eyes

A problem with eyes that had undergone vitrectomy can be posed by residual silicone oil, which can move into the interior chamber and there cause damage to the corneal endothelium or increase the IOP. In this location, silicone oil can both negatively influence the laser's imaging system, for instance, the OCT, and impair the delivery of the laser pulses. To detect such oil particles, meticulous preoperative gonioscopy and/or anterior segment OCT is advised. It is also recommended to inject blue dye into the anterior chamber to stain the anterior capsule, which makes it easier to verify the integrity and completeness of the capsulotomy in these eyes. [1] That these eyes can, despite all difficulties, be operated successfully on has been, among others, shown by Grewal et al. in two cases. [30]

In a study by Wang et al., it was documented that there were no differences in postoperative visual acuity in eyes that had previously undergone vitrectomy between those who had laser cataract surgery and those who had phacoemulsification. Striking was the difference in the need for Nd:YAG treatment for posterior capsule opacification (PCO): 16% in the LCS group versus 48% in the phacoemulsification group. It has to be noted that the authors – who described a trend to better intraoperative and postoperative outcomes after LCS – compared the last 25 surgeries in postvitrectomy eyes before the acquisition of a femtosecond laser with the first 25 surgeries after the device's installation, which means these good results were even achieved while being at the beginning of the surgical learning curve. [31]

Eyes After Radial Keratotomy

Another challenge in an eye with a surgical history is performing LCS in a patient who had – probably in the pioneering days of refractive surgery – undergone radial keratotomy. Just like in posttrabeculectomy eyes (as described above), there are some areas that the surgeon would try to avoid – in this case, the (usually) six or eight radial keratotomy incisions (Fig. 34.14). The excellent imaging system of modern laser platforms, surgical skill, and a certain amount of patience make LCS possible even in these cases (Fig. 34.15). We have described a small number of postkeratotomy eyes whose anterior segments were visualized with the femtosecond laser's integrated three-dimensional optical coherence tomography. Guided by this precise imaging, it was then possible to position the laser corneal incisions between the radial keratotomy incisions. None of these patients suffered complications like corneal perforation, anterior capsular tears, or discontinuities (Fig. 34.16). A note of caution should be added, though. Our group was small and we (and, more importantly, the patients) may have been exceptionally lucky. There are personal reports from other surgeons who described LCS in post-RK eyes as less than promising. It has to be kept in mind that this is a group of patients who will in the near future increase in numbers in our practices and will certainly pose a challenge. They have been the first generation of patients in modern refractive, having undergone such a procedure in the 1980s and 1990s. These individuals are now reaching the age in which cataract surgery will become a necessity. [32]

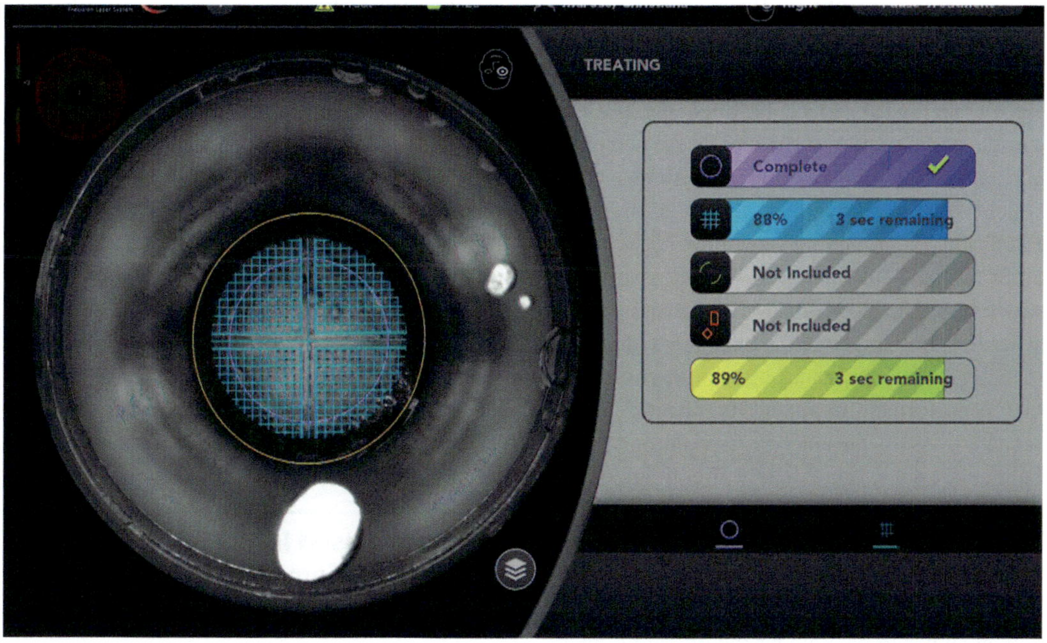

Fig. 34.15 Femtosecond laser capsulotomy and lens fragmentation in an eye with eight radial keratotomies (view of the screen of the laser system)

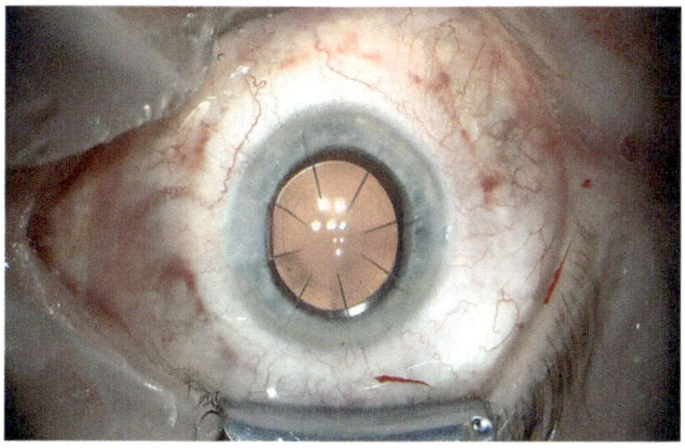

Fig. 34.16 End of the LCS procedure in a post-RK eye (intraoperative view through the microscope)

Alport Syndrome

Alport syndrome is a relatively rare genetic disease whose ocular manifestations – renal failure and deafness are its main features – include anterior lenticonus and diverse retinal abnormalities. Femtosecond laser cataract surgery with intraoperative aberrometry led to a safe and successful intervention in a 38-year-old patient, as Orts-Vila et al. have recently reported. Since the laser platform's OCT cannot precisely identify the anterior capsule, because in these eyes, the normal pattern recognition does not work, the imaging systems will be operated manually. Intraoperative aberrometry was in this case also used to verify the positioning of the axis of the toric IOL that the patient received. In eyes of Alport patients, a higher fragility of the anterior capsule can be expected; capsulotomy in these cases can benefit from the consistency and predictability that the laser provides. [33] A similar case, a 25-year-old man with bilateral progressive vision loss due to anterior lenticonus and anterior polar cataract, was reported by Hipolito-Fernandes et al.; following LCS and IOL implantation in the capsular bag, the patient had an uncorrected visual acuity of 20/20 one month postoperatively [34].

Posterior Capsulotomy

The introduction of the femtosecond laser into cataract surgery was, however, a game-changer not only for performing (anterior) capsulotomy, corneal incisions, and lens fragmentation but also potentially for what we now call primary posterior laser capsulotomy (PPLC). We used the integrated spectral-domain optical coherence tomography (SD-OCT) of a laser system to study the size of the Berger space (space between the posterior capsule and the anterior hyaloid) at the end of surgery after IOL implantation. The Berger space, which is essential for the success and effect of PPLC since it provides a separation between posterior capsule and anterior hyaloid membrane, was larger than 400 mm in 72% of the patients. After IOL implantation, the patient is redocked to the laser and the primary posterior laser capsulotomy is performed (treatment time from 2.4 to 2.6 seconds). As in an anterior capsulotomy, small bubbles are seen. Immediately after treatment, the posterior capsule disk started to contract (triangularly, quadrangularly, pentagonally, or hexagonally), a process that can be followed on the laser system's screen. The eye is undocked and the patient swiveled back under the operating microscope to determine whether the posterior capsulotomy was well centered and free-floating for 360 degrees. No further manipulations are made. In our group of 65 eyes that received PPLC, results did not significantly differ from standard phacoemulsification in the occurrence of macular edema, IOP, laser flare values, visual acuity, and IOL centration. Primary posterior laser capsulotomy currently represents off-label treatment; laser software and IOL design have not been adjusted or optimized. Preliminary results give hope that PCO formation can be significantly reduced by this intervention. [35, 36]

When Really Not to Resort to LCS

There are some genuine contraindications to the employment of the femtosecond laser in cataract surgery. Certain anatomical features of some patients (fortunately only a tiny minority) render contact of the interface with the ocular surface difficult or outright impossible like deep-set eyes and/with small interpalpebral fissures. The special situation the patient finds himself or herself on the treatment bed, in a rather constricted space, unable or rather not permitted to move even slightly, precludes LCS for people who tend to suffer from claustrophobia and related forms of anxiety. Conditions with a more or less constant tremor like Parkinson's disease may prohibit the use of the femtosecond laser, the same applies to individuals with restless legs syndrome. Very obese people might not be properly placed on the treatment bed and under the laser's interface. Severe deformations of the spine like an advanced kyphosis might also prohibit laying down on the platform's treatment bed. Regarding corneal opacities, their location and density decides whether the laser can be employed – as shown above – or not; dense opacities may significantly alter the transmission of laser energy.

Evidence-Based Indications of Using the Femtosecond Laser in Cataract Surgery

Better (slightly) visual acuity compared to regular phacoemulsification

Better (probably) corneal recovery due to reduction/zero ultrasound energy

Thus: To be preferred in eyes with cornea guttata with less endothelial cell loss compared to standard treatment

Better (more circular, more precise) anterior capsulotomy

Thus: To be preferred when premium IOL is to be implanted

When avoidance of posterior capsule rupture is of concern

Pediatric cataract (though regularly listed as a contraindication)

Eyes with modest corneal astigmatism, which can be corrected without much additional effort during the same session [37].

Evidence-Based Contraindications Against Using the Femtosecond Laser in Cataract Surgery

Anatomical situations like deep-set eyes, small lid margin, protruding orbital features, very deep set eyes

Restless patients and those with tremors

Patient with phobias in restricted spaces

Skeletal anomalies like a pronounced kyphosis

Eyes with previous cataract or glaucoma surgery

Corneal scars depending on their extent (experienced surgeons might consider this an obstacle that can be overcome) [38].

Conclusion

Femtosecond laser cataract surgery can be performed with excellent chances of success in eyes with a wide variety of ocular comorbidities. Meticulous planning is essential as is the surgeon's experience and his or her knowledge of the potentials as well as the limits of LCS. Like always in surgical medicine, a "Plan B" should be at hand. Not everybody can be treated with the femtosecond laser – but those who can are an ever-growing number of medically and morphologically diverse patients who deserve the best possible treatment. Which the laser, more often than not, offers.

Take-Home Notes

- A number of case series have demonstrated the feasibility of LCS even in complicated cases like, for instance, in patients with corneal pathologies like paracentral scars and postkeratoplasty eyes.
- The significant reduction in effective phacoemulsification time (EPT) seems to result in a remarkable decrease of endothelial cell loss, which might be particularly beneficial in eyes with a low preoperative endothelial cell count like in cases of cornea guttata and Fuchs dystrophy.
- In posttrabeculectomy eyes, administering brimonidine locally reduces the likelihood of bleeding during docking.
- In glaucoma patients, pressure spike during docking might occur. This IOP rise is comparatively mild when a liquid interface is used.
- In eyes that had previously undergone vitrectomy, detecting remnants of silicone oil in the anterior chamber is essential to prevent damage to the corneal endothelium and make sure the laser and its imaging system can work properly.

References

1. Basti S, Talati RK. Femtosecond laser-assisted cataract surgery in ocular comorbidities. In: Dick HB, Gerste RD, Schultz T, editors. Femtosecond laser surgery in ophthalmology. New York: Thieme Publishers; 2018. p. 167–77.
2. Grewal DS, Basti S, Grewal SP. Customizing femtosecond laser-assisted cataract surgery in a patient with a traumatic corneal scar and cataract. J Cataract Refract Surg. 2014;40:1926–7.
3. Hou JH, Crispim J, Cortina MS, et al. Image-guided femtosecond laser-assisted cataract surgery in Peters anomaly type 2. J Cataract Refract Surg. 2015;41:2353–7.
4. Martin AI, Hodge C, Lawless M, et al. Femtosecond laser cataract surgery: challenging cases. Curr Opin Ophthalmol. 2014;25:71–80.
5. Nagy ZZ, Takacs AI, Filkorn T, et al. (2013) Laser refractive cataract surgery with a femtosecond laser after penetrating keratoplasty: case report. J Refract Surg. 2013;29:8.
6. Conrad-Hengerer I, Al Juburi M, Schultz T, et al. (2013) Corneal endothelial cell loss and corneal thickness in conventional compared with femtosecond laser-assisted cataract surgery: three-month follow-up. J Cataract Refract Surg. 2013;39:1307–13.
7. Hatch K, Talamo JH. Laser-assisted cataract surgery: benefits and barriers. Curr Opin Ophthalmol. 2014;25:54–61.
8. Yong WWD, Chai HCC, Shen L, et al. Comparing outcomes of phacoemulsification with femtosecond laser-assisted cataract surgery in patients with Fuchs endothelial dystrophy. Am J Ophthalmol. 2018;196:173–80.
9. Hatch KM, Schultz T, Talamo JH, Dick HB. Femtosecond laser-assisted compared with standard cataract surgery for removal of advanced cataracts. J Cataract Refract Surg. 2015;41:1833–8.
10. Schultz T, Dick HB. Laser-assisted mini-capsulotomy: a new technique for intumescent white cataracts. J Refract Surg. 2014;30:742–5.

11. Conrad-Hengerer I, Hengerer FH, Joachim SC, et al. Femtosecond laser-assisted cataract surgery in intumescent white cataracts. J Cataract Refract Surg. 2014;40:44–50.
12. Dick HB, Gerste RD. Laser Cataract Surgery: Curse if the small pupil. J Refract Surg. 2013;29:662.
13. Dick HB, Schultz T. Laser-assisted cataract surgery in small pupils using mechanical dilation devices. J Refract Surg. 2014;29:858–62.
14. Bali SJ, Hodge C, Lawless M, et al. Early experience with the femtosecond laser for cataract surgery. Ophthalmology. 2012;119:891–9.
15. Schultz T, Joachim SC, Kuehn M, Dick HB. Changes in prostaglandin levels in patients undergoing femtosecond laser-assisted cataract surgery. J Refract Surg. 2013;29:742–7.
16. Schultz T, Joachim SC, Szuler M, et al. NSAID Pretreatment Inhibits Prostaglandin Release in Femtosecond Laser-Assisted Cataract Surgery. J Refract Surg. 2015;31:791–4.
17. Szepessy Z, Takacs A, Kranitz K, et al. Intraocular femtosecond laser use in traumatic cataract. Eur J Ophthalmol. 2014;24:623–5.
18. Conrad-Hengerer I, Dick HB, Schultz T, et al. Femtosecond laser-assisted capsulotomy after penetrating injury of the cornea and lens capsule. J Cataract Refract Surg. 2014;40:153–6.
19. Titiyal JS, Kaur M, Rathi A, et al. Femtosecond laser-assisted successful management of subluxated cataractous lens with vitreous in anterior chamber. Indian J Ophthalmol. 2019;67:155–7.
20. Schultz T, Ezeanosike E, Dick HB. Femtosecond laser-assisted cataract surgery in pediatric Marfan syndrome. J Refract Surg. 2013;29:1–3.
21. Gerten G, Schultz M, Oberheide U. Treating capsule contraction syndrome with a femtosecond laser. J Cataract Refract Surg. 2016;42:1255–61.
22. Abell RG, Allen PL, Vote BJ. Anterior chamber flare after femtosecond laser-assisted cataract surgery. J Cataract Refract Surg. 2013;39:1321–6.
23. Conrad-Hengerer I, Hengerer FH, Al Juburi MA, et al. Femtosecond laser-induced macular changes and anterior segment inflammation in cataract surgery. J Refract Surg. 2014;30:222–6.
24. Day AC, Gore DM, Bunce C et al. (2016) Laser-assisted cataract surgery versus standard ultrasound phacoemulsification cataract surgery. Cochrane Database Syst Rev. 7.
25. Enz TJ, Faes L, Bachmann LM, et al. Comparison of macular parameters after femtosecond laser-assisted and conventional cataract surgery in age-related macular degeneration. J Cataract Refract Surg. 2018;44:23–7.
26. Schultz T, Conrad-Hengerer I, Hengerer FH, Dick HB. Intraocular pressure variation during femtosecond laser-assisted cataract surgery using a fluid-filled interface. J Cataract Refract Surg. 2013;39:22–7.
27. Renones de Abajo J, Jorge BE, Martin JMG, et al. Effect of femtosecond laser-assisted lens surgery of the optic nerve head and the macula. Int J Ophtalmol. 2019;12:961–6.
28. Manning S, Barry P, Henry Y, et al. Femtosecond laser-assisted cataract surgery versus standard phacoemulsification cataract surgery: Study from the European Registry of Quality Outcomes for Cataract and Refractive Surgery. J Cataract Refract Surg. 2016;42:1779–90.
29. Shah AA, Ling J, Nathan NR, et al. Long-term intraocular pressure changes after femtosecond laser-assisted cataract surgery in healthy eyes and glaucomatous eyes. J Cataract Refract Surg. 2019;45:181–7.
30. Grewal DS, Singh Grewal SP, Basti S. Incomplete femtosecond laser-assisted capsulotomy and lens fragmentation due to emulsified silicone oil in the anterior chamber. J Cataract Refract Surg. 2014;40:2143–7.
31. Wang EF, Worsley A, Polkinghome PJ. Comparative study of femtosecond laser-assisted cataract surgery and conventional phacoemulsification in vitrectomized eyes. Clin Exp Ophthalmol. 2018;46:624–9.
32. Noristani R, Schultz T, Dick HB. Femtosecond laser-assisted cataract surgery after radial keratotomy. J Refract Surg. 2016;32:426–8.
33. Orts-Vila P, Amparo F, Rodriguez-Prats JL, et al. Alport syndrome and femtosecond laser-assisted cataract surgery. J Ophthalmic Vis Res. 2020;15:264–9.
34. Hipolito-Fernandes D, Elisa-Luis M, Alves N, et al. Femtosecond laser-assisted cataract surgery for bilateral anterior lenticonus. J Cataract Refract Surg. 2020;46:789–91.
35. Schojai M, Schultz T, Haeussler-Sinangin Y, et al. Safety of femtosecond laser–assisted primary posterior capsulotomy immediately after cataract surgery. J Cataract Refract Surg. 2017;43:1171–6.
36. Dick HB, Schultz T. Primary posterior laser-assisted capsulotomy. J Refract Surg. 2014;30:128–33.
37. Levitz LM, Dick HB, Scott W, et al. The latest evidence with regards to femtosecond laser-assisted cataract surgery and its use post 2020. Clin Ophthalmol. 2021;15:1357–63.
38. Dick HB, Schultz T. A review of laser-assisted versus traditional phacoemulsification cataract surgery. Ophthalmol Ther. 2017;6:7–18.

35 Complications of Femtosecond Laser-Assisted Cataract Surgery

H. Burkhard Dick

Bullet Points

- In general, laser cataract surgery (LCS) has an excellent safety record. The same holds true, however, for the established procedure it is inevitably measured against, conventional phacoemulsification.
- The docking process, in particular the suction, can lead to a rise in intraocular pressure (IOP). This seems to be, according to numerous publications, a short-term and reversible effect.
- The application of the laser can lead to a prostaglandin release. A pharmacological prophylaxis has proven to be extremely effective: administering nonsteroidal anti-inflammatory drugs (NSAIDs), one eye drop three times on the day of surgery before initiating treatment.
- Anterior capsule tears and incomplete capsulotomy are complications of LCS, though they are relatively rare, with incidences in the range of about 1–2%.
- The most frequent side effect seems to be conjunctival hemorrhages due to the docking process, but they are generally harmless.

Everything so far has gone well for the 70-year-old lady and her surgeon during femtosecond-laser-assisted cataract surgery, although she had remarkably deep-set eyes and a narrow lid margin. Laser capsulotomy was successfully performed, and lens fragmentation was almost complete when the patient abruptly and for no reason moved. The suction ring of the laser platform's interface lost adhesion to the sclera and before the laser automatically stopped as programmed for such situations, for a fraction of a second, a number of shots were still fired (Fig. 35.1). The patient's eye was examined under the operating microscope, revealing a number of displaced laser spots in the periphery of the corneal stroma. The operation proceeded without further laser application, the nucleus was removed without applying any ultrasound, and a 3-piece IOL was implanted. Six weeks later, the patient's visual acuity was 20/20; remnants of the fragmentation grid in the corneal stroma were visible during slit-lamp examination. The patient did not report any problems such as glare or

H. Burkhard Dick (✉)
Ruhr University Eye Clinic, Bochum, Germany
e-mail: burkhard.dick@kk-bochum.de

J. L. Alió et al. (eds.), *Cataract Surgery*, Essentials in Ophthalmology,
https://doi.org/10.1007/978-3-030-94530-5_35

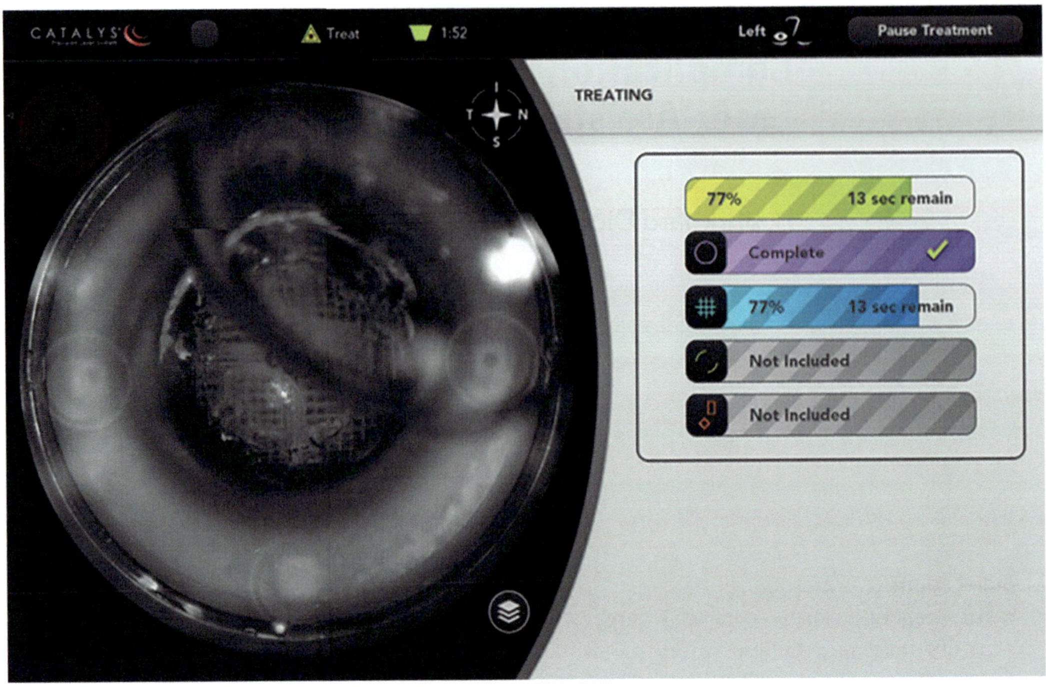

Fig. 35.1 Suction loss of the personal interface during lasing with air ingress into the optical pathway

disturbing optical phenomena and expressed complete satisfaction with the overall outcome [1]. Therefore, it is tempting to quote Shakespeare: all's well that ends well.

There is no surgical procedure, no invasive technology that does not carry risks and can lead to complications: laser cataract surgery (LCS) is no exception. The above example of a sudden suction loss is one of the relatively frequent mishaps that can happen during the application of the laser. The emphasis is on "relatively." More than 10 years after the introduction of the femtosecond laser into cataract surgery, an increasing number of studies and in particular of comparisons with conventional phacoemulsification have been published and both methods' efficacy and safety evaluated. Therefore, the excellent safety record of LCS – as well as, of course, of standard cataract surgery – has by now been well established. A German group recently published a review of 73 studies comprising 12,769 eyes treated with LCS and 12,274 undergoing conventional phacoemulsification. Among the benefits of LCS were better uncorrected and corrected distance visual acuity 1–3 months postoperatively and the application of less phacoemulsification energy; there was less endothelial cell loss and more accurate capsulotomies in the laser group. The one distinct disadvantage was the higher occurrence of anterior capsule ruptures during laser cataract surgery. Even here, the overall numbers are small: 78 events out of 8022 eyes (0.97%) treated with laser compared with 16 ruptures out of 7951 eyes undergoing phacoemulsification (0.20%). In posterior capsule ruptures, the difference between LCS (0.42%) and phacoemulsification (0.27%) was not significant [2].

.There can be no doubt, however, that in the words of Gerd U. Auffarth, the reported benefits of laser cataract surgery necessitate that a surgeon undergoes an adequate familiarization and clinical experience with the technology [3]. Experience with the technology is indeed the key to minimize complications. This has already been documented by Zoltan Z Nagy, who introduced the femtosecond laser into cataract surgery. About 5 years later, in 2014, Nagy et al. analyzed the complications of his first 100 cataract surgeries with the laser. These were: conjunctival redness or hemorrhage in 34%, miosis in 32%, capsule tags and bridges in 20%, anterior tears in 4%, endothelial damage due to a laser cut within this layer in 3% and a suction break – as described in the case above – in 2%. Even within this limited number of surgeries, the effect of the learning curve was evident and the authors stated clearly that during the learning curve period, increased surgical vigilance is needed. They described most complications as predictable and largely preventable [4].

Preoperative Complications

Diligent patient selection is probably the best way to avoid complications in laser cataract surgery. Therefore, the preoperative evaluation and identification of patients who are not suited to undergo femtosecond laser treatment is essential. The surgeon should refrain from LCS – or use the technology only with the greatest caution – in patients with deep-set eyes, with narrow lid margins, protruding eyebrows, anterior synechiae. The preoperative application of NSAID eye drops is an appropriate measure to prevent a small pupil. The prostaglandin release described below seems to be lower with the Ziemer platform (LDV Z8; Ziemer Ophthalmic Systems, Switzerland), which uses a lower energy than the other femtosecond laser systems employed in cataract surgery.

The docking process is the cause of what is probably the most frequent complication after femto-cataract surgery, yet it is a relatively harmless one. There are differences between the femtosecond laser systems with the Catalys (Johnson & Johnson, USA), Ziemer and LensAR (Lensar Inc., USA) platforms using fluid-filled non-applanating interfaces, the Victus (Bausch & Lomb, USA), an applanating fluid-filled interface, and the LenSx (Alcon, USA), a curved contact lens for applanation. In general, a curved interface will cause less bulbus deformation than a flat applanating contact lens [5].

.The frictions associated with the docking process and other steps of handling the eye's surface can result in subconjunctival hemorrhages, which in a case series of 162 eyes were observed in 71 eyes (43.8%) [6]. This is in accordance with another observation, in which 7 out of 21 patients developed what was described as fine subconjunctival hemorrhage and eye redness [7]. In a population of 1105 eyes that were operated by 18 different surgeons (most or at least some of them on the early steps of the learning curve), the incidence of subconjunctival hemorrhage was 26.2% [8]. It might be added that in clinics with experienced surgeons, the incidence of subconjunctival hemorrhage tends to be much lower. It can be prevented by a precise docking, by making sure that there is no lose conjunctiva involved; additionally, a hard headrest is preferable to a soft one that might permit head movement during laser application [3].

Intraoperative Complications

Anterior capsule tears are a complication of laser-performed capsulotomies. Abell et al. found 15 such cases among 804 laser-treated eyes (1.87%) of which 7 extended all the way to the posterior capsule, while in the phacoemulsification group of almost the same size, there was just one such case in 822 eyes (0.12%) [9]. Other study groups reported different incidences, but a capsule tear and capsule tag/slider (Fig. 35.2) and bridge can occur after laser capsulotomy, although the incidence is generally low. Their number has initially been relatively high (20%) like in the aforementioned study by Nagy et al. from 2014. Kohnen et al. have concluded that a soft contact lens interface results in a lower rate of tags and bridges than a rigid interface [10]. The risk of anterior capsule tears can also be significantly reduced by optimized laser settings, particularly with an increased vertical spacing:

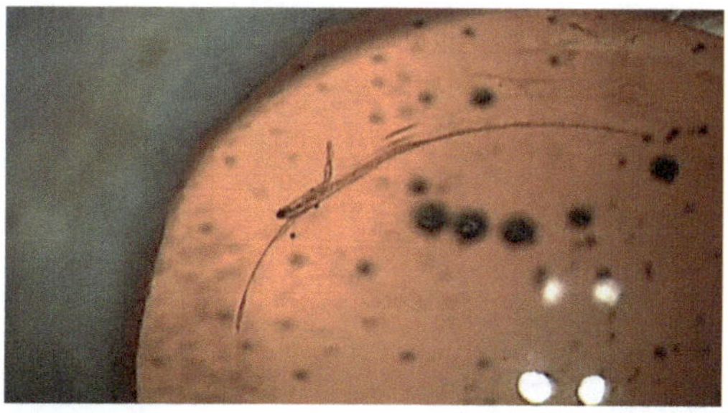

Fig. 35.2 Capsulotomy slider indicates aberrant laser shots and represents a risk factor for a potential anterior capsule tear

setting this to 20 μm resulted in a capsule tear rate of 0.09% compared to 0.79% with a spacing of 10 μm and to 0.35% with a spacing of 15 μm. Remarkable again is how small the overall numbers are [11]. If such a tear happens, it is essential to keep the anterior chamber deep and stable, using OVD and irrigation generously. In this situation, the surgeon will be primarily concerned with preventing the spreading of the tear to the posterior capsule.

Posterior capsule tears are also rare. In a recent randomized controlled trial from the UK, among 392 patients assigned to the LCS, there were two posterior capsule tears, while none occurred among the 393 patients undergoing conventional cataract surgery [12]. Femtosecond laser cataract surgery, on the other hand, can successfully be employed in cases with a posterior capsulotomy following, for instance, blunt trauma [13].

.A decentration of the capsulotomy can be prevented be taking into account the IOL design and adjusting the capsulotomy position intraoperatively according to the chosen reference like pupil edges, limbus, or lenticular capsule curvatures (anterior and posterior; "scanned capsule") as well as checking, for example, an inhomogeneous pupil dilation (Figs. 35.3 and 35.4). In case of an inhomogeneous pupil dilation in a pupil width of greater than 5.2 mm, the lens capsule position serves as the better landmark for the capsulotomy position (Figs. 35.5 and 35.6). Another typical example of the LCS learning curve is to immediately stop lasing in case of initial presentation of gas bubbles in the anterior chamber during the lasing of an intrastromal arcuate incision (Figs. 35.7 and 35.8). Gas bubbles inside or behind the lens which may not move anteriorly seem to occur more frequently in our observations with the LensAR. Rarely, migration of sub-

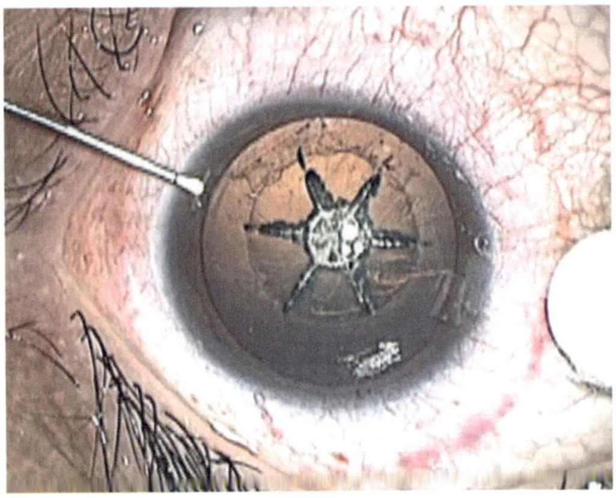

Fig. 35.4 Inferiorly decentered capsulotomy before lens removal with lens cuts in place (same eye as in Fig. 35.3, view through OR microscope)

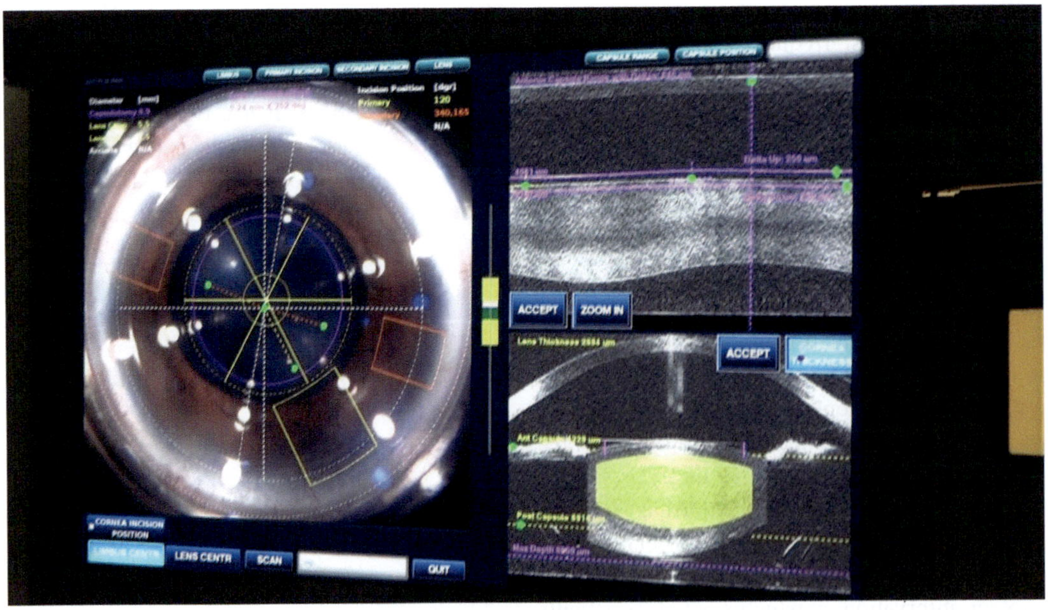

Fig. 35.3 Inhomogeneous pupil dilation during the intraoperative treatment planning pronounced in the 6–12 o'clock direction (photograph of the laser system screen), resulting in an inferiorly located capsulotomy

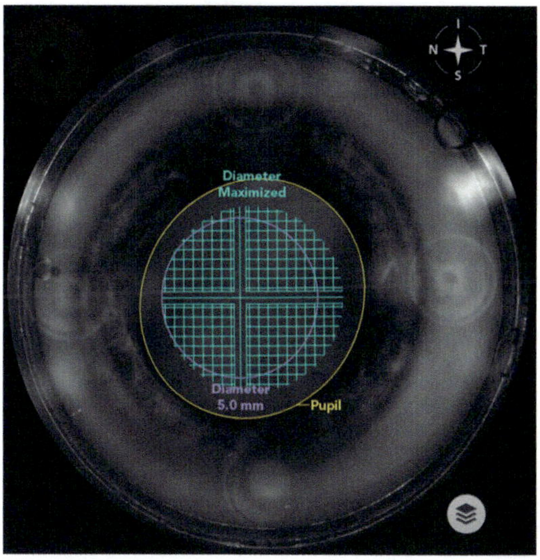

Fig. 35.5 The laser system suggests the capsulotomy position (violet) based on the scanned capsule information and the lens fragmentation pattern position based on pupil edge detection (green): a greater difference can be depicted because of an obviously more nasally located lens (right eye)

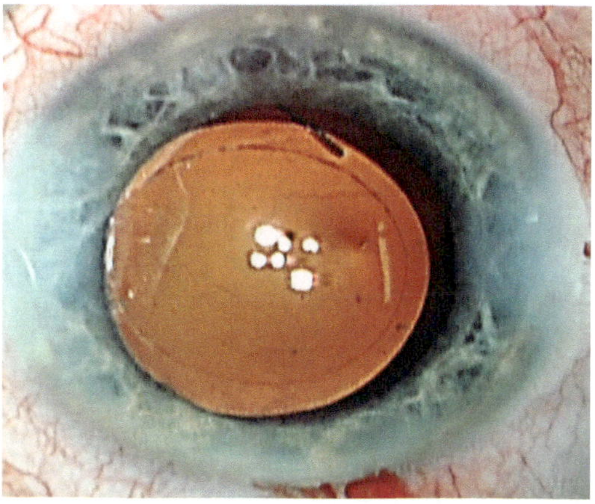

Fig. 35.6 After three-piece IOL implantation (AR 40e, Johnson & Johnson), the scanned capsule-based capsulotomy is well centered with a 360° capsule overlap on the optic (same eye as in Fig. 35.6, view through OR microscope)

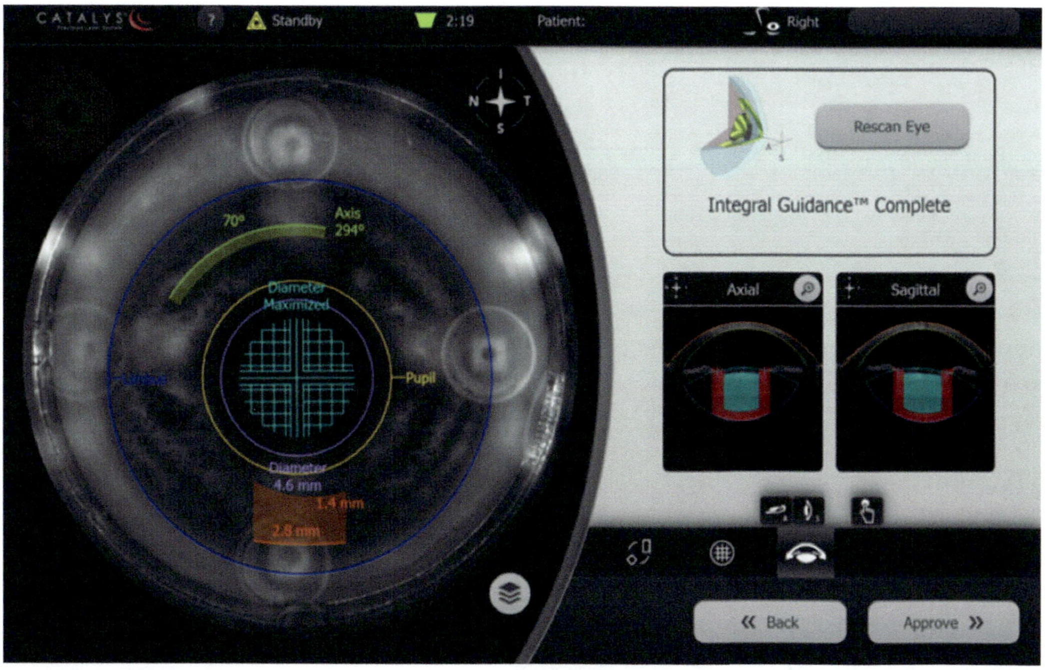

Fig. 35.7 Intraoperative treatment screen based on the 3D SD-OCT anatomic results with the suggested position of an inferiorly located intrastromal arcuate incision

epithelial gas bubbles from the arcuate incision to another unlasered corneal area can (partially) block the lasering of the area to be layered afterward during the procedure (Fig. 35.9). Depending on the laser system used, areas underneath the layered area may be left uncut (Fig. 35.10).

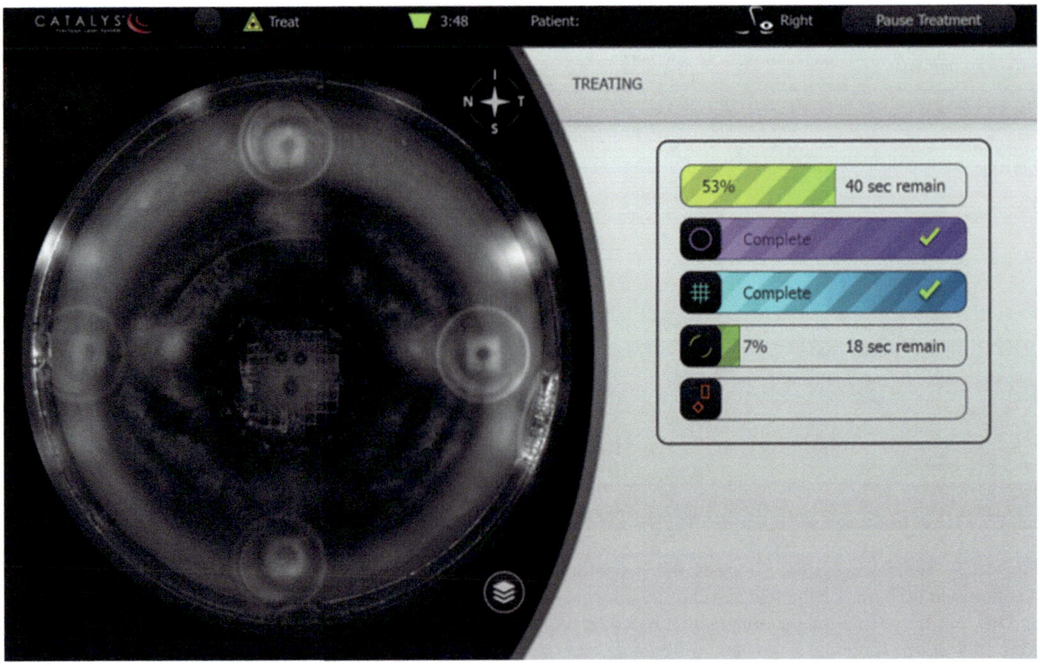

Fig. 35.8 Gas bubbles in the anterior chamber after commencing the lasing of the arcuate incision indicating a deeper than planned laser spot position (screenshot)

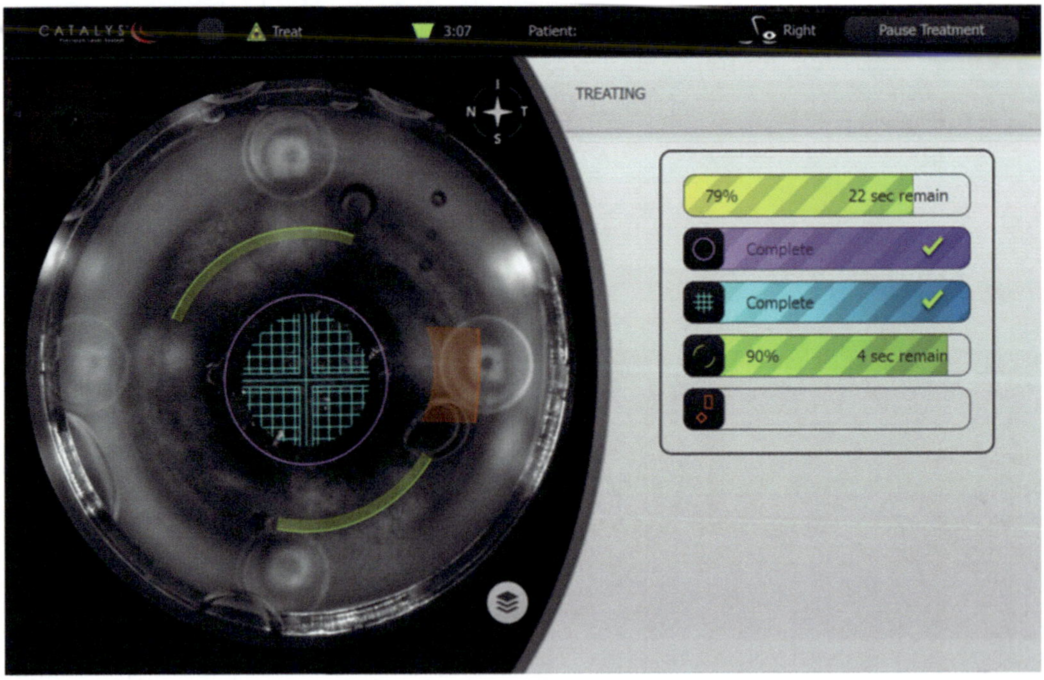

Fig. 35.9 Subepithelial gas bubble deriving from the superior arcuate incision that will not allow a correct intended lasing of the main incision (right eye)

Unexpected undocking during the treatment as in the case described above, though rare, can happen. It can be caused, for instance, by an unexpected head movement; other causes may be excessive pressing of the lids or because the conjunctiva is very loose. While the laser systems in

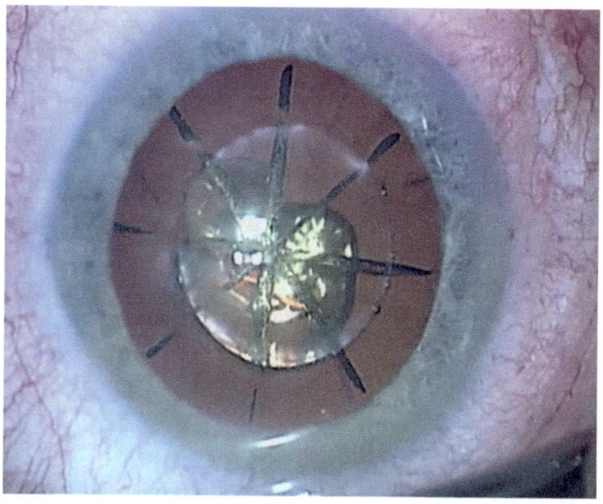

Fig. 35.10 Incomplete lens cuts due to a laser beam blockage by the already performed capsulotomy edge (lens fragmentation followed the capsulotomy)

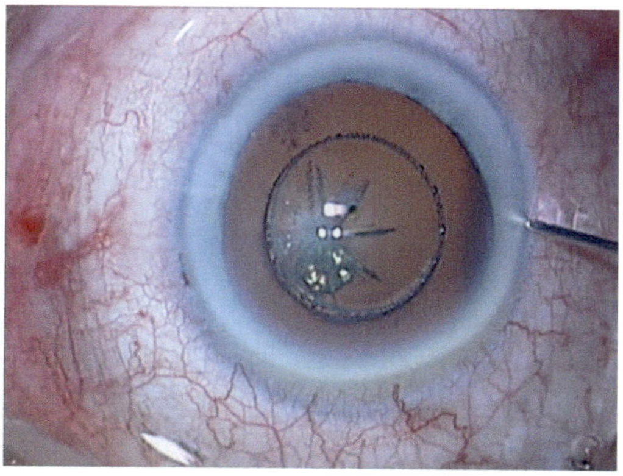

Fig. 35.11 Displacement of laser shots because of a suction loss during lasing of the lens: fragmentation pattern is displaced nasally, whereas the capsulotomy is well centered

such a case of suction loss automatically stop the treatment, the high repetition rate of the laser nevertheless may result in some displaced laser shots in the fraction of a second that passes between suction loss and shutdown (Figs. 35.11 and 35.12). A loss during capsulotomy might lead to incomplete cutting; in this case, redocking and choosing a larger capsulotomy diameter is a potential rescue maneuver as is proceeding with manual capsulorhexis. Though very unlikely, damage to some tissues like the cornea or the iris cannot completely be ruled out. Latest updates in advanced laser systems come with faster processors and a separate suction control line that initiate an automatic stop after suction loss almost immediately and thus prevent this rare potential damage [14].

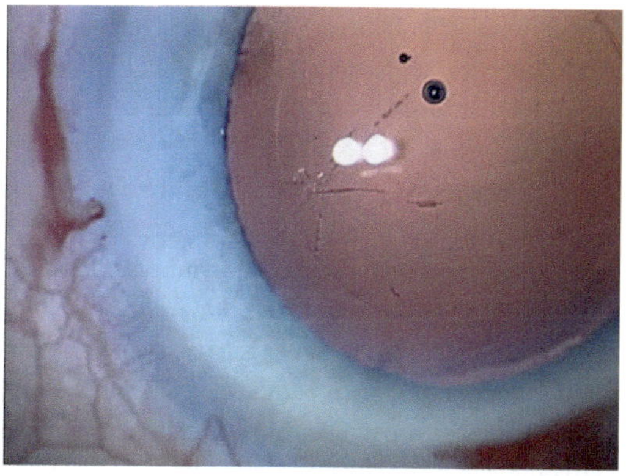

Fig. 35.12 Intracorneal inadvertent laser shots (fragmentation pattern) after a suction loss with the laser firing without immediate stopping after release of the foot pedal (same eye as in Fig. 35.11, view through OR microscope)

.An extremely rare complication described in older patients with mature cataracts is the capsular block syndrome (CBS) caused by the gas bubbles, which are one of the most visible signs of laser treatment [15] Of note: this case was described less than 2 years after the introduction of the femtosecond laser into cataract surgery. CBS has also been reported as an extremely rare complication years after successful conventional cataract surgery [16]. We have not observed a single CBS using the Catalys Laser platform in more than 9000 LCS procedures.

Khandelwal and Koch recommend to closely monitor the fragmentation procedure, because any irregularities to the anterior capsule during this procedure can lead to a radial tear of the capsule. Damage to the posterior capsule during fragmentation, however, is fortunately virtually impossible. It is deemed essential to conduct a careful circumferential irrigation at the end of surgery with balanced salt solution, since some small "chips," fragments of the nucleus, might hide behind the iris [17].

.Postoperative Complications

The application of the laser can lead to the release of prostaglandins, mainly from the nonpigmented epithelial layer of the ciliary body. In samples of aqueous humor from 113 patients undergoing LCS and from 107 patients from a control group on which conventional cataract surgery was performed, the average level of a specific prostaglandin, PGE_2, was about tenfold higher in the laser surgery group: 182 pg/ml versus 17.3 pg/ml. This prostaglandin release can induce an intraoperative miosis, which might constitute a problem for the surgeon during lens removal and IOL implantation and can result in higher complication rates [18]. One way to avoid this effect of the prostaglandin release is speed: continuing the operation immediately after laser treatment before the prostaglandins exert their effect on the sphincter muscle. A pharmacological prophylaxis has proven to be extremely effective: administering nonsteroidal anti-inflammatory drugs (NSAIDs), one eye drop three times on the day of surgery before initiating treatment. This pretreatment led to significantly lower prostaglandin levels in the aqueous humor (65.3 pg/ml) compared to patients who did not receive NSAID eye drops preoperatively (294.4 pg/ml) [19]. The intracameral injection of epinephrine or other measures are recommended to dilate the pupil if a prostaglandin release-induced miosis occurs in LCS.

The short-term release of pro-inflammatory substances like prostaglandins does obviously not lead to an increase in postoperative inflammations of the posterior segment like cystoid macular edema (CME) [20]. This has been confirmed in 2020, when Kolb et al. in a meta-analysis did not find a significantly higher incidence of (CME) after laser cataract surgery [2].

.A rise in intraocular pressure (IOP) has repeatedly been mentioned as a possible complication of LCS. Indeed, we could early on in the development of femtosecond laser cataract surgery demonstrate that the application of vacuum during the docking process leads to a temporary IOP rise: in 100 eyes, the mean preoperative IOP was 15.6 mm Hg, which rose to 25.9 mm Hg after employing the suction ring and was relatively constant during the entire procedure. After removal of the suction ring, the mean IOP decreased to 19.1 mm Hg and was back to normal 1 hour postoperatively [21]. IOP rise or fluctuations during and following LCS have been quite intensely discussed over the last years. Kolb et al., for instance, reported no elevated IOP within 24 hours after surgery in their review in comparison to conventional cataract surgery. Another recent study that assigned 110 eyes either to laser cataract surgery or conventional phacoemulsification found a statistically higher IOP in the laser group on the first postoperative day – though not by much, the mean IOP had risen from 18.6 mm Hg to 20.6 mm Hg, while it was almost constant in the phaco group. The authors conclude that data on the persistence of IOP changes after LCS in the literature are still not sufficient [22].

Conclusion

Laser cataract surgery is an extremely safe procedure though – like in any medical intervention – the risk is not zero. Surgical experience, optimized settings, up-to-date software, and meticulous planning seem to be the best safeguards against any unwanted events during and after this highly effective method to treat cataract and restore the best possible vision.

Take-Home Notes

- Among the benefits of LCS, according to some studies, are better uncorrected and corrected distance visual acuity and the application of less ultrasound energy, the latter contributing to less endothelial cell loss than in conventional cataract surgery that applies a larger amount of ultrasound energy.
- There is a learning curve in LCS as can be evidenced by the reduction of ultrasound energy that comes with growing experience.
- Different laser systems can cause slightly different complications depending on, for example, the integrated software, way of docking, kind of visualization (Scheimpflug, OCT) as well as speed, energy, and pattern of the lasing (Table 35.1).
- The short-term release of pro-inflammatory mediator like prostaglandins can be countered by pharmacological

Table 35.1 Characteristics of the femtosecond laser platforms available for cataract surgery

Parameter	LenSx	Catalys	LensAR	Victus	Ziemer LDV Z8
Patient docking	Applanating: Curved contact lens applanation	Non-applanating: Liquid optic interface with annular vacuum flange onto sclera, 300–700 mmHg vacuum pressure	Non applanating: 2 piece fluid-filled docking device (Robocone immersion lens)	Applanating curved patient interface	Non-applanating: Liquid optic interface with annular vacuum flange onto sclera
Ocular surface identification	Manual	Automatic or user-adjustable	Automatic	Manual	Automatic edge detection and surface mapping
Intraoperative imaging	Spectral domain OCT (wavelength 820–880 nm (± 5 nm))	Spectral domain OCT (820–920 nm, resolution 15 microns lateral, 30 microns axial)	3D-confocal structured illumination (CSI) with automatic biometry, Scheimpflug based	Spectral domain online OCT	Spectral domain OCT
Footprint	152 × 183 cm (no integrated bed)	115 × 164 × 87 cm (integrated bed)	81 × 152 × 145 cm (no integrated bed)	82.7 × 32.5 × 65.9 inches (integrated bed)	101 × 100 × 139 cm (no integrated bed)
Maximum pulse energy	15 μJ (± 1.5 μJ)	3–10 μJ	15 μJ (± 3%)	0.86 W	15 μJ; usually nanojoule range of <1 μJ
Laser wavelength	1030 nm (± 5 nm)	1030 (±5 nm)	1030 (± 2 nm)	1040 (± 25 nm)	1030 nm
Laser pulse width (duration)	600–800 fs (± 50 fs)	<600 fs	1.5 ps	290–550 fs	200–350 fs
Laser type		Diode pumped solid-state, mode-locked		Diode-pumped solid laser	Mode-locked, diode-pumped oscillator

prophylaxis and, under such precaution, is unlikely to lead to an increase in postoperative inflammations of the posterior segment like cystoid macular edema (CME).
- An extremely rare complication described in older patients with mature cataracts is the capsular block syndrome (CBS) caused by the gas bubbles, which are one of the most visible signs of laser treatment.

References

1. Schultz T, Dick HB. Suction loss during femtosecond laser-assisted cataract surgery. J Cataract Refract Surg. 2014;40:493–5.
2. Kolb CM, Shajari M, Mathys L, et al. Comparison of femtosecond laser-assisted cataract surgery and conventional cataract surgery: meta-analysis and systematic review. J Cataract Refract Surg. 2020;46:1075–85.
3. Auffarth GU, Son HS, Gavrilovic B (2018) Pitfalls: femtosecond laser-induced complications. In: H. Burkhard Dick, Ronald D. Gerste, Tim Schultz: Femtosecond laser surgery in ophthalmology. New York Thieme. 191–197.
4. Nagy ZZ, Takacs AI, Filkorn T, et al. Complications of femtosecond laser-assisted cataract surgery. J Cataract Refract Surg. 2014;40:20–8.
5. Grewal DS, Schultz T, Basti S, Dick HB. Femtosecond laser assisted cataract surgery – current status and future directions. Surv Ophthalmol. 2016;61:103–31.
6. Chang JS, Chen IN, et al. Initial evaluation of a femtosecond laser in cataract surgery. J Cataract Refract Surg. 2014;40:29–36.
7. Nejat F, Sarahati S, Nobari SM, et al. Preliminary results of femtosecond laser-assisted cataract surgery in a private clinic in Iran. J Ophthalmic Vis Res. 2017;12:39–43.
8. Chee SP, Yang Y, Ti E. Clinical outcomes in the first two years of femtosecond laser-assisted cataract surgery. Am J Ophthalmol. 2015;159:714–9.
9. Abell RG, Davies PE, Phelan D, et al. Anterior capsulotomy integrity after femtosecond laser-assisted cataract surgery. Ophthalmology. 2014;121:17–24.
10. Kohnen T, Klaproth OK, Ostovic M, et al. Morphological changes in the edge structures following femtosecond laser capsulotomy with varied patient interfaces and energy settings. Graefes Arch Klin Exp Ophthalmol. 2014;252:293–8.
11. Scott WJ, Tauber S, Eck CD, et al. The clinical relationship of anterior capsular tears and vertical spacing in the femtosecond laser capsulotomy procedure. J Refract Surg. 2019;35:280–4.
12. Day AC, Burr JM, Bennett K, et al. Femtosecond laser-assisted cataract surgery versus phacoemulsification cataract surgery (FACT). Ophthalmology. 2020;127:1012–9.
13. Prager AJ, Basti S. Femtosecond laser-assisted cataract surgery in management of posterior capsule tear following blunt trauma: case report and review of literature. Am J Ophthalmol Case Rep, published online May 16;2020:19:100742. https://doi.org/10.1016/j.ajoc.2020.100742.
14. Dick HB (2018) The basics of femtosecond laser cataract surgery. In: H. Burkhard Dick, Ronald D. Gerste, Tim Schultz: Femtosecond laser surgery in ophthalmology. New York Thieme 118–122.
15. Roberts TV, Sutton G, Lawless MA. Capsular block syndrome associated with femtosecond laser-assisted cataract surgery. J Cataract Refract Surg. 2011;37:2068–70.
16. Sandhaus S, Fletcher JG, Mick AE. Case series: late postoperative capsular block syndrome causing reduced vision years after uncomplicated cataract surgery. Optom Vis Sci. 2019;96:710–5.
17. Khandelwal SS, Koch DD (2018) Crucial steps II: lens fragmentation. In: H. Burkhard Dick, Ronald D. Gerste, Tim Schultz: Femtosecond laser surgery in ophthalmology. New York Thieme 142–145.
18. Schultz T, Joachim SC, Kuehn M, Dick HB. Changes in prostaglandin levels in patients undergoing femtosecond laser-assisted cataract surgery. J Refract Surg. 2013;29:742–7.
19. Schultz T, Joachim S, Szuler M, et al. NSAID pretreatment inhibits prostaglandin release in femtosecond laser-assisted cataract surgery. J Refract Surg. 2015;31:791–4.
20. Conrad-Hengerer I, Hengerer FH, Al Juburi MA, et al. Femtosecond laser-induced macular changes and anterior segment inflammation in cataract surgery. J Refract Surg. 2014;30:222–6.
21. Schultz T, Conrad-Hengerer I, Hengerer FH, Dick HB. Intraocular pressure variation during femtosecond laser-assisted cataract surgery using a fluid-filled interface. J Cataract Refract Surg. 2013;39:22–7.
22. Dzhaber D, Mustafa OM, Alsaleh F, et al. Visual and refractive outcomes and complications in femtosecond laser-assisted versus conventional phacoemulsification cataract surgery: findings from a randomized controlled trial. Br J Ophthalmol. 2020;104:1869–600.

Hard Cataract Management with Modern Extracapsular Cataract Surgery

36

Abhay R. Vasavada and Vaishali Vasavada

- Hard cataracts require special attention at every stage, including preoperative evaluation, patient counselling, surgical strategy, and postoperative evaluation.
- The concept of "phases" of surgery and the need for different technique as well as machine parameters during phacoemulsification are highlighted.
- Complete division of the leathery base plate in hard cataracts is often one of the most difficult aspects, which prevents surgeons from performing phacoemulsification in these cataracts. The multilevel chopping technique described in the chapter allows surgeons to completely divide the nucleus, irrespective of whether they are using horizontal or vertical chopping technique.
- Safe and predictable removal of the cataract along with refractive precision is the goal of modern cataract surgery in hard cataracts. The chapter highlights surgical strategies that will ensure good outcomes on postoperative day 1 consistently.
- Latest advances in phacoemulsification and manual small incision cataract surgery that have made surgery safer and more effective are discussed.
- The role of newer technologies like femtosecond laser and devices like the MiLoop are highlighted and discussed.

Introduction

Despite all the technical and technological advancements, cataract surgery in dense cataracts continues to pose challenges to surgeons the world over. Having a surgical technique that is effective, yet safe and predictable, is important to ensure consistent outcomes time after time. This chapter aims to highlight and discuss surgical strategies for effectively and safely removing dense cataracts, as well as preventing complications during surgery. It will describe the modern extracapsular surgical techniques for removing these cataracts in a manner that ensures good technical and functional outcomes on postoperative day one.

Supplementary Information The online version contains supplementary material available at [https://doi.org/10.1007/978-3-030-94530-5_36].

A. R. Vasavada (✉) · V. Vasavada
Iladevi Cataract & IOL Research Centre, Raghudeep Eye Hospital, Ahmedabad, India
e-mail: icirc@abhayvasavada.com;
https://www.raghudeepeyehospital.com

J. L. Alió et al. (eds.), *Cataract Surgery*, Essentials in Ophthalmology,
https://doi.org/10.1007/978-3-030-94530-5_36

Preoperative Evaluation in Dense Cataracts

A detailed examination with and without maximal pupillary dilation should be performed for all patients. Often, subtle changes of pseudoexfoliation or zonular weakness may be detected. Documenting corneal endothelial cell density and morphology is important in these cases as there are greater chances of postoperative corneal edema. It is important with hard cataracts to counsel the patients and their caregivers regarding the potential intraoperative and postoperative difficulties. Getting reliable axial length is often a challenge in these cases, although newer machines with swept source OCT technology are able to penetrate most dense cataracts.

Anesthesia in Dense Cataract Surgery

The choice of anesthesia depends on several factors including the surgical technique (phacoemulsification versus ECCE), surgeon's preference as well as patient co-operation. However, as more and more surgeons perform phacoemulsification for dense cataracts, topical or subtenon's anesthesia are often preferred over injection anesthesia.

Phacoemulsification in Dense Cataracts

Today, phacoemulsification is the standard of care for cataract extraction in most parts of the world. However, an encounter with a dense cataract can be demanding for both the surgeon and the patient, and it is for this reason that phacoemulsification is often not preferred in very dense cataracts. The major difficulties in successful phacoemulsification for hard cataracts are poor visibility, stressful rotation, and incomplete division of the leathery lens fibers. There is an increased risk of thermal damage to the incision (wound site thermal injury) and corneal endothelium by the use of excessive ultrasound energy as well as hard fragments repeatedly hitting the endothelium [1]. The key factors that will often define outcomes in dense cataract emulsification are as follows: achieving a complete division of the leathery lens fibers, maintaining a posterior plane of emulsification, and judicious use of ultrasound energy. To achieve these, the procedure should be governed by the following paradigms:

Incision and Anterior Capsulorhexis

The smallest incision compatible with the surgeon's phaco tip and instrumentation should be created. A square or nearly square configuration of the main incision is crucial in order to for it to be self-sealing (Fig. 36.1). Often, in very hard cataracts, the red reflex is poor, and in such cases, staining the anterior capsule with a vital dye such as trypan blue improves visualization of the capsular flap (Fig. 36.2). Sizing of the anterior continuous curvilinear capsulorhexis is also important – a very small capsulorhexis may increase the chances of anterior capsule split during subsequent maneuvers with the chopper or phaco probe. On the other hand, too large a capsulorhexis may result in fluid-current-induced propulsion of the divided fragments out of the bag, and sometimes dangerously close to the endothelium. Surgeons should aim for an ACCC around 5–5.5 mm in diameter, since this would

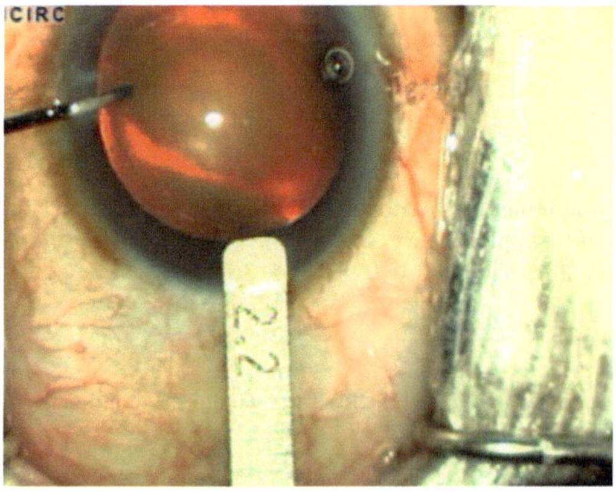

Fig. 36.1 2.2 mm clear corneal temporal incision with internal length and width being similar

confine the mobile nuclear fragments within the capsular bag and facilitate posterior plane emulsification.

Cortical Cleaving Hydrodissection

In hard cataracts, the nucleus is bulky, and often there is not much space within the capsular bag. A forceful cortical cleaving hydrodissection can lead to sudden blow-out of the posterior capsule [2], since the bulky nucleus does not allow egress of the fluid, especially in eyes, where the capsulorhexis is small [3]. In these eyes, careful and gentle cortical-cleaving hydrodissection should be performed. Further, dense cataracts may have strong corticocapsular adhesions [4], making rotation difficult and potentially stressful to the capsulozonular complex. Performing multiquadrant hydrodissection helps surgeons to cleave the corticocapsular adhesions without causing a sudden rise in hydraulic pressure, thereby making nucleus rotation easier.

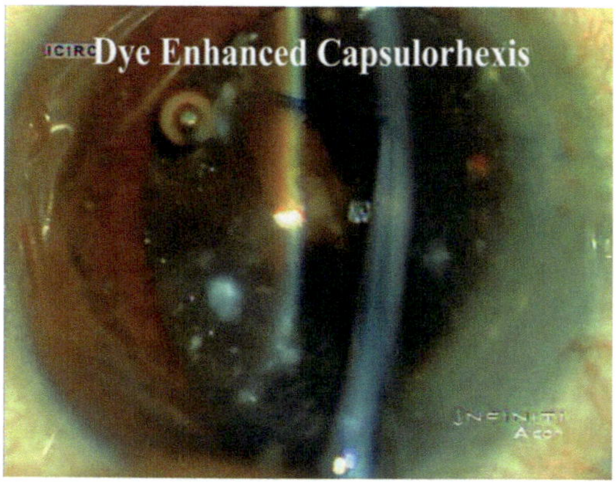

Fig. 36.2 Trypan blue dye injected to enhance visualization of anterior capsule in extremely hard cataract

Principles for Nucleus Division and Fragment Removal

The process of nucleus division and emulsification should be divided into distinct phases, e.g., sculpting, chopping, and fragment removal, depending on the surgeon's preference of technique. This distinction is important to make, since each phase requires a different set of ultrasound and fluidic parameters. Chop techniques, both horizontal and vertical, and their many modifications are very effective for dense cataract emulsification, since they allow complete division of the nuclear fibers. Table 36.1 represents the typical parameters that we prefer during each stage, in terms of ultrasound settings, vacuum, and aspiration flow rate.

Sculpting

The anterior chamber is formed by injecting ophthalmic viscosurgical device (OVD). We prefer the soft shell technique [5], where a dispersive OVD is injected first, followed by a cohesive OVD, which pushes the dispersive OVD toward the corneal endothelium. This helps to protect the

Table 36.1 Representation of the parameters used for emulsification of cataract with dense nuclear sclerosis of ≥ grade 5, on the Centurion Vision System® (Alcon Laboratories, USA)

Surgical parameters			
Stage of surgery	Parameters		
	Torsional ultrasound amplitude – burst mode %	Aspiration flow rate cc / minute	Vacuum mm hg
Sculpting ↓ Approach posterior	70 preset amplitude with linear control, 300 milliseconds on time ↓ 60 amplitude	25 ↓ 20	120 ↓ 60
Chopping	70 preset amplitude with linear control, 300 milliseconds on time	20	650 + (maximum machine vacuum)
1st fragment removal ↓ Last fragment removal	70–80 preset amplitude with linear control, 300 milliseconds on time ↓ 60 ↓ 60	25 ↓ 20 ↓ 18	450 ↓ 300 ↓ 150

endothelium from damage caused by energy dissipation or mechanical trauma. Sculpting creates a central space in the bulky nucleus that acts as a recess for emulsifying the initial fragments within its confines. An ideal space is deep, wide, and steep walled with a very thin posterior plate and is confined within the area of the capsulorhexis (Fig. 36.3). While carrying out sculpting, it is advisable not to mechanically push the nucleus but to scrape the layers gently using optimal energy. A bent tip is better suited to achieve a deep sculpting without undue zonular stress, since it minimizes incision distortion when sculpting is performed in the depths of the crater.

During sculpting, we use ultrasound (U/S) energy in an interrupted mode, with linear foot pedal control, using a preset amplitude of 70–80%. It is important that the surgeon must intermittently change the foot-pedal position from the third to the second position, in order to allow cooling of the phaco tip. The aspiration flow rate is preset to 25–30 cc/min. The end point of sculpting is indicated by a red glow that is visible through the thinned-out posterior plate. An adequate sculpting with a deep, central space is the sheet anchor for dense cataract emulsification.

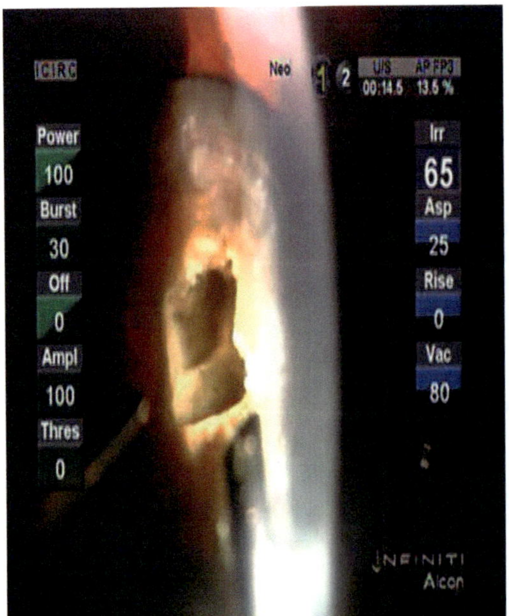

Fig. 36.3 Central, deep trench created in a dense cataract

Chopping

A dense cataract characteristically has extraordinarily tenacious and cohesive leathery fibers that are difficult to separate. Separation of these fibers with forceful lateral movements may produce stress on the capsular bag and the zonules. Also incomplete separation results in multiple fragments held together like the petals of a flower. Fragments attached centrally make posterior plane emulsification extremely difficult and risky and increase the possibility of anterior capsular split, posterior capsular rupture, and prolonged U/S energy dissipation close to the endothelium.

Direct Chop

The direct, or horizontal, chop, originally described by Nagahara, is a very effective technique for division of dense nuclei [6]. No sculpting or trenching is required here. The phaco tip is impaled beyond the midpoint of the nucleus, and a complete vacuum seal is achieved. A sharp tipped chopper is introduced underneath the capsulorhexis margin beyond the lens equator. Once preset vacuum is achieved, the chopper is then moved toward the phaco tip to initiate a crack. However, we have found that using a blunt tipped chopper is equally effective, and yet reduces the risk of mechanical injury to the equatorial posterior capsule. It is important that maximal or supramaximal vacuum is used along with appropriate U/S energy for achieving an effective vacuum seal.

Step-by-Step Chop In Situ and Separation Technique

Our technique of division [7] involves a judicious combination of chop in situ and lateral separating movements. This technique comprises five steps:

Step 1: Vacuum seal – Following a small, central sculpt, the foot pedal is depressed to the third position and the phaco tip is buried inside the trench. If the wall of the trench is arbitrarily divided into 3 equal parts, the tip is buried at the junction of the anterior one-third and posterior two-thirds of the trench (Fig. 36.4). The foot-pedal immediately switches from the third position to the second position and remains there till occlusion (indicated by the machine audio) is achieved.

Step 2: Chop in situ: Initiating a crack – The chopper is placed within the capsulorhexis, just in front of and lateral to the phaco tip. The vertical element of the chopper is depressed posteriorly (toward the optic nerve) (Fig. 36.4). The aim is to only initiate a partial thickness crack and not to divide the nucleus at a single stroke.

Step 3: Lateral separation: In hard cataracts, the initial crack seldom reaches the bottom. Therefore, the chopper is progressively repositioned in the depths of the cracked nucleus (Fig. 36.4) and also repositioned from periphery to the center. Thus, the crack is gently extended from superficial to deep and from periphery to the center. This maneuver allows complete separation of the nuclear fragments without undue zonular stress.

Multilevel Chopping

Often the very dense cataracts will resist complete division of nuclear fragments. In such cases, a multilevel chop technique comes in very handy [8]. For techniques using modifications of the vertical chop technique, an initial crack is initiated, and no attempt is made to extend the crack to the depth. Subsequently, the phaco tip is occluded at a deeper plane, and with each occlusion, fibers adjacent to the tip are chopped with minimal lateral separating movements. This progressive deeper occlusion of the phaco tip allows

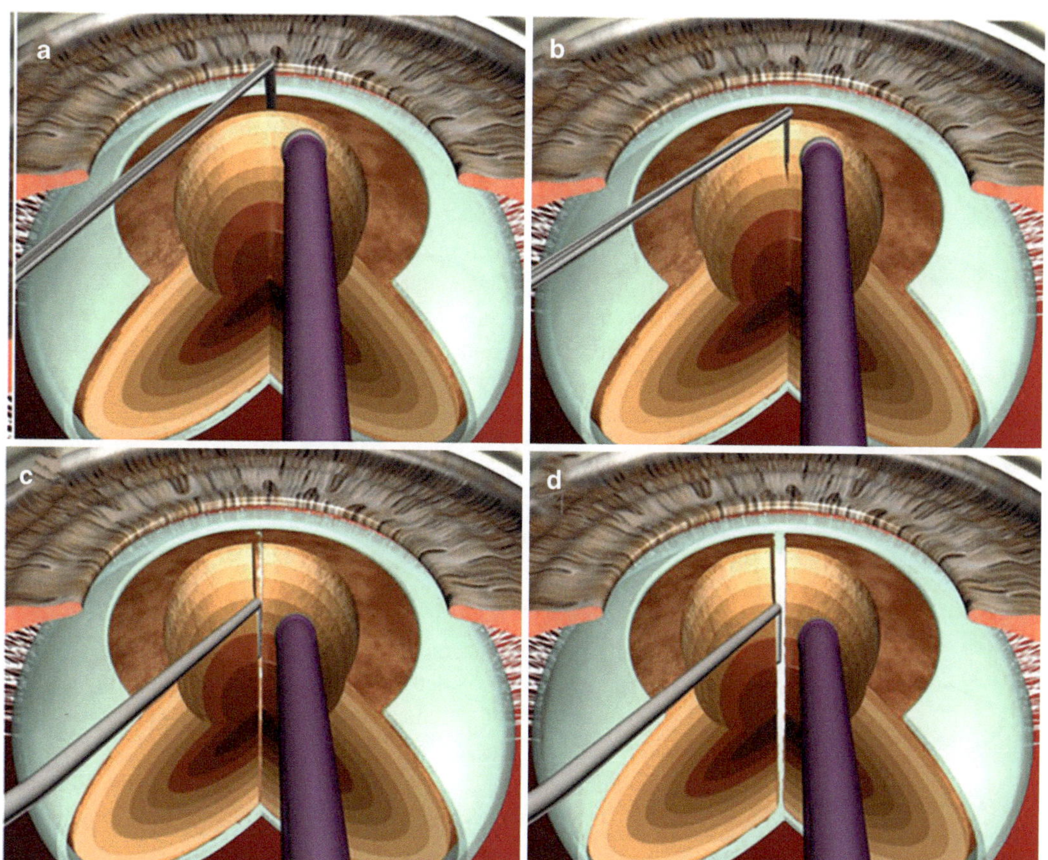

Fig. 36.4 (**a**) Phaco tip buried in the vertical wall of the trench. (**b**) Chopper being placed just in front of and lateral to the phaco tip. (**c**) Initial vertical movement of chopper, aimed at creating a partial thickness crack. (**d**) The chopper is positioned in the depth of the crack, and lateral separating movements are performed

a better vacuum seal and division of the nucleus adjacent to the tip. This facilitates complete division of posterior plate without the need for excessive separation movements. Multiple fragments can be created by repeating this technique every 1–2 clock hours (Video 36.1). The advantages of this technique are safety and efficacy in division of dense, leathery cataracts. The same technique can also be used with direct chop. Here, the phaco tip is first impaled in the periphery and a crack initiated with horizontal movement of the chopper (Fig. 36.5). Subsequently, the phaco tip is brought centrally and occlusion achieved. The crack that was initiated is then extended centrally. The technique can also be employed in cataracts with weak zonules, pseudoexfoliation, subluxated cataracts, hypermature cataracts, as well as in small pupils.

Nuclear Fragment Removal

Creating as many small fragments as possible allows surgeons to emulsify them easily (Fig. 36.6). Surgeons must try to perform emulsification at a posterior plane, in order to avoid thermal and mechanical damage to the corneal endothelium (Fig. 36.7). However, emulsification in the posterior plane increases the risk of inadvertent aspiration of the posterior capsule and iris, especially if a very high vacuum and aspiration flow rate (AFR) are used while removing the last fragments or epinucleus. Therefore, we suggest lowering the vacuum and AFR as progressively more fragments are removed and the posterior capsule is exposed [9, 10]. This allows surgeons to continue emulsifying at a posterior plane without the risk for posterior capsule rupture.

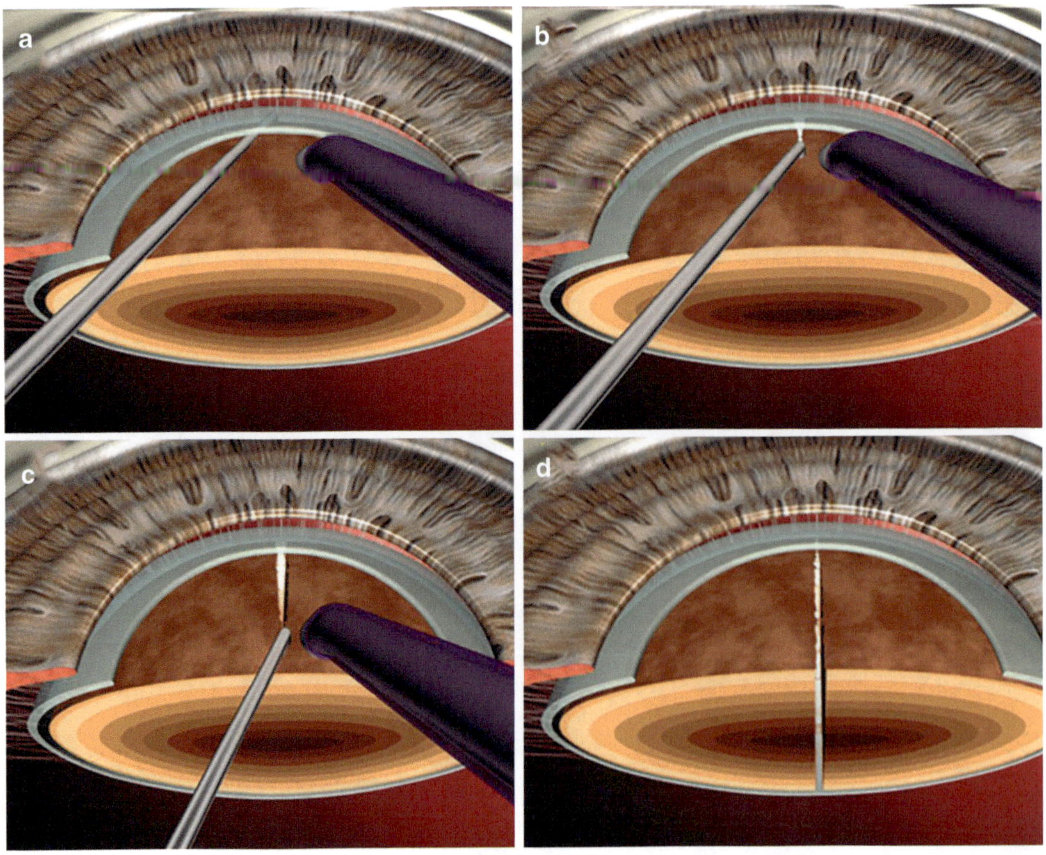

Fig. 36.5 Multiple, small fragments, which become easy to remove during phacoemulsification. (**a**) Phaco tip is occluded beyond the midpoint of the nucleus and chopper inserted beyond the equator. (**b**) The chopper is moved centrally in a horizontal chop action to initiate a crack. At this time, no attempt is made to extend the crack to the centre. (**c**) The phaco tip is then re-occluded more centrally and the initial crack extended more centrally. (**d**) Thus, multilevel chopping ensures complete nucleus division without undue capsulo-zonular stress even in dense, leathery cataracts

Optimal utilization of U/S energy is important for efficient emulsification. Whether longitudinal or torsional ultrasound is used, it is advisable to use interrupted energy as compared to continuous energy. This allows intermittent cooling of the phaco tip, which reduces the chances of wound site thermal injury and corneal endothelial injury. With longitudinal ultrasound, there is a conflict between aspiration forces, on the one hand, which attract the nuclear material, and U/S energy on the other, which tends to repel the fragments. However, with the torsional ultrasound, since there is a constant oscillatory motion at the phaco tip, there is a seamless cutting with minimal repulsion (chatter) of lens material. This makes the U/S energy more efficient, especially in hard cataracts [11, 12]. Whatever the technique or technology used, it is very important to repeatedly inject dispersive OVD during fragment removal to protect the corneal endothelium (Fig. 36.8). It is of utmost importance to closely inspect the incision at the end of surgery to look out for incision distortion / WSTI. In case of doubt, the incision should be sutured.

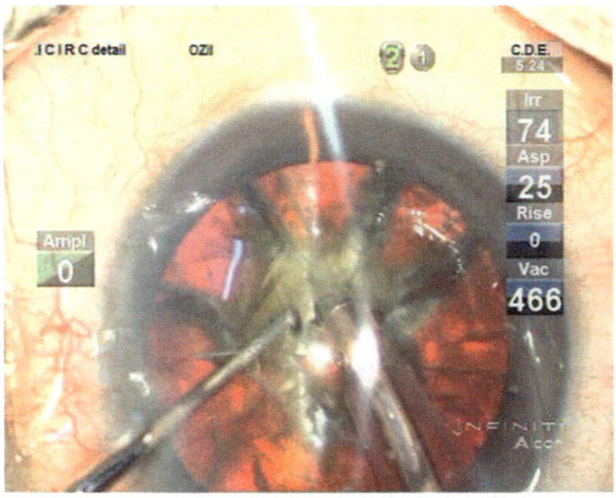

Fig. 36.6 Horizontal multilevel chopping. The phaco tip is first impaled beyond the center of the nucleus and a crack initiated. Subsequently, the tip is occluded more centrally, and the crack is extended centrally, to achieve complete nucleus division without undue capsulozonular stress

Extracapsular Cataract Extraction (ECCE) and Manual Small Incision Cataract Surgery (MSICS) for Dense Cataract Emulsification

Despite the advances in phacoemulsification techniques, there still is a place for ECCE, especially in removal of the very hard cataracts. Not only can this technique be a fallback in cases where phacoemulsification poses difficulties, but it can also be the primary technique of choice in these difficult cases. The disadvantage of ECCE is the large incision required, inability to maintain a closed chamber during surgery, and the need for multiple sutures, with resultant postoperative astigmatism.

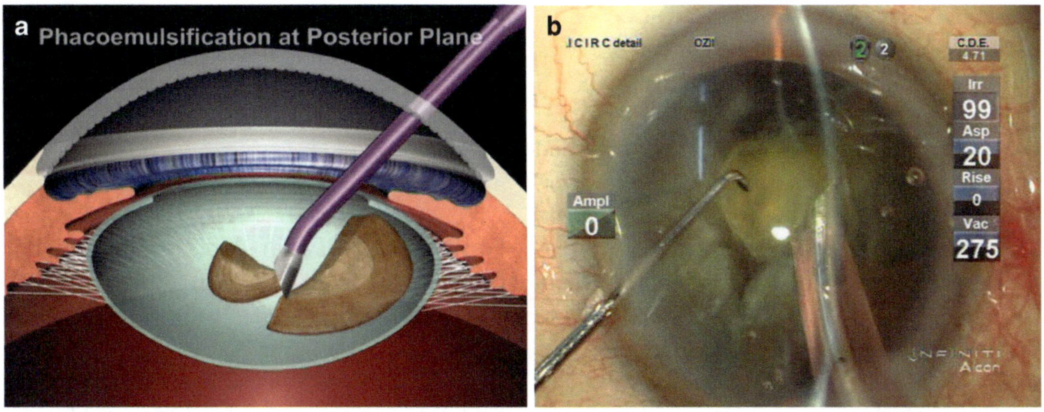

Fig. 36.7 (**a** and **b**) Animation and clinical picture showing dense nuclear fragment being removed away from the corneal endothelium

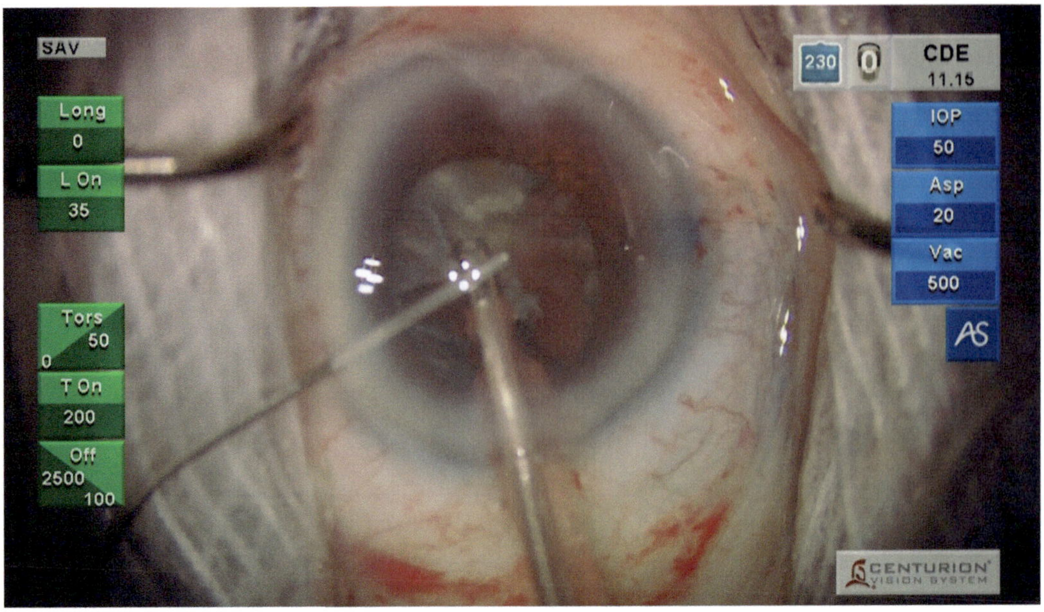

Fig. 36.8 Dispersive OVD being supplemented during fragment removal to protect the corneal endothelium

On the other hand, with MSICS, a self-sealing, 5–6 mm scleral tunnel incision is created. The incision may be superior or temporal. Following a relatively large ACCC, the nucleus is prolapsed into the anterior chamber and subsequently removed from the eye. Now, several modifications such as the use of irrigating wire vectis, nuclear snare, nucleus glides, visco-expression, nucleus fracture, and nucleus bisection are employed by surgeons in order to reduce the size of the nucleus and make delivery out of the eye easier and safer.

There are several published studies in literature that compare outcomes following MSICS and phacoemulsification, and most of the recent ones show that both techniques are safe and effective [13–21]. MSICS and ECCE, however, are more cost effective than phacoemulsification and not dependent on technology. This is the reason why these techniques are often favored in developing nations. Therefore, it would be left to the surgeon's surgical skill and experience, availability of machines, as well as economic viability to choose which is the best surgical strategy in their hands.

Newer Techniques/Devices for Dense Cataract Surgery

Endocapsular Manual Nucleus Fragmentation in Phacoemulsification

Recently, the miLoop, a disposable manual device, has been introduced for endocapsular manual nuclear fragmentation during cataract surgery. Initial reports suggest that this device is safe and effective and that corneal endothelial cell loss as well as intraoperative complications are comparable when performing traditional phacoemulsification versus using the miLoop device [22, 23].

Femtosecond-Laser-Assisted Cataract Surgery (FLACS) – Role in Dense Cataract Removal

With the advent of femtosecond laser technology for cataract surgery, it has been approved for creating corneal incisions, capsulotomy, and nuclear

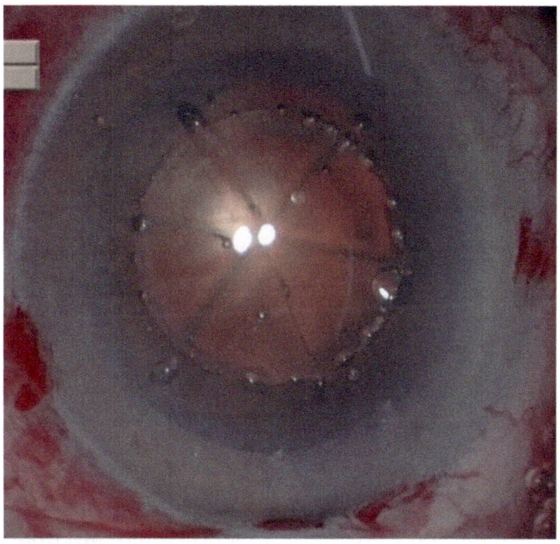

Fig. 36.9 Femtosecond cataract surgery in a dense cataract, capsulorhexis, and chop pattern of nucleus division performed

division. Both the temporal incision and paracenteses incisions can be customized and positioned based on a real-time anterior segment optical coherence tomography view. A centric anterior capsulotomy of a desired size can be created, even in the absence of a good red reflex (Fig. 36.9). Contrary to the initial expectations from the laser, FLACS is able to create various patterns of nucleus division, and even though the division may not extend to the complete depth in very leathery cataracts, it may be useful in reducing the U/S energy consumption during sculpting and chopping. Thus, as this technology continues to evolve, and becomes more cost effective, it may find more use in the surgeons' armamentarium, especially to manage dense cataracts [24–26].

Complications During Dense Cataract Surgery

Common complications that might arise during dense cataract surgery are enlisted below. Although most of them could occur with any technique, some are specific to phacoemulsification or extracapsular cataract surgery:

- Corneal endothelial trauma: surgery in dense cataracts can potentially cause increased endothelial cell loss or even corneal decompensation causes for excessive endothelial cell loss include excessive and continuous use of U/S energy during phacoemulsification, as well as mechanical trauma caused by nuclear fragments/entire nucleus rubbing with the corneal endothelium.

  Preventive measures: repeated use of dispersive OVD to coat the corneal endothelium, being conscious about the plane of emulsification, and the use of interrupted U/S energy delivery/ torsional U/S.
- Incisional thermal damage: caused by excessive and continuous use of U/S energy, especially with a tight wound construction. In ECCE / MSICS, an irregular wound construction can lead to collagen distortion and irregular wound healing.

  Preventive measures: During phacoemulsification, surgeons must make sure to use interrupted U/S energy, which allows for intermittent cooling of the phaco tip. Further a higher AFR should be used during sculpting, so as to allow continuous cooling of the phaco tip. Also, it is very important to create an incision that is not too tight. There should be no compression of the phaco tip at the incision, so that the irrigation flow around the phaco tip is not compressed. For example, if a surgeon uses 2.2 mm incision routinely, he or she should perform a 2.4 mm incision to avoid oar locking and tight wound geometry.
- Posterior capsule rupture: often occurs due to the use of very high flow rate and vacuum settings in these eyes, which may have fragile capsular bags to begin with.

  Preventive measures: adhering to the principles of closed chamber technique and the use of modestly low vacuum and AFR settings will allow the surgeon to avoid inadvertent rupture of the posterior capsule as well as injury to the iris tissue.
- Zonular dialysis/weakness: dense cataracts are very often associated with pre-existing

zonular weakness. Also, stressful surgical maneuvers such as nucleus rotation, excessive lateral separation movements, or forceful nucleus delivery during phacoemulsification / ECCE / MSICS may lead to iatrogenic zonular defects. Many times, dense cataracts may be associated with comorbidities such as glaucoma or pseudoexfoliation syndrome, which can further predispose to zonular weakness.

Preventive measures: it is important for surgeons to detect any zonular weakness preoperatively by performing a thorough and full dilated slit-lamp evaluation.

Conclusion

Dense cataract management has improved dramatically over time. However, technique and technology must complement each other for consistent and predictable outcomes. Surgeons need to be extra careful during preoperative evaluation, paying special attention to the corneal endothelial health, pupillary dilatation, and zonular weakness. During surgery, the judicious use of U/S energy, adhering to posterior plane phacoemulsification, optimal use of U/S energy such as the use of torsional U/S, interrupted energy, and repeated use of dispersive OVDs will ensure intraoperative efficacy and safety and good postoperative outcomes (Fig. 36.10).

- Hard cataracts pose two major challenges to surgeons during surgery: (a) effective division of the lens and (b) safe and predictable removal of fragments without causing any damage to the corneal endothelium or uveal tissues.
- Both manual extracapsular cataract surgery and phacoemulsification are viable options in hard cataract management. Surgeons should choose their approach based on surgical experience, comfort, and availability of technology.
- Chop techniques tend to work better during phacoemulsification of hard cataracts. Select a technique that ensures complete nucleus division before the fragments are removed.
- Understanding your machine and modulating the ultrasound energy and fluidic parameters will help surgeons optimize their technique.
- The use of adjuncts, such as dispersive ophthalmic viscosurgical devices during surgery, is critical to ensure least corneal endothelial damage.

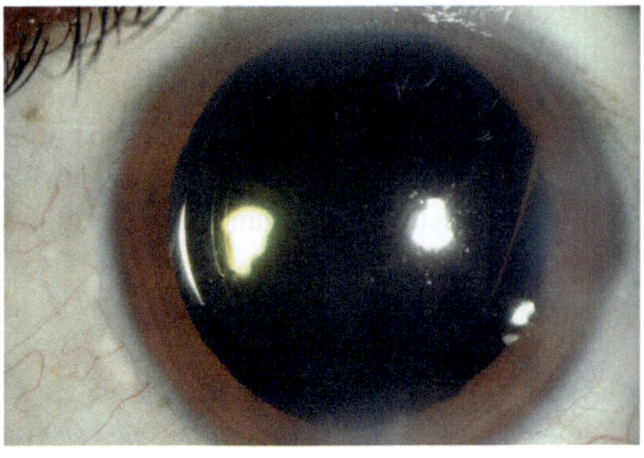

Fig. 36.10 Clear cornea on postoperative day 1 in a dense cataract

Financial Disclosures Dr. Abhay R. Vasavada receives research support grant from Alcon Laboratories, USA. Dr. Vaishali Vasavada has no financial disclosures.

References

1. Singh R, Vasavada AR. Phacoemulsification of brunescent and black cataracts. J Cataract Refract Surg. 2001;27:1762–9.
2. Fine IH. Cortical cleaving Hydrodissection. J Cataract Refract Surg. 1992;18:508–12.
3. Yeoh R. The 'pupil snap' sign of posterior capsule rupture with hydrodissection in phacoemulsification (letter). Br J Ophthalmol. 1996;80:486.
4. Vasavada AR, Goyal D, Shastri L, Singh R. Cortico capsular adhesions and their effect during cataract surgery. J Cataract Refract Surg. 2003;29:1–6.
5. Arshinoff SA. Dispersive-cohesive viscoelastic soft shell technique. J Cataract Refract Surg. 1999;25:167–73.
6. Can I, Takmaz T, Cakici F, Ozgul M. Comparison of Nagahara phaco-chop and stop-and-chop phacoemulsification nucleotomy techniques. J Cataract Refract Surg. 2004;30:663–8.
7. Singh R, Vasavada AR. Step-by-step chop in situ and separation of very dense cataracts. J Cataract Refract Surg. 1998;24:156–9.
8. Vasavada AR, Raj SM. Multilevel chop technique. J Cataract Refract Surg. 2011;37:2092–4.

9. Vasavada AR, Raj S. Step down technique. J Cataract Refract Surg. 2003;29:1077–9.
10. Osher RH. Slow motion phacoemulsification approach. J Cataract Refract Surg. 1993;19:667.
11. Liu Y, Zeng M, Liu X, et al. Torsional mode versus conventional ultrasound mode phacoemulsification: randomized comparative clinical study. J Cataract Refract Surg. 2007;33:287–92.
12. Vasavada AR, Raj SM, Patel U, et al. Comparison of torsional (Ozil) versus microburst longitudinal (traditional) phacoemulsification – a prospective, randomized, masked clinical trial. In press, Ophthalmic Surg Lasers Imaging. 2010;41(1):109–14.
13. Minassian DC, Rosen P, Dart JK, Reidy A, Desai P, Sidhu M. Extracapsular cataract extraction compared with small incision surgery by phacoemulsification: a randomised trial. Br J Ophthalmol. 2001;85:822–9.
14. Gogate PM, Wormald RP, Deshpande M, Deshpande R, Kulkarni SR. Extracapsular cataract surgery compared with manual small incision cataract surgery in community eye care setting in Western India: a randomized controlled trial. Br J Ophthalmol. 2003;87:673–9.
15. Gogate PM, Wormald RP, Deshpande M. Is manual small incision cataract surgery affordable in the developing countries? A cost comparison with extracapsular cataract extraction. Br J Ophthalmol. 2003;87:841–4.
16. Gogate PM, Kulkarni SR, Krishnaiah S, Deshpande RD, Joshi SA, Palimkar A, et al. Safety and efficacy of phacoemulsification compared with manual small incision cataract surgery by a randomized controlled clinical trial: six weeks results. Ophthalmology. 2005;112:869–74.
17. Gogate PM, Deshpande MD, Nirmalan P. Why do phacoemulsification? Manual small incision cataract surgery is almost as effective and more economical. Ophthalmology. 2007;114:965–8.
18. Venkatesh R, Muralikrishnan R, Balent LC, Prakash SK, Prajna V. Outcomes of high volume cataract surgeries in a developing country. Br J Ophthalmol. 2005;89:1079–83.
19. Madurai NG. Manual small incision cataract surgery: an alternative technique to instrumental phacoemulsification. Mandurai: Aravind Publication; 2000.
20. Henning A, Kumar J, Yorston D, Foster A. Sutureless cataract surgery with nucleus extraction: outcome of a prospective study in Nepal. Br J Ophthalmol. 2003;87:266–70.
21. Ruit S, Tabin G, Chang D, Bajracharya L, Kline DC, Richheimer R, et al. A prospective randomized clinical trial of phacoemulsification vs. manual sutureless small incision extracapsular cataract surgery in Nepal. Am J Ophthalmol. 2007;143:32–8.
22. Ianchulev T, Chang DF, Koo E, MacDonald S, Calvo E, Tyson FT, Vasquez A, Ahmed IIK. Microinterventional ensocapsular nucleus disassembly : novel technique and results of first-in human randomized controlled study. Br J Ophthalmol. 2019;103(2):176–80.
23. Ianchulev T, Chang DF, Koo E, MacDonald S. Microinterventional endocapsular nucleus disassembly for phacoemulsification-free full-thickness fragmentation. J Cataract Refract Surg. 2018;44(8):932–4.
24. Roberts HW, Day AC, O'Brart DP. Femtosecond laser-assisted cataract surgery: a review. Eur J Ophthalmol. 2020;30(3):417–29.
25. Chen X, Xiao W, Ye S, Chen W, Liu Y. Efficacy and safety of femtosecond laser-assisted cataract surgery versus conventional phacoemulsification for cataract: a meta-analysis of randomized controlled trials. Sci Rep. 2015;13(5):13123.
26. Taravella MJ, Meghpara B, Frank G, Gensheimer W, Davidson R. Femtosecond laser-assisted cataract surgery in complex cases. J Cataract Refract Surg. 2016;42(6):813–6.

Managing Complications During Cataract Surgery

37

Robert H. Osher, Graham D. Barrett, Lucio Buratto, and Arjan Hura

Bullet Point

- Every cataract surgeon will encounter a wide range of complications in his or her career.
- Fortunately, complications are infrequent and usually well managed.
- Understanding the reason that the complication occurs and preparing in advance for how to manage these adrenaline-provoking events will yield the highest chances for a successful outcome.

Supplementary Information The online version contains supplementary material available at [https://doi.org/10.1007/978-3-030-94530-5_37].

R. H. Osher (✉)
Cincinnati Eye Institute, University of Cincinnati, Cincinnati, OH, USA
e-mail: rhosher@cvphealth.com

G. D. Barrett
University of Western Australia, Centre for Ophthalmology and visual Science, Lions Eye Institute, Sir Charles Gairdner Hospital, Perth, WA, Australia

L. Buratto
CAMO Centro Ambrosiano Oftalmico – Milano, Milan, Italy

A. Hura
Cleveland Eye Clinic, Brecksville, OH, USA

It is difficult to write a concise chapter on a topic which deserves an entire book. However, we will try to address a spectrum of complications in far less detail than each deserves. Therefore, the purpose of this chapter is to provide an overview, one that allows the reader to get his arms around the subject. A deeper understanding of the rescue techniques described can be attained by viewing surgical videos from different sources, for example, the Video Journal of Cataract, Refractive, and Glaucoma Surgery (www.vjcrgs.com) [1].

Anesthesia Complications

Regardless of whether the surgeon performs retrobulbar, peribulbar, or topical anesthesia, complications can occur [2]. Certainly, topical anesthesia may be the safest but it is not uncommon for superficial punctate keratopathy to obscure the surgeon's view [2, 3]. Moreover, photophobia may be intense and can be managed by intracameral anesthetic agents in addition to operating under low illumination [4]. Discomfort may be reduced by additional topical or intracameral medication, lowering the infusion pressure, which places less stress on the zonules, and frequent reassurance. Occasionally, it is necessary to supplement with a subconjunctival or subtenon's injection, which can be spread into the sensitive area with a muscle hook for more effective anesthesia.

J. L. Alió et al. (eds.), *Cataract Surgery*, Essentials in Ophthalmology,
https://doi.org/10.1007/978-3-030-94530-5_37

Retrobulbar and peribulbar injections can have consequences due to the needle [5]. If a subconjunctival hemorrhage occurs and it is significant enough to elevate the limbal tissue which interferes with visualization, a cut-down can be made with scissors to allow egress of blood and the bleeding vessel can be cauterized [6]. If the hemorrhage originates from a more posterior source, then the surgeon should be concerned about the effect of increasing volume within a confined bony orbit that may lead to positive pressure. If a retrobulbar hemorrhage is suspected, the surgeon should differentiate between a venous and an arteriole bleed. The venous bleed is more benign and can be diagnosed by a lack of progressive proptosis, limitation of the bleeding, mobility of the lids, and easy retropulsion of the globe. By contrast, an arteriole bleed spreads rapidly, pushing the globe forward and creating enough additional volume that the lids become tight and the globe cannot be easily retropulsed [7]. The former condition may lead to slight positive pressure, but the latter condition may lead to blindness. A venous bleed can be managed by gentle intermittent digital pressure, while a retrobulbar arteriolar hemorrhage is a sight-threating emergency. Surgery should be cancelled and the intraocular pressure should be recorded and monitored. Ophthalmoscopy will reveal whether perfusion has been interrupted, and, if so, the surgeon should consider decompressing the orbit. Various recommendations include a lateral canthotomy, an inferior cantholysis, plunging a scissors into each quadrant to express blood, and even disinsertion of the lids [7]. In a severe case, the patient should be admitted to the hospital and intravenous steroids should be initiated [8]. Sadly, we have witnessed a permanent loss of all useful vision, despite prompt oculoplastic intervention, due to an ischemic optic neuropathy.

Adverse reaction to the intravenous sedative is also possible. We have seen patients become acutely nauseated and puke from fentanyl. More commonly, the anesthesia person will over-sedate a patient who then becomes disoriented or abruptly moves during surgery. For this reason, it is recommended that the surgeon emphasize to the anesthesia team that it is safer to perform cataract surgery when the patient is minimally sedated, awake, and easily communicating. We are not reluctant to tell the anesthesia person that the best anesthesia is not general or local, but rather vocal! [9].

Dr. Barrett's comment: *The choice of anesthesia in patients with high myopia undergoing cataract surgery may be challenging. Retrobulbar or peribulbar anesthesia poses a greater risk of needle injury, which is greater with long axial lengths exceeding 26 mm, but topical anesthesia may be uncomfortable even with intracameral lignocaine as reverse pupillary block is more common. General anesthesia is a useful alternative in this context and in complex cases requiring intrascleral lens fixation.*

The Incision

Scleral, near-clear, and clear corneal incisions share in common certain rules that must be respected. A premature entry is conducive to iris damage or prolapse, while too long of an incision will cause corneal distortion and compromised visibility. The effect on the incision by different instruments may also cause an additional endothelial cell loss and even positive pressure as the ultrasound or I&A handpiece compress the globe. Too narrow of an incision may compromise the infusion and cause a thermal injury, while the "oar-locking" restricts movement of the tip [10]. Too large of an incision allows wound leak, chamber instability, iris prolapse, and more induced astigmatism than anticipated.

The construction of the incision must be meticulous and precise [11, 12]. One-plane incisions may slide more than a two-plane incision, which begins with a groove. Dr. Osher prefers a three-plane incision beginning with a groove, uphill tunnel, and a final downward angle toward the pupil forming a carpenter's "lap joint." [13] After introducing micro-coaxial phacoemulsification through a 2.2 mm incision, Dr. Osher published the idea of an internal flare architecture [14]. By slightly flaring the internal incision to 2.4 mm, several benefits are realized. First, the temperature within the incision is lower; second, there is greater maneuverability of the ultrasound and I&A handpiece; and third, there is less resistance when injecting a foldable lens when using the incision as an extension of the cartridge [14].

Careful construction of the incision will always pay dividends by preventing annoying and sometimes serious complications. Should the incision leak despite adequate hydration, a watertight closure should be achieved with sutures or an ophthalmic sealant [15, 16].

Dr. Buratto's comment: *Too peripheral an incision may lead to corneal distortion and compromise visualization. Moreover, long tunnels restrict movement of the phaco and a greater risk of wound burn. An incision that is too peripheral may also permit premature entry into the anterior chamber resulting in a short tunnel, which may allow iris prolapse and fail to be watertight at the end of the procedure.*

Dr. Barrett's comment: *The location of the incision is relevant and a constant temporal location is preferred. This provides better access and less surgically induced astigmatism. The latter is quite variable and keeping the incision to less than 2.4 mm at a constant location and using toric IOLs is more predictable than attempting to perform on axis incisions to reduce corneal astigmatism.*

The Constricting Pupil

It is well recognized that visualization of anatomic detail is essential in cataract surgery. Suboptimal pupillary dilatation should be noted during the office examination, and either pharmacologic or mechanical pupillary dilatation should be anticipated in the surgical plan. Patients with pseudoexfoliation, posterior synechiae, diabetic neuropathy, and the aging process alone may prevent a widely dilated pupil, and management of these conditions has been discussed elsewhere in this book [17–20]. Yet it is different when the pupil starts out well dilated and then begins to progressively constrict as the operation is proceeding. This behavior is typical of the patient who has been taking Flomax (or a similar alpha-blocking drug) [21]. Moreover, when either lens nucleus or fragments come in contact with iris or when fluidic turbulence exists, a prostaglandin release from the iris may occur which results in pupillary constriction [22].

The surgeon has a number of options from which to choose if the pupil begins to constrict. While the highly experienced surgeon may simply continue, the injection of a retentive viscoelastic agent like Healon5 will produce viscomydriasis [23, 24]. Alternatively, intracameral epinephrine, Shugarcaine, or Omidria (phenylephrine and ketorolac) can be used for pharmacologic dilatation [25–27]. In rare cases, the pupil might constrict so much that a mechanical pupil stretch technique or even a device like a Malyugin ring should be injected [28, 29], although the surgeon must be careful to avoid damage to the border of the anterior capsulotomy. Rather than risk tearing the capsulorhexis margin, the anterior capsule should be displaced with the OVD prior to either stretching the pupil or using a device [30]. Once the pupil has been adequately widened, the risk of subsequent complications will have been reduced.

Descemet's Tear or Detachment

Every time the surgeon introduces an instrument or injects an OVD into the anterior chamber, there is a risk of damaging Descemet's membrane. There are few more dramatic videos than watching an inexperienced surgeon continue to inject OVD as Descemet's membrane is being cleaved from the corneal stroma [31]. Moreover, it is not uncommon to observe small tears in Descemet's membrane at the site of the main or stab incision during the course of an operation. For this reason, it is absolutely necessary to depress the incision when an instrument is being introduced which avoids contact with and damage to Descemet's membrane. The same holds true with the introduction of a cannula, and neither the balanced salt solution nor OVD should be injected until the tip of the cannula is safely beyond the internal opening of the incision [32].

Should a Descemet's tag occur, it is usually unnecessary to repair [33, 34]. By contrast, the surgeon should try to remove the trapped OVD, if it has caused a significant Descemet's detachment. This can be accomplished by either a small cut in Descemet's or a stab into the OVD pocket through clear cornea followed by raising the intraocular pressure with a forceful OVD injection. An air bubble, intraocular gas, or passing full-thickness corneal sutures will reapproximate the Descemet's membrane to the corneal stroma in most cases, although occasionally surgical re-intervention is necessary [35–37]. Prevention by careful technique is vastly preferred to managing this complication.

Dr. Barrett's comment: *One strategy that may be helpful is to deepen the eye with viscoelastic prior to introducing the phacoemulsification tip and then commencing infusion rather than inserting the phaco tip with the infusion on to simultaneously inflate the anterior chamber.*

Dr. Buratto's comment: *A Descemet's tear can be avoided by using sharp blades to enter the anterior chamber. The phaco tip should be introduced parallel to the corneal tunnel. Instrument entry should avoid stressing the interior edge of the incision. If construction of the first tunnel is poor, do not hesitate to construct a second tunnel. Never force an IOL through a corneal tunnel of inadequate size.*

Complications of Hydrodissection

While it seems like such an innocuous procedure, hydrodissection can actually cause several problems. A forceful stream injected from a 30 g cannula can actually "water pick" through the capsule. The surgeon should use a larger cannula, at least 27 g, and inject gently. A forceful injection may also prolapse the entire nucleus through the pupil releasing prostaglandins, which cause pupillary constriction. If the nucleus prolapses forward, it is best to gently retro place it back into the capsular bag using OVD. Incomplete hydrodissection is another problem that may result in poor rotation of the nucleus during the emulsification and place excessive force on the zonules. The surgeon should consider performing hydrodissection in several meridia if the nucleus does not easily rotate. If dense cortical capsule adhesions prevent hydrodissection, the surgeon may consider viscodissection [38, 39]. Alternatively, a deep central groove followed by a cracking maneuver will create an escape path for additional hydrodissection beneath OVD. Finally, it is not uncommon to loosen the entire posterior cortex as a sheet, which prevents easy cortical removal. This posterior plate if engaged results in residual stringy equatorial cortex, which must be patiently removed.

There are two situations, which require additional considerations when using hydrodissection. The first condition is the mature brunescent cataract where the capsule is tightly adherent to a large "bowling ball." Routine hydrodissection may create a fluid wave, which elevates the lens against the capsulorhexis edge trapping fluid in the confined space behind the lens. If the surgeon continues to inject, the inelastic posterior capsule can break [40]. The best prophylaxis is to dribble or ballot the lens as the fluid is injected which allows it to return and escape into the anterior chamber. An alternate strategy previously mentioned is to defer the hydrodissection until a central crack is made which provides an escape route for fluid preventing a posterior capsule rupture.

The second situation deals with the posterior polar cataract, which has a thin, fragile central posterior capsule. In some cases, the posterior capsule is even open [41–45]. Hydrodissection is contraindicated because the stream of fluid may tear the capsule. The surgeon should instead perform hydrodelineation mobilizing the fetal nucleus, which can be emulsified. Aspirating the epi-nucleus and cortex across from the incision creates the escape route to allow late hydrodissection in order to free the remaining epi-nucleus, which can then be either emulsified or aspirated.

Another serious complication that can occur during hydrodissection will be covered later in this chapter under the heading of a Fired Cannula.

Dr. Buratto's comment: *A rapid increase in the volume of the bag due to injecting too much or too rapidly may result in capsular rupture jeopardizing subsequent phacoemulsification. Rupture of the posterior capsule can occur because of excessive fluid pressure on the poste-*

rior capsule: there is inadequate exit for the amount and force of the fluid. The situation can be aggravated by a small anterior capsulorhexis. Inadequate hydrodissection results in inadequate cleaving of cortical adhesions to the capsular bag. Attempted rotation of the nucleus during phacoemulsification exerts excessive stress on the zonules and may result in a dialysis. If the nucleus appears stuck due to persistent posterior adhesions, phaco must be interrupted and a small amount of OVD should be cautiously injected to achieve 360 degrees of viscodissection.

Anterior Capsule Complications

The anterior capsule must be respected even before the surgeon begins the capsulorhexis. If a patient has a shallow anterior chamber, peripheral anterior synechiae, or iris bombe, it is possible to inadvertently injure the capsule when the main or stab incision is being made. The surgeon should consider injecting a retentive OVD after the main incision is constructed prior to plunging a knife into the chamber for the second incision. A helpful trick for finding the nearly invisible stab is to select a vessel and make the second incision where it can be easily located, always aiming the knife toward the center of the pupil.

Just like the construction of the main incision, the capsulorhexis should be precisely centered and sized. After placing the eye in the primary position, Dr. Osher uses the Purkinje images on the Lumera microscope to facilitate centration. He places a trephine on the corneal surface, which leaves an epithelial imprint that can be traced with the bent 22-gauge needle on the anterior capsule. This technique helps to achieve a capsulorhexis size of 4.75 mm, which assures that the optic will be covered. If the rhexis size is too small or slightly eccentric, it can be enlarged after the IOL has been implanted by filling the chamber with OVD, making an angled snip in the margin with an intracameral scissors, and then performing a secondary capsulorhexis with intraocular forceps (Video 37.1).

When making the original capsulorhexis, a number of things can go wrong [46]. If the surgeon finishes the rhexis inside the starting point, a notch is created and is more likely to break at some point in the procedure. The notch can be excised by injecting OVD, making a slanted cut, and then performing a secondary rhexis around the notch.

The capsulorhexis edge may also begin to run peripherally which occurs if the chamber shallows, or more notably with an intumescent cataract. Another situation that deserves mention is the aniridic anterior capsule which instead of being the normal 14–20 microns thick, may only be a few microns thick, and therefore, more likely to rupture [47]. If the surgeon has the luxury of observing only minimal peripheral extension, it is a good idea to inject OVD to flatten the lens bow, which mitigates the downhill tendency of the capsular edge to run peripherally. The flap can be unfolded and redirected (the Little Maneuver) [48] or the surgeon may start the rhexis elsewhere and encircle the leading edge of the capsular extension [46]. On the other hand, if the edge is too peripheral, the surgeon should be extremely cautious because there is a risk of the tear going around the equator and through the posterior capsule. Any force applied to the capsular bag may encourage this "wrap-around" tear, so the surgeon should be familiar with the technique of in situ phacoemulsification [46]. It is also important to reduce turbulence, so parameters should be lowered consistent with the concept of slow motion phacoemulsification [49].

Because most anterior capsular tears will stop in the anterior zonules, the surgeon may still implant an intraocular lens into the capsular bag [46]. A forceful lens injection or excessive rotation should be avoided. We prefer to fill the capsular bag with Healon5, and then the IOL will remain folded allowing atraumatic rotation before the haptics open [46]. The orientation should be 90 degrees from the axis of the tear, and then the anterior capsular opening can be altered safely with a scissors or a vitrector, if a flap of capsule is close to or involving the visual axis.

The anterior capsule of the intumescent cataract requires more explanation, and the reader is referred to the chapter by Figueiredo and

Figueiredo. Excellent visualization is the key to all surgery and these capsules must be stained with a dye like trypan blue [50]. Flattening the anterior capsule with a retentive OVD like Healon5 will counteract the elevated intralenticular pressure [51]. It should be emphasized that a relative nuclear block creates an elevation in both the anterior and posterior cortical compartments, requiring immediate balloting or posterior voiding as soon as the anterior capsule is opened [51]. This will decompress the posterior compartment and prevent the Argentinian flag sign some occurring [51]. A smaller capsulorhexis, which can be enlarged later in the procedure, has also been recommended (Video 37.2).

An anterior capsular tear represents a serious complication and the best strategy is prevention. The surgeon must be cognizant whenever a sharp instrument is introduced into the anterior chamber, and care should be taken to avoid hitting the capsular edge with the ultrasonic needle, especially if the bevel of the torsional needle is perpendicular to the capsular edge. It is helpful to demarcate the edge of the capsulorhexis by removing the underlying anterior cortex just to the edge of the capsular margin prior to beginning the emulsification of the nucleus. With vigilance and meticulous technique, this complication is rare, but the surgeon should have an action plan formulated in advance if an anterior capsular tear occurs.

Dr. Buratto's comment: *A tear of the capsulorhexis margin may occur during phacoemulsification when there is contact with the phaco tip or second instrument during cracking or chopping maneuvers. The tear can be divided into three categories:* (1) *partial tear not reaching the equator or zonules,* (2) *full tear reaching to but not through the equator and the zonules, and* (3) *full tear that goes beyond the equator and involves the posterior capsule. The surgeon should inject OVD above and below the capsular tear to counteract centripetal forces. The capsulorhexis that results is eccentric and asymmetric but can still resist phacoemulsification forces. The capsule may also tear during cortical aspiration, especially with sub-incisional removal when the view through the cornea may be distorted. I prefer a bimanual approach using a Buratto style I/A cannula separating infusion and aspiration in order to eliminate any stress on the capsulorhexis margin.*

Dr. Barrett's comment: *There are many maneuvers recommended to avoid extension of the rhexis with an intumescent cataract. A mini dose of mannitol 0.25 g per kilo is extremely helpful in these cases. It reduces pressure in the posterior segment and may even help reduce intralenticular pressure. The smaller dose is effective in this context as well as reducing vitreous pressure in very short eyes with shallow anterior chambers. As long as the patient voids prior to surgery, catheterization is not required, and the impact on the cardiovascular system is significantly less than the typical dose of 0.5 to 1 gram/kilo, which is often recommended.*

Iris Prolapse

While this complication used to be quite common, smaller incisions and improved wound construction have reduced the incidence of iris prolapse [52]. It may still occur with certain conditions, namely, intraoperative floppy iris syndrome and nanophthalmos [21, 53, 54]. In the former condition, there are pharmacologic agents that will reduce the likelihood of iris prolapse [55–57]. In the latter condition, intravenous mannitol in combination with intermittent compression of the globe to dehydrate the vitreous will reduce the tendency for iris prolapse. Naturally, making the incision the correct size and avoiding a premature entry are essential [53].

When iris prolapse does occur, the surgeon should resist the knee-jerk reflex to shove the iris back into the anterior chamber. This action serves to traumatize the iris and usually results in persistent prolapse throughout the case. If the anterior chamber is filled with an OVD, the pressure gradient can be reduced by aspirating the OVD through a separate site and then repositing the iris [52]. If high infusion pressure is contributing, the bottle should be lowered. If the incision is faulty, it may be closed and another site selected to continue the surgery. If the iris prolapse is the result of positive posterior pressure, the surgeon should not hesitate to view the retina and consider the possibility of choroidal expansion. Using an Osher surgical fundus lens (Ocular Instruments) with the operating microscope or an indirect ophthalmoscope, the surgeon can make the diagnosis of a significant choroidal hemorrhage, effusion, or even an infolding of the sclera.

An excellent technique to manage routine iris prolapse is to place an OVD cannula through the second incision and sweep the iris back into the anterior chamber (Video 37.3). Through the same cannula, the OVD can be injected to create iris concavity which should then allow the safe introduction of the ultrasound needle, the I&A handpiece, or the intraocular lens [52]. Rarely, the cannula must remain over the iris to prevent recurrent prolapse. Before withdrawing the ultrasound or I&A tip, the infusion pressure should always be lowered, allowing the intraocular pressure to approach atmosphere, which prevents recurrent iris prolapse. An intracameral miotic can be injected through the stab incision after the intraocular lens is in place, which further reduces any tendency for iris prolapse.

When iris prolapse is properly managed, it is no longer necessary to perform the once popular large iridectomy which caused glare and cosmetic disfigurement [52]. In fact, the pupil will remain functional and the only postoperative evidence of iris prolapse may be some transillumination defects. However, it should be reemphasized that a careful preoperative history regarding Flomax-like drug usage and meticulous incision construction are worth the time in predicting and preventing this annoying complication.

Dr. Buratto's comment: *Iris root detachment (iridodialysis) can occur when entering the anterior chamber with the phaco tip, especially in a shallow anterior chamber, and can lead to pupil distortion, posterior synechia, and iris atrophy. When pinching or catching the iris in the phaco tip occurs, especially with small pupils and/or in floppy iris syndrome, deepening the anterior chamber with an OVD, lowering the infusion bottle, and reducing the vacuum/aspiration rate parameters are recommended.*

Thermal Injury

One of the few drawbacks of phacoemulsification is that the ultrasound needle generates heat as it vibrates back and forth [58]. Longitudinal ultrasound generates more heat than torsional ultrasound, although any needle is capable of creating a thermal injury under certain conditions [59, 60]. The tip is cooled by the movement of fluid both inside and around the needle, which, if obstructed, can cause a rapid rise in temperature. It only takes a few seconds for a thermal injury to occur which is characterized by a milky appearance to the lens particles at the tip and a rapid shrinkage of the collagen surrounding the ultrasound needle [61, 62]. Although sleeves and bypass holes have been designed to minimize this risk, the surgeon must be aware of the warning bells on the machine which indicate that there is an obstruction at the tip [61]. Moreover, the surgeon must avoid constructing a tight incision that retards leakage around the tip, while forceful compression of the sleeve against the walls of the incision should also be avoided.

If a thermal injury is observed, at the very least, the surgeon should expect a leaky incision throughout the procedure. Even a subtle burn may prevent a watertight seal and require a special suturing technique to close the incision [63]. A standard suturing method does not work well when tissue shrinkage has occurred. Dr. Osher has described a horizontal gape closure where the back of the roof of the tunnel is approximated to the front of the floor which "adds tissue." [64] A vertical suturing technique can also be effective by sewing the roof of the tunnel to the floor of the incision, rather than passing the needle to the posterior lip (Video 37.4). The surgeon should consider reinforcing the incision with a tissue sealant like ReSure. In severe cases, it may even be necessary to mobilize and advance a scleral flap or utilize a scleral patch graft [65].

If the surgeon is aware of the warning sounds and early clinical signs, promptly discontinuing ultrasound may prevent a thermal injury. More often than not, a transient viscoelastic obstruction can be eliminated by increasing the vacuum and then safely resuming ultrasound. Fortunately, the once dreaded thermal injury has become an infrequent complication of phacoemulsification.

Dr. Barrett's comment: *One of the most common causes of thermal burns is the commencement of phacoemulsification before aspiration of viscoelastic and establishment of flow within the AC. This is particularly important with higher density viscoelastic such as Healon5.*

Nuclear Chip Management

A nuclear chip is capable of escaping from the surgeon's view and remaining hidden in the eye until it is detected in the postoperative period. While a soft chip can be absorbed, the hard chip may cause prolonged inflammation, elevated intraocular pressure, and corneal edema [66–70]. Therefore, the surgeon should prioritize removing a chip as soon as it is seen rather than procrastinate until later in the procedure. While it may seem counterintuitive, reducing the ultrasound energy may also reduce the chatter and repulsion allowing for more efficient chip removal. It is important to always check the second stab incision where a chip may be found before withdrawing the phaco tip from the eye. If a chip is identified within the OVD, it can be either emulsified or aspirated more easily through the larger opening of the phaco tip than with the smaller I&A port.

When a chip is identified during cortical removal, it may be too hard to aspirate, so a second instrument can be introduced through the side port incision to crush the chip as it is being held against the port by the vacuum. If a chip has been hiding in the angle or in the posterior chamber and is identified after the IOL has been implanted, the surgeon should not hesitate to reintroduce the phaco tip and remove it. It should be mentioned that if an opening in the posterior capsule is present, a chip may be trapped in the anterior chamber by injecting a retentive OVD behind it. If the chip does fall back into the vitreous, the surgeon should not be tempted to chase it into the posterior segment where more severe complications can occur. An honest and reassuring explanation to the patient followed by a referral to a vitreoretinal surgeon will likely result in an excellent outcome.

Posterior Capsule Tear

There is no question that an entire book could be devoted to the management of the torn posterior capsule. It is certainly the most frequent significant complication that cataract surgeons experience. The management of the tear depends on a number of factors including when it occurs, whether it extends to the periphery, and whether or not nucleus, cortex, or vitreous is present [71, 72]. This section will review several important principles.

When a tear occurs, it is essential not to remove the phaco or the I&A tip, essentially taking the "finger out of the dike." If this happens, the anterior chamber will immediately shallow and vitreous will prolapse forward toward the incision. The anterior hyaloid face will rupture and vitreous will be present in the anterior chamber, or worse, in the incision [71]. It is critical to leave the ultrasound or I&A tip plugging the incision while the other hand is able to inject OVD filling the chamber. This will prevent chamber collapse while also tamponading vitreous prolapse. Once the posterior capsule is concave and the chamber is deep, the instrument can be safely removed [71] (Video 37.5).

If lens fragments are present, it is possible to inject a retentive OVD behind them and convert to either a slow motion phaco or an extracapsular expression by enlarging the incision [49, 73]. If the tear occurs during the cortex removal, the surgeon can convert to a dry aspiration technique using a curved and a straight 27-gauge cannula on a 3-cc syringe filled with 1 cc of balanced salt solution [74]. It is important to engage only the most proximal anterior cortex in order to strip cortical fibers cleanly from the capsule (Video 37.6). To prevent chamber shallowing, OVD can be generously replaced. The surgeon should consider injecting a dispersive OVD like Viscoat into the tear for vitreous tamponade while using a cohesive OVD like Healon in the bag for easier cortical removal.

Converting a linear posterior capsular tear to a posterior capsulorhexis is another excellent technique [75]. The capsule should be stabilized within a sandwich of OVD, and then using an intracameral micro-forceps, the edge of the tear is grasped and guided to create a posterior capsulorhexis. This is more difficult than an anterior capsulorhexis because the posterior capsule is much thinner than the anterior capsule measuring only 3 or 4 microns. In the case of a posterior polar cataract, the capsule may be only 1 or even 0 microns thick! [41]

When a posterior capsular tear occurs, the key mission is to remove nucleus and cortex safely without losing lens material into the posterior segment. Some surgeons have advocated inserting the intraocular lens behind nuclear fragments to act as a scaffold, while a dispersive viscoelastic agent may also be effective [73]. Should nuclear fragments dislocate into the posterior segment, the surgeon should absolutely not attempt to retrieve them, but should meticulously clean up the anterior segment in preparation for a referral to a vitreoretinal surgeon.

The cataract surgeon must be able to manage vitreous in the anterior segment and the vitrectomy technique is quite important. Performing the vitrectomy through the incision with a separate infusion is a valid approach, although there is always a risk of pulling vitreous forward and enlarging the tear [76]. Visualizing vitreous can be facilitated using triamcinolone, a technique developed by Scott Burk MD, PhD when he was a Fellow with Dr. Osher [77]. A pars plana vitrectomy with anterior infusion facilitates complete vitreous removal from the anterior segment without enlarging the tear. It is essential that the surgeon does not exert traction on the vitreous so a high cutting speed is mandatory. In addition, the surgeon should stop aspiration prior to discontinuing the cutting as the vitrector is withdrawn. The anterior segment should be free of vitreous and cortical removal should then be completed.

The intraocular lens may be placed safely into the capsular bag, if either enough capsular support exists or a posterior capsulorhexis has been achieved. If a single-piece lens is being used, it can also be placed into the torn capsular bag, and the optic can be prolapsed forward in order to achieve reverse optic capture [78] (Video 37.7). Alternatively, a three-piece lens can be placed into the ciliary sulcus prolapsing the optic back through the capsulorhexis opening achieving traditional optic capture [79] (Video 37.8). It is also possible to fixate the IOL by sewing the lens to iris or sclera [80–82]. Recently, there has been interest in intrascleral haptic fixation utilizing an Agarwal glued IOL or a Yamane technique [83–85], or the flanged haptic technique of Canabrava [86]. Regardless of the IOL location, when the posterior capsule is open, patients are at a greater risk for postoperative pressure rise, inflammation, corneal edema, cystoid macular edema, and retinal tear/detachment [71, 87, 88]. There is also a greater risk for endophthalmitis so the appropriate anti-infective, anti-inflammatory, and IOP-lowering prophylactic medications should be administered at the end of the case and in the early postoperative period [71, 87–89].

Since there is always an adrenaline response when the posterior capsule tears which may prevent clear thinking, it is important to rehearse the appropriate steps for managing this complication ahead of time, both in the surgeon's mind and with the OR team. Knowledgeable and skilled management of the torn posterior capsule will usually reward the surgeon with an excellent visual outcome.

Dr. Buratto's comment: *There are a number of clinical signs indicating a posterior capsular rupture that the surgeon should recognize. The pupil snap sign is a sudden change in pupillary diameter. A sudden increase in the anterior chamber depth, an unexpected tumbling of the nucleus, and a lateral/posterior dislocation of the nucleus are ominous signs. Vitreous prolapse may displace the iris, interfere with normal emulsification/cortical aspiration, or cause a sudden and prominent red reflex.*

Dr. Barrett's comment: *Although pars plana vitrectomy has several advantages, a 25-gauge vitrectomy probe can be inserted through a 1-mm sideport incision together with irrigation* via *a 19-gauge or 20-gauge infusion cannula from a bimanual IA set so that the chamber is well sealed. The 25-gauge vitrectomy probe can even be directed with care through a tear to avoid dragging vitreous into the anterior chamber.*

Dropped Nucleus

Sooner or later, every ophthalmologist who operates will encounter one of the most dreaded complications guaranteed to weaken the knees of even the strongest and most experienced cataract surgeons. Situations that raise the risk of nucleus loss include the posterior polar cataract, the mature cataract, and the eye with previous trauma. The explanation for the posterior polar cataract is obvious since these capsules are fragile and occasionally open [41–45]. The explanation for the mature cataract is less obvious but important to understand. When the nucleus is hard and the lens is extremely thick, the surrounding capsule is taut. When the surgeon begins to hydrodissect, the fluid wave goes around the equator and behind the nuclear/cortical complex, lifting the complex forward against the anterior capsular opening. As the surgeon injects more fluid to achieve a thorough hydrodissection, there is absolutely no "give" in the capsule and no place for this fluid to escape. The result is that the posterior capsule blows out and the surgeon is unaware that this complication has occurred [90, 91]. Somewhere in the middle of the phacoemulsification, the nucleus begins to descend, and the surgeon's heart stops!

There was a time when surgeons attributed this posterior capsular tear to the sharp edges of the hard-nuclear fragments, but a Grand Prize-winning video produced by Dr. Osher and his son James in 1997 disproved this myth [92]. The mechanism by which the capsule ruptures is actually an intracapsular block caused by persistent hydrodissection [40]. The best prevention is a gentle posterior ballottement of the mature nucleus, which allows escape of the injected fluid from behind the nuclear/cortical complex back around and out of the bag. An alternate approach would be to simply avoid the initial hydrodissection, waiting until a deep groove in the nucleus has been sculpted. The hemispheres or quadrants are gently separated producing a deep crack. At this point, hydrodissection can be performed safely allowing fluid to escape back through the crack.

If the surgeon notices that the nucleus is beginning to descend, he can immediately alter the pressure dynamics by pulling the phaco tip out of the eye and quickly injecting OVD behind the nucleus. Dr. Charles Kelman described a technique for rescuing the nucleus utilizing a stab incision through the pars plana, elevating the nucleus with an instrument which he called posterior-assisted levitation [93] (Video 37.9). Once the nucleus is stable and perched upon a retentive OVD, which Dr. David Chang has called Visco Trap, the surgeon can elect to either continue phacoemulsification (which is challenging), open the incision to express the nucleus, or implant the IOL beneath the nucleus which acts as a protective scaffold as described by Dr. Amar Agarwal [73, 94].

There is one inviolate rule that must be obeyed. As mentioned in the last section on the torn posterior capsule, the anterior segment surgeon must resist the temptation to chase a nucleus back into the posterior segment. This is where surgical disasters can occur. It is best to proceed by cleaning up the cortex and any vitreous that has prolapsed into the anterior segment, and then either implanting an intraocular lens or leaving that task to the vitreoretinal surgeon. An honest and reassuring explanation to the patient and a prompt referral to the vitreoretinal surgeon can lead to an excellent outcome.

Dr. Barrett's comment: *If a tear in the posterior capsule occurs and the nucleus is subluxated posteriorly, conversion to manual extraction with a Vectus can be attempted. However, it may be preferable to continue phacoemulsification as long as vitreous is not present, remove as much lens material as feasible letting the nucleus dislocate posteriorly, and then perform an anterior vitrectomy and insert a lens with optic capture if possible. The eye remains closed with a small incision throughout the procedure, and a vitreoretinal surgeon can effectively deal with the dropped nucleus* via *the pars plana. Overall, the eye sustains less damage than that incurred with enlarging the incision, which may bleed, resulting in desperate attempts to retrieve a dropped nucleus with endothelial damage.*

Zonular Dialysis

Most problems with the zonules are either congenital or traumatic in origin. Yet indelicate surgery may also result in damage to the zonules. The surgeon may be expecting weak zonules if several signs are observed on the initial examination. The iris border of the dilated pupil will normally appear to come into contact with the anterior lens capsule, but if a significant space is observed, this is known as the gap sign signifying zonular weakness [95]. Another clinical sign is focal iridodonesis, where vitreous is bumping the back of the iris through an opening in the zonules [95]. Another subtle sign is displacement of the fetal nucleus. More obvious signs like phacodonesis or the visibility of the lens equator should also serve as a warning to the surgeon [95]. In the operating room, there may be excessive movement of the anterior capsule during the capsulorhexis or the capsule may misbehave as a result of poor countertraction. Decentration or wobbling of the lens may be noticed during the phacoemulsification or cortical stripping. The unexpected appearance of the lens equator or vitreous prolapse may also surprise the surgeon.

Iatrogenic zonular damage [96] may be caused by excessive movement of the lens during the emulsification or inadvertent traction placed on the capsular bag during cortical removal. A mild to moderate zonular weakness can be managed by injecting a dispersive OVD into the dialysis which will tamponade vitreous and prevent prolapse. Then the capsular bag may be widely expanded with a cohesive OVD to allow the atraumatic injection or insertion of a capsular tension ring or segment [97]. The management of a severe zonular dialysis is beyond the scope of this chapter and has been covered elsewhere in this book. The surgeon, however, should be familiar with the use of capsular retractors which will stabilize the bag for nuclear and cortical removal. It has been stated that the IOL should be oriented perpendicular to the dialysis, but with a capsular tension ring in place, the orientation probably does not matter.

On the other hand, the management of vitreous prolapse is very important and may be necessary at any time, even near the end of the procedure if a strand suddenly presents between loose zonules in a patient with previous trauma, pseudo-exfoliation, high myopia, or a congenital zonulopathy. The surgeon may elect to perform the vitrectomy by an anterior approach with separate infusion, either placing the vitreous cutter into the zonular dialysis or carefully severing vitreous strands (Video 37.10). Alternatively, a pars plana vitrectomy may be performed by aspirating and cutting vitreous behind the anterior segment. Triamcinolone may facilitate visualization of the vitreous. The surgeon should always prevent chamber shallowing by injecting OVD, balanced salt solution, or air before withdrawing instruments. This sequence will avoid chamber shallowing and additional vitreous prolapse.

There are many devices for managing severe zonulopathies and the surgeon should be familiar with the insertion of a CTR or segment [98–100]. He should also be comfortable performing alternate IOL fixation techniques which may be necessary if the capsular bag has lost zonular support. While careful surgical technique will avoid an iatrogenic zonulysis, one never knows when zonular damage from a preexisting condition will surprise the surgeon and require a device or a modified technique. It is a good idea to always expect the unexpected.

Dr. Barrett's comment: *One scenario that is not uncommon is where the nucleus fails to rotate easily despite what appears to have been an adequate hydrodissection. This may be seen with a vertical chop technique, particularly with a large nucleus in an elderly patient. Rather than vigorously trying to rotate the nucleus, it is preferable to direct the phaco tip obliquely after the first crack is successful and perform another crack. Removal of this segment typically reduces nuclear volume, which can then be rotated with less tension on the zonules.*

Anterior Chamber Shallowing and Positive Pressure

The laws of physics suggest that there should always be an equilibrium between infusion, aspiration rate, and vacuum. If the infusion is not enough to maintain the chamber depth, the result will be shallowing of the anterior chamber. Either increasing the infusion or decreasing the aspiration rate and/or vacuum level will balance the equation [101]. The anterior chamber will also shallow if there is excessive fluid leakage from a poorly constructed incision, which must either be corrected or closed and moved.

The anterior chamber may also shallow as part of the syndrome of positive pressure, which increases the risk of complications. When the posterior capsule becomes convex, it is vulnerable to rupture if it comes into contact with the ultrasound needle. Cortex becomes very difficult to remove when the entrance to the capsular bag is narrowed or closed. To manage the shallow chamber caused by positive pressure, the surgeon may need to inject a retentive OVD and enter with the ultrasound tip "dry" without infusion [102]. Once the emulsification is underway, a second dull instrument may be used to hold the posterior capsule back, while the nuclear removal takes place directly above this restraining instrument. It may also be necessary to remove cortex in a "dry" OVD-filled chamber using a straight and a curved 27-gage cannula on a 3-cc syringe filled with 1 cc of balanced salt solution. Alternatively, a bimanual system working through two stab incisions within a "closed" chamber may be helpful.

When severe chamber shallowing is present, lens implantation may need to be aborted or require surgical gymnastics, whereby the lens is placed into the OVD-filled anterior chamber followed by manipulation of the haptics into the capsular bag. If extreme positive pressure threatens IOL contact with the corneal endothelium, the injection of an air bubble may prove to be an urgent rescue technique. Once the incision has been hydrated or sealed until watertight, the air bubble can be removed in small aliquots through the stab incision, exchanging it for either acetylcholine or balanced salt solution. A special cannula (Bausch + Lomb) for removing air, which curves upward toward the dome of the cornea without distorting the stab incision, has been designed by Dr. Osher (Video 37.11).

The surgeon should have a differential diagnosis of positive pressure in his mind. Extrinsic factors like tight lids, severe adipose tissue prolapse, or a speculum compressing the globe can act like two thumbs indenting a balloon. A similar behavior might occur with scleral collapse in a very young patient or with scleromalacia, extreme myopia, or when associated with a collagen vascular disease. Scleral thickening associated with nanophthalmos may also cause positive pressure [103].

Intrinsic factors can also cause progressive chamber shallowing, for example, when hydration of the vitreous space occurs as balanced salt solution enters through a posterior capsule tear or a zonular dialysis [104]. The choroidal volume may be increased by any Valsalva mechanism such as coughing or straining. The most serious expansion of the choroidal space would be a progressive hemorrhage, a true emergency requiring prompt closure of the incision, digital pressure over the incision, and possibly a cut-down into the suprachoroidal space to allow blood to escape [105, 106]. The surgery is terminated, hypotensive medications are initiated, and the patient can return safely to the operating room at a later date.

Anterior chamber shallowing with or without positive pressure is a situation that every cataract surgeon should be prepared to manage knowledgably and effectively.

Dr. Buratto's comment: *Flow leaving the eye is also dependent on other factors not directly under control of the equipment, such as the relationship between the sleeve diameter and the corneal incision size. In various steps of lens emulsification and aspiration, occlusion of the tip by lens material leads to blockage of fluid aspiration with increased vacuum levels in the tubing, which is associated with a subtle but critical contraction of the tubing. When the occlusion clears, the tubing rapidly expands back to its original diameter. Fluid is momentarily aspirated which leads to surge. A sudden shallowing of the anterior chamber is accompanied by a forward movement of the posterior capsule causing contact with the phaco tip, which can tear the capsule. Newer phaco machines may minimize surge, but the surgeon must always be aware of fluctuations in chamber depth.*

The Excessively Deep Chamber

The technique of phacoemulsification is safest when the ultrasound tip is engaging nucleus in a direction away from the posterior capsule. Yet when the chamber is extremely deep, the ultrasound tip is angled posteriorly which elevates the risk of posterior capsule tear. The surgeon may reduce the infusion pressure or increase the aspiration rate which may help reduce the chamber depth. However, in highly myopic eyes and in those which have undergone previous vitrectomy, there is a specific condition called lens-iris diaphragm retropulsion syndrome (LIDRS) which is very important to understand [107–109]. The infusion stream expands the anterior segment and displaces the iris posteriorly so that the peripupillary iris comes in contact with the anterior capsule. Also known as "reverse pupillary block," this barrier prevents fluid from reaching the circular compartment that extends 360 degrees behind the iris. The constant infusion pressure has limited access to a reduced space driving the posterior capsule back to the occipital lobes! Not only is the phaco tip pointed toward the posterior capsule, but also the port on the I&A tip is unable to come in contact with the posterior capsule which prevents vacuuming. Moreover, extreme dilation of the pupil occurs, the eye may appear aniridic, and sphincter ruptures have even been reported [110].

Fortunately, if the surgeon recognizes this condition, it is very easy to reverse [109]. By simply elevating the iris or depressing the anterior capsule, a rush of fluid will fill the retro-irideal space, and the chamber immediately shallows as the pupil returns to a more physiologic dilatation. While some surgeons prefer to lift the iris, this can cause some pigment dispersion and transillumination defects, so it may be a better technique to simply depress the anterior capsule allowing fluid to rush into the accessible space behind the iris (Video 37.12). By utilizing this maneuver, the surgery can proceed with less risk of a capsular rupture.

Fired Cannula

Anytime the surgeon is injecting fluid or OVD into the eye, there is the potential for turning the cannula into a flying missile with the consequence of severe damage to any intraocular structure. The literature provides examples of penetrating injuries to the cornea, iris, ciliary body, capsule, and even to the retina [32, 111–113]. The surgeon should take the following measures to minimize this complication. First, he should instruct his team to always secure the cannula and test it, even if it is a lure-lock, prior to actual use. Second, the surgeon should always pinch the hub of the cannula between his fingers as the plunger is being depressed. By assuming that every cannula can forcefully detach, this technique will allow the surgeon to "catch" a cannula before it can cause damage. Third, the surgeon should aim the cannula tip toward the lateral wall of the incision when hydrating at the end of the procedure. It is far better for the cannula to strike the wall of the incision rather than enter the eye. Being aware of this complication and utilizing these preventive measures, the anterior segment surgeon can avoid a serious cannula injury.

Acute Corneal Clouding

There is always the potential for a rare complication to occur which is why the experienced surgeon will stay focused and attentive for every second of the procedure, even after the IOL has been implanted. For example, if acetylcholine (Miochol) is being injected to constrict the pupil at the end of the operation, the cornea may suddenly cloud. The likely cause is inadequate mixture of the diluent and the lyophilized powder leaving the injected fluid hypotonic. The surgeon should immediately place the I&A handpiece into the anterior chamber and irrigate until the cornea clears. Again, proper education for the nursing team will prevent this type of complication from occurring.

Hemorrhage

Hemorrhage can occur from several different locations during cataract surgery. The most common place for bleeding to occur is from the incision. Patients who have a long history of contact lens wear with corneal neovascularization, a previous corneal disease, or those who are on anticoagulation drugs are at greater risk. The incision can be moved more anteriorly, although many surgeons prefer a near-clear rather than a pure corneal location. Persistent bleeding which either causes blood to reenter the eye, interferes with visualization, or persists during the entirety of the case must be addressed. Simply holding a Weck cell sponge against the hemorrhaging vessel with some pressure may expedite coagulation. However, if unsuccessful, the surgeon should have access to a fine-tipped wet field cautery, which will not cause contraction of collagen, since any thermal damage can result in an incompetent incision.

Bleeding may also occur from the iris or from the angle due to either trauma or hypotony. Raising the pressure in the eye with balanced salt solution or OVD should stop the hemorrhage, but gravity may allow blood to accumulate in the capsular bag. It should be emphasized that blood should not be left behind the IOL within the capsular bag because a clot may form and compromise vision following surgery. Rarely, we have had to reoperate and inject TPA into the capsular bag to hemolyze the clot. This could have been avoided by simply reintroducing the I&A handpiece, decentering the IOL, and removing the blood during the initial surgery. Bleeding from the ciliary body was occasionally seen when a three-piece IOL with stiff haptics was placed into the ciliary sulcus. With the introduction of single-piece lenses implanted into the capsular bag, this source of bleeding has disappeared. Similarly, when large incision extracapsular surgery was the standard of care, prolonged hypotony would increase the risk of a choroidal hemorrhage. Sudden pain with acute positive pressure, iris prolapse, and chamber shallowing signaled this catastrophic event. Fortunately, smaller incisions which maintain some intraocular pressure have made a choroidal hemorrhage a rare event. Still, the surgeon should understand that he must immediately close the eye, apply pressure to tamponade the hemorrhage [114], suture or seal the incision, confirm the location and size using ophthalmoscopy, abort the procedure, and monitor/treat the IOP. Placing an incision into the suprachoroidal space for drainage is a more controversial maneuver. However, should disaster strike, it is always recommended that the operating surgeon solicit prompt assistance from a subspecialist with expertise in glaucoma and/or vitreoretinal surgery. Once the risk of an expulsive hemorrhage has been eliminated, the surgeon will likely be able to return to the operating room at a later time to safely complete the procedure.

Patient Movement

Performing cataract surgery under the high magnification of a microscope is incompatible with either a moving eye or a moving patient. Proper anesthesia will deal the former, while the latter can be managed depending upon whether the patient movements are expected or unexpected. Certain neurologic conditions like Parkinson's disease are associated with head movements which can be dampened by wrapping cloth tape around the patient's forehead and head of the bed. Unexpected movements like restless legs syndrome or a sudden head jerk due to oversedation can catch the surgeon by surprise. It is essential to emphasize to the person administering the anesthesia that the patient should be kept "light" and under no circumstances allowed to fall asleep. The surgeon should also explain to the patient that a small movement under the microscope is equivalent to an earthquake for the surgeon. It is a good practice to explain that a question should be answered with a verbal "yes or no" rather than a head nod. If the patient expresses concern about claustrophobia, the drape should be lifted off the patient's face, and the touch of a nurse's hand in combination with reassurance from the surgeon may avert a panic attack. Coughing can be addressed by quickly giving the patient a cough drop. The surgeon should make it a top priority to communicate with and often reassure the patient throughout the procedure.

IOL Problems

Entire chapters have been written on this topic, which encompasses either the management of intraoperative or late complications. Situations that the surgeon might encounter during surgery include an injection malfunction, misbehavior of a haptic, damage to an optic, or lens malposition. A haptic that is stuck in the cartridge can sometimes be freed by slicing the tip of the cartridge with a knife. The haptic, which is stuck to the optic, can be squeezed at the end with a forceps freeing the haptic. If a haptic has been disinserted on a three-piece lens, the surgeon may actually harvest a haptic from another lens and insert it into the optic. By contrast, a disinserted haptic on a single piece lens can either be substituted by a suture or explanted. A damaged optic requires judgment by the surgeon since a peripheral gash or impurity may be visually insignificant. On the other hand, a scratch or a gash in a central optic requires exchange. Suboptimal placement, for example, one haptic in the capsular bag and the other in the ciliary sulcus, should be corrected in order to avoid late decentration. The same holds true if a single-piece lens is inserted into the ciliary sulcus. If a lens is inserted backwards, the surgeon may not need to perform intraocular gymnastics if the IOL is uniplanar and the power is approximately the same. However, toric, presbyopia-correcting, and intraocular lenses with angled haptics should be "summersaulted" using two hooks and a chamber full of OVD. If the IOL finds its way through a posterior capsular tear or a zonular dialysis, it must be recovered in combination with anterior vitrectomy and refixated by either optic capture or a lasso suture sewn to the sclera or iris, or explanted and exchanged. A posterior luxation with loss of the lens requires prompt referral to a vitreoretinal surgeon.

There are a multitude of reasons why an IOL should be exchanged days, weeks, months, or even years after the original surgery. The most common cause is a refractive surprise, which the surgeon deems unacceptable. It is quite easy to reopen the capsular bag and exchange the lens through a small incision with OVD protection of the cornea and the capsule. A variety of explantation techniques are available; Dr. Paul Ernest introduced the intraocular lens refolding technique [115] (Video 37.13); Dr. Shuichlo Eguchi introduced the "Pac-man" technique [116] (Video 37.14); Dr. Jack Dodick developed the partial transection [117, 118]; Dr. Amar Agarwal used a second intraocular lens as a scaffold [119]; and Dr. Michael Snyder and I developed a set of instruments for fixating the lens through the stab incision (Geuder, CrestPoint Instruments) and then trisecting the lens with a micro scissors through the main incision [120] (Video 37.15). There are certainly other techniques that allow for a small incision explantation and lens exchange. Alternatively, one could perform laser vision correction. If the capsular bag has fibrosed or the posterior capsule is open, there may be enough room in the ciliary sulcus to consider implantation of a secondary piggyback lens [121].

Late IOL repositioning or exchange may be required when the lens is decentered or subluxed. A number of techniques including reopening the capsular bag, passing a lasso suture, sulcus fixation, suturing the lens to the iris [80] or sclera [82], or more recently intrascleral haptic fixation [85] have all been used to manage malpositioned intraocular lenses. Other late complications including persistent UGH syndrome from lens-iris contact, chronic inflammation from *P. acnes*, intolerable dysphotopsia [122], damage from the YAG laser [123–125], or opacification/calcification of the lens are rare but require aggressive management. Lens exchange may be reserved for those patients who fail more conservative management, for example, an intensive anti-inflammatory regime which causes confluent KP on the optic to vanish.

Most surgeons do not have a great deal of experience managing these complications, and it is often prudent to refer the patient to a surgeon with more experience with these unusual cases.

Conclusion

Every cataract surgeon who operates, regardless of his or her skill and experience, will infrequently encounter complications. What differentiates the good from the excellent surgeon is the way these complications are recognized and managed. The well-prepared surgeon has rehearsed in advance the maneuvers necessary to achieve a successful outcome.

In closing, please allow a few final words of advice. Always be honest with the patient. If a complication occurs, patiently explain the situation with eye-to-eye contact and reassurance. Try to avoid placing blame on the machine, on the nurse, or on the patient himself. Whenever possible, develop a corrective plan, which can be explained to the patient, and then either execute it or refer the patient in a timely manner. By combining preparation, skill, honesty, and empathy, both the patient and the surgeon will likely live happily ever after.

Take-Home Note

- The only way to completely avoid complications is to stop operating!
- Complications are best managed by early recognition, understanding the corrective options, and skillful execution of the rescue technique by a well-prepared surgeon.

References

1. Osher RH. Video Journal of Cataract, Refractive, & Glaucoma Surgery. https://vjcrgs.com/.
2. Patel BCK, Burns TA, Crandall A, et al. A comparison of topical and retrobulbar anesthesia for cataract surgery. Ophthalmology. Published online 1996. https://doi.org/10.1016/S0161-6420(96)30522-8.
3. Jacobi PC, Dietlein TS, Jacobi FK. Comparative study of topical vs retrobulbar anesthesia in complicated cataract surgery. Arch Ophthalmol. Published online 2000. https://doi.org/10.1001/archopht.118.8.1037.
4. Seo H, Nam DH, Lee JY, et al. Macular photostress and visual experience between microscope and intracameral illumination during cataract surgery. J Cataract Refract Surg. Published online 2018. https://doi.org/10.1016/j.jcrs.2017.11.016.
5. Weiss JL, Deichman CB. A Comparison of retrobulbar and periocular anesthesia for cataract surgery. Arch Ophthalmol. Published online 1989. https://doi.org/10.1001/archopht.1989.01070010098035.
6. Avakian A, Osher RH. Rescue technique for salvaging toric intraocular lens alignment. J Cataract Refract Surg. Published online 2012. https://doi.org/10.1016/j.jcrs.2012.08.019.
7. Cionni RJ, Osher RH. Retrobulbar hemorrhage. Ophthalmology. Published online 1991. https://doi.org/10.1016/S0161-6420(91)32158-4.
8. Winterton J V., Patel K, Mizen KD. Review of management options for a retrobulbar hemorrhage. J Oral Maxillofac Surg. Published online 2007. https://doi.org/10.1016/j.joms.2005.11.089.
9. Pandey SK, Werner L, Apple DJ, Agarwal A, Agarwal A, Agarwal S. No-anesthesia clear corneal phacoemulsification versus topical and topical plus intracameral anesthesia: Randomized clinical trial. J Cataract Refract Surg. Published online 2001. https://doi.org/10.1016/S0886-3350(01)00793-3.
10. Osher RH. Shark fin: A new sign of thermal injury. J Cataract Refract Surg. Published online 2005. https://doi.org/10.1016/j.jcrs.2004.11.034.
11. Fine IH. Architecture and construction of a self-sealing incision for cataract surgery. J Cataract Refract Surg. Published online 1991. https://doi.org/10.1016/S0886-3350(13)80682-7.
12. Fine IH, Hoffman RS, Packer M. Profile of clear corneal cataract incisions demonstrated by ocular coherence tomography. J Cataract Refract Surg. Published online 2007. https://doi.org/10.1016/j.jcrs.2006.09.016.
13. Langerman DW. Architectural design of a self-sealing corneal tunnel, single-hinge incision. J Cataract Refract Surg. Published online 1994. https://doi.org/10.1016/S0886-3350(13)80052-1.
14. Osher RH. Internal flare: Modification of wound construction for microincisional cataract surgery.

J Cataract Refract Surg. Published online 2012. https://doi.org/10.1016/j.jcrs.2012.01.011.
15. Hovanesian JA, Karageozian VH. Watertight cataract incision closure using fibrin tissue adhesive. J Cataract Refract Surg. Published online 2007. https://doi.org/10.1016/j.jcrs.2007.03.060.
16. Masket S, Hovanesian JA, Levenson J, et al. Hydrogel sealant versus sutures to prevent fluid egress after cataract surgery. J Cataract Refract Surg. Published online 2014. https://doi.org/10.1016/j.jcrs.2014.03.034.
17. Zaczek A, Zetterström C. Cataract surgery and pupil size in patients with diabetes mellitus. Acta Ophthalmol Scand. Published online 1997. https://doi.org/10.1111/j.1600-0420.1997.tb00407.x.
18. Hayashi K, Hayashi H. Pupil size before and after phacoemulsification in nondiabetic and diabetic patients. J Cataract Refract Surg. Published online 2004. https://doi.org/10.1016/j.jcrs.2004.04.045.
19. Akman A, Yilmaz G, Oto S, Akova YA. Comparison of various pupil dilatation methods for phacoemulsification in eyes with a small pupil secondary to pseudoexfoliation. Ophthalmology. Published online 2004. https://doi.org/10.1016/j.ophtha.2004.02.008.
20. Winn B, Whitaker D, Elliott DB, Phillips NJ. Factors affecting light-adapted pupil size in normal human subjects. Investig Ophthalmol Vis Sci. Published online 1994.
21. Chang DF, Campbell JR. Intraoperative floppy iris syndrome associated with tamsulosin. J Cataract Refract Surg. Published online 2005. https://doi.org/10.1016/j.jcrs.2005.02.027.
22. Abdel-Latif AA. Release and effects of prostaglandins in ocular tissues. Prostaglandins. Leukot Essent Fat Acids. Published online 1991. https://doi.org/10.1016/0952-3278(91)90186-9.
23. Jhanji V, Sharma N, Vajpayee RB. Management of intraoperative miosis during pediatric cataract surgery using healon 5. Middle East Afr J Ophthalmol. Published online 2011. https://doi.org/10.4103/0974-9233.75888.
24. Osher RH. Healon 5 in IFIS. Video J Cataract Refract Surg. 2005;21(2). https://www.aao.org/clinical-video/achieving-viscomydriasis-with-healon5.
25. Osher RH, Ahmed IIK, Demopulos GA. OMS302 (phenylephrine and ketorolac injection) 1%/0.3% to maintain intraoperative pupil size and to prevent postoperative ocular pain in cataract surgery with intraocular lens replacement. Expert Rev Ophthalmol. Published online 2015. https://doi.org/10.1586/17469899.2015.1026806.
26. Donnenfeld ED, Whitaker JS, Jackson MA, Wittpenn J. Intracameral ketorolac and phenylephrine effect on intraoperative pupil diameter and postoperative pain in cataract surgery. J Cataract Refract Surg. 2017. https://doi.org/10.1016/j.jcrs.2017.02.030.
27. Gurbaxani A, Packard R. Intracameral phenylephrine to prevent floppy iris syndrome during cataract surgery in patients on tamsulosin. Eye. Published online 2007. https://doi.org/10.1038/sj.eye.6702172.
28. Malyugin B. Small pupil phaco surgery: a new technique. Ann Ophthalmol. Published online 2007. https://doi.org/10.1007/s12009-007-0023-8.
29. Chang DF. Use of Malyugin pupil expansion device for intraoperative floppy-iris syndrome: Results in 30 consecutive cases. J Cataract Refract Surg. Published online 2008. https://doi.org/10.1016/j.jcrs.2008.01.026.
30. Malyugin B. The Malyugin ring in FLACS. The Ophthalmologist. Published 2015. Accessed 10 Aug, 2020. https://theophthalmologist.com/subspecialties/the-malyugin-ring-in-flacs.
31. Hoover DL, Giangiacomo J, Benson RL. Descemet's membrane detachment by sodium hyaluronate. Arch Ophthalmol. Published online 1985. https://doi.org/10.1001/archopht.1985.01050060065027.
32. Osher RH. Iris damage by inadvertent cannula injection. J Cataract Refract Surg. Published online 2007. https://doi.org/10.1016/j.jcrs.2006.08.063.
33. Andres Benatti C, Tsao JZ, Afshari NA. Descemet membrane detachment during cataract surgery: etiology and management. Curr Opin Ophthalmol. Published online 2017. https://doi.org/10.1097/ICU.0000000000000332.
34. Samarawickrama C, Beltz J, Chan E. Spontaneously resolving descemet's membrane detachment caused by an ophthalmic viscosurgical device during cataract surgery. Saudi J Ophthalmol. Published online 2015. https://doi.org/10.1016/j.sjopt.2015.07.003.
35. Osher RH, Cionni RJ, Burk SE, Chang DF. Cataract Surgery. In: Cataract Surgery. 3rd ed. Elsevier; 2010.
36. Marcon AS, Rapuano CJ, Jones MR, Laibson PR, Cohen EJ. Descemet's membrane detachment after cataract surgery: management and outcome. Ophthalmology. Published online 2002. https://doi.org/10.1016/S0161-6420(02)01288-5.
37. Assia EI, Levkovich-Verbin H, Blumenthal M. Management of Descemet's membrane detachment. J Cataract Refract Surg. Published online 1995. https://doi.org/10.1016/S0886-3350(13)80573-1.
38. Mackool RJ, Nicolich S, Mackool R. Effect of viscodissection on posterior capsule rupture during phacoemulsification. J Cataract Refract Surg. Published online 2007. https://doi.org/10.1016/j.jcrs.2006.08.066.
39. Vasavada V, Vasavada VA, Werner L, Mamalis N, Vasavada AR, Crandall AS. Corticocapsular cleavage during phacoemulsification: Viscodissection versus hydrodissection Miyake-Apple view analysis. J Cataract Refract Surg. Published online 2008. https://doi.org/10.1016/j.jcrs.2008.03.026.
40. Miyake K, Ota I, Ichihashi S, Miyake S, Tanaka Y, Terasaki H. New classification of capsular block syndrome. J Cataract Refract Surg. Published online 1998. https://doi.org/10.1016/S0886-3350(98)80017-5.

41. Osher RH, Yu BCY, Koch DD. Posterior polar cataracts: A predisposition to intraoperative posterior capsular rupture. J Cataract Refract Surg. Published online 1990. https://doi.org/10.1016/S0886-3350(13)80724-9.
42. Siatiri H, Moghimi S. Posterior polar cataract: Minimizing risk of posterior capsule rupture. Eye. Published online 2006. https://doi.org/10.1038/sj.eye.6702023.
43. Allen D, Wooda C. Minimizing risk to the capsule during surgery for posterior polar cataract. J Cataract Refract Surg. Published online 2002. https://doi.org/10.1016/S0886-3350(02)01244-0.
44. Fine IH, Packer M, Hoffman RS. Management of posterior polar cataract. J Cataract Refract Surg. Published online 2003. https://doi.org/10.1016/S0886-3350(02)01616-4.
45. Vasavada AR, Raj SM, Vasavada V, Shrivastav S. Surgical approaches to posterior polar cataract: a review. Eye. Published online 2012. https://doi.org/10.1038/eye.2012.33.
46. Marques FF, Marques DMV, Osher RH, Osher JM. Fate of anterior capsule tears during cataract surgery. J Cataract Refract Surg. Published online 2006. https://doi.org/10.1016/j.jcrs.2006.05.013.
47. Schneider S, Osher RH, Burk SE, Lutz TB, Montione R. Thinning of the anterior capsule associated with congenital aniridia. J Cataract Refract Surg. Published online 2003. https://doi.org/10.1016/S0886-3350(02)01602-4.
48. Little BC, Smith JH, Packer M. Little capsulorhexis tear-out rescue. J Cataract Refract Surg. Published online 2006. https://doi.org/10.1016/j.jcrs.2006.03.038.
49. Osher RH. Slow Motion Phacoemulsification Approach. J Cataract Refract Surg. Published online 1993. https://doi.org/10.1016/S0886-3350(13)80025-9.
50. Melles GRJ, De Waard PWT, Pameyer JH, Beekhuis WH, Van Vroonhoven CCJ. Trypan blue capsule staining to visualize the capsulorhexis in cataract surgery. J Cataract Refract Surg. Published online 1999. https://doi.org/10.1016/S0886-3350(99)80004-2.
51. Figueiredo CG, Figueiredo J, Figueiredo GB. Brazilian technique for prevention of the Argentinean flag sign in white cataract. J Cataract Refract Surg. Published online 2012. https://doi.org/10.1016/j.jcrs.2012.07.002.
52. Allan BDS. Mechanism of iris prolapse: A qualitative analysis and implications for surgical technique. J Cataract Refract Surg. Published online 1995. https://doi.org/10.1016/S0886-3350(13)80507-X.
53. Tint NL, Dhillon AS, Alexander P. Management of intraoperative iris prolapse: Stepwise practical approach. J Cataract Refract Surg. Published online 2012. https://doi.org/10.1016/j.jcrs.2012.08.013.
54. Osher RH. Association between IFIS and Flomax. J Cataract Refract Surg. Published online 2006. https://doi.org/10.1016/j.jcrs.2006.01.008.
55. Shugar JK. Use of epinephrine for IFIS prophylaxis. J Cataract Refract Surg. Published online 2006. https://doi.org/10.1016/j.jcrs.2006.01.110.
56. Masket S, Belani S. Combined preoperative topical atropine sulfate 1% and intracameral nonpreserved epinephrine hydrochloride 1:2500 for management of intraoperative floppy-iris syndrome. J Cataract Refract Surg. Published online 2007. https://doi.org/10.1016/j.jcrs.2006.10.059.
57. Shugar JK. Prophylaxis for IFIS. J Cataract Refract Surg. Published online 2007. https://doi.org/10.1016/j.jcrs.2007.02.011.
58. Sippel KC, Pineda R. Phacoemulsification and thermal wound injury. Semin Ophthalmol. Published online 2002. https://doi.org/10.1076/soph.17.3.102.14776.
59. Ernest P, Rhem M, McDermott M, Lavery K, Sensoli A. Phacoemulsification conditions resulting in thermal wound injury. J Cataract Refract Surg. Published online 2001. https://doi.org/10.1016/S0886-3350(01)00908-7.
60. Osher RH, Injev VP. Thermal study of bare tips with various system parameters and incision sizes. J Cataract Refract Surg. Published online 2006. https://doi.org/10.1016/j.jcrs.2005.06.054.
61. Sugar A, Schertzer RM. Clinical course of phacoemulsification wound burns. J Cataract Refract Surg. Published online 1999. https://doi.org/10.1016/S0886-3350(99)00021-8.
62. Scleral and corneal burns during phacoemulsification with viscoelastic materials. Health Devices. Published online 1988.
63. Haldar K, Saraff R. Closure technique for leaking wound resulting from thermal injury during phacoemulsification. J Cataract Refract Surg. Published online 2014. https://doi.org/10.1016/j.jcrs.2014.07.016.
64. Osher, Robert H., Osher JM. Wound gape: two closure techniques. Cataract Refract Surg Today. Published online June 2011:73–4. https://crstoday.com/wp-content/themes/crst/assets/downloads/crst0611_feature_osher.pdf.
65. Khodabakhsh AJ, Zaidman G, Tabin G. Corneal surgery for severe phacoemulsification burns. Ophthalmology. Published online 2004. https://doi.org/10.1016/j.ophtha.2003.06.004.
66. Bohigian GM, Wexler SA. Complications of retained nuclear fragments in the anterior chamber after phacoemulsification with posterior chamber lens implant. Am J Ophthalmol. Published online 1997. https://doi.org/10.1016/S0002-9394(14)70181-3.
67. Hui JI, Fishler J, Karp CL, Shuler MF, Gedde SJ. Retained Nuclear Fragments in the Anterior Chamber after Phacoemulsification with an Intact Posterior Capsule. Ophthalmology. Published online 2006. https://doi.org/10.1016/j.ophtha.2006.03.066.
68. Zavodni ZJ, Meyer JJ, Kim T. Clinical Features and Outcomes of Retained Lens Fragments in the Anterior Chamber after Phacoemulsification. Am

J Ophthalmol. Published online 2015. https://doi.org/10.1016/j.ajo.2015.08.019.
69. Mokhtarzadeh A, Kaufman SC, Koozekanani DD, Meduri A. Delayed presentation of retained nuclear fragment following phacoemulsification cataract extraction. J Cataract Refract Surg. Published online 2014. https://doi.org/10.1016/j.jcrs.2014.02.013.
70. Oliveira C, Liebmann JM, Dodick JM, Topilow H, Cykiert R, Ritch R. Identification of retained nucleus fragment in the posterior chamber using ultrasound biomicroscopy. Am J Ophthalmol. Published online 2006. https://doi.org/10.1016/j.ajo.2005.12.013.
71. Osher RH, Cionni RJ. The torn posterior capsule: Its intraoperative behavior, surgical management, and long-term consequences. J Cataract Refract Surg. Published online 1990. https://doi.org/10.1016/S0886-3350(13)80805-X.
72. Gimbel H V., Sun R, Ferensowicz M, Anderson Penno E, Kamal A. Intraoperative management of posterior capsule tears in phacoemulsification and intraocular lens implantation. Ophthalmology. Published online 2001. https://doi.org/10.1016/S0161-6420(01)00716-3.
73. Chang DF, Packard RB. Posterior assisted levitation for nucleus retrieval using Viscoat after posterior capsule rupture. J Cataract Refract Surg. Published online 2003. https://doi.org/10.1016/S0886-3350(03)00216-5.
74. Akura J, Hatta S, Kaneda S, Ishihara M, Matsuura K, Tamai A. Management of posterior capsule rupture during phacoemulsification using the dry technique. J Cataract Refract Surg. Published online 2001. https://doi.org/10.1016/S0886-3350(00)00838-5.
75. Castaneda VE, Legler UFC, Tsai JC, et al. Posterior Continuous Curvilinear Capsulorhexis: An Experimental Study with Clinical Applications. Ophthalmology. Published online 1992. https://doi.org/10.1016/S0161-6420(92)32014-7.
76. Eller AW, Barad RF. Miyake analysis of anterior vitrectomy techniques. J Cataract Refract Surg. Published online 1996. https://doi.org/10.1016/S0886-3350(96)80221-5.
77. Burk SE, Da Mata AP, Snyder ME, Schneider S, Osher RH, Cionni RJ. Visualizing vitreous using Kenalog suspension. J Cataract Refract Surg. Published online 2003. https://doi.org/10.1016/S0886-3350(03)00016-6.
78. Jones JJ, Oetting TA, Rogers GM, Jin GJC. Reverse optic capture of the single-piece acrylic intraocular lens in eyes with posterior capsule rupture. Ophthalmic Surg Lasers Imaging. Published online 2012. https://doi.org/10.3928/15428877-20120830-02.
79. Gimbel H V., DeBroff BM. Intraocular lens optic capture. J Cataract Refract Surg. Published online 2004. https://doi.org/10.1016/j.jcrs.2003.11.035
80. Menezo JL, Martinez MC, Cisneros AL. Iris-fixated Worst claw versus sulcus-fixated posterior chamber lenses in the absence of capsular support. J Cataract Refract Surg. Published online 1996. https://doi.org/10.1016/S0886-3350(96)80151-9.
81. Güell JL, Barrera A, Manero F. A review of suturing techniques for posterior chamber lenses. Curr Opin Ophthalmol. Published online 2004. https://doi.org/10.1097/00055735-200402000-00009.
82. Michaeli A, Assia EI. Scleral and iris fixation of posterior chamber lenses in the absence of capsular support. Curr Opin Ophthalmol. Published online 2005. https://doi.org/10.1097/00055735-200502000-00010.
83. Kumar DA, Agarwal A. Glued intraocular lens: A major review on surgical technique and results. Curr Opin Ophthalmol. Published online 2013. https://doi.org/10.1097/ICU.0b013e32835a939f.
84. Kumar DA, Agarwal A, Agarwal A, Prakash G, Jacob S. Glued intraocular lens implantation for eyes with defective capsules: A retrospective analysis of anatomical and functional outcome. Saudi J Ophthalmol. Published online 2011. https://doi.org/10.1016/j.sjopt.2011.04.001.
85. Yamane S, Sato S, Maruyama-Inoue M, Kadonosono K. Flanged Intrascleral intraocular lens fixation with double-needle technique. Ophthalmology. 2017. https://doi.org/10.1016/j.ophtha.2017.03.036.
86. Canabrava S, Canedo Domingos Lima AC, Arancibia AEL, Bicalho Dornelas LF, Ribeiro G. Novel double-flanged technique for managing Marfan syndrome and microspherophakia. J Cataract Refract Surg. Published online 2020. https://doi.org/10.1097/j.jcrs.0000000000000116.
87. Hong AR, Sheybani A, Huang AJW. Intraoperative management of posterior capsular rupture. Curr Opin Ophthalmol. Published online 2015. https://doi.org/10.1097/ICU.0000000000000113.
88. Wu MC, Bhandari A. Managing the broken capsule. Curr Opin Ophthalmol. Published online 2008. https://doi.org/10.1097/ICU.0b013e3282f2a9d5.
89. Nakaguma S, Matsumoto K, Hirata A, Inada K, Negi A. Bacterial endophthalmitis following cataract surgery. Japanese J Clin Ophthalmol. Published online 2003. https://doi.org/10.1007/978-3-540-68119-9_8.
90. Hurvitz LM. Posterior capsular rupture at hydrodissection. J Cataract Refract Surg. Published online 1991. https://doi.org/10.1016/S0886-3350(13)80433-6.
91. Yeoh R. The "pupil snap" sign of posterior capsule rupture with hydrodissection in phacoemulsification [2]. Br J Ophthalmol. Published online 1996. https://doi.org/10.1136/bjo.80.5.486-a.
92. Osher RH., Osher JM. The mature cataract and its sharp edges: fact or fiction. 1997. https://vjcrgs.com/volume31-issue2/the-mature-cataract-and-its-sharp-edges-fact-or-fiction-1997.
93. Kelman C. PAL Technique. Video J Cataract Refract Surg. 1996.
94. Kumar DA, Agarwal A, Prakash G, Jacob S, Agarwal A, Sivagnanam S. IOL scaffold technique for posterior capsule rupture. J Refract Surg. Published online 2012. https://doi.org/10.3928/1081597X-20120413-01.

95. Marques DMV, Marques FF, Osher RH. Subtle signs of zonular damage. J Cataract Refract Surg. Published online 2004. https://doi.org/10.1016/j.jcrs.2003.09.071.
96. Munshi V, Sampat V, Pagliarini S. Zonular dialysis and vitreous loss with a J-shaped hydrodissection cannula during phacoemulsification. J Cataract Refract Surg. Published online 2005. https://doi.org/10.1016/j.jcrs.2004.06.043.
97. Cionni RJ, Osher RH. Management of profound zonular dialysis or weakness with a new endocapsular ring designed for scleral fixation. J Cataract Refract Surg. Published online 1998. https://doi.org/10.1016/S0886-3350(98)80218-6.
98. Weber CH, Cionni RJ. All about capsular tension rings. Curr Opin Ophthalmol. Published online 2015. https://doi.org/10.1097/ICU.0000000000000118.
99. Menapace R, Findl O, Georgopoulos M, Rainer G, Vass C, Schmetterer K. The capsular tension ring: Designs, applications, and techniques. J Cataract Refract Surg. Published online 2000. https://doi.org/10.1016/S0886-3350(00)00446-6.
100. Hasanee K, Butler M, Ahmed IIK. Capsular tension rings and related devices: current concepts. Curr Opin Ophthalmol. Published online 2006. https://doi.org/10.1097/01.icu.0000193069.32369.e1.
101. Osher RH. Causes and management of intraoperative shallowing of the anterior chamber. Am Intra-Ocular Implant Soc J. Published online 1984. https://doi.org/10.1016/S0146-2776(84)80025-7.
102. Khng C, Osher RH. Surgical options in the face of positive pressure. J Cataract Refract Surg. Published online 2006. https://doi.org/10.1016/j.jcrs.2006.06.011.
103. Wu W, Dawson DG, Sugar A, et al. Cataract surgery in patients with nanophthalmos: Results and complications. J Cataract Refract Surg. Published online 2004. https://doi.org/10.1016/j.jcrs.2003.07.009.
104. Bellucci R. Vitreous hydration: often a hidden complication of cataract surgery. Cataract Refract Surg Today. Published 2006. http://crstoday.com/wp-content/themes/crst/assets/downloads/CRST0806_01.pdf.
105. Speaker MG, Guerriero PN, Met JA, Coad CT, Berger A, Marmor M. A Case-control study of risk factors for intraoperative suprachoroidal expulseve hemorrhage. Ophthalmology. Published online 1991. https://doi.org/10.1016/S0161-6420(91)32316-9.
106. Ling R, Cole M, James C, Kamalarajah S, Foot B, Shaw S. Suprachoroidal haemorrhage complicating cataract surgery in the UK: Epidemiology, clinical features, management, and outcomes. Br J Ophthalmol. Published online 2004. https://doi.org/10.1136/bjo.2003.026138.
107. Zauberman H. Extreme deepening of the anterior chamber during phacoemulsification. Ophthalmic Surg. Published online 1992. https://doi.org/10.3928/1542-8877-19920801-12.
108. Wilbrandt HR, Wilbrandt TH. Pathogenesis and management of the lens-iris diaphragm retropulsion syndrome during phacoemulsification. J Cataract Refract Surg. Published online 1994. https://doi.org/10.1016/S0886-3350(13)80043-0.
109. Cionni RJ, Barros MG, Osher RH. Management of lens-iris diaphragm retropulsion syndrome during phacoemulsification. J Cataract Refract Surg. Published online 2004. https://doi.org/10.1016/j.jcrs.2004.01.030.
110. Osher RH, Osher JM, Cionni RJ. Multifocal iris sphincter ruptures: New sign of the lens-iris diaphragm retropulsion syndrome. J Cataract Refract Surg. Published online 2010. https://doi.org/10.1016/j.jcrs.2009.06.045.
111. Rumelt S, Kassif Y, Koropov M, et al. The spectrum of iatrogenic intraocular injuries caused by inadvertent cannula release during anterior segment surgery. Arch Ophthalmol. Published online 2007. https://doi.org/10.1001/archopht.125.7.889.
112. Saha N, Price NC. Iatrogenic retinal tear and vitreous haemorrhage with Rycroft cannula during phacoemulsification cataract surgery [9]. Eye. Published online 2003. https://doi.org/10.1038/sj.eye.6700284.
113. Kahawita S, Cugati S, Casson R. Cyclodialysis cleft with late hypotony maculopathy after inadvertent cannula detachment during cataract surgery. J Cataract Refract Surg. Published online 2015. https://doi.org/10.1016/j.jcrs.2015.04.002.
114. Osher MS. Emergency treatment of vitreous bulge and wound gaping Complicating cataract surgery. Am J Ophthalmol. Published online 1957. https://doi.org/10.1016/0002-9394(57)92778-2.
115. Ernest PH. Explantation of foldable lenses - intraocular re-folding. Video J Cataract Refract Surg. 1997;XII(4).
116. Eguchi S. Quadrantotomy. Video J Cataract Refract Surg. 2000;Volume XVI(1). https://vjcrgs.com/archive/2000.
117. Batlan SJ, Dodick JM. Explantation of a foldable silicone intraocular lens. Am J Ophthalmol. Published online 1996. https://doi.org/10.1016/s0002-9394(14)72024-0.
118. Batlan S, Doddick J. Explantation of foldable lenses - partial lensectomy. Video J Cataract Refract Surg. 1997;XII(4).
119. Narang P, Steinert R, Little B, Agarwal A. Intraocular lens scaffold to facilitate intraocular lens exchange. J Cataract Refract Surg. Published online 2014. https://doi.org/10.1016/j.jcrs.2014.07.015.
120. IOL Explantation Set According to Snyder/Osher. Geuder https://www.geuder.de/produkte/instrumente/iol-explantation-nach-snyder-osher/.
121. Basarir B, Kaya V, Altan C, Karakus S, Pinarci EY, Demirok A. The use of a supplemental sulcus fix-

ated IOL (HumanOptics Add-On IOL) to correct pseudophakic refractive errors. Eur J Ophthalmol. Published online 2012. https://doi.org/10.5301/ejo.5000156.
122. Davison JA. Positive and negative dysphotopsia in patients with acrylic intraocular lenses. J Cataract Refract Surg. Published online 2000. https://doi.org/10.1016/S0886-3350(00)00611-8.
123. Smith SG, Holladay J, Knoll R. YAG laser injury of intraocular lenses. Eur J Implant Refract Surg. Published online 1992. https://doi.org/10.1016/S0955-3681(14)80009-9.
124. Bath PE, Hoffer KJ, Aron-Rosa D, Dang Y. Glare disability secondary to YAG laser intraocular lens damage. J Cataract Refract Surg. Published online 1987. https://doi.org/10.1016/S0886-3350(87)80076-7.
125. Mamalis N, Craig MT, Price FW. Spectrum of Nd:YAG laser-induced intraocular lens damage in explanted lenses. J Cataract Refract Surg. Published online 1990. https://doi.org/10.1016/S0886-3350(13)80806-1.

Dislocated IOLs

38

Ken Hayashi, Motoaki Yoshida,
and Koichi Yoshimura

Bullet Points

- IOL dislocation is divided into 2 types: in-the-bag and out-of-the-bag dislocation. Out-of-the bag dislocation due mainly to complicated surgery occurs in the early postoperative period, while in-the-bag IOL dislocation due to a slowly progressive dehiscence of the zonules occurs several years after cataract surgery.
- In-the-bag IOL dislocation progresses vertically according to the degree of the remaining zonular or capsular support. According to the progression of IOL dislocation, we classified the dislocation sites into the 5 categories.
- Before explantation of the dislocated IOL, lifting up onto the iris is performed using 1 of 3 techniques based on the dislocation site; (1) pulling up through 2 limbal side ports, 2) pushing up from the pars plana to the posterior chamber, or (3) lifting up from the retinal surface.
- The dislocated IOL onto the iris is explanted via a clear corneal incision or scleral incision. Polymethyl methacrylate and silicone IOLs are explanted though a 6.0- or 6.5-mm scleral incision having a width equal to the optic diameter. Hydrophobic and hydrophilic acrylic IOLs can be explanted thorough an incision almost half the width of the optic diameter by folding or cutting the optic.
- We only perform anterior vitrectomy through limbal side ports, except for cases in which an IOL has dropped onto the retina. Before scleral fixation of the IOL, we insert a vitreous cutter through the side port and remove a minimal amount of the vitreous body that has prolapsed in the anterior chamber.

Introduction

Late dislocation of an intraocular lens (IOL) is a serious complication following cataract surgery [1–4]. Many surgical techniques are applied for managing dislocated IOLs, including exchanging or repositioning of the IOL with suturing to the

Supplementary Information The online version contains supplementary material available at [https://doi.org/10.1007/978-3-030-94530-5_38].

K. Hayashi (✉) · M. Yoshida · K. Yoshimura
Hayashi Eye Hospital, Fukuoka, Japan
e-mail: hayashi-ken@hayashi.or.jp

J. L. Alió et al. (eds.), *Cataract Surgery*, Essentials in Ophthalmology,
https://doi.org/10.1007/978-3-030-94530-5_38

sclera or iris, which are performed with pars plana vitrectomy or anterior vitrectomy [5–15]. The surgeon's preference usually dictates the technique. In general, posterior segment surgeons prefer the posterior approach with repositioning of the IOL and pars plana vitrectomy [5–13], while anterior segment surgeons prefer the anterior approach with exchange of the IOL through limbal incisions and anterior vitrectomy [4, 14, 15]. Most of the IOLs in use currently are 1-piece acrylic IOLs without rigid loops, making them unsuitable for repositioning by suturing to the sclera or iris in eyes without adequate capsular support. As a result, IOL repositioning procedures have gradually become less commonly performed, and IOL exchange procedures are now the predominant technique.

Many studies have reported various sites of dislocated IOL based on the horizontal position determined by slit-lamp microscopy with the patient upright [4, 12, 14], but there is currently no classification system. A dislocation site classification system based on the vertical position as observed under an operating microscope with the patient in a supine position would provide useful information for planning the surgical repair. Although pars plana vitrectomy is performed in most previous cases [5–8, 13], several reports suggest that anterior vitrectomy is adequate even for eyes with IOLs posteriorly dislocated to the vitreous cavity [4–12]. We recently developed a classification system for IOL dislocation sites based on the vertical position determined under an operating microscope, and specially considered the requirement for pars plana vitrectomy [16].

In-the-Bag and out-of-the-Bag Dislocation of the IOL

IOL dislocation is divided into two types: in-the-bag and out-of-the-bag dislocation (Fig. 38.1). Until the 1980s, IOL dislocation usually occurred outside of the capsule, such as in sunset or sunrise syndrome [17, 18]. Because out-of-the bag dislocation is due predominantly to asymmetrical fixation of the IOL or to complicated surgery, it occurs early in the postoperative period [17, 18]. The type of IOL dislocation has markedly changed, since the 1990s, however, when continuous curvilinear capsulorrhexis and in-the-bag

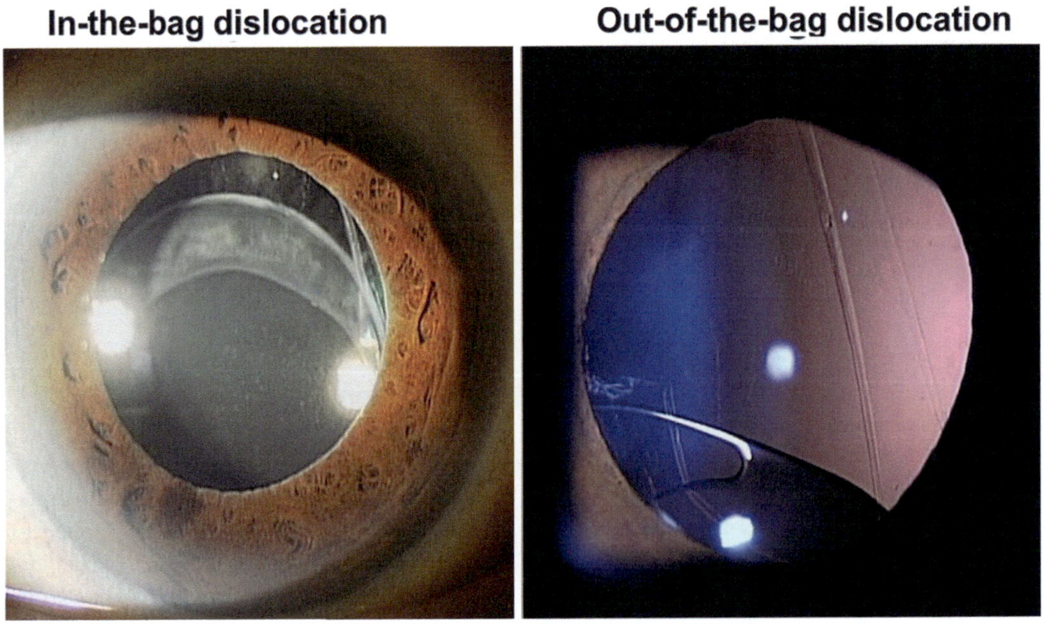

Fig. 38.1 In-the-bag and out-of-the-bag IOL dislocation

implantation of the IOL became the standard technique for cataract surgery. Many cases of IOL dislocation within the capsular bag have been reported, and pseudoexfoliation syndrome, allergic conjunctivitis associated with atopic dermatitis, chronic uveitis, trauma, postvitrectomy status, and long axial length are considered predisposing factors [19–24]. In-the-bag IOL dislocation usually occurs several years after cataract surgery and, thus, results from a slowly progressive dehiscence of the zonules.

Classification System of IOL Dislocation Sites

In-the-bag IOL dislocation progresses vertically according to the degree of the remaining zonular or capsular support (Fig. 38.2). Zonule or capsule deterioration leads to pseudophakodonesis or tilting and sinking of the IOLX, in which the IOL is observed within the pupillary area. When large portions of the zonules break, the IOL dangles from the remaining zonules like a trap door in the

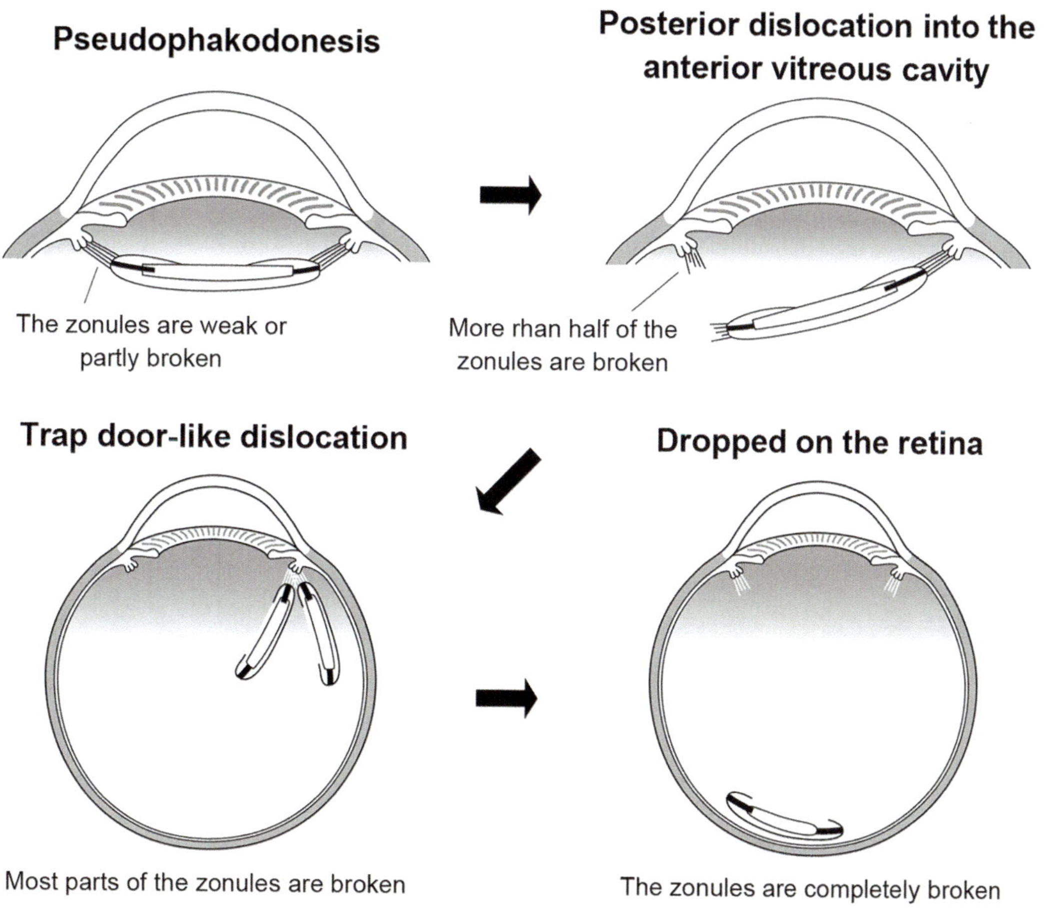

Fig. 38.2 Schema of progression of in-the-bag IOL dislocation [16]. In-the-bag IOL dislocation progresses according to the number of the remaining zonules. When the zonules become weak or partly broken, pseudophakodonesis begins. When more than half of the zonules are broken, the IOLs become tilted or sink into the vitreous cavity. When most of the zonules are broken, the IOL dangles while connected to the remaining zonules in the peripheral vitreous cavity, like a trap door. When the connection with the zonules or capsules breaks completely, the IOL drops onto the retina

peripheral vitreous cavity (i.e., trap-door-like dislocation). A perpendicularly dangling IOL is rarely observed within the pupillary area when the patient is in a supine position, but when the upper zonules remain, the IOL may be seen within the pupillary area on slit lamp microscopy with the patient in a sitting position. Complete disconnection of the IOL from the zonules or capsules allows the IOL to drop onto the retina. According to this progression of IOL dislocation, we classified the dislocation sites into the following five categories (Fig. 38.3): (1) prolapse into the anterior chamber, (2) pseudophakodonesis, (3) posterior dislocation in the anterior vitreous cavity within the pupillary area, (4) trap-door-like dislocation, and (5) being dropped onto the retina [24]. Classification according to this system should be determined under an operating microscope with the patient in the supine position. Prolapse of the IOL into the anterior chamber usually occurs after rubbing or compressing the eye (Fig. 38.4).

This classification system determined under microscope is useful for anterior segment surgeons who do not usually perform pars plana vitrectomy. The first 4 categories, namely, (1) anterior chamber prolapse, (2) pseudophakodonesis, (3) posterior dislocation within the pupillary area, (4) trap-door-like dislocation, can be managed without performing pars plana vitrectomy, because the IOL remains in the upper part of the eye. We first use this classification to distinguish whether the IOL remains in the upper part of the eye. To look for the dislocated IOL under microscope is also useful for determining

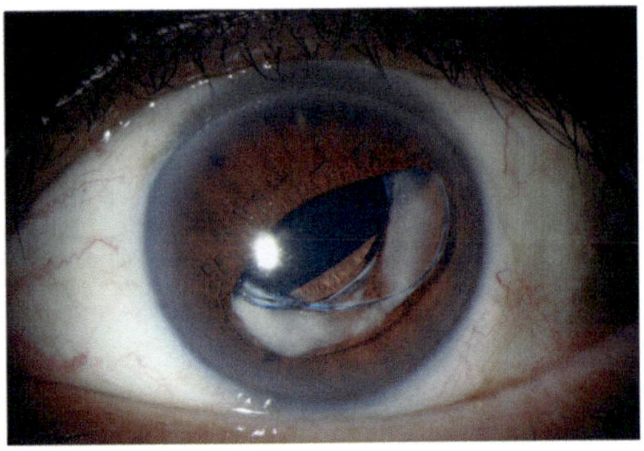

Fig. 38.4 Anterior prolapse of the in-the-bag IOL dislocated to the anterior chamber

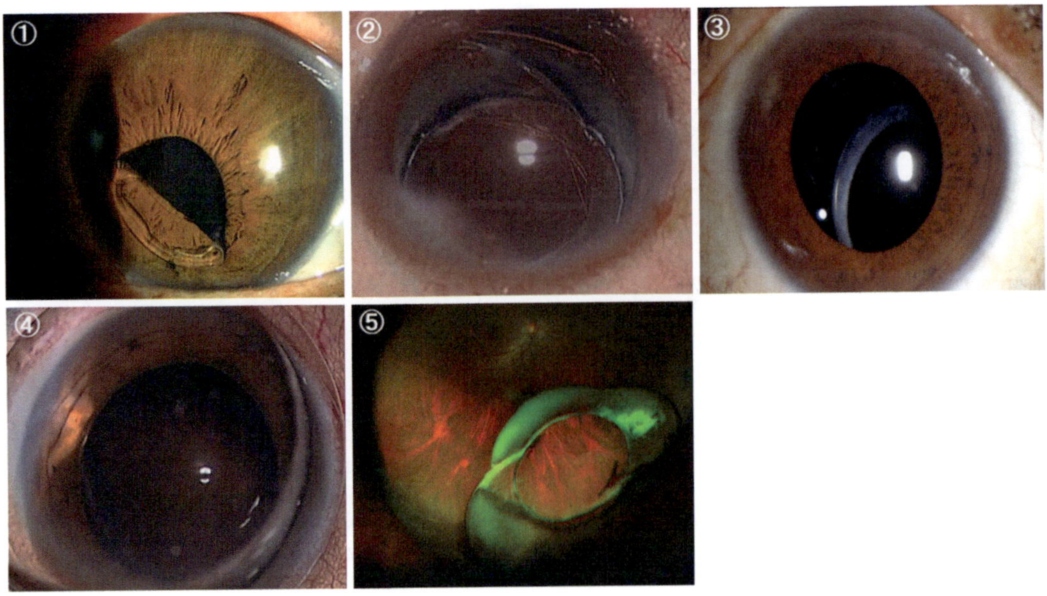

Fig. 38.3 Classification system for IOL dislocation sites [16]. The dislocation sites were classified into the following five categories: ① prolapse into the anterior chamber, ② pseudophakodonesis, ③ posterior dislocation in the anterior vitreous cavity within the pupillary area, ④ trap-door-like dislocation, and ⑤ being dropped onto the retina

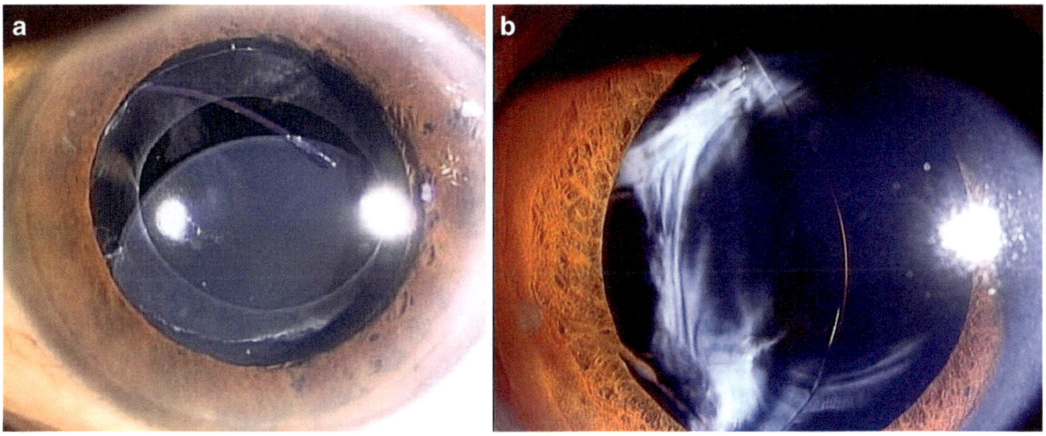

Fig. 38.5 Out-of-the bag IOL dislocation due to posterior capsule rupture in the early postoperative period (**a**) and in the late postoperative period (**b**)

the position of the pars plana on which a trocar for pushing up the IOL should be placed.

Progression of out-of-the-bag IOL dislocation differs from that of in-the-bag dislocation. Out-of-the-bag dislocation is predominantly due to complicated surgery after posterior capsule rupture or anterior capsule tears and, therefore, usually occurs in the immediate or early postoperative periods (Fig. 38.5). When the out-of-the-bag dislocation occurs late after surgery, rubbing or compressing the eye is the likely cause. Because the IOL rapidly luxates with no capsular support in out-of-the-bag dislocation, the IOL is frequently detected on the retina. When an out-of-the-bag dislocated IOL dangles in the peripheral vitreous cavity, one side of the haptic is suspected to be attached to the sclera.

IOL Dislocation Sites

We evaluated 269 eyes of 240 patients who consecutively underwent IOL exchange surgery due to IOL dislocation between April 2006 and June 2013. Of these eyes, 39 were excluded from analysis and 230 eyes were analyzed. Of the 230 eyes (Table 38.1), the major dislocation sites were posterior dislocation in the anterior vitreous cavity in 109 eyes (47.4%), pseudophakodonesis in 44 (19.1%), and trap-door-like dislocation in 37 (16.1%). Of the 209 eyes with in-the-bag dislocation, the major dislocation sites were posterior dislocation in the anterior vitreous in 104 eyes (49.8%), pseudophakodonesis in 42 (20.1%), and trap-door-like dislocation in 36 (17.2%). Of the 21 eyes with out-of-the-bag dislocation, the major dislocation sites were being dropped onto the retina in 10 eyes (47.6%) and dislocation in the anterior vitreous cavity in 5 (23.8%). The incidence of the dislocation sites differed significantly between the in-the-bag and out-of-the-bag dislocation groups ($p < 0.0001$).

Explantation of Dislocated IOLs

In most cases, we explant the dislocated IOL and fixate a new posterior-chamber IOL to the sclera [4]. We prefer not to implant an anterior-chamber IOL, because corneal endothelial cell injury is a serious concern, or to suture the IOL to the iris because of chronic inflammation, which leads to cystoid macular edema. Before explantation, lifting up the dislocated IOL onto the iris is performed using 1 of 3 techniques based on the dislocation site: (1) pulling up through 2 limbal side ports, (2) pushing up from the pars plana to the posterior chamber, or (3) lifting up from the retinal surface. For eyes with pseudophakodonesis, prolapse into the anterior chamber, or slight posterior dislocation of the IOL into the vitreous, the IOLs are lifted up

Table 38.1 Comparison in-the-bag and out-of-the-bag IOL dislocation sites [16]

	In-the-bag dislocation	Out-of-the-bag dislocation	Overall dislocation sites
	Group (n = 209)[a]	Group (n = 21)[a]	Group (n = 230)
1. Prolapse into the AC	25 (12.0%)	3 (14.3%)	28 (12.2%)
2. Pseudophakodonesis	42 (20.1%)	2 (9.5%)	44 (19.1%)
3. Posterior dislocation into the anterior vitreous cavity	104 (49.8%)	5 (23.8%)	109 (47.4%)
4. Trap door-like dislocation	36 (4.8%)	1 (4.8%)	37 (16.1%)
5. Dropped onto the retina	2 (1.0%)	10 (47.6%)	12 (5.2%)

AC anterior chamber
[a]Statistically significant difference in the distribution of IOL dislocation sites between the in-the-bag and out-of-the-bag dislocation groups ($p < 0.0001$)

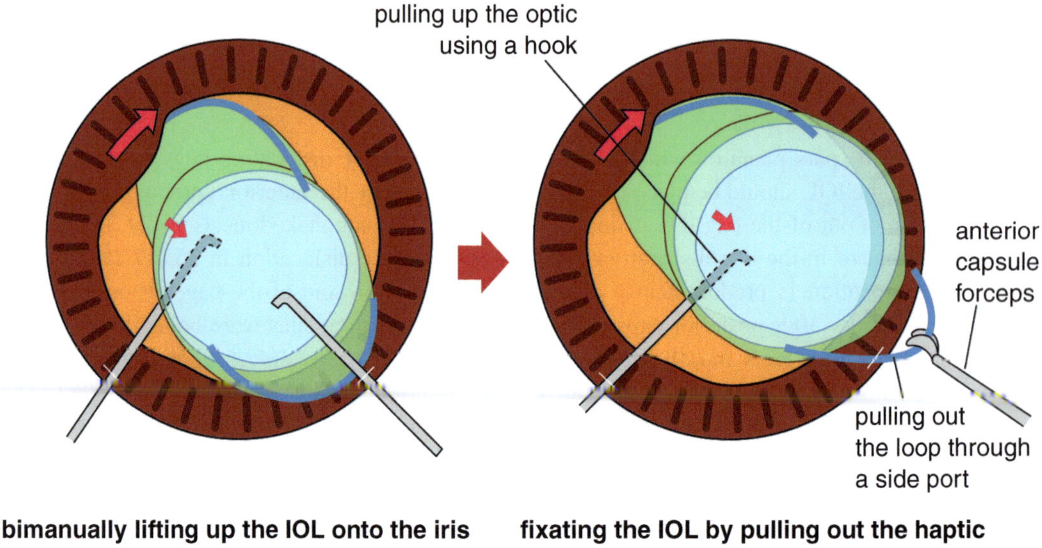

Fig. 38.6 Schema for bimanual pulling up of a dislocated IOL onto the iris using a hook, an anterior capsule forceps, and an IOL explantation forceps

onto the iris by holding the haptic or optic using a bimanual hook, anterior capsule forceps, or IOL explantation forceps (Fig. 38.6). For eyes with a trap-door-like dislocation and deep posterior dislocation into the vitreous, a 25 or 23 G trocar for vitrectomy is inserted in the pars plana where the zonules remain, and the IOL is pushed up into the posterior chamber using a pick, and then pulled up onto the iris using a hook, anterior capsule forceps, or IOL forceps through the limbus (Figs. 38.7 and 38.8). For eyes in which the IOL has dropped onto the retina, 3-port pars plana vitrectomy is performed first, and the IOL haptic is grasped and pulled up to the posterior chamber using internal limiting membrane peeling (ILM) forceps or a pick, and then fixed onto the iris through the limbal side ports using a hook, anterior capsule forceps, or IOL forceps. For grasping and pulling up the IOL, we recommend the Max-Grip ILM forceps (Alcon Laboratories, Fort Worth, Texas, USA). When an in-the-bag dislocated IOL is difficult to grasp because of an intact capsule, scraping away part of the capsule around the haptic using a vitreous

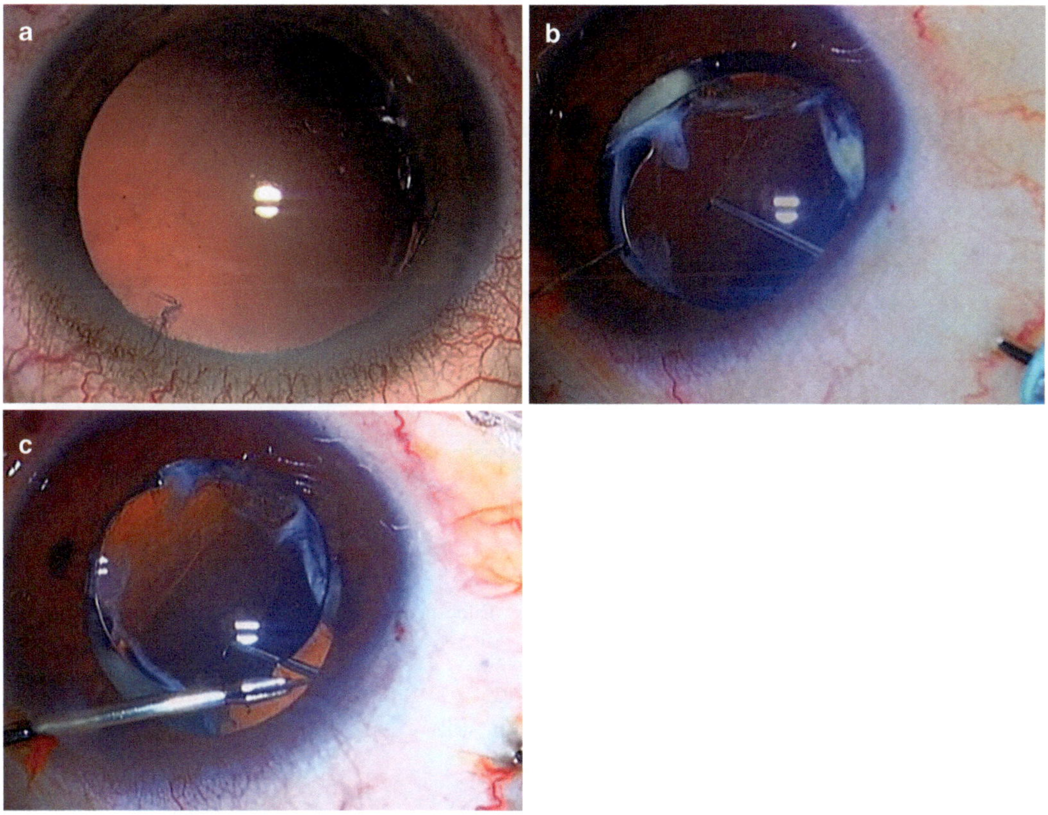

Fig. 38.7 Lifting an IOL with a trap-door-like dislocation up onto the iris (**a**) Under an operating microscope, the IOL was difficult to see within the pupillary area, because the IOL was dangling in the peripheral vitreous while connected to the remaining zonules at the 10 o'clock meridian. After placing a trocar for 25-gauge vitrectomy into the pars plana at the 10 o'clock meridian, (**b**) the vertically dangling IOL was pushed up to the posterior chamber using a pick, and (**c**) was lifted onto the iris using an anterior capsulotomy forceps

cutter will make it easier to grasp. Thus, IOL dislocation at sites 1 through 4 according to our classification system is repaired using an anterior approach, and only IOLs that have dropped onto the retina are repaired using a posterior approach.

After pulling the dislocated IOL onto the iris, it is explanted via a clear corneal incision or scleral tunnel incision. Polymethyl methacrylate and silicone IOLs are explanted though a 6.0- or 6.5-mm scleral tunnel incision having a width equal to the optic diameter. At this time, any regenerated lens within the capsule, namely Soemmering's ring, should be explanted together as a whole. Hydrophobic and hydrophilic acrylic IOLs can be explanted thorough an incision almost half the width of the optic diameter by folding or cutting the optic. In eyes with in-the-bag IOL dislocation, we prefer folding the optic over cutting it, because Soemmering's ring can be explanted as a whole. To fold the optic in the anterior chamber, a hook is inserted under the IOL from a side port opposite the main incision, IOL folding forceps are inserted through the main incision, and the IOL is folded using the IOL folding forceps and a hook (Fig. 38.9). The folded IOL and regenerated lens fiber complex are explanted through approximately 3.5- to 4.0-

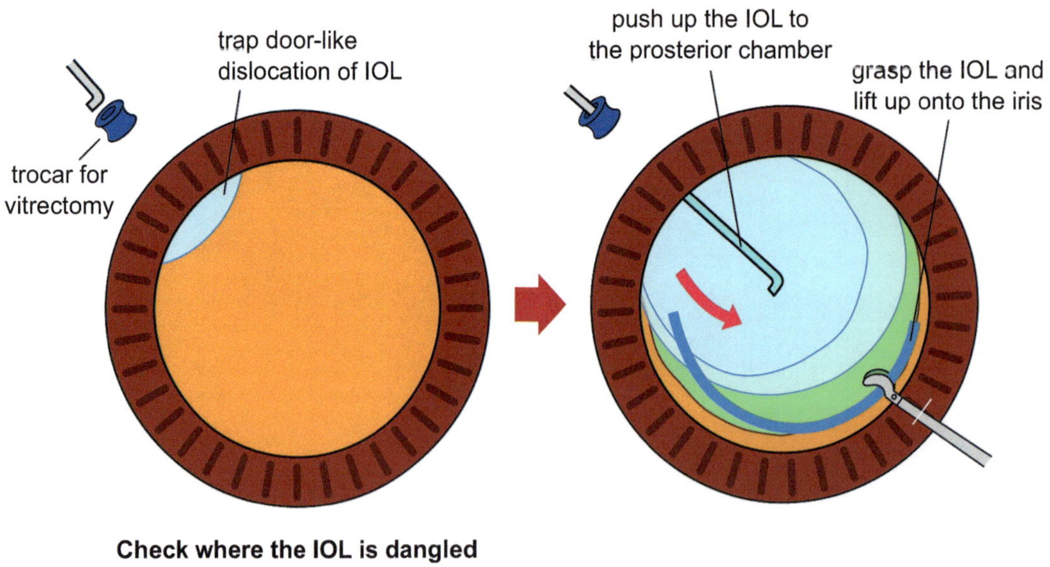

Fig. 38.8 Schema for lifting up an IOL with a trap-door-like dislocation onto the iris

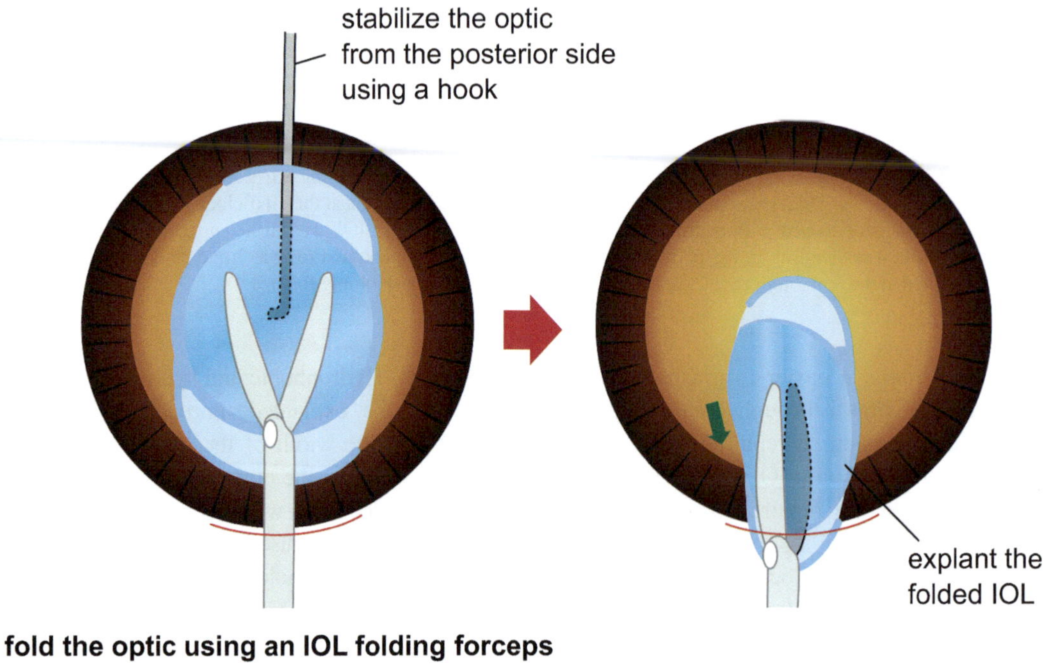

Fig. 38.9 Schema for explanting an acrylic IOL by folding the optic using IOL folding forceps and a hook

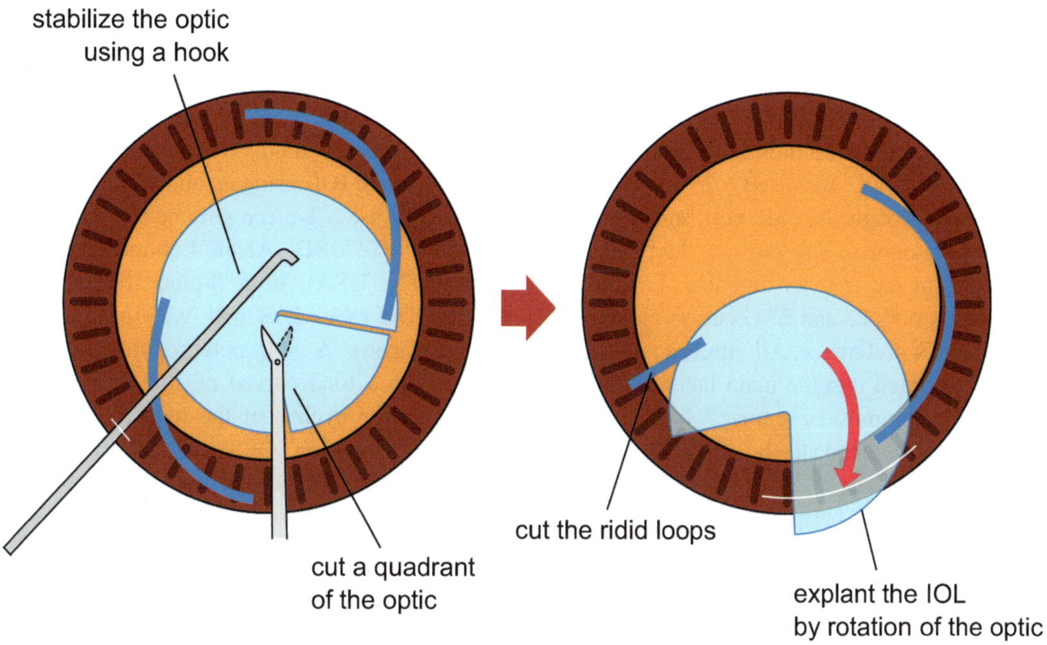

Fig. 38.10 Schema for explanting an acrylic IOL by cutting the optic

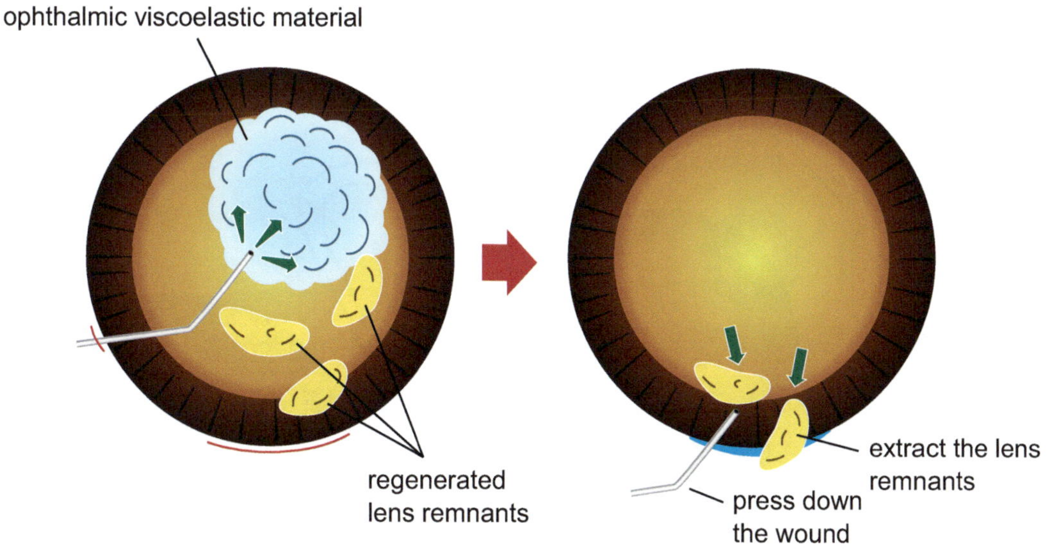

Fig. 38.11 Schema for extracting the remnants of Soemmering's ring by a pressure of ophthalmic viscoelastic materials

mm clear corneal incision. In eyes with an out-of-the-bag IOL dislocation, the IOL can be cut and explanted through the main incision (Fig. 38.10). If the capsule is ruptured during explantation, and regenerated lens fibers remain in the anterior chamber, the lens remnants should be extracted by the pressure of ophthalmic viscoelastic device (Fig. 38.11).

Vitrectomy

We only perform anterior vitrectomy through limbal side ports, except for cases in which an IOL has dropped onto the retina. Before scleral fixation of the IOL, we insert a 23 or 25 G vitreous cutter through the side port, and remove a minimal amount of the vitreous body that has prolapsed in the anterior chamber. For anterior vitrectomy, both 23 and 25 G cutters can be used by surgeon's preference. All vitreous strands that are incorporated into the main incision and side ports, however, must be removed. Iatrogenic retinal holes/tears tend to be developed during removing the peripheral vitreous. Because iatrogenic holes in the peripheral retina may not be sufficiently treated, however, excessive amount of the vitreous should not be removed. For an IOL that has dropped onto the retina, 3-port pars plana vitrectomy is performed. After pars plana vitrectomy, the dropped IOL is picked up from the retinal surface using a pick or internal limiting membrane forceps, and then lifted up onto the iris.

Scleral Fixation of IOL

Because many surgical techniques are available for scleral fixation of IOLs, surgeons may select their preferred method. We prefer transscleral suturing of the IOL using an ab-externo method. We usually use a 1-piece polymethyl methacrylate IOL (CZ70BD; Alcon Laboratories, Fort Worth, TX, USA), or a 3-piece hydrophobic acrylic IOL (YA-65BB and VA70AD; HOYA, Tokyo, Japan). A 9–0 polypropylene looped-suture with a long curved or straight needle is hitched to the eyelets of the loop of the polymethyl methacrylate IOL or directly to the loop of the hydrophobic acrylic IOL. After piercing the sclera using a 26- or 27-gauge catheter needle at the ciliary sulcus approximately 1.5-mm posterior to the limbus, the end of a long needle is inserted into the lumen of the catheter needle, and then both needles are pulled out together from the eye (Fig. 38.12). The IOL is then inserted into the posterior chamber, and the bilateral sutures are drawn tight until the IOL is well centered. Another superficial suture bite is taken

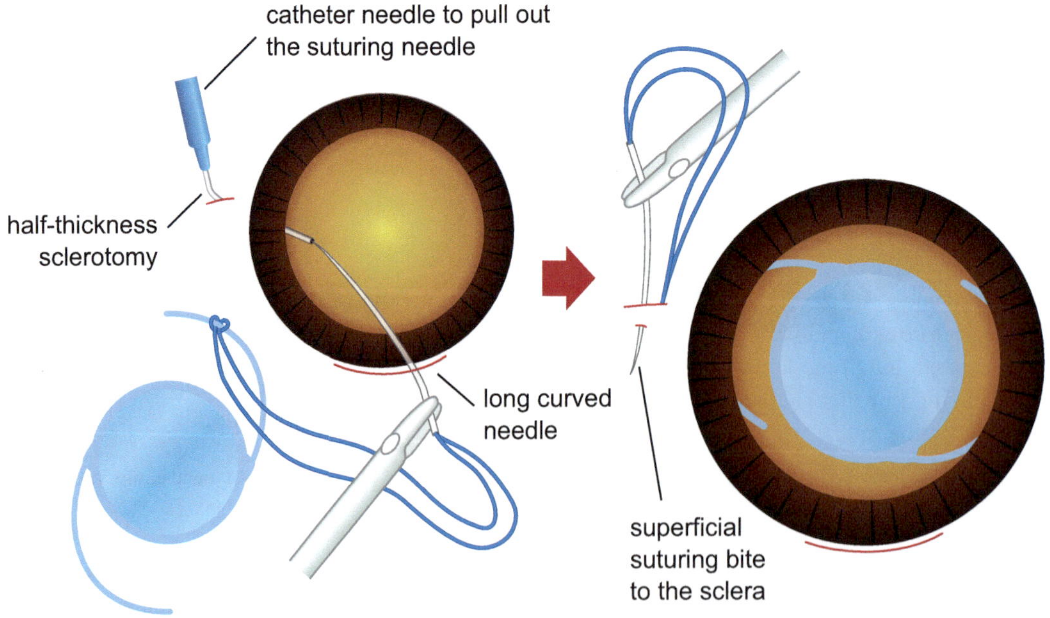

Fig. 38.12 Schema of an ab-externo method of scleral suturing of the IOL

in the sclera, and then one arm of the suture is cut and tied to the other arm of the suture; this is done on both sides. After instilling a miotic agent, the vitreous that has prolapsed into the anterior chamber is removed using a 23 or 25 G vitreous cutter and the vitreous strand is swept using a hook until the pupil becomes round. Both loops of the 3-piece hydrophobic acrylic IOL are externalized from the sclerotomy sites using fine forceps or 24-gauge needles. The ends of the loops are buried in the half-thickness sclerotomy sites. We also perform intrascleral fixation of the IOL without sutures. The IOL used for intrascleral fixation is a 7.0-mm hydrophobic acrylic IOL with polyvinylidene difluoride loops (X-70 and NX-70; Santen, Osaka, Japan). It is also possible to perform iris suturing of the anterior chamber lens by surgeon's preference.

Take-Home Notes

- According to the progression of IOL dislocation, we classified the dislocation sites into five categories: (1) prolapse into the anterior chamber, (2) pseudophakodonesis, (3) posterior dislocation in the anterior vitreous cavity within the pupillary area, (4) trap-door-like dislocation, and (5) being dropped onto the retina.
- To make surgical plan, dislocation site should be determined according to this classification system under an operating microscope with the patient in the supine position.
- Before explantation, lifting up the dislocated IOL onto the iris is performed using 1 of 3 techniques based on the dislocation site; (1) pulling up through 2 limbal side ports, (2) pushing up from the pars plana to the posterior chamber, or (3) lifting up from the retinal surface.
- The dislocated IOL onto the iris is explanted via a clear corneal incision or scleral tunnel incision. Polymethyl methacrylate and silicone IOLs are explanted though an approximately 6.0-mm scleral incision having a width equal to the optic diameter. Hydrophobic and hydrophilic acrylic IOLs can be explanted through a clear corneal incision almost half the width of the optic diameter by folding or cutting the optic.
- We only perform anterior vitrectomy through limbal side ports, except for cases in which an IOL has dropped onto the retina.

References

1. Lee GI, Lim DH, Chi SA, Kim SW, Shin DW, Chung TY. Risk factors for intraocular lens dislocation after phacoemulsification: a nationwide population-based cohort study. Am J Ophthalmol. 2020;214:86–96. https://doi.org/10.1016/j.ajo.2020.03.012.
2. Pueringer SL, Hodge DO, Erie JC. Risk of late intraocular lens dislocation after cataract surgery, 1980-2009: a population-based study. Am J Ophthalmol. 2011;152:618–23. https://doi.org/10.1016/j.ajo.2011.03.009.
3. Krėpštė L, Kuzmienė L, Miliauskas A, Janulevičienė I. Possible predisposing factors for late intraocular lens dislocation after routine cataract surgery. Medicina (Kaunas). 2013;49:229–34.
4. Hayashi K, Hirata A, Hayashi H. Possible predisposing factors for in-the-bag and out-of-the-bag intraocular lens dislocation and outcomes of intraocular lens exchange surgery. Ophthalmology. 2007;114:969–75. https://doi.org/10.1016/j.ophtha.2006.09.017.
5. Dalby M, Drolsum L, Kristianslund O. Repositioning surgery of different intraocular lens designs in eyes with late in-the-bag intraocular lens dislocation. J Cataract Refract Surg. 2021; https://doi.org/10.1097/j.jcrs.0000000000000588.
6. Fan KC, Smiddy WE. Rescuing an akreos 4-point haptic intraocular lens: a novel surgical technique. Retina. 2021; https://doi.org/10.1097/IAE.0000000000003159.
7. Goemaere J, Trigaux C, Denissen L, Dragnea D, Hua MT, Tassignon MJ, et al. Fifteen years of IOL exchange: indications, outcomes, and complications. J Cataract Refract Surg. 2020;46:1596–603. https://doi.org/10.1097/j.jcrs.0000000000000349.
8. Czajka MP, Frajdenberg A, Johansson B. A technique for sutured scleral fixation of one-piece hydrophobic acrylic intraocular lenses dislocated into the vitreous. Retina. 2020; https://doi.org/10.1097/IAE.0000000000003008.

9. Sella S, Rubowitz A, Sheen-Ophir S, Ferencz JR, Assia EI, Ton Y. Pars plana vitrectomy for posteriorly dislocated intraocular lenses: risk factors and surgical approach. Int Ophthalmol. 2021;41:221–9. https://doi.org/10.1007/s10792-020-01570-7.
10. Yang S, Nie K, Jiang H, Feng L, Fan W. Surgical management of intraocular lens dislocation: a meta-analysis. PLoS One. 2019;14:e0211489. https://doi.org/10.1371/journal.pone.0211489.
11. Yamane S, Sato S, Maruyama-Inoue M, Kadonosono K. Flanged intrascleral intraocular lens fixation with double-needle technique. Ophthalmology. 2017;124:1136–42. https://doi.org/10.1016/j.ophtha.2017.03.036.
12. Lorente R, de Rojas V, de Parga PV, Moreno C, Landaluce ML, Domínguez R, et al. Management of late spontaneous in-the-bag intraocular lens dislocation: retrospective analysis of 45 cases. J Cataract Refract Surg. 2010;36:1270–82. https://doi.org/10.1016/j.jcrs.2010.01.035.
13. Al-Halafi AM, Al-Harthi E, Al-Amro S, El-Asrar AA. Visual outcome and complications of pars plana vitrectomy for dislocated intraocular lenses. Saudi J Ophthalmol. 2011;25:187–92. https://doi.org/10.1016/j.sjopt.2011.01.013.
14. Shingleton BJ, Yang Y, O'Donoghue MW. Management and outcomes of intraocular lens dislocation in patients with pseudoexfoliation. J Cataract Refract Surg. 2013;39:984–93. https://doi.org/10.1016/j.jcrs.2013.01.044.
15. Fernández-Buenaga R, Alio JL, Pérez-Ardoy AL, Larrosa-Quesada A, Pinilla-Cortés L, Barraquer R, et al. Late in-the-bag intraocular lens dislocation requiring explantation: risk factors and outcomes. Eye (Lond). 2013;27:795–801. https://doi.org/10.1038/eye.2013.95.
16. Hayashi K, Ogawa S, Manabe S, Hirata A, Yoshimura K. A classification system of intraocular lens dislocation sites under operating microscopy, and the surgical techniques and outcomes of exchange surgery. Graefes Arch Clin Exp Ophthalmol. 2016;254:505–13. https://doi.org/10.1007/s00417-016-3273-6.
17. Böke WR, Krüger HC. Causes and management of posterior chamber lens displacement. J Am Intraocul Implant Soc. 1985;11:179–84. https://doi.org/10.1016/s0146-2776(85)80022-7.
18. Smith SG, Lindstrom RL. Malpositioned posterior chamber lenses: etiology, prevention, and management. J Am Intraocul Implant Soc. 1985;11:584–91. https://doi.org/10.1016/s0146-2776(85)80139-7.
19. Jehan FS, Mamalis N, Crandall AS. Spontaneous late dislocation of intraocular lens within the capsular bag in pseudoexfoliation patients. Ophthalmology. 2001;108:1727–31. https://doi.org/10.1016/s0161-6420(01)00710-2.
20. Masket S, Osher RH. Late complications with intraocular lens dislocation after capsulorhexis in pseudoexfoliation syndrome. J Cataract Refract Surg. 2002;28:1481–4. https://doi.org/10.1016/s0886-3350(01)01267-6.
21. Brilakis HS, Lustbader JM. Bilateral dislocation of in-the-bag posterior chamber intraocular lenses in a patient with intermediate uveitis. J Cataract Refract Surg. 2003;29:2013–4. https://doi.org/10.1016/s0886-3350(03)00226-8.
22. Shigeeda T, Nagahara M, Kato S, Kunimatsu S, Kaji Y, Tanaka S, et al. Spontaneous posterior dislocation of intraocular lenses fixated in the capsular bag. J Cataract Refract Surg. 2002;28:1689–93. https://doi.org/10.1016/s0886-3350(01)01178-6.
23. Yamazaki S, Nakamura K, Kurosaka D. Intraocular lens subluxation in a patient with facial atopic dermatitis. J Cataract Refract Surg. 2001;27:337–8. https://doi.org/10.1016/s0886-3350(00)00499-5.
24. Yasuda A, Ohkoshi K, Orihara Y, Kusano Y, Sakuma A, Yamaguchi T. Spontaneous luxation of encapsulated intraocular lens onto the retina after a triple procedure of vitrectomy, phacoemulsification, and intraocular lens implantation. Am J Ophthalmol. 2000;130:836–7. https://doi.org/10.1016/s0002-9394(00)00630-9.

39 Management of Dropped Nucleus in Complicated Cataract Surgery

Marta S. Figueroa and Andrea Govetto

Bullet Points

- Dropped nucleus management involves both medical and surgical strategies.
- The surgeon must identify risk factors for dropped nucleus prior to the surgery.
- Addressing the issue from both anterior and posterior approaches is critical to achieve good anatomical and functional results.
- Different techniques may be used to remove the nucleus from the vitreous chamber.
- A suboptimal management of dropped nucleus may have serious consequences on the visual potential of the eye.

Supplementary Information The online version contains supplementary material available at [https://doi.org/10.1007/978-3-030-94530-5_39].

M. S. Figueroa
Ophthalmology Department, Ramon y Cajal University Hospital, Alcala de Henares University, Madrid, Spain

A. Govetto (✉)
Oftalmico Hospital, ASST-Fatebenefratelli-Sacco, Milan, Italy

Introduction

Dropped nucleus is one of the most feared and severe complications of modern cataract surgery [1]. It is defined as the dislocation of part of the crystalline lens, or rarely the whole lens, to the vitreous cavity. The lens material may drop through iatrogenic breaks of the posterior capsule. In some cases, the whole lens may fall back due to zonular weakness or dialysis.

The correct clinical and surgical management of a dropped lens is critical to achieve good functional and anatomical results for the patients, and to lower the risk of further complications such as intraocular inflammation, intraocular pressure rise, corneal edema, cystoid macular edema, and retinal detachment [1].

This chapter will give guidance in the treatment of such complex cases, with a particular focus on the vitreoretinal point of view.

Dropped Nucleus: Causes and Preoperative Risk Factors

The dislocation of lens material into the vitreous chamber has a reported incidence, which may vary between 0.3% and 1.1% according to the published literature [1–4]. Some preoperative factors that may increase the risk of dropped nucleus are as follows:

J. L. Alió et al. (eds.), *Cataract Surgery*, Essentials in Ophthalmology,
https://doi.org/10.1007/978-3-030-94530-5_39

- Inexperienced surgeon
- Advanced age
- Undilated pupil
- Pseudoexfoliation
- Increased axial length
- Posterior polar cataract
- Zonular disruption
- Traumatic cataract
- Hollow orbit
- Previous vitrectomy surgery
- Intraoperative floppy iris syndrome (IFIS)

Knowing such risk factors may allow surgeons to predict complications more accurately prior to surgery, plan more effectively, and counsel patients who are at risk.

Not surprisingly, the level of expertise of a surgeon is inversely correlated with the likelihood to experience dropped nucleus, and previous reports confirmed that the learning curve is associated with a higher level of complications [3].

Phacoemulsification technique (divide and conquer versus phaco-chop) is not associated with a higher incidence of this complication, but peripheral sculpting was reported to be a high-risk maneuver, as the lens is thinner in the periphery and the phaco-tip may touch the posterior capsule more likely if compared to central sculpting [3].

Fluctuating anterior chamber depth, caused by increased movement of the lens-iris diaphragm, is common in vitrectomized eyes. Such phenomenon may increase the risk of touching the posterior capsule with the phaco-probe.

Dropped Nucleus: What to Do?

Anterior Segment

The basic principle of complication management in any surgical setting

must be to reduce the risk of further complications. The surgical strategy in case of posterior capsule rupture with vitreous loss and dropped nucleus must follow an ordinated step-by step set of procedures to increase the odds to achieve satisfactory functional and anatomical results.

In a dropped nucleus situation, leaving vitreous incarcerated to surgical incision or in the anterior chamber leads to an increased rate of cystoid macular edema, retinal detachment, and postoperative endophthalmitis. Further, any attempt to remove posteriorly dislocated lens material from the anterior segment may result in vitreous traction, retinal tear, hemorrhages, and retinal detachment.

The goal of the anterior segment surgery must be to deliver a clean anterior chamber, free of vitreous and lens remnants, and possibly to implant a sulcus three-piece intraocular lens in case of preserved anterior capsule.

The first step is to reduce vitreous traction. Drop in anterior chamber pressure may cause a gradient allowing the posterior vitreous to flow into the anterior chamber, potentially causing significant traction over the retina and possibly the creation of retinal breaks and detachment [5]. Continued irrigation alone may help to prevent the creation of such gradient and allows to remove the second instrument and to inject a dispersive ophthalmic viscoelastic device (OVD) [5]. This may tamponade the vitreous and support the remaining lens material and gives time to the surgeon to assess the situation and plan the following steps.

Once the prolapse of the vitreous and the displacement of further lens material are prevented, the second step is to remove the vitreous from the anterior chamber. This can be done with bimanual vitrectomy, with the vitreous cutter inserted through the main incision and the irrigation probe placed through the service incision, which may need to be enlarged. The use of a vitreous cutter is preferable as the phaco-probe cannot cut vitreous gel, causing vitreoretinal traction at the level of the vitreous base.

Even with a vitreous cutter, lower cut rate and high vacuum increase vitreous traction [6]. As showed by Teixeira et al., traction is directly correlated to the vacuum and inversely correlated to the cut rate and distance from the retina [6]. Therefore, high cut rate and lower vacuum should be preferred when performing anterior vitrectomy. This procedure may be performed with the aid of intracamerular triamcinolone, which would enhance the visibility of vitreous remnants.

Once the anterior chamber is free from vitreous, it may be useful to insert the vitreous cutter through the posterior capsule tear and to perform a limited posterior vitrectomy. This should further reduce the risk of vitreous prolapse into the anterior chamber.

If the anterior chamber is preserved, the implant of a three-piece intraocular lens may be recommended. This may guarantee the isolation of the anterior and posterior compartments of the eye and facilitates the next surgical steps, which involve a vitreoretinal approach. At the end of the procedure, it is important to check for any possible residual vitreous strain. Injection of a myotic agent like acetylcholine may be useful. A regular, reactive, and round pupil normally indicates that there is no vitreous incarceration.

However, whether to implant an IOL at the time of nucleus drop is a controversial issue. Von Lany et al. in a large survey carried out in the United Kingdom found that the primary IOL was left in situ after the secondary procedure in only 23% of eyes. In other words, approximately three quarters of the eyes in which an IOL was implanted simultaneously at the time of the complicated cataract surgery had the IOL replaced during the secondary vitreoretinal procedure [2]. In our experience, best surgical results are achieved when the anterior segment surgeon is able to implant a sulcus IOL during the first surgery so that the vitreoretinal surgeon may focus on the posterior segment only.

If there is not adequate capsular support, the strategy shifts toward a secondary intraocular lens implant (scleral-fixated versus iris-claw lenses) to be performed in a separate surgical act.

Posterior Segment

In case of dislocation of lens material into the vitreous chamber, the anterior segment surgeon should not try to pursue it with the phaco-probe. This may lead to significant retinal damage. A vitreoretinal approach via pars plana should be preferred instead [7].

However, it may not be necessary to perform a pars plana vitrectomy if the dropped fragment is small, if it is unnoticed by the patient (i.e., not involving the visual axis), and if it is not causing significant inflammation. Published research suggests performing pars plana vitrectomy for dropped nucleus fragments, which may block the visual axis, in case of lens-induced uveitis and glaucoma, size of the dropped lens fragment >2 mm or 25% of the lens size, retinal tear, and detachment due to dropped nucleus [8].

If the anterior segment surgeon is not experienced in vitreoretinal surgery, the procedure may be delayed. Until then, it is critical to manage inflammation and possible rise in intraocular pressure. Corneal edema must be controlled with the use of topical corticosteroids and intraocular pressure lowered with both topical and systemic treatment [9–11]. In such cases, topical beta-blockers and carbonic anhydrase inhibitors may be preferred to prostaglandins due to lower risk of inflammatory reactions. If needed, oral acetazolamide may also be used.

There is not a consensus regarding a precise timeframe for the vitreoretinal procedure, although an expedite procedure is likely to provide the best outcomes.

Previous evidence suggested that delayed vitrectomy may increase the incidence of retinal detachment and intraocular pressure elevation and resulted in a worse visual prognosis [12]. On the contrary, other studies have reported that there is no difference in visual acuity between early and late vitrectomy [13].

The vitreoretinal procedure is performed as follows. Complete core and peripheral vitrectomy is performed, and the dropped lens material is freed from the vitreous and mobilized. In case of soft lens and cortical material, the use of the vitreous cutter may be enough to remove it from the vitreous chamber. In such cases, low cut rate and high vacuum may be used, and the procedure is time consuming.

Importantly, if the posterior hyaloid is still attached to the retina, it is critical to achieve a complete posterior vitreous detachment. This step must be performed prior to any attempt to remove the nuclear material from the back of the eye. Intravitreal triamcinolone may be used to enhance vitreous visualization.

The popularization of microincision vitreous surgery (MIVS) has led to the use of 25-, 23-, and even 27-gauge systems for vitreous surgery that would formerly have been performed with a 20-gauge system. However, with the decrease in vitreous cutter diameter, the suction aperture in the vitreous cutters used in MIVS has also decreased, making it difficult to deal with hard fragments of nucleus that have dropped into the vitreous cavity. Further, with high-speed cuts, the duty cycle is reduced as well as the suction flow volume, lowering the efficiency of vitreous probes in removing lens fragments [14].

In our experience, 23-gauge cutters may be a good compromise in dropped nucleus surgery. A wider port may allow to remove lens material in a quicker and more efficient way if compared to 25-gauge or 27-gauge probes.

In all cases, the lens material should be divided into smaller fragments, which are moving freely into the vitreous cavity due to the intraocular currents produced by the infusion. It is challenging for the vitreoretinal surgeon to chase all the fragments as when the guillotine of the cutter is moving, the port often loses grip with the fragment, which then falls back. This problem may be partially overcome by newer double-port probes, in which the port is never occluded, granting constant aspiration flow [15].

In case of harder nucleus, the use of a phacofragmentation probe may be necessary. The disadvantage of this technique is that it requires a wider scleral incision to be inserted if a 25-G system is used, with the risk of leaks through the wider sclerotomy. In such cases, a 23-G system may be preferred as there are fragmatomes of the same size available in the market. This would allow the surgery to perform the nucleus removal through standard 23-G port.

Ultrasounds delivered directly into the vitreous chamber may increase the risk of postoperative inflammation such as cystoid macular edema [16].

Some authors advocate the use of perfluorocarbon liquids (PFCLs) as adjuvant in these kinds of surgeries [17]. The perfluorocarbon may be injected into the vitreous chamber to float the lens material up to the anterior chamber, where it can be removed by traditional phacoemulsification techniques. The perfluorocarbon liquids may also be used to protect the posterior pole from possible damage due to scattering lens fragments in motion. However, in our experience, the convex shape of the perfluorocarbon bubble may induce the lens material to displace from the center toward the periphery of the bubble, closer to the retina, where they may be challenging to chase. There is not a consensus on whether perfluorocarbon fluids may or may not be used. Previous research favors the use of PFCL for this indication, whereas others have reported comparable success without its use.

At the end of the surgery, a careful check of the retinal periphery with 360° indentation must be performed to avoid possible pre-existing or iatrogenic breaks, which may increase the risk of postoperative retinal detachment.

Take-Home Messages

- A complete removal of any vitreous remnant from the anterior chamber and the placement of a three-piece intraocular lens into the sulcus may create compartmentalization and facilitate the posterior segment surgery.
- It is important to control intraocular inflammation and to prevent corneal edema with topical and systemic anti-inflammatory drugs. Hypotensive therapy may reduce the incidence of postoperative intraocular pressure spikes and corneal edema.
- A complete posterior vitreous detachment must be achieved prior to removal of any nuclear fragment from the vitreous chamber.
- A phacofragmentation probe may be used for harder nuclear fragments. However, most of the times, smaller fragments may be removed with the aid of a 23-G cutter only.
- A careful 360° peripheral retinal examination mush be performed at the end of all cases.

References

1. Karadag R, Aydin B. Management of the dropped nuclear fragments. Br J Ophthalmol. 2013;97:2–4.
2. Von Lany H, Mahmood S, James CR, Cole MD, Charles SJ, Foot B, Gouws P, Shaw S. Displacement of nuclear fragments into the vitreous complicating phacoemulsification surgery in the UK: clinical features, outcomes and management. Br J Ophthalmol. 2008;92:493–5.
3. Narendran N, Jaycock P, Johnston RL, et al. The Cataract National Dataset electronic multicentre audit of 55,567 operations: risk stratification for posterior capsule rupture and vitreous loss. Eye (Lond). 2009;23(1):31–7.
4. Pande M, Dabbs TR. Incidence of lens matter dislocation during phacoemulsification. J Cataract Refract Surg. 1996;22:737–42.
5. Osher RH, Yu BC, Koch DD. Posterior polar cataracts. A predisposition to intraoperative posterior capsular rupture. J Cataract Refract Surg. 1990;16:157–62.
6. Teixeira A, Chong LP, Matsuoka N, et al. Vitreoretinal traction created by conventional cutters during vitrectomy. Ophthalmology. 2010;117(7):1387–92.
7. Stewart MW. Managing retained lens fragments: raising the bar. Am J Ophthalmol. 2009;147:569–70.
8. Monshizadeh R, Samiy N, Haimovici R. Management of retained intravitreal lens fragments after cataract surgery. Surv Ophthalmol. 1999;43:397–404.
9. Lai TY, Kwok AK, Yeung YS, et al. Immediate pars plana vitrectomy for dislocated intravitreal lens fragments during cataract surgery. Eye. 2005;19:1157–62.
10. Stewart MW. Management of retained lens fragments: can we improve? Am J Ophthalmol. 2007;144:445–6.
11. Kwok AK, Li KK, Lai TY, et al. Pars plana vitrectomyin the management of retained intravitreal lens fragments after cataract surgery. Clin Exp Ophthalmol. 2002;30:399–403.
12. Merani R, Hunyor AP, Playfair TJ, et al. Pars plana vitrectomy for the management of retained lens material after cataract surgery. Am J Ophthalmol. 2007;144:364–70.
13. Scott IU, Flynn HW Jr, Smiddy WE, et al. Clinical features and outcomes of pars plana vitrectomy in patients with retained lens fragments. Ophthalmology. 2003;110:1567–72.
14. Watanabe A, Tsuzuki A, Arai K, Gekka T, Tsuneoka H. Treatment of dropped nucleus with a 27-gauge twin duty cycle vitreous cutter. Case Rep Ophthalmol. 2016;7(1):44–8.
15. Pavlidis M. Two-Dimensional Cutting (TDC) vitrectome: in vitro flow assessment and prospective clinical study evaluating core vitrectomy efficiency versus standard vitrectome. J Ophthalmol. 2016;2016:3849316.
16. Chiang A, Garg SJ, Alshareef RA, Pitcher JD 3rd, Hu AY, Spirn MJ, Hsu J, Lane RG, Regillo CD, Ho AC, Schwartz SD. Removal of posterior segment retained lens material using the OZil phacoemulsification handpiece versus Fragmatome during pars plana vitrectomy. Retina. 2012;32(10):2119–26.
17. Verma L, Gogoi M, Tewari HK, Kumar A, Talwar D. Comparative study of vitrectomy for dropped nucleus with and without the use of perfluorocarbon liquid. Clinical, electrophysiological and visual field outcomes. Acta Ophthalmol Scand. 2001;79(4):354–8.

The Miscalculated IOL: Postoperative Refractive Surprise

40

Ehud I. Assia, Adi Levy, and Tal Sharon

In this chapter, we shall discuss the leading factors related to errors in IOL power calculations:

1. Preoperative measurements of the eye (axial length and keratometry).
2. Choosing the right formula (including formulas for unusual eyes).
3. Previous corneal refractive surgery (LVC and RK).
4. Toric IOLs power calculation.
5. Ocular pathologies – dry eyes, corneal ecstatic disorders, and adnexa.

Cataract surgery is the most common and one of the most successful operations in medicine.

The introduction of intraocular lenses (IOLs) 70 years ago and the improvement in IOL power calculation provided spectacle independence, for at least one focal plane, in most of the cases. In recent years, new generations of specialized "premium" lenses were developed, including toric lenses to treat corneal astigmatism and a variety of multifocal lenses such as bifocals, trifocals, and extended depth of focus (EDOF) IOLs. Today, modern cataract surgery using premium lens implantation may provide not only removal of lens opacity and clearing of the visual axis, but also to achieve emmetropia, correct corneal astigmatism, and provide optical multifocality for all practical distances – far, intermediate and near.

Not so long ago, miscalculation of IOL power was a leading cause for IOL explantation. To date, new diagnostic devices and improved fourth- and fifth- generation IOL power calculation formulas provide high precision of refractive prediction, even in eyes with high ametropia, corneal pathologies, and post-refractive surgery. Patients' expectations are accordingly increasing, and the tolerance to optical errors is decreasing [1].

Yet, occasionally, postoperative refractive surprises may still occur because of a misplaced or a miscalculated IOL. This chapter deals with the common causes of IOL miscalculation and the means to prevent it.

Supplementary Information The online version contains supplementary material available at https://doi.org/10.1007/978-3-030-94530-5_40.

E. I. Assia (✉) · T. Sharon
Center for Applied Eye Research, Department of Ophthalmology, Meir Medical Center, Kfar Saba, Israel, affiliated with the Sackler School of Medicine, Tel Aviv University, Tel Aviv, Israel

Ein-Tal Eye Center, Tel Aviv, Israel
e-mail: assia@eintal.com; assia@netvision.net.il

A. Levy
Ein-Tal Eye Center, Tel Aviv, Israel

J. L. Alió et al. (eds.), *Cataract Surgery*, Essentials in Ophthalmology,
https://doi.org/10.1007/978-3-030-94530-5_40

Preoperative Measurements of the Eye

To correctly predict the optical power needed to focus light on the retina, one should accurately estimate the effective lens position (ELP), which is theoretically deduced from axial length of the globe, anterior chamber depth, corneal features, and more [2]. Several formulas were developed to precisely forecast the ELP, each taking into account different ingredients of the measurements. Main components of these calculations are the axial length (AL) and the keratometry.

Axial Length

Half of the errors in IOL power calculation are attributed to axial length measurements error: An error of 100 μm in AL measurements leads to 0.28D of postoperative error; therefore, accurate measurements are extremely important. Though modern biometric instruments are very accurate, and technical failure is rare, errors may still occur. Common mistakes in AL measurements stem from an opaque media (e.g., when a corneal scar or opacity is present in the visual axis, in case of optically dense cataract or a significant vitreous hemorrhage), changes in intraocular media density (as in silicone oil filling the vitreous cavity), fixation errors (such as in nystagmus, significant tropias, or in a very low cooperation of the patient), detached retina, and more [3].

Optical measurement is far more accurate than ultrasonic devices, which are done by direct contact with the globe or by immersion techniques. Pressing the ultrasonic probe against the cornea may affect measurement accuracy and lead to a significant error. Current optical machines are very accurate and can measure axial length also in eyes with advanced cataract. Ultrasonic measurement, preferably by immersion, is reserved today for cases when optical devices are not available or optical measurement cannot be obtained (such as very opaque lenses), especially in short eyes [4, 5]. Sonographic measurement may be influenced not only by the pressure exerted on the globe, but also by the density and sonographic reflectivity of the media (e.g., density of cataract, silicone oil filling, etc.), probe position, gaze direction, and more. A mean difference of 0.14 mm (corresponding to 0.35 D) was found between contact and immersion ultrasonic biometry [6].

Even when measured by the most advanced optical instruments, it is highly advised to compare AL measurements of the two fellow eyes and maintain strict validation criteria. In case of a significant difference in AL between the two eyes (greater than 0.3 mm), data needs to be reconfirmed. Axial measurement should also correlate with clinical refraction to corroborate the results. An error should be suspected if there is a mismatch between axial length and refraction (a long eye and hypermetropia or short eye and myopia), or significant anisometropia previously unknown. Obviously, such a mismatch can be explained by other pathologies such as zonulolysis and forward movement of the lens or lenticular myopic shift; or because of very steep or very flat cornea, however, the accuracy of the measurement must first be confirmed. In high myopic eyes, it is important to also verify the fixation because of a possible posterior staphyloma. The fovea is then not located at the most distant point from the central cornea. If an error is suspected, axial length measurement can be rechecked using the same device to confirm repeatability; however, it is advisable to use another biometric device and compare results. Repeated results by a second biometer strongly support the validity of the measurement. Studies have shown that comparing measurement using different devices revealed almost identical results, indicating the high accuracy and repeatability of modern machines [4, 7].

In some circumstances which require extra caution, we recommend a routine policy of measuring the axial length (and keratometry) using at least two different biometers. Those include high myopia and hypermetropia, postrefractive surgery, calculation of multifocal lenses, low signal, and high anisometropia [8].

Keratometry

The cornea provides about two-thirds of the eye's refractive power. Therefore, estimating corneal power correctly has a great influence on calculating the IOL's power. When the cornea is largely spherical and curvature is within the normal scale, calculations tend to be accurate using most calculation equations. However, corneal irregularities, asymmetry, and a variety of corneal pathologies may significantly affect corneal power evaluation, especially in atypical eyes. Accuracy of corneal curvature and symmetry and regularity is important in all eyes, but it may be critical in eyes with high astigmatism or for considering advanced IOLs [9]. Browne and Osher demonstrated that multiple K readings by manual and autokeratometers reduced the number of outliers and increased the accuracy of measurement as compared to a single device measurement [10].

As a general rule, it is recommended to routinely repeat preoperative measurement by the same machine or, even better, to use two different devices in eyes with short (<21.0 mm) or long (>26.0 mm) axial length, flat (<41.0 D) or steep (> 47.0 D) K readings, high astigmatism (> 2.50 D), or high differences in axial length (> 0.3 mm), or keratometry (> 1.0 D) between two eyes.

Example: Case #1 (Fig. 40.1)
A 68-year-old woman with myopia and left eye amblyopia underwent cataract surgery in her left eye with a + 3 nuclear cataract. Preoperative biometry using Tomey OA-2000 revealed keratometry of 46.49 / 46.81 D in her right eye and 43.95 / 45.67 D in her left eye. Axial length was 25.79 mm in the right eye and 25.92 mm in the left eye. She was implanted with an IOL targeted for mild myopia in the range of −1.50 to −2.00 D. Postoperatively, the spherical equivalent on the left eye was −7.00 D! Note that the placido image on the cornea is not centered, indicating poor fixation, and the SNR is 36. On repeated biometry by the same machine, postoperatively, the axial length was 27.23 mm and the SNR was 402.

Contact lenses Failure to remove contact lenses (CL) either soft or hard, long enough before the biometry can greatly contribute to IOL miscalculation, since prolonged wear of contact lenses may have long-term effects on corneal morphology. Soft contact lenses should be removed for at least 7–10 days and rigid contact lenses should be removed for 2–4 weeks prior to keratometry; otherwise, a mistake of 1.0D and higher in IOL power prediction and toric correction is not uncommon. In one study, changes in spherical equivalent and lens toricity were demonstrated in more than one-half of the patients [11].

Example: case #2 (Fig. 40.2)
Biometry of a myopic patient was taken 2 hours after removal of soft contact lenses. Keratometric readings on the right eye: 43.63 / 45.60 D @ 124 ° and left eye: 46.30 / 46.57 D @ 157°. Two weeks after removal of the contact lenses, the keratometry values were as follows: right eye, 43.47 / 45.45 @ 122 °; left eye, 46.84 / 48.00 @ 86 °. The keratometric measurements did not change on the right eye but were 1.0 D steeper, with almost 1.0 D higher astigmatism and 70 ° shift of axis on the left eye. This demonstrates the inconsistent and unpredictable effects of contact lenses on corneal measurement and may lead to significant error in IOL power calculation.

Ocular surface and dry eye Ocular surface diseases, including dry eye, blepharitis, and meibomian glands dysfunction, are common, especially in the senile cataract age group. Many patients are often not aware of their ocular surface abnormalities and may not contribute relevant information unless asked specifically targeted questions.

Corneal topography is actually a tear film topography. Lacrimal dysfunction and poor quality of the oily layer of the tears film can be associated with surface irregularities and incorrect

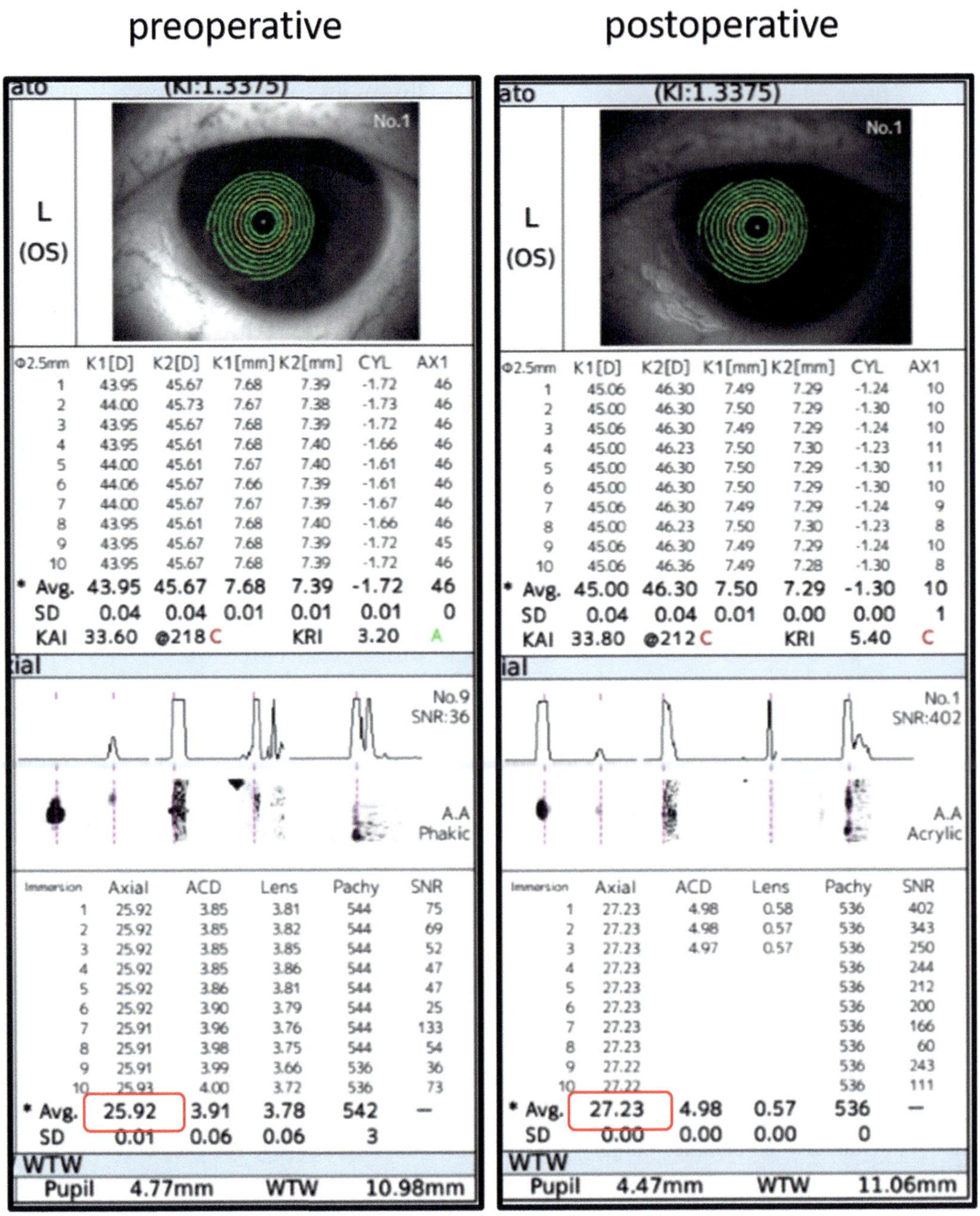

Fig. 40.1 Left eye amblyopia underwent cataract surgery

measurement of corneal surface power. The technician must keep the cornea moisture during the entire measurement and not allow it to dry when the eye is opened for more than a few seconds. Also, dry eye symptoms such as burning sensation, itching, red eye, and blurring of vision are very common following surgery and are aggravated by the postoperative inflammatory response.

Two **hours** after removal of CL

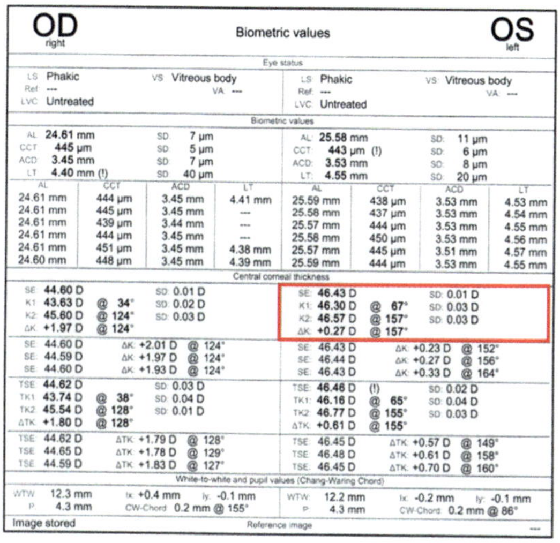

Two **weeks** after removal of CL

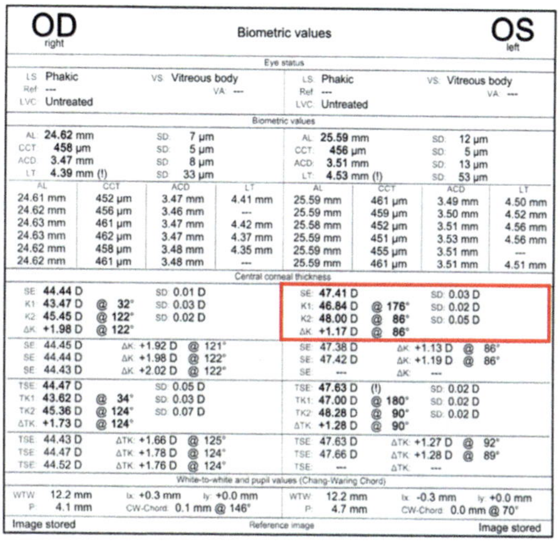

Fig. 40.2 Biometry of a myopic patient

"Dry eyes" is probably the most common complaint after surgery and often associated with unsatisfactory visual quality. This can be mistaken as incorrect IOL calculation; therefore, tear film dysfunction should be recognized preoperatively and treated aggressively.

Example # 3 (Fig. 40.3)

A patient with partially treated dry eyes was suspected of having a clinically significant astigmatism that may require toric IOL. After intensive wetting of the cornea, the measured astigmatism was significantly lower and toric lens was not required. All other parameters did not change.

Choosing the Right Formula

Third-generation formulas including SRK/T, Holladay I, and Hoffer Q provide good IOL power prediction in eyes within the normal range of axial length (22.0–24.5 mm). About 75% of all eyes fall within this category and all 3 formulas predict IOL power within 0.5 diopters of the target refraction in about 75% of the patients [12]. A source of error is utilizing the manufacturers' constants (A constant, SF, and ACD, respectively) for all eyes. Personalized modification of each constant for each IOL by each surgeon is recommended to fine-tune the IOL prediction to the specific surgical technique. The User group for Laser Interference Biometry (ULIB) provides a cumulative information of A constants reported by multiple users worldwide. This, however, should not replace the personalized fine-tuning by the individual surgeon.

Clinical experience demonstrated that the lowest mean absolute error was achieved with the Hoffer Q formula in the hyperopic group (axial length < 20.0 mm) and with the SRK/T formula for the myopic eyes (axial length > 27.0 mm). Koch adjustment further improved clinical results for high myopic eyes [12].

Fourth-generation formulae were developed in the early years of the current century and provide improved performance, especially in irregular eyes. Those include Holladay II, Haigis, Olsen, and Barrett formulas. Good predictability was reported in hyperopia using Haigis, Hoffer Q, and Holladay II formulas and in myopic eyes using Barrett Universal II, Haigis, SRK/T, and Olsen formulas [13]. Further development in recent years is recognized as the fifth generation of IOL formulas and includes the combined Hoffer H-5 formula, Hill Radial Basis Function (Hill RBF) – a machine-learned formula, the FullMonte method based on a mathematical algorithm, the Ladas Super formula, which is

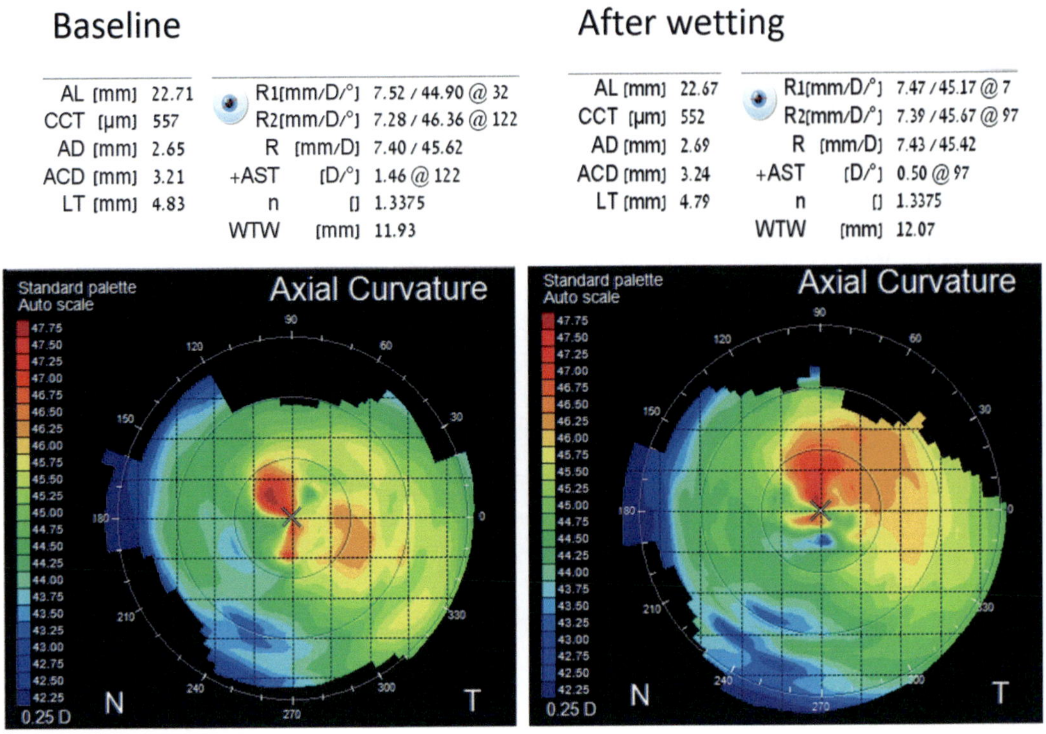

Fig. 40.3 Corneal topography

based on multiple earlier formulas, the Kane formula, which incorporates theoretical optics, regression analysis, and artificial intelligence and the Emmetropia Verifying Optical formula (EVO) based on the theory of emmetropization. Numerous studies have demonstrated the highest IOL power prediction rate using the Barrett Universal II formula for a variety of normal and abnormal eyes; however, accumulating clinical reports demonstrate equivalent results by some of the other latest formulas. Melles et al. compared the accuracy of 10 formulas including most of the fifth-generation formulas in 18,500 eyes and found that the Kane formula was the most accurate overall; however, Olsen, Barrett, EVO, and Hill RBF formulas were also highly effective [14].

The current benchmark of IOL power prediction in normal eyes is approximately 85–90% within a mean error of ±0.5 diopter. It should be noted that IOL power calculating formulas can be accurate only as much as the measurement are accurate. The common cause of wrong power calculation is often mismeasured parameters. No formula can compensate, for example, for wrong axial length measurement in a long eye with posterior staphyloma. On the other hand, accurate measurement may not suffice to precisely predict postoperative refraction in high myopic eyes. In a group of patients with axial length exceeding 26.0 mm, most formulas were adequate for IOLs of 6.0 diopters and higher; however, for IOLs lower than 6.0 diopters, only Barrett Universal II and axial length adjusted Holladay-1 and Haigis formulas yield accurate refractive results that met current benchmark criteria [7].

Steep and flat K's Most of the modern IOL power calculation formulas usually demonstrate a reasonable agreement in eyes with normal corneal curvature (around 44.0D). In eyes with steep corneas (average curvature greater than 46.0D) or flat corneas (less than 42.0D), myopic or hyperopic mistakes are much more common. Some formulas are more sensitive to the corneal effect than the others. Generally, for steep corneas, it is advisable to utilize Barrett Universal II, Haigis, Hill-RBF, Holladay 2, or Olsen-A formulas. For flat corneas, most new-generation formulas meet the benchmark criteria of up to 0.5D error [15].

All formulas calculate IOL power for in-the-bag placement. Positioning the IOL in the ciliary sulcus is often associated with slight myopia; therefore, an IOL planned for sulcus fixation should be approximately 0.5 D weaker than calculated for capsular fixation. Another cause of refractive surprise is related to capsular block syndrome and anterior displacement of the implanted IOL by ophthalmic viscosurgical device (OVD) injected to inflate the capsular bag for a safe implantation but not completely removed afterwards. The OVD may retain in the lens capsule for months and induce myopia. It can be easily evacuated by miniature Nd:YAG capsule puncture peripheral to the IOL optic, either in the anterior or posterior capsule.

Miscalculated IOL power may require additional surgical intervention such as IOL exchange, Laser Bioptics, or Piggyback IOL implantation. However, it is usually advisable to delay surgery by at least 3 months, especially in abnormal eyes such as post Laser-assisted in situ keratomileusis (LASIK) or eyes with corneal ectatic pathology. Refraction is often unstable for a long period of time and final refraction may be achieved only 3–6 months postoperatively. Also, patients may consider a – 0.75 diopters deviation from planned refraction as a catastrophe 3 days after surgery, but a comfortable compromise at 3 months postoperatively.

Previous ocular surgery may also affect postoperative refraction. Pars plana vitrectomy can be associated with a myopic surprise, most probably because of a change in the ELP, even in eyes in which ACD remained unchanged.

Previous Corneal Refractive Surgery

Laser Vision Correction

Laser refractive corneal surgeries are common, and the number of cataract patients after a previous refractive procedure is constantly increasing. Many of the patients who were operated 2–3 decades ago have now matured to develop age-related cataract. Patients with ametropia, and especially high myopia, tend to develop cataract more often and at a younger age than emmetropic patients. Many of these patients, who were willing to perform a costly eye surgery at a young age to reduce spectacle dependence, are often more demanding and have high expectations to maintain spectacle independence also after cataract surgery. On the other hand, most of the basic IOL power formulas were developed before refractive surgery was popularized. The refractive surgery changes the basic structure and anatomical relationship of the virgin corneas on which most of the power calculation formulas are based. There are generally several sources of errors: The natural relationship between the anterior and posterior corneal curvatures and between the central and paracentral corneas considerably changes during surgery; therefore, some of the basic optical assumptions of most formulas (e.g., a fixed relation between anterior and posterior corneal curvatures) are no longer valid. Using regular formulas that were developed for the normal corneas will usually result in 1–3 diopters of ametropia.

Keratometer index errors Keratometers measure anterior corneal surface and assume a constant ratio of anterior to posterior corneal curvature. Since the corneal stroma is ablated during a laser surgery, this correlation is altered. The amount of error is generally proportional to the amount of tissue ablated, leading to overestimation of the mean keratometry power. This will potentially lead to a hyperopic surprise after a myopic correction and to postoperative myopia in hyperopic correction [16, 17].

Radius errors A mistake in calculations may occur when the keratometry measurements are not taken at the center of the cornea. As the cornea is not a perfect sphere, the surface curvature, the refractive power, and the correlation between anterior and posterior surfaces change in different areas of the cornea. Following an ablative corneal surgery, these differences become much more pronounced and significant. This is especially relevant in cases of small or decentered treatments, where the corneal radius may be measured on the periphery of the treated zone, or over an irregular central cornea.

IOL formula errors Using the third-generation IOL power formulas (Hoffer Q, Holladay 1, and SRK/T) may lead to incorrect estimation of the effective lens position (ELP), thus leading to IOL miscalculation and refractive surprise. In normal eyes, corneal steepness correlates with the anterior chamber depth; that is, steep cornea usually indicates a deep anterior chamber and a flat cornea is related to a shallow anterior chamber. Following corneal refractive surgery, only the anterior cornea is flattened; thus, the K values, which are used to predict the ELP, no longer represent the eye's geometry. Using standard formulas, the "new" flat anterior corneal curvature is falsely linked to erroneous calculation of the ELP, leading to a hyperopic refractive shift in patients after myopic laser correction and a myopic shift after hyperopic correction [15–17].

Rosen et al. [18] compared 8 IOL power calculation formulas, including fourth-generation formulas, and demonstrated significant changes in predictive values over time for all formulas. They concluded that it is inadequate to evaluate the performance of IOL power formulas in less than 3 months postoperatively.

Topography Corneal topography should be done in all patients with a history of previous corneal refractive surgery. Occasionally, patients do not know if they were far-sighted or near-sighted and what kind of laser treatment they underwent. Topography or tomography maps can easily differentiate between central and peripheral flattening and localized changes in corneal thickness. They can also help detect other sources of refractive errors including instability and regression of the refractive correction, corneal ectasia, decentered ablation, etc.

Calculation of IOL power for eyes with a history of corneal refractive surgery must be done using designated formulas for post laser-refractive surgeries. Those are generally divided into two groups:

1. Formulas using previous corneal data (prior to refractive surgery) – such as Barrett True-K, Masket, modified-Masket, Adjusted Atlas 9000, etc. These formulas use the nominal anterior-posterior cornea correlation constant to estimate the original curvature of posterior cornea, by considering anterior curvature and the power corrected by the laser surgery. Until recently, these formulas were considered the gold-standard for postrefractive calculations, meeting the old benchmark of prediction errors (55% of the eyes within 0.5D and 85% within 1D from target refraction).
2. Formulas not dependent on previous data. Those include Wang-Koch-Maloney (WKM), Shammas, Haigis-L, Galilei, Potvin-Hill Pentacam, Barrett True-K (no history), and others. These formulas rely only on current (postrefractive surgery) measurements and require more detailed data, usually obtained by scheimpflug technology, such as curvature in different areas of the cornea and accurate actual corneal power. This data exhibits the true correlation between anterior and posterior corneal power and helps accurately estimate the true total corneal refractive power. Recently, it became clinically evident that the "no-history" formulas may provide an even better predictability than the "prior-data" formulas, with Barrett True-K (no history) and Haigis-L giving the best results with lowest prediction errors.

All formulas mentioned above can be easily accessed online on the ASCRS website for a free use. In general, since the calculation of postrefractive IOL power is prone to numerous mistakes and is still a significant challenge, it is highly advised to use highly reliable measurements, as many parameters as could be obtained, and averaging the results of several formulas. Additionally, a greater "security margin" with a slight deviation to the higher power (more myopic) IOLs should be considered, to avoid an unwanted hyperopic result [19, 20]. Nevertheless, mismatch between formulas is still common and postoperative refractive surprises are not rare. The importance of preoperative discussion with postrefractive patients cannot be overemphasized. A refractive error is expected in many cases and should not be regarded as a complication.

Optical results are far less than the excellent prediction we now experience in virgin eyes (approximately 90% within ±0.50D). It is therefore debatable whether multifocal IOLs should be used in patients after refractive surgery. Since emmetropia cannot be guaranteed, patients may still require spectacle optical correction for quality vision and would not benefit from the main advantages of the multifocal IOL, namely, spectacle independence. Moreover, changes in corneal stroma, corneal haze, or scars may further aggravate photic phenomena such as glare, halos, and decreased contrast sensitivity. Many surgeons are currently reluctant to use multifocal IOLs in patients after refractive laser correction and the debate is expected to intensify within the next years [16–21].

Prior Radial Keratectomy (RK)

Calculating IOL power after radial keratectomy (RK) may be even more challenging than the calculation for postlaser ablation surgery. Manual keratectomy is a far less accurate procedure as compared to the high precision of automated, topography-guided laser surgery. Surgical results are affected by the number of keratectomies, length and depth of the incisions, and the distance from corneal center. In contrast to ablation procedures, the relationship between anterior and posterior corneas is preserved (since no stroma was removed); therefore, ELP calculation is less of a problem. However, the surgical results are much less predictable and irregular astigmatism is quite common. Optical stability is a major concern and refraction may keep changing even years after the procedure in matters of days and even hours. Moreover, cataract surgery in these eyes is challenging since intraoperative and postoperative complications are not uncommon, as radial cuts are prone to rupture even years after the RK surgery, which may require suturing of the corneal wound, and affect final refraction. In addition, cornea may decompensate, and refractive fluctuations may aggravate following a cataract removal. Many surgeons prefer using a scleral tunnel to avoid tension on the weakened corneal cuts; however, corneal rupture may still occasionally occur, especially during IOL implantation. Clear corneal incisions can be done in between previous radial cuts when only 4 or 8 keratotomy incisions have been made; however, the main incision should never intersect a previous radial cut. The surface of the anterior cornea is often scarred, leading to a clinical irregular and asymmetrical astigmatism. Surgical correction of the astigmatism using toric lenses is unpredictable and often not practical.

Toric lenses can be considered for high astigmatism in eyes with a relatively regular and symmetrical topographic pattern. Multifocal lenses, including extended depth of focus lenses, are usually contraindicated after RK surgery [17, 20, 21].

Example: case #4 (Fig. 40.4)
A 53-year-old man had BCVA of 0.4 LogMAR and nuclear cataract in his left eye and underwent 4-cuts radial keratotomy and 2-cuts astigmatic keratotomy many years earlier. Corneal astigmatism of 3.00 D against-the-rule was demonstrated on corneal topography with no component of posterior corneal astigmatism. Because of the regular and relatively symmetric anterior corneal astigmatism, a toric SN6AT8 IOL was implanted. At 1 month, his corrected vision (−0.25–0.50 × 137°) was 0.18 LogMAR. Toric IOLs can be used in selected cases also following RK.

Toric IOLs

Refractive surprises after toric IOL implantation are not uncommon. Toric calculation is multifactorial and can be significantly affected by corneal symmetry and regularity, surgical technique, and IOL rotational stability. Comparing different measurement devices and toric calculators Abulafia et al. [22] found that the combination of Barrett toric calculator and optical low-coherence reflectometry (Lenstar LS 900) provided the most accu-

Preoperative corneal tomography

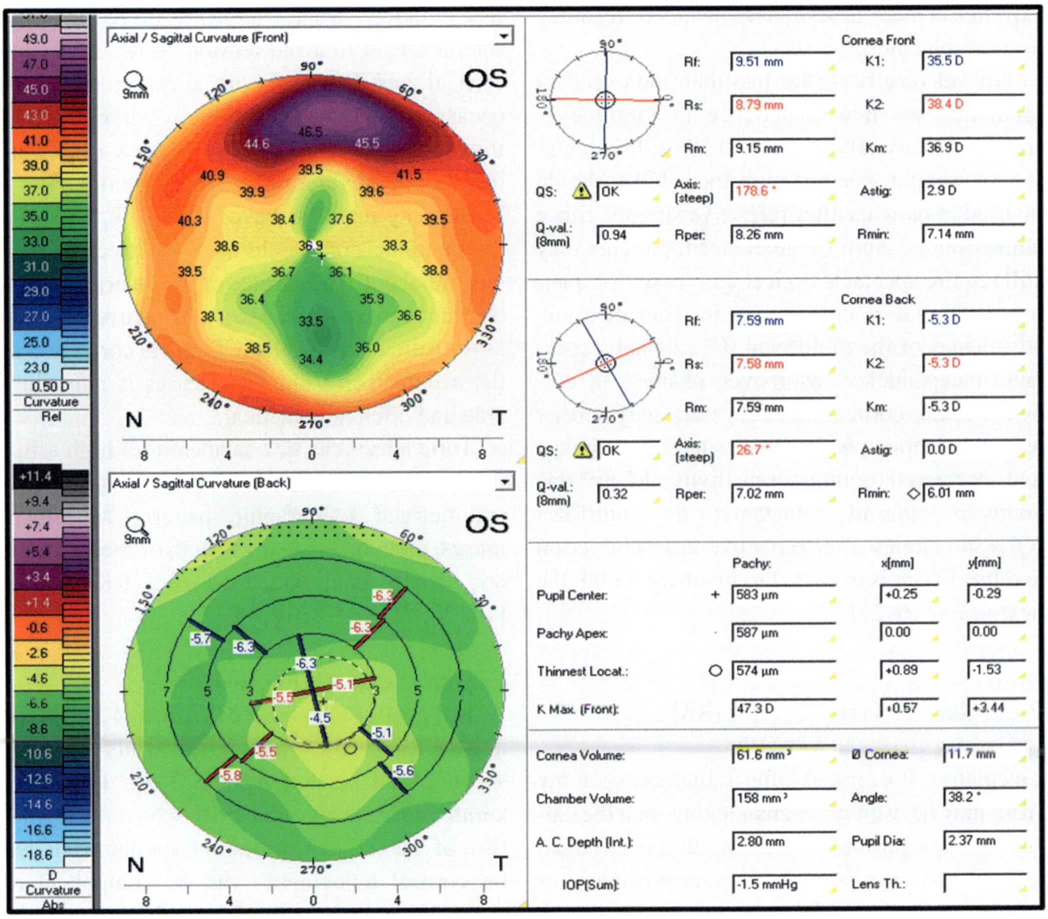

Fig. 40.4 Corneal astigmatism – on corneal topography Please query all caption in proof

rate results; however, they compared the Lenstar to the older version of the IOL Master 500. Using the IOL Master 700, Kurian et al. found measurement accuracy at least similar to the Lenstar in terms of agreement and repeatability [23].

Surgically induced astigmatism (SIA) can be influenced by various factors, including location (in meridians and distance from limbus), size, and architecture of the cataract main incision. It is also affected by the preoperative corneal astigmatism, corneal thickness, and probably by individual biological properties and scarring response. Recognizing personal SIA is mandatory for toric IOL power calculation; however, studies suggest that its significance is lower than previously considered, especially in small incision surgery.

Posterior corneal astigmatism The total refractive power of the cornea is the difference between the anterior corneal power and the posterior corneal power. Whereas normally, calculations take into consideration the average difference between anterior and posterior cornea, in some cases, mostly when calculating a toric correction, this correlation might introduce an erroneous result, which may lead to overcorrection (in cases of with-the-rule (WTR) astigmatism) or undercorrection (in the case of against-the-rule (ATR) astigmatism). Recent study proved this is less of an issue in oblique astigmatism [24]. Measuring the posterior corneal astigmatism is part of the routine biometric evaluation by some biometers or can be measured by scheimpflug or OCT tomography and manually inserted to a toric power calculator [25]. Normal corneas typically shift toward ATR astigmatism with time; therefore, it is generally advised to undercorrect preoperative WTR astigmatism and overcorrect ATR astigmatism (and shift axis to slight WTR astigmatism). Koch et al. suggested the Baylor toric IOL nomogram to calculate toric correction in eyes with WTR / ATR astigmatism [26]. Reitblat et al. compared methods to consider posterior corneal curvature and found that a method based on vector summation of both anterior and posterior astigmatism provided the best median simulated residual astigmatism [27].

Intraoperative aberrometry can help surgeons corroborate or fine-tune IOL power in challenging cases such as long and short eyes, eyes with keratoconus (KC), or following laser vision correction. This is especially valuable for toric lenses in these challenging eyes. In case of discrepancy between preoperative calculations and intraoperative aberrometry, many surgeons recommend to err on the side of the intraoperative measurement.

IOL misalignment, which may result from inaccurate preoperative prediction of the axis of IOL alignment, from failure to implant the IOL in the accurate meridian or postoperative rotation of the IOL (usually within first postoperative hours to days), can be one of the main reasons for postoperative refractive error and of suboptimal visual outcomes after toric IOL implantation. One degree of misalignment causes a loss of approximately 3% of the effective cylinder power, and the entire toric effect is lost in cases of 30° of misalignment [28]. Optimal timing for surgical correction of misaligned toric IOL is usually between 1 week and 1 month. Earlier rotation may result in a repeated IOL rotation, whereas a later surgery may require surgical release of adhesions between the anterior and posterior capsules and may risk capsular integrity.

Ocular Pathologies

Keratoconus and Other Ectatic Disorders

Ectatic diseases of the cornea, the most common of which is keratoconus (KC), are characterized by weakening of the collagenous stroma, resulting in irregular steepening and thinning of the cornea. Surgical intervention performed in advanced cases such as collagen cross-linking, intrastromal corneal ring segment, lamellar or penetrating corneal transplant, etc., may further add to the irregularity of the corneal curvature.

The common error in IOL Power calculation for eyes with KC is typically toward a hyperopic result, and the offset is generally larger in eyes with a more severe disease. Using the total corneal refractive power (anterior and posterior), rather than measurements of the anterior surface only, may improve calculation precision ability. The preferred location of the corneal measurements is still not clear because of the shift of the steep curvature away from the optical center in the visual axis. Various formulas suggest modifications for KC eyes; however, according to a recent review by Ghiasian et al. in 2019, SRK II formula provided the best accuracy in eyes with mild keratoconus [29]. A literature review by Garzon et al. in 2020 suggests that SRK/T provided the best outcome [30]; however, the newest fourth and fifth generations were not tested and may further improve IOL power prediction.

Incision location may also affect postoperative astigmatism and corneal stability. Some surgeons advocate scleral tunnel also in KC eyes. In advanced cases, corneal transplant is a valid option at some point of time. In these eyes, using an average corneal curvature for IOL power calculation has been proposed.

Toric correction of the high astigmatism characteristic of KC is currently being recognized as highly effective in selected cases with relatively regular corneal pattern and acceptable symmetry. Several studies have demonstrated a significant reduction of preoperative astigmatism (ranging between 2 to 7 diopters) to an average of 1.0 diopter. This is less than the results obtained in non-KC eyes; however, in most patients, an effective final corrected visual acuity of 0.2–0.3 LogMAR was achieved [31, 32]. In our personal experience in a series of 38 selected eyes of 26 patients implanted with toric IOLs, 76% of patients achieved 0.3 LogMAR (6/12) uncorrected distance vision and 92% achieved 0.3 LogMAR best distant corrected vision [33].

Other Corneal and Ocular Pathologies

Pterygium (an elastotic change of the conjunctival and corneal tissues), Salzman's nudules, corneal dystrophies, and other corneal lesions and diseases may influence corneal surface, refractive power, and astigmatism and may also cause difficulty in keratometry. Thus, corneal lesions may cause unexpected refractive surprises and residual astigmatism, especially if corneal abnormality progresses after IOL implantation. Therefore, it is preferable to first treat any corneal pathology as needed prior to cataract surgery. After removal of the lesion, the astigmatism is likely to change (both in power and axis), and accordingly the toric power calculation. Keratometry and biometric measurements should be performed only after corneal stabilization, and no changes are recorded in repeated measurements. This is usually achieved after 3 months from corneal surgery. Corneal dystrophies, such as map-dot-fingerprint surface dystrophy, must also be recognized and addressed prior to biometry. Corneal astigmatism of as much as 4 diopters may be evident when the pathology is apical; however, the astigmatism vanishes following superficial keratectomy. Salzmann's nodules should be scraped 2–3 months prior to keratometry. IOL power calculation is done only after K readings are stable and consistent.

Some extraocular conditions, such as ptosis, eyelids lesions (such as tumors or chalazia), meibomian dysfunction, palpebral conjunctival papillae, and others, may affect corneal topography and may lead to misinterpretation of keratometry. As a general rule, eyelid pathology should be addressed and treated before cataract surgery (and long enough before measurements) in order to avoid errors and surprises [34–36].

Conclusion

Miscalculation of IOL power and postoperative surprises are uncommon using modern technology and advanced IOL power calculation formulas. Improved prediction can be achieved by practicing strict validation criteria and double check of measurements in any case of doubt. Premium lenses such as toric and multifocal lenses require extra caution, and retrieval of more data is recommended. Calculation of IOL following refractive surgery is complex, but excellent results can be achieved using specialized new formulas. Nevertheless, prediction error may still occur, and surgeons should recognize means to diagnose and manage postoperative surprises.

Take-Home Messages

- Validation criteria of preoperative measurements should be carefully maintained, especially for premium IOLs. Multiple measurements by different devices increase accuracy.
- Using modern formulas (fourth to fifth generations) in normal and unusual eyes provides high power prediction rate (current benchmark approximates 90% within ±0.5D).
- In eyes following refractive surgery, only designated formulas should be used to calculate IOL power.
- Toric power calculation should consider surgically induced astigmatism and posterior corneal curvature, especially in eyes with keratoconus.
- Dry eyes and other ocular pathologies may lead to significant prediction errors unless properly managed.

Financial Disclosure Ehud I Assia MD: Hanita Lenses, Biotechnology General, Vision Care Technologies, APX Ophthalmology, IOPtima, VisiDome, CorNeat.

Adi Levy: None.

Tal Sharon: None.

References

1. Olson RJ. Perspective – cataract surgery from 1918 to the present and future—just imagine! Am J Ophthalmol. 2018;185:10–3.
2. Yoo YS, Whang WJ, Kim HS, Joo CK, Yoon G. Preoperative biometric measurements with anterior segment optical coherence tomography and prediction of postoperative intraocular lens position. Medicine. 2019;98:50.
3. Lee D, Kim M, Kim WJ, Kim MM. Changes in refractive error and axial length after horizontal muscle surgery for strabismus. J AAPOS. 2019;23:20.
4. Dong J, Zhang Y, Zhang H, Jia Z, Zhang S, Wang X. Comparison of axial length, anterior chamber depth and intraocular lens power between IOLMaster and ultrasound in normal, long and short eyes. PLoS One. 2018;2018:13(3).
5. Haigis W, Lege B, Miller N, Schneider B. Comparison of immersion ultrasound biometry and partial coherence interferometry for intraocular lens calculation according to Haigis. Graefes Arch Clin Exp Ophthalmol. 2000;238:765–73.
6. Olsen T, Nielsen PJ. Immersion versus contact technique in the measurement of axial length by ultrasound. Acta Ophthalmol. 1989;67(1):101–2.
7. Abulafia A, Barrett GD, Rotenberg M, Kleinmann G, Levy A, Reitlat O, Koch DD, Wang L, Assia EI. Intraocular lens power calculation for eyes with an axial length greater than 26.0 mm: comparison of formulas and methods. J Cat Refract Surg. 2015;41(3):548–56.
8. Reitblat O, Assia EI, Kleinmann G, Levy A, Barrett G, Abulafia A. Accuracy of predicted refraction with multifocal IOLs using two biometry measurement devices and multiple IOL power calculation formulas. Clin Exp Ophthalmol. 2015;43(4):328–49.
9. Ofir S, Abulafia A, Kleinmann G, Reitblat O, Assia EI. Surgically induced astigmatism assessment: comparison between three corneal measuring devices. J Refract Surg. 2015;31(4):244–7.
10. Browne AW, Osher RH. Optimizing precision in Toric lens selection by combining keratometry techniques. J Refract Surg. 2014;30(1):67–72.
11. Meyer JJ, Kim MJ, Kim T. Effects of contact lens Wear on biometry measurements for intraocular lens calculations, eye and contact lens 2017. Eye Contact Lens. 2018;44(Suppl 1):S255–8.
12. Siddiqui AA, Devgan U. Intraocular lens calculations in atypical eyes. Indian J Ophthalmol. 2017;65:1289–93.
13. Hoffer KJ, Savini G. IOL power calculation in short and long eyes. Asia-Pac J Ophthalmol. 2017;6:330–1.
14. Melles RB, Kane JX, Olsen T, Chang WJ. Update on intraocular lens calculation formulas. Ophthalmology. 2019;126(9):1334–5.
15. Reitblat O, Levy A, Kleinmann G, Lerman TT, Assia EI. Intraocular lens power calculation for eyes with high and low average keratometry readings: comparison between various formulas. J Cataract Refract Surg. 2017;43(9):1149–56.
16. Savini G, Hoffer KJ. Intraocular lens power calculation in eyes with previous corneal refractive surgery. Eye Vision. 2018;5:18.
17. Abulafia A, Hill WE, Wang L, Reitblat O, Koch DD. Intraocular lens power calculation in eyes after laser in situ keratomileusis or photorefractive keratectomy for myopia. Asia Pac J Ophthalmol (Phila). 2017;6(4):332–8.
18. Rosen DB, Heiland MB, Tingey M, Liu HY, Kang P, Buckner B, Ronquillo YC, Hoopes PC, Moshirfar M. Intraocular lens calculation after refractive surgery: a long-term retrospective comparison of eight formulas. Med Hypothesis Discov Innov Ophthalmol. 2019;8(3):121–8.
19. von Mohrenfels W, Gabler B, Lohmann CP. Optical biometry before and after excimer laser epithelial keratomileusis (LASEK) for myopia. Eur J Ophthalmol. 2003;13(3):257–9.
20. Seitz B, Langenbucher A. Intraocular lens calculations status after corneal refractive surgery. Curr Opin Ophthalmol. 2000;11:35–46.
21. Montes de Oca I, Gokce SE, Hallahan K, Wang L, Koch DD. IOL calculations in short, long, and postrefractive eyes. Int Ophthalmol Clin. 2016;56(3):49–70.
22. Abulafia A, Barrett GD, Kleinmann G, Ofir S, Levy A, Marcovich AL, Michaeli A, Koch DD, Wang L, Assia EI. Prediction of refractive outcomes with toric intraocular lens implantation. J Cataract Refract Surg. 2015;41(5):936–44.
23. Kurian M, Negalur N, Das S, Puttaiah NK, Haria D, Tejal SJ, Thakkar MM. Biometry with a new swept-source optical coherence tomography biometer: repeatability and agreement with an optical low-coherence reflectometry device. J Cataract Refract Surg. 2016;42:577–81.
24. Sheen Ophir S, LaHood B, Goggin M. Refractive outcome of toric intraocular lens calculation in cases of oblique anterior corneal astigmatism. J Cataract Refract Surg. 2020;46:688–93.
25. Koch DD, Ali SF, Weikert MP, Shirayama M, Jenkins R, Wang L. Contribution of posterior corneal astigmatism to total corneal astigmatism. J Cataract Refract Surg. 2012;38:2080–7.
26. Koch DD, Jenkins RB, Weikert MP, Yeu E, Wang L. Correcting astigmatism with toric intraocular lenses: effect of posterior corneal astigmatism. J Cataract Refract Surg. 2013;39:1803–9.
27. Reitblat O, Levy A, Kleinmann G, Abulafia A, Assia EI. Effect of posterior corneal astigmatism on power

calculation and alignment of toric intraocular lenses: comparison of methodologies. J Cataract Refract Surg. 2016;42:217–25.
28. Kaur M, Shaikh F, Falera R, Titiyal JS. Optimizing outcomes with toric intraocular lenses. Indian J Ophthalmol. 2017;65:1301–13.
29. Ghiasian L, Abolfathzadeh N, Manafi N, Hadavandkhani A. Intraocular lens power calculation in keratoconus; a review of literature. J Curr Ophthalmol. 2019;31:127–34.
30. Garzón N, Arriola-Villalobos P, Felipe G, Poyales F, Garcıa-Montero M. Intraocular lens power calculation in eyes with keratoconus. J Cataract Refract Surg. 2020;46:778–83.
31. Alió JL, Peña-García P, Guliyeva FA, Soria FA, Zein G, Abu-Mustafa SK. MICS with toric intraocular lenses in keratoconus: outcomes and predictability analysis of postoperative refraction. Br J Ophthalmol. 2014;98(3):365–70.
32. Mol IE, Van Dooren BT. Toric intraocular lenses for correction of astigmatism in keratoconus and after corneal surgery. Clin Ophthalmol. 2016;10:1153–9.
33. Ton Y, Barrett G, Kleinmann G, Levy A. Assia EI: Toric intraocular lens power calculation in cataract patients with keratoconus. J Cataract Refract Surg. 2021;1:47(11):1389–97.
34. Jin KW, Shin YJ, Hyon Y. Effects of chalazia on corneal astigmatism large-sized chalazia in middle upper eyelids compress the cornea and induce the corneal astigmatism. BMC Ophthalmol. 2017;17:36.
35. Bagheri A, Hasani HR, Karimian F, Abrishami M, Yazdani S. Effect of chalazion excision on refractive error and corneal topography. Eur J Ophthalmol. 2009;19(4):521–6.
36. Savino G, Battendieri R, Riso M, Traina S, Poscia A, D'Amico G, Caporossi A. Corneal topographic changes after eyelid ptosis surgery. Cornea. 2016;35:501–5.

MIGS in Special Cases

41

John Liu, Jingyi Ma, Jeb Alden Ong, and Iqbal Ike Ahmed

Bullet Points

In this chapter, we will discuss the following:

- The coincident problem of glaucoma and age-related cataract.
- Common microinvasive glaucoma surgery (MIGS) devices.
- The effects of cataract surgery alone on lowering intraocular pressure.
- The effect of phacoemulsification and MIGS on endothelial cell density.
- Efficacy of combined cataract extraction with filtering surgery compared with standalone filtering surgery.

Introduction

Glaucoma is the leading cause of irreversible blindness worldwide, and significantly increases in prevalence with age across all ethnic groups [1–3] With a rapidly aging population, the prevalence of glaucoma is expected to increase by 50% from 2020 to 2040 [2]. The current prevalence of glaucoma is 3.5% in people between 40 and 80 years of age [4], while the prevalence of cataracts varies from 3.9% in people aged 55–64 years of age to 92.6% in people ≥ 80 years of age [5]. Given these trends and the association of these conditions together, ophthalmologists will likely face the coincident problem of treating age-related cataract and glaucoma within the same patient and potentially the combined surgical treatment of these conditions together. In treating glaucoma and preventing progression of the disease, lowering intraocular pressure (IOP) is a mainstay of therapy, whether that is accomplished medically or surgically. Effective IOP control can slow glaucoma progression and reduce further visual field loss [6, 7].

A recent major development in glaucoma surgery is a new class of devices called microinvasive glaucoma surgery (MIGS) [8]. MIGS is a group of surgical procedures that are conjunctival sparing, minimally traumatic, and increase aqueous humor outflow by directly accessing Schlemm's canal, or by redirecting fluid from the anterior chamber to the suprachoroidal or subconjunctival space [9]. A meta-analysis showed that MIGS was effective in lowering both IOP and medication burden, with a good safety profile [10]. Given their ab interno approach, MIGS can

Supplementary Information The online version contains supplementary material available at [https://doi.org/10.1007/978-3-030-94530-5_41].

J. Liu (✉) · J. Ma · J. A. Ong · I. I. Ahmed
Department of Ophthalmology and Vision Sciences, Faculty of Medicine, University of Toronto, Toronto, ON, Canada
e-mail: ike@prismeye.ca

J. L. Alió et al. (eds.), *Cataract Surgery*, Essentials in Ophthalmology,
https://doi.org/10.1007/978-3-030-94530-5_41

easily be combined with cataract surgery by utilizing the same clear corneal incision that would be created for phacoemulsification.

In this chapter, we will present the utility of three common MIGS devices in the cataract population, discuss the IOP-lowering effects of cataract surgery alone, as well as touch upon the effect of combined phaco-MIGS on endothelial cell density. Lastly, we will review the efficacy data of combining cataract extraction with filtering surgery versus filtering surgery alone. Table 41.1 at the end of this chapter outlines a brief summary of different MIGS devices available.

Table 41.1 A comparison of microinvasive glaucoma surgery (MIGS) devices

MIGS device	Company	Year commercial use began	Pros	Cons	Level of evidence[a]
Schlemm canal					
iStent	Glaukos	2012 – iStent trabecular micro-bypass 2018 – iStent inject 2020 – iStent inject-W	Excellent safety outcomes Versatile and efficient procedure Shorter learning curve Multiple iStents can be injected for additional IOP-lowering effect	Small device may be prone to under- or overimplantation When using multiple, should ideally be placed apart, which can be technically demanding Less efficacy than subconjunctival approaches	Level I (various randomized controlled trials have demonstrated efficacy)
Hydrus	Ivantis	2018	Excellent safety outcomes Potential for greater IOP reduction with single implant Single implant access >3 clock-hours of distal outflow	Larger device may reduce some of the versatility in different eye anatomies Less efficacy than subconjunctival approaches	Level I (various randomized controlled trials have demonstrated efficacy.)
Kahook dual blade	New World medical	2015	Nonimplant approach	Higher risk of intraoperative and postoperative hyphema Less efficacy than subconjunctival approaches	Level II (evidence from well-designed trials without randomization)
Subconjunctival					
XEN-45 gel stent	Allergan	2017	Allows for implantation without conjunctival/tenons dissection Demonstrated similar efficacy to trabeculectomy	Risks inherent to bleb-forming procedures, such as blebitis and hypotony-related complications High postoperative needling rates.	Level II (evidence from well-designed trials without randomization)
Preserflo microshunt	Santen	2021	Promising efficacy results in treating primary and refractory glaucoma	Ab externo approach requiring conjunctival/tenons dissection Risks inherent to bleb-forming procedures, such as blebitis and hypotony-related complications Newer device with less evidence available	Level II (evidence from well-designed trials without randomization)

[a]Roughly adapted from the US Preventive Services Task Force (USPSTF) definitions of levels of evidence

iStent

The iStent (Glaukos, San Clemente, CA) is an ab interno trabecular microbypass stent that has been demonstrated to effectively and safely reduce intraocular pressure when implanted alone, or in combination with phacoemulsification. It is a heparin-coated, nonferromagnetic titanium device first approved by the US Food and Drug Administration (FDA) in June 2012 [11], and has since quickly gained popularity. A study evaluating long-term data of combined cataract surgery with iStent implantation demonstrated a significant IOP decrease of 3.16 ± 3.9 mmHg after 53 months of follow-up, with good safety outcomes and no serious adverse events related to iStent implantation [12]. Various randomized controlled trials (RCTs) ranging from 12 to 24 months of follow-up have all demonstrated a statistically significant reduction in mean IOP and number of pressure-lowering medications when undergoing combined phacoemulsification with iStent implantation compared to phacoemulsification only, with comparable safety profiles [13–16]. Multiple iStents can also be implanted in a single eye at once to allow titration to achieve target pressure [17]. Currently, there are several iterations of the iStent that exist on the market: the original iStent trabecular microbypass stent and the iStent inject, which is slowly being replaced by the iStent inject W.

Hydrus Microstent

The Hydrus Microstent (Ivantis, Irvine CA) is an ab interno Schlemm's canal MIGS device designed to enhance aqueous outflow into Schlemm's canal and into the distal outflow system. It is an 8-mm flexible, nonluminal open structure, made from nitinol (55% nickel, 45% titanium alloy), and first received FDA approval in 2018 for its use in combination with phacoemulsification [18]. Various prospective and retrospective studies have demonstrated the Hydrus to lower IOP ranging from 2.8 mmHg to 9.0 mmHg from a baseline IOP at a follow-up ranging from 12 to 24 months in both standalone cases and when combined with phacoemulsification with a good safety profile [18–22]. A few RCTs have demonstrated similar efficacy and, when compared to similar RCTs performed for the iStent, imply that the Hydrus may result in greater complete success with less medication dependence and a similar safety profile compared to the iStent inject [23–26]. A 2019 review of the Hydrus microstent concluded that it is able to reproducibly lower IOP to the mid-high teens and reduce medication burden. However, long-term efficacy of the Hydrus will be required to further determine its position along the continuum of glaucoma management [18].

Kahook Dual Blade

The Kahook Dual Blade (KDB, New World Medical, Rancho Cucamonga, CA) is a goniotomy blade introduced in 2015 that is designed to achieve almost complete removal of the trabecular meshwork (TM) through a minimally invasive approach, in order to minimize surrounding tissue damage. In contrast to gonioscopy-assisted transluminal trabeculotomy (GATT) and the trabectome, KDB has less residual trabecular meshwork leaflets and is thought to lead to less fibrosis overtime, thereby producing better long-term outcomes [27]. Additionally, it is a single-use disposable surgical instrument with no implant related risks.

Since its introduction, several studies have assessed its effectiveness in intraocular pressure (IOP) reduction, whether alone or in combination with phacoemulsification. Dorairaj et al. conducted a prospective multicenter study of 52 eyes that underwent KDB combined with phacoemulsification [28]. At 1 year, they found an IOP reduction of 26.2% ($p < 0.001$). Additionally, 63.5% of patients used at least one fewer IOP-lowering medications. Similarly, Greenwood et al. found that 58.3% of patients achieved at least 20% IOP reduction and 61.7% had at least one medication reduction at 6 months [29]. In a retrospective study assessing the efficacy and safety of KDB at 18 months, 93 eyes underwent phaco-KDB and 23 eyes underwent standalone KDB [30]. There was no statistically significant difference in IOP between the two cohorts at 18 months (standalone 14.4 +/− 3.7 vs. combined 16.7 +/− 7.6, $p = 0.5$). In terms of medication use, the combined group had a significantly lower number of drops (1.3 +/− 1.2 vs. 3.3 +/− 1.2, $p < 0.05$). However, this difference also existed at baseline (2.4 +/− 1.2 vs. 2.9 +/− 1.0, $p < 0.05$). A larger retrospective study of 197 eyes also compared outcomes of standalone KDB ($n = 32$) to phaco-KDB ($n = 165$) at 1 year. Surgical success was defined as at least 20% IOP reduction from baseline. This was achieved in 68.8% of eyes in the standalone KDB cohort and in 71.8% in the phaco-KDB cohort (no p-value given). Both groups also showed a significant IOP and medication reduction from baseline.

Cataract Extraction and Effect on Intraocular Pressure

It has been shown that cataract surgery in glaucoma patients can reduce intraocular pressure (IOP). However, the extent of IOP reduction and the value of cataract surgery as a treatment option to lower IOP is dependent on a few different factors. A 2017 systematic review of 32 studies examined IOP change at a final follow-up period of 12 months or longer in eyes with open-angle glaucoma (OAG), chronic angle-closure glaucoma (ACG), and pseudoexfoliation glaucoma (PXG). It revealed that IOP reduction following cataract extraction in ACG resulted in a decrease of 6.4 mmHg (95% CI: 9.4 to 3.4), while for OAG, it resulted in a decrease of 2.7 mmHg (95% CI: 3.7 to 1.7). For PXG, an IOP drop of 5.8 mmHg (95% CI: 9.5 to 2.0) was determined, but it was acknowledged that further research was required to arrive at an adequate conclusion as this was only based on four studies [31]. It concluded that overall, the effect of cataract surgery on IOP reduction is marked in ACG, moderate in PXG, and small in OAG.

Cataract Extraction and Angle Closure Glaucoma

IOP reduction is more significant in eyes with narrow or closed angles compared to eyes with open angles; as a result, cataract surgery is acknowledged as a valuable glaucoma intervention for those with ACG. Cataract surgery in ACG will deepen the anterior chamber and open the angle [32–35]. In particular, the EAGLE study, which randomized both primary angle closure (PAC) and primary angle closure glaucoma (PACG) patients to receive either clear-lens extraction or standard care with laser peripheral iridotomy and topical medications, concluded that clear-lens extraction was more cost effective and showed greater efficacy. More specifically, lens extraction demonstrated an additional mean IOP reduction of 1.18 mmHg lower versus peripheral iridotomy [36]. This purported clear-lens extraction to be a viable first-line treatment option for PAC and PACG patients. In eyes that have had a history of acute angle closure, the IOP reduction is even greater. A study that compared treatment with cataract surgery against peripheral iridotomy in patients after acute angle closure showed that the mean IOP for those who received cataract surgery was 12.6 ± 1.9 mmHg for the cataract surgery group versus 15.0 ± 3.4 mmHg for the peripheral iridotomy group. Additionally, at 18 months, only 3% of the cataract surgery group developed an IOP rise postoperatively (defined as IOP > 21 mmHg) versus 46.7% in the LPI group [32]. The IOP-lowering effect of phacoemulsification in angle closure cases is likely secondary to reopening of the angle and allowing for outflow via the conventional pathway.

Cataract Extraction and Pseudoexfoliation Glaucoma

Additionally, in eyes with PXG, cataract extraction has also been shown to significantly reduce

IOP. One study showed that the mean IOP dropped from 17.45 ± 3.32 mmHg to 12.57 ± 1.58 mmHg in eyes with PXG after cataract surgery [37]. Pseudoexfoliative material accumulates in the trabecular meshwork, thereby reducing aqueous humor outflow, and can subsequently increase intraocular pressure and lead to glaucoma. With the removal of the lens as well as the central anterior capsule, pseudoexfoliative matter and pigment release is thought to be significantly reduced. There is also likely to be a "washout" effect of fibrillar material during the surgery itself [38, 39].

Despite the purported benefits of cataract surgery in PXG, it is important to remember that these eyes are at increased risk of complications due to the higher incidence of zonular weakness. However, with proper preoperative detection and careful examination for donesis, the astute surgeon can plan accordingly in order to maximize good surgical outcome [38].

Cataract Extraction and Open Angle Glaucoma

The relatively modest reduction in IOP after cataract surgery in OAG has resulted in debate on its value as a glaucoma procedure for eyes with open angles and no pseudoexfoliation syndrome [40]. A 2002 meta-analysis found that cataract extraction usually reduced IOP by 2–4 mmHg; however, the evidence was graded as "weak" as there were no randomized clinical trials and no untreated control groups among the studies [41]. Criticism of using cataract surgery as a treatment method for open angle glaucoma arises from the fact that the studies are often retrospective and many use only a single pressure measurement for the preoperative value. Additionally, many of the studies did not include gonioscopy, which lends to the possibility that angle closure cases had been unintentionally included [40].

Although the mechanism for lowered IOP in ACG and PXG is more straightforward, the mechanism for patients with open angles is poorly understood [42]. A few mechanisms have been proposed for how IOP is lowered in open angle glaucoma. It has been suggested that phacoemulsification increases the postoperative aqueous outflow facility, and cultured trabecular meshwork cells have been found to release interleukins and tumor necrosis factors. This could cause increased synthesis of matrix metalloproteinases in the trabecular meshwork [43].

Despite this modest IOP-lowering effect, there are other reasons why one may choose to perform cataract surgery early in glaucomatous patients – especially if they are at high risk of eventually needing glaucoma surgery. It is well known that glaucoma surgery can cause a cataract to mature soon after. Intraocular lens power calculations and astigmatism correction are also less accurate in situations of hypotony following glaucoma surgery and cataract surgery after a filtering bleb can increase risk of infections. Cataract surgery post filtration surgery can also have deleterious effects on bleb health. As a result, although IOP reduction is modest in eyes with open angle glaucoma, there could be a multitude of reasons why a surgeon would elect to perform cataract surgery early in a glaucomatous patient [40].

Furthering Our Understanding

Clearly, the amount of IOP reduction in patients after cataract surgery varies based on the type of glaucomatous disease, with particular attention to angle anatomy and the existence of pseudoexfoliation syndrome – although it is unclear if there other factors that come into play as well. Increasing evidence has suggested that the magnitude of IOP reduction following cataract extraction has been shown to be positively correlated to the elevation of preoperative IOP. However, it has also been argued that this could be accounted for due to the statistical phenomenon of regression toward the mean [42]. Additionally, a method for predicting the degree of IOP reduction has been proposed based on a ratio of the preoperative IOP and anterior chamber depth (ACD), measured in mm. One study consistently demonstrated that a greater than 4 mmHg reduction in IOP was found in patients with a pressure-to-ACD ratio of more than 7. In these patients who had presumed normal anterior chamber anatomy, the anterior chamber depth was found to decrease on average by 1.10 mm postoperatively [44].

Although current evidence to date suggests that IOP is indeed reduced following cataract surgery, the exact patient-specific factors that determine the magnitude and duration of the IOP-lowering effects require further investigation.

MIGS and Endothelial Cell Density

In 2018, a MIGS device known as the CyPass Micro-Stent (Alcon, Texas, United States) was voluntarily withdrawn from the manufacturer [45], and was later recalled by the US Food and Drug Administration [46]. The CyPass Micro-Stent was a 6.35 mm-long fenestrated device with 3 retention rings and a collar at the proximal tip. It was intended for supraciliary placement. The removal was due to concerns of progressive loss of endothelial cell loss (ECL) caused by CyPass Micro-Stent implantation. The COMPASS XT trial demonstrated that at 60 months, endothelial cell density (ECD) had reduced by 20.4% in the CyPass Micro-Stent group (which had eyes that underwent phacoemulsification and CyPass implantation) and by 10.1% in the control group (which had eyes that underwent phacoemulsification only) [47, 48]. Additionally, the proportion of subjects with >30% ECL, which is what most surgeons consider clinically significant, was 27.2% in the CyPass Micro-Stent group compared to 10.0% in the control group.

It is important to note that the same study identified device position as the only factor in the analysis that correlated with ECL. When two or three retention rings were visible in the anterior chamber angle, the yearly ECL rate was 6.96% versus 1.39% when no rings were visible. Additionally, the angulation of the device within the chamber likely plays a role as well; some patients with two or more visible rings did not see a significant ECL [3]. Although it is possible that there are other variables that can affect the ECL (such as material, change in aqueous flow, reflux flow, etc.), there is no evidence of this yet. Further, due to the strong correlation with mechanical positioning of the implant in the anterior chamber with deeper implants having similar ECL levels to controls, this is unlikely [49].

The current recommendation in patients who received the CyPass Micro-Stent is screening with a complete slit-lamp examination including gonioscopy to assess the device's position. In case of clinically apparent or functionally significant changes, such as worsening ECD/pachymetry and/or corneal edema, the intervention of choice is proximal end trimming with microforceps and microscissors. Device explantation is currently not recommended as firm attachments often develop to surrounding uveal tissue by the first postoperative month.

Subsequently, increased scrutiny has been applied to MIGS devices and their effect on ECD. By their very nature, these devices are expected to have an excellent safety profile. Thus, we are willing to surgically intervene earlier for a more modest IOP-lowering effect. High-quality long-term data may be lacking, but from experience with tube shunt and trabeculectomy, ECL with traditional filtering surgery does occur and can be significant. ECL rates at 2 years post-trabeculectomy have been reported to be around 10%. One study has shown a 7.8% and 11.8% ECL rate at 2 years postoperatively for 1-site and 2-site phacotrabeculectomies, respectively [50]. With tube shunt surgery (both Ahmed glaucoma valve and Baerveldt glaucoma implant surgery), ECL rates have been reported to range between 8.0% and 18.6% at 2 years [51–54].

There is limited data on the effect of MIGS devices on ECD. A previous study showed that the iStent Inject (Glaukos Corporation, Laguna Hills, California, USA) did not lead to substantial ECL at 1 year compared to phacoemulsification alone [55]. Additionally, by this point, more than 10 year of data is available on the iStent

Inject with no known corneal complications reported. The 3-year results of the HORIZON study, assessing the safety and efficacy of the Hydrus microstent, showed that the addition of the microstent induced a 15% ECL versus 11% in the cataract surgery alone group. The proportion of patients who underwent >30% ECL was 14.2% in the microstent group versus 10% in the cataract surgery alone group. None of these differences were statistically significant. These patients are under continued monitoring for ECL. It is likely that ECD reduction is due to the initial surgical procedure itself, with the extra manipulations required for implantation. The presence of the Hydrus device is not thought to adversely threaten corneal health compared to cataract surgery alone. The iStent and the Hydrus microstent likely differ from the CyPass Micro-Stent in that their inlet lie further from the cornea. The CyPass device follows the curvature of the inner sclera and assumes a more vertical orientation; thus, its proximal tip is located closer to the peripheral cornea. If implanted too anteriorly, the collar can even come into contact with the cornea.

There remains little investigation on long-term effects of subconjunctival MIGS devices, such as the Xen Gel Stent (Allergan) and the PreserFlo MicroShunt (Santen), on the health of corneal endothelial cells. The few studies that have investigated this are small in sample size or investigate short-term effects only [56]. One 2-year study investigating the impact of the Xen Gel Stent on ECD concluded the ECL was similar in amount to standalone phacoemulsification [57].

Standalone Filtering Procedures Versus Combined with Phacoemulsification

Combining glaucoma and cataract surgery offers patients the advantage of having a single surgical experience, reducing risks of repeated surgery, and saving costly operating room time. However, some previous studies have demonstrated that standalone filtering surgeries showed better intraocular pressure (IOP) control than combined glaucoma surgery procedures [58–61]. In a retrospective series of 60 eyes, the IOP was significantly lower in the trabeculectomy group than the phaco-trabeculectomy group (11.08 +/− 2.80 mmHg vs. 15.04 +/− 2.40 mmHg, $p < 0.001$) [58]. Similarly, Kleinmann et al. found a significantly larger percentage reduction in IOP after trabeculectomy alone than after trabeculectomy combined with phacoemulsification (48.5% vs. 31.5%) ($P = 0.0001$) [59]. Bellucci et al. compared 100 trabeculectomies with 200 phaco-trabeculectomies and found that trabeculectomy alone resulted in a larger mean IOP decrease than phaco-trabeculectomy (11.2 mmHg vs. 3.1 mmHg; $P < 0.01$) [60]. In a retrospective cohort study of 40 eyes, Caprioli et al. found that mean IOP decreased more in the trabeculectomy alone group than in the combined phaco-trabeculectomy group (10.3 +/− 7.6 mmHg vs. 6.8 +/− 5.5 mmHg) [61]. They also found that a higher proportion of patients achieved the target pressure in the trabeculectomy alone group (88% vs. 72%). At 2 years, surgical success was achieved in 86% in the trabeculectomy group and in 62% in the phaco-trabeculectomy group. A possible hypothesis for the discrepancy in surgical success seen with combined phaco-trabeculectomy may be that perioperative inflammation associated with phacoemulsification produces negative consequences on bleb survival and IOP [59].

In contrast, other studies have found similar IOP-lowering effects with combined surgery and trabeculectomy alone [62, 63]. In a prospective study, Guggenbach et al. found no significant differences in mean IOP reduction between the two groups [62]. Similarly, in a retrospective analysis of 42 eyes, the mean IOPs (22.8 mmHg vs. 22.9 mmHg) and number of glaucoma medications (2.12 vs 0.2.26) were similar for phaco-trabeculectomy and standalone trabeculectomy, respectively [63]. No p-values were given for this study. At 4 years, Wachtl et al. also found that phaco-trabeculectomy had similar outcomes as trabeculectomy alone in terms of lowering IOP and reducing glaucoma medications [64]. In patients with primary angle closure glaucoma (PACG), there were no significant differences in mean IOP ($p = 0.42$), number of glaucoma medications ($p = 0.85$), or logMAR visual acuity ($p = 0.42$) between the trabeculectomy and phaco-trabeculectomy groups after 12 months [65]. However, it is important to mention that the IOP-lowering effect of phacoemulsification alone in angle closure cases has previously been documented and could well be a confounder in this latter study [32–35].

In a prospective case series of patients with refractory glaucoma, El Wardani et al. compared the efficacy and safety of standalone Baerveldt glaucoma implant (BGI) to combined phacoemulsification and BGI implantation [66]. They found a significantly higher failure rate in the combined group at 3 years (37% vs. 15%, $p = 0.02$). Additionally, a greater proportion of patients in the standalone BGI group had significantly lower IOP at 3 years. However, there were no significant differences in glaucoma medications or complications between the two groups. These results suggest that combined surgery may have negative long-term effects on bleb survival, and that a staged approach of separating phacoemulsification and tube surgery should be considered.

Rai et al. conducted a retrospective cohort study to compare the efficacy of phacoemulsification combined with either Ahmed glaucoma valve (AGV) or BGI [67]. A total of 57 eyes underwent phaco-AGV and 47 eyes underwent phaco-BGI. At 2 years, 44% of the phaco-AGV group and 23% of the phaco-BGI group failed ($p = 0.02$). To the best of our knowledge, all other reports on combined phacoemulsification and tube shunt implantation have been noncomparative with small sample sizes [68–70]. As a result, the studies were only powered to show very large differences in failure rates. With these limitations in mind, all noncomparative studies have shown a significant reduction in IOP from baseline in eyes undergoing combined phacoemulsification and AGV or BGI.

A systematic review by Friedman et al. concluded that strong evidence of efficacy only exists for better IOP control with combined glaucoma and cataract surgery compared with cataract surgery alone. Otherwise, there seems to be weak evidence when comparing IOP control in combined cataract extraction and trabeculectomy versus trabeculectomy alone, or when looking at the deleterious effects of cataract surgery on preexisting filtering blebs [71].

Although primarily considered blebless procedures, MIGS devices have begun to enter traditional filtering surgery territory with the advent of subconjunctival MIGS, such as the Preserflo MicroShunt (Santen) and the XEN Gel Stent (Allergan), while presumably retaining some of the increased safety profile known to MIGS. It has previously been demonstrated that trabecular bypass MIGS combined with cataract surgery lowers IOP and hypotensive medication used compared to cataract surgery alone [24, 23, 72, 73]. However, it is not yet clear whether subconjunctival MIGS combined with cataract surgery presents the same synergistic effect.

Several studies have compared the effectiveness of standalone XEN to combined XEN and phacoemulsification [74]. In a retrospective series comparing 200 cases of standalone XEN to 39 cases of phaco-XEN, Hengerer et al. found no significant differences between the two groups in terms of mean IOP at 1 year (standalone 14.3 +/− 4.2 mmHg vs. combined 13.9 +/− 2.5 mmHg) [75]. Similarly, Karimi et al. evaluated XEN standalone ($n = 187$) versus combined ($n = 72$) at 12 months [76]. They found no significant difference in outcomes between the two groups, and both cohorts had similar needling and complication rates. In a single center prospective study with 6 months of follow-up, 46.9% of XEN standalone eyes ($n = 81$) and 53.3% of phaco-XEN eyes ($n = 30$) achieved complete success [65]. There were no significant intergroup differences. In a 2-year, prospective, multicenter study, Reitsamer et al. compared 120 standalone eyes to 98 combined eyes [77]. The mean changes in IOP from baseline were − 6.4 +/− 5.2 mmHg in standalone and – 5.9 +/– 4.6 mmHg in combined eyes, with no statistically significant differences between the two groups. Additionally, Fea et al. compared 298 standalone eyes to 56 combined eyes at 1 year in a prospective, multicenter study [78]. The mean IOP at 1 year was 15.8 mmHg in the combined group and was 15.4 mmHg in the standalone group. There was a significantly lower IOP in the standalone group at the postoperative week 1 visit ($p = 0.04$), but no statistically significant differences at the subsequent follow-up visits. In terms of qualified and complete success, there were no significant differences between the two groups with IOP thresholds of ≤18 and 16 mmHg. However, with an IOP threshold of ≤14 mmHg, the standalone group achieved a significantly higher success rate (41.6% vs. 22.9%, $p = 0.03$).

The only study to find a significant difference between XEN standalone and phaco-XEN was by Mansouri et al. in a prospective, interventional case series that compared the safety and efficacy of XEN standalone ($n = 40$) and combined ($n = 109$) at 1 year [79]. The median percentage IOP reduction was 40% in the XEN standalone group and 22.9% in the phaco-XEN group. Their primary endpoint, a 20% or more decrease from baseline IOP, was achieved in 81.0% of standalone eyes and in 56.1% of combined eyes ($p = 0.04$). However, it is important to note that the XEN standalone group had a higher median preoperative IOP (20 vs. 18 mmHg) and more advanced glaucoma than the XEN combined group. Additionally, more needling procedures were performed in XEN standalone eyes (45% vs. 34%), possibly contributing to a more pronounced IOP reduction.

In a review of previously published studies comparing XEN as a standalone procedure to combined with phacoemulsification, the authors acknowledged the heterogeneity of study design, inclusion and exclusion criteria, and statistical analysis for studies included in their review [74]. The authors themselves also disagree on whether XEN demonstrates better efficacy as a standalone or combined procedure, illustrating the clinical nuance of this question.

Take-Home Messages

- With a global population that is rapidly aging, ophthalmologists are likely going to face an impending burden of coincident age-related cataract and glaucoma patients in their practice.
- The iStent, Hydrus Microstent, and Kahook Dual Blade are some examples of microinvasive glaucoma surgery (MIGS) devices that can be combined with cataract surgery and can lower intraocular pressure (IOP) with minimal trauma to the eye.
- Cataract surgery alone can lower IOP and can be used as a treatment to lower IOP in certain cases; however, the extent to which it is lowered depends on specific patient factors and the type of preexisting glaucomatous disease.
- MIGS devices are expected to have a very high safety profile; as a result, there is ongoing research into how MIGS devices affect endothelial cell density.
- There is evidence that standalone filtering surgeries demonstrate better IOP control than filtering surgeries combined with cataract extraction; however, the extent of this difference and the exact type of filtering surgeries where this is observed may require further investigation.

References

1. Congdon N, O'Colmain B, Klaver CCW, Klein R, Muñoz B, Friedman DS, et al. Causes and prevalence of visual impairment among adults in the United States. Arch Ophthalmol. 2004;122(4):477–85.
2. Tham Y-C, Li X, Wong TY, Quigley HA, Aung T, Cheng C-Y. Global prevalence of glaucoma and projections of glaucoma burden through 2040. Ophthalmology. 2014;121(11):2081–90.
3. Friedman DS, Wolfs RCW, O'Colmain BJ, Klein BE, Taylor HR, West S, et al. Prevalence of open-angle glaucoma among adults in the United States. Arch Ophthalmol. 2004;122(4):532–8.

4. Jonas JB, Aung T, Bourne RR, Bron AM, Ritch R, Panda-Jonas S. Glaucoma. Lancet. 2017;390(10108):2183–93.
5. Liu Y-C, Wilkins M, Kim T, Malyugin B, Mehta JS. Cataracts. Lancet. 2017;390(10094):600–12.
6. Heijl A. Reduction of intraocular pressure and glaucoma progression: results from the early manifest glaucoma trial. Arch Ophthalmol. 2002;120(10):1268.
7. The advanced glaucoma intervention study (AGIS): 7. The relationship between control of intraocular pressure and visual field deterioration. Am J Ophthalmol. 2000;130(4):429–40.
8. Samples JR, Ahmed IK. Surgical innovations in glaucoma. New York: Springer; 2013.
9. Saheb H, Ahmed IIK. Micro-invasive glaucoma surgery: current perspectives and future directions. Curr Opin Ophthalmol. 2012;23(2):96–104.
10. Lavia C, Dallorto L, Maule M, Ceccarelli M, Fea AM. Minimally-invasive glaucoma surgeries (MIGS) for open angle glaucoma: a systematic review and meta-analysis. PLoS One. 2017;12(8):e0183142.
11. Wellik S, Dale E. A review of the iStent® trabecular micro-bypass stent: safety and efficacy. OPTH. 2015;9:677.
12. Arriola-Villalobos P, Martínez-de-la-Casa JM, Díaz-Valle D, Fernández-Pérez C, García-Sánchez J, García-Feijoó J. Combined iStent trabecular micro-bypass stent implantation and phacoemulsification for coexistent open-angle glaucoma and cataract: a long-term study. Br J Ophthalmol. 2012;96(5):645–9.
13. Craven RE, Katz JL, Wells JM, Giamporcaro JE. Cataract surgery with trabecular micro-bypass stent implantation in patients with mild-to-moderate open-angle glaucoma and cataract: two-year follow-up. J Cataract Refract Surg. 2012;38(8):1339–45.
14. Samuelson TW, Katz LJ, Wells JM, Duh Y-J, Giamporcaro JE. Randomized evaluation of the trabecular micro-bypass stent with phacoemulsification in patients with glaucoma and cataract. Ophthalmology. 2011;118(3):459–67.
15. Fernández-Barrientos Y, García-Feijoó J, Martínez-de-la-Casa JM, Pablo LE, Fernández-Pérez C, García SJ. Fluorophotometric study of the effect of the glaukos trabecular microbypass stent on aqueous humor dynamics. Invest Ophthalmol Vis Sci. 2010;51(7):3327–32.
16. Fea AM. Phacoemulsification versus phacoemulsification with micro-bypass stent implantation in primary open-angle glaucoma: randomized double-masked clinical trial. J Cataract Refract Surg. 2010;36(3):407–12.
17. Belovay GW, Naqi A, Chan BJ, Rateb M, Ahmed IIK. Using multiple trabecular micro-bypass stents in cataract patients to treat open-angle glaucoma. J Cataract Refract Surg. 2012;38(11):1911–7.
18. Samet S, Ong JA, Ahmed IIK. Hydrus microstent implantation for surgical management of glaucoma: a review of design, efficacy and safety. Eye Vis. 2019;6(1):32.
19. Gandolfi SA, Ungaro N, Ghirardini S, Tardini MG, Mora P. Comparison of surgical outcomes between Canaloplasty and Schlemm's canal scaffold at 24 months' follow-up. J Ophthalmol. 2016;2016:3410469.
20. Fea AM, Rekas M, Au L. Evaluation of a Schlemm canal scaffold microstent combined with phacoemulsification in routine clinical practice: two-year multicenter study. J Cataract Refract Surg. 2017;43(7):886–91.
21. Fea AM, Ahmed IIK, Lavia C, Mittica P, Consolandi G, Motolese I, et al. Hydrus microstent compared to selective laser trabeculoplasty in primary open angle glaucoma: one year results: Hydrus *versus* SLT efficacy in glaucomatous patients. Clin Exp Ophthalmol. 2017;45(2):120–7.
22. Al-Mugheiry TS, Cate H, Clark A, Broadway DC. Microinvasive Glaucoma Stent (MIGS) surgery with concomitant Phakoemulsification cataract extraction: outcomes and the learning curve. J Glaucoma. 2017;26(7):646–51.
23. Pfeiffer N, Garcia-Feijoo J, Martinez-de-la-Casa JM, Larrosa JM, Fea A, Lemij H, et al. A randomized trial of a Schlemm's canal microstent with phacoemulsification for reducing intraocular pressure in open-angle glaucoma. Ophthalmology. 2015;122(7):1283–93.
24. Samuelson TW, Chang DF, Marquis R, Flowers B, Lim KS, Ahmed IIK, et al. A Schlemm canal microstent for intraocular pressure reduction in primary open-angle glaucoma and cataract: the HORIZON study. Ophthalmology. 2019;126(1):29–37.
25. Ahmed IIK, Fea A, Au L, Ang RE, Harasymowycz P, Jampel HD, et al. A prospective randomized trial comparing hydrus and iStent microinvasive glaucoma surgery implants for standalone treatment of open-angle glaucoma. Ophthalmology. 2020;127(1):52–61.
26. Ahmed IIK, Rhee DJ, Jones J, Singh IP, Radcliffe N, Gazzard G, et al. Three-year findings of the HORIZON trial: a Schlemm canal microstent for pressure reduction in primary open-angle glaucoma and cataract. Ophthalmology. 2020;128:857.
27. Seibold LK, SooHoo JR, Ammar DA, Kahook MY. Preclinical investigation of ab Interno trabeculectomy using a novel dual-blade device. Am J Ophthalmol. 2013;155(3):524–529.e2.
28. Dorairaj SK, Seibold LK, Radcliffe NM, Aref AA, Jimenez-Román J, Lazcano-Gomez GS, et al. 12-month outcomes of goniotomy performed using the Kahook dual blade combined with cataract surgery in eyes with medically treated glaucoma. Adv Ther. 2018;35(9):1460–9.
29. Greenwood MD, Seibold LK, Radcliffe NM, Dorairaj SK, Aref AA, Román JJ, et al. Goniotomy with a single-use dual blade: short-term results. J Cataract Refract Surg. 2017;43(9):1197–201.
30. Wakil SM, Birnbaum F, Vu DM, McBurney-Lin S, ElMallah MK, Tseng H. Efficacy and safety of a single-use dual blade goniotomy: 18-month results. J Cataract Refract Surg. 2020;46(10):1408–15.

31. Masis M, Mineault PJ, Phan E, Lin SC. The role of phacoemulsification in glaucoma therapy: a systematic review and meta-analysis. Surv Ophthalmol. 2018;63(5):700–10.
32. Lam DSC, Leung DYL, Tham CCY, Li FCH, Kwong YYY, Chiu TYH, et al. Randomized trial of early phacoemulsification versus peripheral Iridotomy to prevent intraocular pressure rise after acute primary angle closure. Ophthalmology. 2008;115(7):1134–40.
33. Jacobi P. Primary phacoemulsification and intraocular lens implantation for acute angle-closure glaucoma historical image. Ophthalmology. 2002;109(9):1597–603.
34. Lai JSM, Tham CCY, Chan JCH. The clinical outcomes of cataract extraction by Phacoemulsification in Eyes With Primary Angle-Closure Glaucoma (PACG) and co-existing cataract: a prospective case series. J Glaucoma. 2006;15(1):47–52.
35. Vizzeri G, Weinreb RN. Cataract surgery and glaucoma. Curr Opin Ophthalmol. 2010;21(1):20–4.
36. Azuara-Blanco A, Burr J, Ramsay C, Cooper D, Foster PJ, Friedman DS, et al. Effectiveness of early lens extraction for the treatment of primary angle-closure glaucoma (EAGLE): a randomised controlled trial. Lancet. 2016;388(10052):1389–97.
37. Vahedian Z, Salmanroghani R, Fakhraie G, Moghimi S, Eslami Y, Zarei R, et al. Pseudoexfoliation syndrome: effect of phacoemulsification on intraocular pressure and its diurnal variation. J Curr Ophthalmol. 2015;27(1–2):12–5.
38. Desai MA, Lee RK. The medical and surgical management of Pseudoexfoliation Glaucoma. Int Ophthalmol Clin. 2008;48(4):95–113.
39. Kristianslund O, Østern AE, Råen M, Sandvik GF, Drolsum L. Does cataract surgery reduce the long-term risk of glaucoma in eyes with pseudoexfoliation syndrome? Acta Ophthalmol. 2016;94(3):261–5.
40. Brown RH, Zhong L, Lynch MG. Lens-based glaucoma surgery: using cataract surgery to reduce intraocular pressure. J Cataract Refract Surg. 2014;40(8):1255–62.
41. Friedman DS, Jampel HD, Lubomski LH, Kempen JH, Quigley H, Congdon N, et al. Surgical strategies for coexisting glaucoma and cataract. Ophthalmology. 2002;109(10):1902–13.
42. Shrivastava A, Singh K. The effect of cataract extraction on intraocular pressure. Curr Opin Ophthalmol. 2010;21(2):118–22.
43. Wang N, Chintala SK, Fini ME, Schuman JS. Ultrasound activates the TM ELAM-1/IL-1/NF-κB response: a potential mechanism for intraocular pressure reduction after phacoemulsification. Invest Ophthalmol Vis Sci. 2003;44(5):1977.
44. Issa SA. A novel index for predicting intraocular pressure reduction following cataract surgery. Br J Ophthalmol. 2005;89(5):543–6.
45. Alcon announces voluntary global market withdrawal of CyPass Micro-Stent for surgical glaucoma [Internet]. Novartis. [cited 2021 Jan 20]. Available from: https://www.novartis.com/news/media-releases/alcon-announces-voluntary-global-market-withdrawal-cypass-micro-stent-surgical-glaucoma
46. Health C for D and R. Potential eye damage from Alcon CyPass micro-stent used to treat open-angle glaucoma: FDA safety communication. FDA [Internet] 2018 Mar 11 [cited 2021 Jan 20]; Available from: https://www.fda.gov/medical-devices/safety-communications/potential-eye-damage-alcon-cypass-micro-stent-used-treat-open-angle-glaucoma-fda-safety
47. Reiss G, Clifford B, Vold S, He J, Hamilton C, Dickerson J, et al. Safety and effectiveness of CyPass supraciliary micro-stent in primary open-angle glaucoma: 5-year results from the COMPASS XT study. Am J Ophthalmol. 2019;208:219–25.
48. Lass JH, Benetz BA, He J, Hamilton C, Von Tress M, Dickerson J, et al. Corneal endothelial cell loss and morphometric changes 5 years after phacoemulsification with or without CyPass micro-stent. Am J Ophthalmol. 2019;208:211–8.
49. Durr G, Ahmed IIK. Endothelial Cell Loss and MIGS: What We Know and Don't Know [Internet]. Glaucoma Today. Bryn Mawr Communications; [cited 2021 Feb 14]. Available from: https://glaucomatoday.com/articles/2018-sept-oct/endothelial-cell-loss-and-migs-what-we-know-and-dont-know
50. Buys YM, Chipman ML, Zack B, Rootman DS, Slomovic AR, Trope GE. Prospective randomized comparison of one- versus two-site Phacotrabeculectomy two-year results. Ophthalmology. 2008;115(7):1130–1133.e1.
51. Lee E-K, Yun Y-J, Lee J-E, Yim J-H, Kim C-S. Changes in corneal endothelial cells after Ahmed glaucoma valve implantation: 2-year follow-up. Am J Ophthalmol. 2009;148(3):361–7.
52. Kim KN, Lee SB, Lee YH, Lee JJ, Lim HB, Kim C. Changes in corneal endothelial cell density and the cumulative risk of corneal decompensation after Ahmed glaucoma valve implantation. Br J Ophthalmol. 2016;100(7):933–8.
53. Tan AN, Webers CAB, Berendschot TTJM, de Brabander J, de Witte PM, Nuijts RMMA, et al. Corneal endothelial cell loss after Baerveldt glaucoma drainage device implantation in the anterior chamber. Acta Ophthalmol. 2017;95(1):91–6.
54. Tojo N, Hayashi A, Consolvo-Ueda T, Yanagisawa S. Baerveldt surgery outcomes: anterior chamber insertion versus vitreous cavity insertion. Graefes Arch Clin Exp Ophthalmol. 2018;256(11):2191–200.
55. Arriola-Villalobos P, Martínez-de-la-Casa JM, Díaz-Valle D, García-Vidal SE, Fernández-Pérez C, García-Sánchez J, et al. Mid-term evaluation of the new Glaukos iStent with phacoemulsification in coexistent open-angle glaucoma or ocular hypertension and cataract. Br J Ophthalmol. 2013;97(10):1250–5.
56. Olgun A, Duzgun E, Yildiz AM, Atmaca F, Yildiz AA, Sendul SY. XEN gel stent versus trabeculectomy: short-term effects on corneal endothelial cells. Eur J Ophthalmol. 2020;26:112067212092433.

57. Gillmann K, Bravetti GE, Rao HL, Mermoud A, Mansouri K. Impact of phacoemulsification combined with XEN gel stent implantation on corneal endothelial cell density: 2-year results. J Glaucoma. 2020;29(3):155–60.
58. Noben KJ, Linsen MC, Zeyen TG. Is combined phacoemulsification and trabeculectomy as effective as trabeculectomy alone? Bull Soc Belge Ophtalmol. 1998;270:85–90.
59. Kleinmann G, Katz H, Pollack A, Schechtman E, Rachmiel R, Zalish M. Comparison of trabeculectomy with mitomycin C with or without phacoemulsification and lens implantation. Ophthalmic Surg Lasers. 2002 Apr;33(2):102–8.
60. Bellucci R, Perfetti S, Babighian S, Morselli S, Bonomi L. Filtration and complications after trabeculectomy and after phaco-trabeculectomy. Acta Ophthalmol Scand Suppl. 1997;224:44–5.
61. Caprioli J, Park HJ, Weitzman M. Temporal corneal phacoemulsification combined with superior trabeculectomy: a controlled study. Trans Am Ophthalmol Soc. 1996;94:451–63; discussion 463–8
62. Guggenbach M, Mojon DS, Böhnke M. Evaluation of phacotrabeculectomy versus trabeculectomy alone. Ophthalmologica. 1999;213(6):367–70.
63. Derick RJ, Evans J, Baker ND. Combined phacoemulsification and trabeculectomy versus trabeculectomy alone: a comparison study using mitomycin-C. Ophthalmic Surg Lasers. 1998;29(9):707–13.
64. Wachtl J, Harms MT, Frimmel S, Kniestedt C. Phacotrabeculectomy equals trabeculectomy in lowering IOP-A 4 years follow-up study. J Clin Exp Ophthalmol [Internet]. 2016; [cited 2021 Feb 22];07(06). Available from: https://www.omicsonline.org/open-access/phacotrabeculectomy-equals-trabeculectomy-in-lowering-iopa-4-yearsfollowup-study-2155-9570-1000622.php?aid=84224
65. Song BJ, Ramanathan M, Morales E, Law SK, Giaconi JA, Coleman AL, et al. Trabeculectomy and combined phacoemulsification-trabeculectomy: outcomes and risk factors for failure in primary angle closure glaucoma. J Glaucoma. 2016;25(9):763–9.
66. El Wardani M, Bergin C, Bradly K, Sharkawi E. Baerveldt shunt surgery versus combined Baerveldt shunt and phacoemulsification: a prospective comparative study. Br J Ophthalmol. 2018;102(9):1248–53.
67. Rai AS, Shoham-Hazon N, Christakis PG, Rai AS, Ahmed IIK. Comparison of the Ahmed and Baerveldt glaucoma shunts with combined cataract extraction. Can J Ophthalmol. 2018;53(2):124–30.
68. Chung AN, Aung T, Wang J-C, Chew PTK. Surgical outcomes of combined phacoemulsification and glaucoma drainage implant surgery for Asian patients with refractory glaucoma with cataract. Am J Ophthalmol. 2004;137(2):294–300.
69. Valenzuela F, Browne A, Srur M, Nieme C, Zanolli M, López-Solís R, et al. Combined phacoemulsification and Ahmed glaucoma drainage implant surgery for patients with refractory glaucoma and cataract. J Glaucoma. 2016;25(2):162–6.
70. Hoffman KB, Feldman RM, Budenz DL, Gedde SJ, Chacra GA, Schiffman JC. Combined cataract extraction and Baerveldt glaucoma drainage implant: indications and outcomes. Ophthalmology. 2002;109(10):1916–20.
71. Friedman DS, Jampel HD, Lubomski LH, Kempen JH, Quigley H, Congdon N, et al. Surgical strategies for coexisting glaucoma and cataract: an evidence-based update. Ophthalmology. 2002;109(10):1902–13.
72. Vold S, Ahmed IIK, Craven ER, Mattox C, Stamper R, Packer M, et al. Two-year COMPASS trial results: supraciliary microstenting with phacoemulsification in patients with open-angle glaucoma and cataracts. Ophthalmology. 2016;123(10):2103–12.
73. Samuelson TW, Sarkisian SR, Lubeck DM, Stiles MC, Duh Y-J, Romo EA, et al. Prospective, randomized, controlled pivotal trial of an Ab interno implanted trabecular micro-bypass in primary open-angle glaucoma and cataract: two-year results. Ophthalmology. 2019;126(6):811–21.
74. Fea AM, Durr GM, Marolo P, Malinverni L, Economou MA, Ahmed I. XEN®gel stent: a comprehensive review on its use as a treatment option for refractory glaucoma. OPTH. 2020;14:1805–32.
75. Hengerer FH, Kohnen T, Mueller M, Conrad-Hengerer I. Ab interno gel implant for the treatment of glaucoma patients with or without prior glaucoma surgery: 1-year results. J Glaucoma. 2017;26(12):1130–6.
76. Karimi A, Lindfield D, Turnbull A, Dimitriou C, Bhatia B, Radwan M, et al. A multi-centre interventional case series of 259 ab-interno Xen gel implants for glaucoma, with and without combined cataract surgery. Eye. 2019;33(3):469–77.
77. Reitsamer H, Sng C, Vera V, Lenzhofer M, Barton K, Stalmans I, et al. Two-year results of a multicenter study of the ab interno gelatin implant in medically uncontrolled primary open-angle glaucoma. Graefes Arch Clin Exp Ophthalmol. 2019;257(5):983–96.
78. Fea AM, Bron AM, Economou MA, Laffi G, Martini E, Figus M, et al. European study of the efficacy of a cross-linked gel stent for the treatment of glaucoma. J Cataract Refract Surg. 2020;46(3):441–50.
79. Mansouri K, Guidotti J, Rao HL, Ouabas A, D'Alessandro E, Roy S, et al. Prospective evaluation of standalone XEN gel implant and combined phacoemulsification-XEN gel implant surgery: 1-year results. J Glaucoma. 2018;27(2):140–7.

Epilogue

A Glance at the Future

Contemporary cataract surgery offers a unique opportunity to improve the quality of vision and quality of life for millions of patients worldwide. As the most frequently practiced surgical procedure on human beings with unprecedented outcomes, one might assume that we have reached the final frontier of cataract surgery. This assumption, however, would be a gross mistake. Cataract surgery has the potential for immense development in the future as we shall predict in this closing chapter of our book.

The authors believe that cataract surgery will witness an explosion of innovations and advances. Burkhard Dick asserts that lasers are in their infancy and that laser energy will be harnessed to achieve effective lens removal enhancing both safety and efficacy.

Jorge Alio predicts that intracapsular liquefaction, aspiration, and injection of a polymer with a calculated power will become a reality. A new generation of multifocal and presbyopia lenses will be designed by applying advanced optics, including solutions for low vision. Lens regeneration is even a possibility as we learn to regulate the lens epithelium. He also predicts that cataract surgery might be practiced in part robotically and a new era of biomorphometry and simulations of outcomes will facilitate decision-making by both surgeon and the patient.

Burkhard Dick agrees that biomorphometrics will also be a key tool in making cataract surgery safer: iris recognition will finally put to rest the age-old nightmare of accidentally operating on the wrong eye. Identifying the target axis during astigmatism surgery will become even more accurate when guided by lasers. Cataract surgery will continue to improve because of simulation technology, which will greatly accelerate the learning curve of trainees.

Jorge Alio anticipates that artificial intelligence will dramatically change the way we diagnose and treat cataracts. Continued development of microscopes including 3D systems and associated procedures like keratopigmentation will proliferate. Physicians and industry will partner to identify ways to increase cost-effectiveness and surgical efficiency. He adds that we should not forget about the potential to help millions of cataract patients in underdeveloped areas who have minimal or no access to adequately trained surgeons, predicting that robotic surgery may provide a solution.

The authors agree that innovative devices associated with cataract surgery will continue to expand indications as physiologic replacements of the cornea, iris, angle structures, and artificial posterior capsules of ultra-thin, elastic, and totally transparent materiales are introduced. Just as refractive surgery has merged with cataract surgery, combining glaucoma and even retinal

J. L. Alió et al. (eds.), *Cataract Surgery*, Essentials in Ophthalmology,
https://doi.org/10.1007/978-3-030-94530-5

procedures will continue to gain popularity. Burkhard Dick is excited about implantable chips that will provide intraocular pressure (IOP) monitoring in real time, while new filtration devices will be designed to permanently lower IOP to safe levels.

Robert Osher has a different vision. "We may envision a day when all people after a certain age will undergo a surgical procedure directed by artificial intelligence that will eliminate all preexisting refractive errors. It will be lens-based and there will be no more myopia, hyperopia, astigmatism, or even presbyopia. That means no more cataract surgery!" He believes that the lens solution will be dynamic with artificial intelligence to correct both distance and near focus. In addition, he predicts that the lens will be empowered to do many more things. For example, it will be associated with a drug delivery system that will deliver the postoperative medications making eye drops obsolete. Posterior capsular opacification will be completely inhibited. In addition to measuring the IOP (which was accomplished by Adatomed years ago), all blood chemistries will be measured. Diabetics will monitor their blood pressure using a scale on the IOL. While optometry and optical shops will vanish, ophthalmic surgeons will be very busy for decades to come.

We close this book with shared confidence and enthusiasm for the unwritten chapters in the future that will introduce brilliant ideas, exciting products, new techniques, and breakthroughs in technology— all aimed at preserving humanity's most precious gift, the gift of Sight.

Index

J. L. Alió et al. (eds.), *Cataract Surgery*, Essentials in Ophthalmology,
https://doi.org/10.1007/978-3-030-94530-5

J

K

L

M

GPSR Compliance

The European Union's (EU) General Product Safety Regulation (GPSR) is a set of rules that requires consumer products to be safe and our obligations to ensure this.

If you have any concerns about our products, you can contact us on ProductSafety@springernature.com

In case Publisher is established outside the EU, the EU authorized representative is:

Springer Nature Customer Service Center GmbH
Europaplatz 3
69115 Heidelberg, Germany

Batch number: 08942889

Printed by Printforce, the Netherlands